PROGRESS IN
CLINICAL MEDICINE

PROGRESS IN CLINICAL MEDICINE

Editors

RAYMOND DALEY

M.A., M.D. Cantab., F.R.C.P.

Physician to the Cardiac Department,
St Thomas's Hospital.
Consultant Cardiologist,
King Edward VII Hospital for Officers.
Consultant Physician and Cardiologist,
Chelsea and Kensington Group of Hospitals

and

HENRY MILLER

M.D., F.R.C.P.

Honorary Consulting Neurologist,
Royal Victoria Infirmary,
Newcastle upon Tyne

SIXTH EDITION

1971

CHURCHILL LIVINGSTONE

EDINBURGH AND LONDON

First Edition	.	.	.	.	.	.	1948
Reprinted	.	.	.	.	.	.	1948
Second Edition	.	.	.	.	.	.	1952
Third Edition	.	.	.	.	.	.	1956
Fourth Edition	.	.	.	.	.	.	1961
Reprinted	.	.	.	.	.	.	1963
Fifth Edition	.	.	.	.	.	.	1966
Reprinted	.	.	.	.	.	.	1967
Sixth Edition	.	.	.	.	.	.	1971

International Standard Book Number 0.7000.1486.1

Printed in Great Britain
by T. & A. CONSTABLE LTD, Edinburgh

Preface to the Sixth Edition

THE purpose of this book has remained unchanged since its first appearance 22 years ago. It aims to describe current developments in internal medicine in a manner intelligible and useful to the general physician and the post-graduate student.

Recent progress has blurred the outline of the traditional disciplines. New developments in genetics and immunology are relevant in every speciality. Psychiatry is increasingly neurochemical, and computerization now begins to permeate every field of medicine.

Our first edition was traditional in concept and arrangement, but like its immediate predecessor this volume bespeaks a constant struggle to embody contributions of basic science into the clinical armamentarium. The reader will find a more extended consideration of medical computerization, a comprehensive review of the invasion of clinical medicine by immunology, and a succinct presentation of the present status of transplant surgery. Where duplication occurs it is entirely intentional: the different approaches of the neurologist and immunologist to myasthenia are illuminating. The more traditional aspects of medicine have not been overlooked, though it would be fair comment to say that the focus of the book is now as biochemical as it is clinical. The editors hope that their pleasure in assembling a series of outstanding reviews will be shared by their readers.

RAYMOND DALEY AND HENRY MILLER
London and Newcastle upon Tyne

Contributors

R. I. S. BAYLISS, M.A., M.D.CANTAB., F.R.C.P.
Physician to H.M. The Queen; Physician and Endocrinologist, Westminster Hospital, London.

R. Y. CALNE, M.A.CANTAB., M.S.LOND., F.R.C.S.ENG.
Professor of Surgery, University of Cambridge; Fellow of Trinity Hall.

C. A. CLARKE, C.B.E., F.R.S., SC.D., M.D., F.R.C.P., F.R.C.O.G.
Professor of Medicine and Director of the Nuffield Unit of Medical Genetics, University of Liverpool; Consultant Physician, Liverpool Royal Infirmary and Broadgreen Hospital, Liverpool.

P. H. CONNELL, M.D., M.R.C.P., D.P.M.
Physician, The Bethlem Royal Hospital and the Maudsley Hospital.

BRIAN CREAMER, M.D.LOND., M.R.C.P.
Physician to St. Thomas's Hospital.

RAYMOND DALEY, M.A., M.D.CANTAB., F.R.C.P.
Physician to the Cardiac Department, St Thomas's Hospital; Consultant Cardiologist, King Edward VII Hospital for Officers; Consultant Physician and Cardiologist, Chelsea and Kensington Group of Hospitals.

G. HAMILTON FAIRLEY, D.M., F.R.C.P.
Director of Imperial Cancer Research Fund, Medical Oncology Research Unit at St Bartholomew's Hospital, London, E.C.1., Consultant Physician, St Bartholomew's Hospital, London, E.C.1., and the Chester Beatty Research Institute, Royal Marsden Hospital, Sutton, Surrey.

MAX. M. GLATT, M.D., M.R.C.P., D.P.M.
Consultant Psychiatrist, St Bernard's Hospital and the Paddington Clinic and Day Hospital; Consultant in Charge, Regional Alcoholism and Addiction Unit of the North-West Metropolitan Regional Hospital Board; Honorary Consultant Physician, Department of Psychological Medicine, University College Hospital, London; Visiting Psychotherapist, H.M. Prison, Wormwood Scrubs.

R. HALL, B.SC.DUNELM, M.D.DUNELM., F.R.C.P.
Professor of Medicine at the University of Newcastle upon Tyne; Physician, Royal Victoria Infirmary, Newcastle upon Tyne.

P. HUDGSON, M.B., M.R.A.C.P.
Consultant Neurologist, The General Hospital and the Royal Victoria
Infirmary, Newcastle upon Tyne.

M. C. G. ISRAËLS, M.D.,MANCH., M.SC., F.R.C.P.
Professor of Clinical Haematology, University of Manchester and
Physician to the United Manchester Hospitals.

D. N. S. KERR, M.B.EDIN., M.SC.WIS.
Professor of Medicine and Physician to the Royal Infirmary, Newcastle
upon Tyne.

E. G. KNOX, M.D., M.R.C.P.
Professor of Social Medicine, University of Birmingham.

M. H. LESSOF, M.A., M.D., F.R.C.P.
Physician and Clinical Immunologist, Guy's Hospital, London.

W. A. LISHMAN, B.SC., M.D., M.R.C.P., D.P.M.
Consultant Psychiatrist, The Bethlem Royal and Maudsley Hospitals;
Senior Lecturer, Institute of Psychiatry, London.

D. M. McLEAN, M.D.MELBOURNE, F.R.C.PATH., F.R.C.P. CANADA.
Professor of Medical Microbiology, University of British Columbia,
Vancouver B.C., Canada.

H. MILLER, M.D., F.R.C.P.
Honorary Consulting Neurologist, Royal Victoria Infirmary, Newcastle
upon Tyne.

A. S. RUSSELL, M.A., M.R.C.P.
Senior Medical Registrar, West London Hospital.

T. B. STRETTON, M.B., CH.B., M.R.C.P.
Consultant Physician and Senior Lecturer in Medicine, the Royal
Infirmary, Manchester.

Contents

PROGRESS IN
CLINICAL MEDICINE

1 Clinical Virology

DONALD M. McLEAN

VIRUS CLASSIFICATION. LABORATORY DIAGNOSIS. MEASLES. RUBELLA. MUMPS

VIRUS CLASSIFICATION

VIRUSES are living organisms whose sizes range from 20 to 300 nanometers (nm) diameter and which replicate only inside living cells of susceptible host tissues. The laboratory cultivation of viruses therefore depends on their ability to induce microscopically visible changes in tissue cultures or characteristic clinical syndromes following inoculation into experimental animals. At present the only transmissible agents causing disease in man which have not been cultivated with certainty in the laboratory are the viruses of infectious hepatitis and serum hepatitis.

The complete infectious unit (virion) is composed of nucleic acid surrounded by a protein shell (capsid) which is composed of subunits (capsomeres) (Pereira and Valentine, 1967). For some viruses, the capsid is surrounded by an outer membrane (envelope), which contains protein and lipid, principally of host origin.

Viruses pathogenic for man are classified among the animal viruses. These comprise one of four main categories of viruses, according to the phylum of hosts which they infect; vertebrate animals, insects, bacteria, angiosperm plants. The animal viruses are subdivided (Andrewes and Pereira, 1967) into groups primarily on the basis of their known physicochemical properties. Within each group they are further subdivided into serotypes or "virus species" according to their antigenic constitution. Individual strains of virus belonging to the same serotype may show important differences in other attributes. For example the development of the disease, mumps, may follow exposure of a susceptible human to a clinical case, but development of antibody occurs without clinical illness after injection with the Jeryl Lynn attenuated strain of mumps vaccine (Weibel et al., 1967). Table 1.1 lists 11 groups of viruses which are pathogenic for man

TABLE 1.1

Classification of Viruses affecting Man according to Chemical and Physical Criteria (adapted from Andrewes and Pereira, 1967)

Virus group	Particle size (nm)	Nucleic acid	Symmetry	Number of capsomers	Enveloped or naked	Common viruses which infect man
Herpesvirus	100–150	DNA	Cubic	162	Enveloped	Herpes simplex, varicella
Adenovirus	70–90	DNA	Cubic	252	Naked	Adenovirus
Papovavirus	30–50	DNA	Cubic	72	Naked	Warts
Poxvirus	200–300	DNA	Helical?	—	Enveloped	Variola, vaccinia
Myxovirus	80–120	RNA	Helical	—	Enveloped	Influenza
Paramyxovirus	140–250	RNA	Helical	—	Enveloped	Mumps, measles
Arbovirus	20–100	RNA	Cubic	?	Enveloped	St Louis, Powassan
Picornavirus	20–30	RNA	Cubic	42	Naked	Poliovirus echovirus
Reovirus	60–90	RNA	Cubic	92	Naked	Reovirus
Rhabdovirus	100–150	RNA	Helical	—	Enveloped	Rabies
Rubella	120–280	RNA	Cubic	?	Enveloped	Rubella

TABLE 1.2

Viruses commonly associated with Syndromes in Man

Syndrome	Viruses found regularly	Virus group
Respiratory tract infection	Influenza	Myxovirus
	Parainfluenza, respiratory Syncytial	Paramyxovirus
	Adenovirus	Adenovirus
	Rhinovirus	Picornavirus
Pleurodynia	Coxsackievirus B	Picornavirus
Mouth lesions	Herpesvirus hominis	Herpesvirus
	Coxsackievirus A	Picornavirus
Rash: maculopapular	Measles	Paramyxovirus
	Rubella	Ungrouped
	Echovirus	Picornavirus
CNS: meningitis	Mumps	Paramyxovirus
	Coxsackievirus B, echovirus	Picornavirus
CNS: encephalitis	St Louis, Powassan	Arbovirus
Tropical fevers	Dengue, chikungunya	Arbovirus
Eye infections	Trachoma, inclusion blenorrhea	Chlamydia
	Vaccinia	Poxvirus
	Herpesvirus hominis	Herpesvirus

according to whether: (i) the virion contains ribonucleic (RNA) or deoxyribonucleic acid (DNA) as the only form of nucleic acid; (ii) the internal protein subunits are arranged in cubic or helical symmetry; (iii) the virion is enveloped or naked.

At the bedside however, the clinician must be familiar with the range of viruses which are likely to be associated with the patient's illness (Table 1.2). In several instances, for example the picornaviruses, one agent such as echovirus 9 may be associated with diverse syndromes such as maculopapular rash and aseptic meningitis. On the other hand, syndromes such as acute laryngotracheobronchitis may be associated with a wide range of agents including myxoviruses such as influenzavirus A2, paramyxoviruses such as parainfluenzavirus 1 and measles virus, and a member of the herpesvirus group, varicella.

REFERENCES

ANDREWES, C. H. & PEREIRA, H. G. (1967). *Viruses of Vertebrates.* 2nd ed. London: Baillière, Tindall and Cassell.

PEREIRA, H. G. & VALENTINE, R. C. (1967). Morphological and antigenic sub-units of viruses. *Brit. med. Bull.,* **23**, 129.

WEIBEL, R. E., STOKES, J., BUYNAK, E. B., WHITMAN, J. E. & HILLEMAN, M. R. (1967). Live, attenuated mumps-virus vaccine. 3. Clinical and serologic aspects in a field evaluation. *New Engl. J. Med.,* **276**, 245.

LABORATORY DIAGNOSIS

Although clinical inspection is frequently sufficient to establish the viral aetiology of conditions such as measles, mumps and chickenpox, knowledge of the syndromes which are usually associated with virus infections, and the particular virus groups which are commonly implicated (Table 1.2), will permit rapid and accurate confirmation of the infecting agent by laboratory procedures. In syndromes such as aseptic meningitis which occurs during winter and in the absence of involvement of the salivary glands, laboratory diagnostic procedures are essential to determine whether the infecting agent is mumps virus or a picornavirus. During the normal winter upsurge of measles and rubella in Temperate Zone communities, it is vitally important to establish by laboratory means whether an exanthem in a child is due to measles or rubella virus, when the mother is in her first trimester of pregnancy. In the Tropics, where undifferentiated fevers due to arboviruses occur commonly, laboratory techniques frequently provide the only means of differentiation between yellow-fever virus which may cause fatal disease in some subjects, and dengue or chikungunya viruses which induce less severe illness.

Laboratory diagnosis of virus infections depends upon two general methods; direct and indirect. Direct methods involve: (i) isolation of virus from the site at which the pathological process is occurring, for example mumps virus from the cerebrospinal fluid (CSF) in cases of aseptic meningitis (McLean et al., 1967); (ii) observation of virions in electron micrographs of secretions or exudates stained negatively with phosphotungstic acid (Doane et al., 1967), for example mumps virus in CSF; or by observation by light microscopy of characteristic changes in epithelial cells from scrapings of vesicles following staining with Giemsa, for example, multinucleate (Tzanck) cells with acidophilic intranuclear inclusions in chickenpox. Direct methods establish the causative virus in the patient's illness immediately, without recourse to tests on additional specimens. Indirect methods involve the demonstration of a conversion of the patient's antibody status against a particular virus from negative to positive during convalescence, or at least a fourfold increment in antibody titre in those subjects who had detectable antibody at the time the initial blood sample was secured.

Suggestive evidence that a particular virus has induced a disease, for example coxsackieviruses in aseptic meningitis (McLean, 1966), may be obtained by the isolation of this agent from a site in the body, such as the faeces, which is remote from the area at which the pathological process is occurring. Since some subjects, especially residents of warm climates, may excrete coxsackieviruses in the faeces without developing overt illnesses (Cook et al., 1969; Pelon et al., 1966), additional confirmatory evidence must be sought, usually by detection of antibody conversion, to show that this virus infected the patient at the time of illness.

Whenever possible, direct methods should be employed to identify the causative virus in an illness. Collection of appropriate specimens depends upon knowledge of the pathogenesis of the disease. In addition, indirect methods should regularly be used as confirmatory evidence when direct methods elucidate the viral aetiology, or to provide suggestive information regarding the type of causative agent if direct methods yield negative results. Selection of the optimum laboratory techniques for virus isolation and serology depends on knowledge of the range of susceptible host tissues and types of antibody detected most readily. The range of laboratory tests for viral infections is shown in Table 1.3.

Specimens for attempts at virus isolation should be collected as soon as possible after onset of illness. These include CSF from any case of suspected involvement of the central nervous system; faeces or rectal swabs plus throat washings from patients with syndromes involving the CNS, serous membranes or musculoskeletal system; throat washings, swabs or nasopharyngeal secretions from cases of respiratory disease; and scrapings of the base of lesions, or samples of vesicle fluid, from subjects with vesicular exanthemata or enanthemata. Serum derived from 1 to 5 ml of whole clotted blood should be obtained from each patient on two occasions—the first as soon as possible after onset of symptoms and the second at least one day after the temperature has returned to normal. This is usually two to seven days after collection of the initial serum sample, but for some tests such as the complement-fixing antibody response to arbovirus infection, it is advisable to collect an additional serum sample three to four weeks after onset of illness.

When the virus laboratory is located geographically close to the patient, all specimens should be delivered unrefrigerated by messenger immediately after their collection. Specimens submitted for attempts at virus isolations may be held at 4°C in refrigerators in the hospital ward or preferably in the virus laboratory, for testing up to 24 hours after their collection. An exception to this rule is a throat swab from a case of respiratory infection which requires inoculation into tissue cultures at the patient's bedside in order to recover respiratory syncytial virus readily (Tobin, 1963). However, if more than one day is likely to elapse between receipt of a specimen by the virus laboratory and start of the test, the specimen should be stored in a deep freeze at −20°C.

When the laboratory is far from the patient, specimens of CSF, throat washings and scrapings of vesicles should be placed in screw-capped bottles which are then stacked into vacuum jars or expanded polystyrene containers to which ice-cubes or re-usable "Sno-Gel" packs have been added. Containers should be sent to the laboratory by the most rapid means available, so as to arrive there within 24 hours. Avoid shipments which are likely to arrive at the laboratory on Fridays, weekends or statutory holidays. If longer periods of transit are anticipated, pieces of dry ice should be used in place of ice-cubes.

REFERENCES

COOK, I., ALLAN, B. C. & WELHAM, S. (1969). Coxsackieviruses in normal children. *Med. J. Aust.*, **2**, 789.

DOANE, F. W., ANDERSON, N., CHATIYANONDA, K., BANNATYNE, R. M., MCLEAN, D. M. & RHODES, A. J. (1967). Rapid laboratory diagnosis of paramyxovirus infections by electron microscopy. *Lancet*, **2**, 751.

MCLEAN, D. M. (1966). Coxsackieviruses and echoviruses. *Amer. J. med. Sci.*, **251**, 351.

MCLEAN, D. M., LARKE, R. P. B., COBB, C., GRIFFIS, E. D. & HACKETT, S. M. R. (1967). Mumps and enteroviral meningitis in Toronto, 1966. *Canad. med. Ass. J.*, **96**, 1355.

TABLE 1.3

Laboratory Tests applicable to Common Virological Syndromes
(adapted from McLean, D. M. et al. (1960), *Canad. J. Pub. Health*, **51**, 94)

Syndrome	Group of causative agent	Virus isolation		Histopathology		Serology	Electron microscopy
		Specimen	Test system	Specimen	Light microscopy		
Central nervous system diseases							
Aseptic meningitis Poliomyelitis	Enterovirus	CSF, faeces, throat swab	Macaca kidney, human amnion, human thyroid, Tissue cultures, Suckling mice	Brain	Perivascular cuffing Neuronophagia	NT, CF, HI	*Enterovirus* non-enveloped, 30 nm virions, 42 capsomers *Mumps* enveloped, 150 nm virions, helical nucleocapsid
Encephalitis	Arbovirus	CSF, blood brain	Suckling mice hamster kidney Swine kidney Chick embryo Fibroblast Tissue cultures Mice	Brain	Perivascular cuffing Neuronophagia Glial knots	NT, CF, HI	*Arbovirus* enveloped, 40 nm virions, cubic symmetry
	Rabies	Brain, saliva	Tissue cultures Mice	Brain	Fluorescence Negri bodies		*Rabies* enveloped, 150 nm virions, complex symmetry
	Herpesvirus	Brain	Macaca kidney Human amnion Continuous line Tissue cultures	Brain	Eosinophilic intranuclear inclusions	NT, CF	*Herpesvirus* enveloped 125 nm virions, 162 capsomeres
Respiratory disease							
Influenza, coryza, croup, bronchiolitis, bronchopneumonia	Myxovirus Paramyxovirus	Throat swab, Throat washing, Nasopharyngeal suction	Macaca kidney, Continuous line tissue cultures Chick embryo (amniotic)			HI, CF, NT	*Myxovirus and paramyxovirus* enveloped 90–180 nm virions, helical nucleocapsid
	Adenovirus	Throat swab, etc.	Continuous line cultures			NT, CF	*Adenovirus* non-enveloped 80 nm virions, 252 capsomeres
	Chlamydia	Throat washing	Chick embryo (yolk sac)			CF	*Chlamydia* enveloped 300 nm particles
Serous membrane affections							
Pleurodynia Pericarditis	Enterovirus	Faeces or throat swab	Macaca kidney cultures Suckling mice			NT	

TABLE 1.3 (cont'd.)

Laboratory Tests applicable to Common Virological Syndromes
(adapted from McLean, D. M. *et al.* (1960), *Canad. J. Pub. Health*, **51**, 94)

Syndrome	Group of causative agent	Virus isolation		Histopathology		Serology	Electron microscopy
		Specimen	Test system	Specimen	Light microscopy		
Exanthemata							
Measles	Paramyxovirus	Throat washing Blood	Human amnion, grivet kidney cultures	Lymph node nasal mucosa	Warthin-Finkeldey giant cells	HI, NT, CF	
Rubella	Rubella	Throat washing	Grivet kidney (primary) Rabbit kidney (continuous)			NT, CF	*Rubella* enveloped, 40 nm virions, cubic symmetry
Varicella	Herpesvirus	Vesicle fluid	Human amnion	Vesicle scraping	Acidophilic intranuclear inclusions	CF	
Herpes	Herpesvirus	Vesicle scraping	Suckling mice Continuous line or human amnion cultures	Vesicle scraping	Acidophilic intranuclear inclusions	NT, CF	
Smallpox	Poxvirus	Throat washing blood, vesicle scraping	Chick embryo (chorioallantoic) Macaca kidney Chick embryo Fibroblast	Vesicle scraping	Acidophilic cytoplasmic inclusions	HI, CF, NT	*Poxvirus* enveloped 200 nm virions, complex symmetry
Eye diseases							
Inclusion blenorrhoea, Trachoma	Chlamydia	Conjunctival scrapings	Chick embryo (yolk sac)	Conjunctival scrapings	Basophilic cytoplasmic inclusions	CF	
Tropical fevers							
Yellow fever Tropical fevers	Arbovirus	Blood, CSF, Liver biopsy	Suckling mice Chick embryo Fibroblast cultures Hamster kidney cultures	Liver (yellow fever)	Midzonal necrosis	CF, HI, NT	
Rickettsial diseases							
Q fever	C. burnetii	Clotted blood	Chick embryo (yolk sac)			CF, A	
Rocky Mountain spotted fever	R. rickettsii	Clotted blood	Male guinea-pig			CF, A	
Rickettsialpox	R. akari	Clotted blood				CF, A	
Typhus	R. prowazekii	Clotted blood				CF, A	
Murine typhus	R. typhi	Clotted blood				CF, A	

Serology: NT = Neutralization test.   CF = Complement-fixation test.   HI = Haemagglutination inhibition test.   A = Agglutination test.

PELON, W., VILLAREJOS, V. M., RHIM, J. S. & PAYNE, F. J. (1966). Coxsackie group B virus infection and acute diarrhoea occurring among children in Costa Rica. *Arch. Dis. Childh.*, **41**, 636.

TOBIN, J. O'H. (1963). The isolation of respiratory viruses from children in hospital in South-East Lancashire. *Proc. roy. Soc. Med.*, **56**, 991.

MEASLES

Differential Diagnosis

Development of a blotchy maculopapular rash involving principally the face and trunk, accompanied by fever and Koplik's spots, nasopharyngeal and conjunctival catarrh, after an incubation period usually of 14 days provide sufficient clinical criteria for the diagnosis of measles (red measles or rubeola). However, laboratory procedures may be required, for example, to establish a diagnosis of measles in an allergic child, a patient taking antibiotics or other medication who develops a rash, in a subject previously vaccinated against measles, or in a leukaemic patient. In the Temperate Zone, during the cooler months, when both measles and rubella spread rapidly through communities, it is often desirable to invoke laboratory tests to distinguish measles from rubella in situations where a pregnant woman or her offspring develops a febrile exanthem.

Haemagglutination inhibition (HI) provides the most convenient procedure for the laboratory diagnosis of measles virus infections. It is essential to collect a serum sample within one day after onset of rash, but even at that early stage of illness, some antibody may be detected (Gresser and Chany, 1963; McLean *et al.*, 1966). Collection of a second serum sample two to four days later, within one day after defervescence, will reveal a fourfold or greater increment of measles antibody. Although measles virus has been recovered by inoculation into tissue cultures of human amnion cells, of the leucocyte fraction of heparinized blood obtained from nine of ten subjects one day after onset of rash (Gresser and Chany, 1963), this procedure is too highly specialized for everyday use.

Complications

(i) General

Despite the low case fatality rate from measles in Toronto, Canada (3/10,000) (Department of Public Health), the United States (1/10,000) (Langmuir, 1962) and Great Britain (2/10,000) (Miller, 1964), and a somewhat higher rate (1·2 per cent) among hospitalized patients in Sydney, Australia (Boughton, 1964a), in Tropical Africa the mortality rate among children hospitalized with measles may range from 5·7 to 21 per cent (Morley, 1969). It seems likely that malnutrition in tropical countries contributes to this high case fatality rate. Complications have been reported in one of 15 cases of measles in Britain (Miller, 1964). Complications frequently involve the respiratory tract and associated structures, giving rise to acute laryngo-tracheobronchitis, otitis media and bronchopneumonia. Of 44 deaths among 3601 Australian patients, 27 were due to pneumonia (Boughton, 1964a); but among 1283 West African children, 604 developed pneumonia and 169 (28 per cent) died (Morley, 1969). Encephalitis may affect about one in 700 cases of measles in the community (Greenberg et al., 1955; Miller, 1964) and 4·7 per cent of cases hospitalized with measles (Boughton, 1964b). Febrile convulsions without encephalitis occur in another one of 700 cases in Britain (Miller, 1964), but in West Africa 1·5 per cent of children hospitalized with measles convulsed before admission and 2·9 per cent had convulsions after admission (Morley, 1969).

(ii) Measles in leukaemia

Conditions affecting the reticuloendothelial system, such as leukaemia, may predispose to unusually severe attacks of measles resulting in giant-cell pneumonia, with (Mitus et al., 1959) or without (Enders et al., 1959) an antecedent rash. A Toronto patient aged five years who had received corticosteroids and antileukaemic chemotherapy for eight months following a diagnosis of leukaemia, developed extensive bilateral nodular infiltration of the lung field, with some areas of confluent alveolar consolidation, particularly in the left lower lobe from which she died three days subsequently. Syncytial giant cells with acidophilic intranuclear inclusions were observed to outline the alveolar air spaces, some of which were filled with exudate containing mononuclear and giant cells. Measles virus was isolated from the lung tissue (McLean et al., 1966).

Administration of 0·2 ml/kg pooled human gammaglobulin to a leukaemic child aged four years under treatment with corticosteroids and antileukaemic chemotherapy immediately after he became febrile, following household contact with measles, was followed two days later by a mild morbilliform rash and a rising measles antihaemagglutinin titre. However no antibody was detected 261 days after onset of rash. Intramuscular injection of leukocytes, derived from 500 ml plasma obtained from a subject who developed measles seven days previously, into a leukaemic child aged two years who developed clinical and radiological evidence of giant-cell pneumonia 20 days after onset of measles, was followed by satisfactory recovery from pneumonia. This patient, who had no measles antihaemagglutinin before administration of human donor leukocytes, developed a low HI antibody level four days later (McLean et al., 1966). Thus administration of pooled human gammaglobulin, or leukocytes from donors who have recently recovered from measles, may be life-saving procedures in patients with suppression of the reticuloendothelial system who contract measles.

(iii) Central nervous system

Encephalitis usually begins two to seven days after onset of the measles rash, and most commonly on the third to the fifth day (Boughton, 1964b; Karelitz and Eisenberg, 1961; McLean et al., 1966). Signs of encephalitis include a temperature exceeding 39°C, drowsiness deepening into stupor or coma, irritability, neck stiffness, and more than 10 lymphocytes per c.mm are found in CSF of 75 per cent of cases. Virtually all cases show diffuse abnormalities of the electroencephalogram. The case fatality rate has varied from zero in Toronto during 1964 and 1965 (McLean, et al., 1966) and Long Island, New York from 1952 to 1959 (Karelitz and Eisenberg, 1961) to 8·8 per cent in Sydney, Australia from 1943 to 1959 (Boughton, 1964b), 15 per cent in New York City from 1949 to 1954 (Greenberg et al., 1955), and 28·6 per cent in Milwaukee, Wisconsin between 1927 and 1951 (Fox et al., 1953). Neurological sequelae including paresis, athetosis, loss of speech and dementia, together with personality changes such as emotional lability and temper tantrums, may be present in 18 to 23 per cent of cases of measles encephalitis upon discharge from hospital (Greenberg et al., 1955; Boughton, 1964b). Personality changes may persist for one year or more, Administration of corticosteroids or adrenocorticotrophic hormone has not significantly increased the recovery rate from measles encephalitis or reduced the incidence of sequelae (Karelitz and Eisenberg, 1961; Swanson, 1956), nor has human gammaglobulin yielded benefit (Greenberg et al., 1955).

Although no significant difference was found between previous attacks of measles, as measured by the presence of measles antihaemagglutinin, and the readiness of first-grade schoolchildren for reading and learning in a homogeneous well-educated middle-class community in north-western U.S.A. (Kogon et al., 1968), performance of readiness tests for reading and learning was slightly lower among children who sustained unmodified measles in an upper middle-class area of the north-eastern U.S.A. (Fox et al., 1968). However in a third area with wide differences of socio-economic and educational status, it seemed likely that measles combined with a poor socio-economic and educational environment reduced performance in tests for reading and learning (Black and Davis, 1968). British observations (Douglas, 1964) showed that, in general, children who have contracted measles do not show any detectable educational or behavioural handicaps.

(iv) Subacute sclerosing panencephalitis

This slowly progressive encephalopathy, which usually terminates fatally within two years, comprises progressive dementia, myoclonic jerks, pyramidal and extrapyramidal signs, an electroencephalogram with regular periodic complexes, and a paretic type of colloidal gold reaction in the CSF (Connolly et al., 1968). Neurones may contain acidophilic intranuclear and cytoplasmic inclusions, there may be neuronal degeneration accompanied by accumulations of astrocytes and microglia, and perivascular cuffing with mononuclear cells is observed, sometimes associated with demyelination. The measles antibody titres in sera of patients with subacute sclerosing panencephalitis were significantly higher than in age-matched controls, and within those patients high measles antibody levels were found in CSF, which suggests synthesis of measles antibody in the central nervous system. All cases had measles several years previously. Foci were observed in neurones of cerebral tissue in patients following staining with fluorescent-labelled measles antiserum (Connolly et al., 1967). The herringbone appearance of measles virus nucleocapsid was observed in brains stained negatively with phosphotungstic acid and examined by electron microscopy (Bouteille et al., 1965). Direct inoculation of triturated cerebral tissue into tissue cultures failed to yield virus. However, when brain from cases was trypsinized lightly and grown in mixed cultures with susceptible continuous lines of human cells, strain HeLa or Hep2, measles virus was recovered (Horta-Barbosa et al., 1969). It therefore seems likely that subacute sclerosing panencephalitis may be a persistent and late manifestation of measles infection. However, the recovery of a slow virus from other cases of this condition suggests that it may be a syndrome resulting from infection with a variety of unrelated viruses, one of which may be measles.

Vaccines

Decline of the peak monthly incidence of measles per 1000 of the population of the United States, from 70 in 1963 at the time of introduction of measles vaccination, to 30 in 1966 and 10 in 1967, has amply demonstrated the protective value of widespread vaccination against measles. This low incidence of measles contrasts sharply with the mean incidence of 90 per 1000 at the peaks during the previous five years (Dull and Witte, 1968).

Live measles vaccine is the only type of vaccine currently recommended for use. Of the varieties available at present, the further attenuated strain (Schwarz, 1962) derived after 77 additional passages in chick embryo tissue cultures of the original Edmonston strain of live measles vaccine (Enders et al., 1960) has shown significantly fewer side-effects than the earlier Edmonston strain (Krugman et al., 1963; Miller et al., 1967). In Honduras during early 1965, of 71 seronegative children who received Schwarz vaccine intramuscularly, 15 per cent developed temperatures exceeding 39·5°C nine to eleven days subsequently and 12 per cent showed a morbilliform rash. This was in contrast to 30 per cent of 83 who became febrile, 27 per cent who developed a rash after the Edmonston vaccine, 3 per cent who developed fever and 10 per cent who showed rashes after a placebo (Miller et al., 1967). Although the geometric mean HI antibody titre was somewhat lower (70·6) in those who received the Schwarz vaccine than following the Edmonston vaccine (111·6), both groups of vaccinated subjects showed antibody conversion rates exceeding 95 per cent. Concomitant administration of 0·2 ml gammaglobulin with a measles neutralizing antibody titre of 400 per 0·1 ml has reduced the incidence of febrile reactions following Schwarz vaccine from 15 to 3 per cent (Krugman *et al.*, 1963) without significant decrease of the antibody response or protection rate against subsequent challenge by natural measles. Despite febrile reactions, vaccinated children were relatively undisturbed in their daily activities following measles vaccine alone (Benson *et al.*, 1964). Currently, there is no justification for the use of gammaglobulin concomitant with live vaccine.

Good evidence of protection against natural challenge by measles virus was observed regularly when live measles vaccine accompanied by gammaglobulin was administered as closely as two to 10 days before exposure of vaccines to the disease. However, virtually no evidence of protection was noted when measles vaccine was administered up to five days after exposure to natural measles (Fulginiti and Kempe, 1963).

Administration of a combined live vaccine for measles, yellow fever and smallpox by jet-gun injector has resulted in antibody conversions exceeding 80 per cent to all three viruses in large numbers of Africans (Meyer *et al.*, 1964).

The recent occurrence of several cases of encephalitis following vaccination with measles strains which were less highly attenuated than the Schwarz strain has prompted the Department of Health and Social Security of Great Britain to recommend the use of the Schwarz strain of measles vaccine exclusively (Department of Health and Social Security, 1969). Previously, it was found that measles vaccine evoked no abnormality in the electro-encephalogram of otherwise normal children (Gibbs *et al.*, 1961).

Reduction of the attack rate per 1000 among a group of British children from 222 in unvaccinated subjects to 13 during two years after one dose of live vaccine (94 per cent protection rate), and to 27 after one dose of killed vaccine followed by one dose of live vaccine (88 per cent protection rate), together with less severe attacks in vaccinated subjects who developed measles, has confirmed the protective efficacy of live measles vaccine (Medical Research Council, 1968). However, the use of killed vaccine to modify febrile reactions following live vaccine is now considered inadvisable on account of the occurrence of unusually severe illnesses accompanied by pneumonia and atypical rashes in 10 children who received killed vaccine five to six years before challenge by natural measles (Fulginiti *et al.*, 1967).

In view of the high degree of protective efficacy of live measles vaccine, the prospects of eradication of measles seem bright following adoption of the four following principles (Dull and Witte, 1968): (1) Routine immunization of all infants at approximately their first birthdays; (2) Immunization of all susceptible children when they enter kindergarten or the first grades of elementary schools; (3) Active surveillance of measles cases; (4) Prompt control of measles epidemics.

REFERENCES

BOUTEILLE, M., FONTAINE, C., VENDREME, C. & DELARUE, J. (1965). Sur un cas d'encéphalite subaignë à inclusions. Etude anatomo-clinique et ultrastructurale. *Rev. Neurol.*, **113**, 454.

BENSON, P. F., BUTLER, N. R., GOFFE, A. P., KNIGHT, G. J., LAWRENCE, G. D., MILLER, C. L. & POLLOCK, T. M. (1964) Vaccination of infants with living attenuated measles vaccine (Edmonston strain), with and without gamma-globulin. *Brit. med. J.*, **2**, 851.

BLACK, F. L. & DAVIS, D. E. M. (1968). Measles and readiness for reading and learning. II. New Haven study. *Amer. J. Epidem.*, **88**, 337.

BOUGHTON, C. R. (1964a). Morbilli in Sydney: a review of 3601 cases with consideration of morbidity, mortality and measles encephalomyelitis. *Med. J. Aust.*, **2**, 859.

BOUGHTON, C. R. (1964b). Morbilli in Sydney: neurological sequelae of morbilli. *Med. J. Aust.*, **2**, 908.

CONNOLLY, J. H. (1967). Measles-virus antibody and antigen in subacute sclerosing panencephalitis. *Lancet*, **1**, 542.

CONNOLLY, J. H., ALLEN, I. V., HURWITZ, L. J. & MILLAR, J. H. D. (1968). Subacute sclerosing panencephalitis. *Quart. J. Med.*, **37**, 625.

DEPARTMENT OF HEALTH AND SOCIAL SECURITY, GREAT BRITAIN (1969). Measles vaccines. *Brit. med. J.*, **1**, 701.

DOUGLAS, J. W. B. (1964). Ability and adjustment of children who have had measles. *Brit. med. J.*, **2**, 1301.

DULL, H. B. & WITTE, J. J. (1968). Progress of measles eradication in the United States. *Publ. Hlth Rep.*, **83**, 245.

ENDERS, J. F., McCARTHY, K., MITUS, A. & CHEATHAM, W. J. (1959). Isolation of measles virus at autopsy in cases of giant-cell pneumonia without rash. *New Engl. J. Med.*, **261**, 875.

ENDERS, J. F., KATZ, S. L., MILOVANOVIC, M. V. & HOLLOWAY, A. (1960). Studies on an attenuated measles-virus vaccine. 1. Development and preparation of the vaccine: technics for assay of effects of vaccination. *New. Engl. J. Med.*, **263**, 153.

FOX, J. P., BLACK, F. L., ELVEBACK, L., KOGON, A., HALL, C. E., TURGEON, L. & ABRUZZI, W. (1968). Measles and readiness for reading and learning. III. Wappingers Central School District study. *Amer. J. Epidem.*, **88**, 345.

FOX, M. J., KUZMAN, J. F. & STUKER, J. D. (1953). Measles encephalomyelitis. *Amer. J. Dis. Child.*, **85**, 444.

FULGINITI, V. A., ELLER, J. J., DOWNIE, A. W. & KEMPE, C. H. (1967). Altered reactivity to measles virus. *J.A.M.A.*, **202**, 1075.

FULGINITI, V. A. & KEMPE, C. H. (1963). Measles exposure among vaccine recipients. *Am. J. Dis. Child.*, **106**, 450.

GIBBS, F. A., GIBBS, E. L. & ROSENTHAL, I. M. (1961). Electroencephalographic study of children immunized against measles with live attenuated virus vaccine. *New Engl. J. Med.*, **264**, 800.

GREENBERG, M., PELLITTERI, O. & EISENSTEIN, D. T. (1955). Measles encephalitis. I. Prophylactic effect of gammaglobulin. *J. Pediat.*, **46**, 642.

GRESSER, I. & CHANY, C. (1963). Isolation of measles virus from the washed leucocytic fraction of blood. *Proc. Soc. exp. Biol. (N.Y.)*, **113**, 695.

HORTA-BARBOSA, L., FUCILLA, D. A., SEVER, J. L. & ZEMAN, W. (1969). Subacute sclerosing panencephalitis: isolation of measles virus from a brain biopsy. *Nature*, **221**, 974.

KARELITZ, S. & EISENBERG, M. (1961). Measles encephalitis. *Pediatrics*, **27**, 811.

KATZ, M., RORKE, L. B., MOSLUND, W. S., KOPROWSKI, H. & TUCKER, S. H. (1968). Transmission of encephalitogenic agent from brains of patients with subacute sclerosing panencephalitis to ferrets. *New Engl. J. Med.*, **279**, 793.

KOGON, A., HALL, C. E., COONEY, M. K. & FOX, J. P. (1968). Measles and readiness for reading and learning. II. Shoreline School District study. *Amer. J. Epidem.*, **88**, 351.

KRUGMAN, S., GILES, J. P., JACOBS, A. M. & FRIEDMAN, H. (1963). Studies with a further attenuated live measles-virus vaccine. *Pediatrics*, **31**, 919.

LANGMUIR, A. D. (1962). Medical importance of measles. *Amer. J. Dis. Child.*, **103**, 224.

McLEAN, D. M., BEST, J. M., SMITH, P. A., LARKE, R. P. B. & McNAUGHTON, G. A. (1966). Viral infections of Toronto children during 1965. II. Measles encephalitis and other complications. *Canad. med. Ass. J.*, **94**, 905.

MEYER, H. M., HOESTLER, D. D., BERNHEIM, B. C., ROGERS, N. G., LAMBIN, P., CHASSORY, A., LABUSQUIERE, R. & SONADEL, J. E. (1964). Response of Volta children to jet inoculation of combined live measles, smallpox and yellow fever vaccines. *Bull. Wld Hlth Org.*, **30**, 783.

MILLER, D. L. (1964). Frequency of complications of measles, 1963. *Brit. med. J.*, **2**, 75.

MILLER, G., GALE, J., VILLAREJOS, V., JAMES, W., ARTEAGA, G. G., CACEY, H. & HENDERSON, D. A. (1967). Edmonston B and a further attenuated measles vaccine—a placebo controlled double blind comparison. *Amer. J. Publ. Hlth.*, **57**, 1333.

MITUS, A., ENDERS, J. F., CRAIG, J. M. & HOLLOWAY, A. (1959). Persistence of measles virus and depression of antibody formation in patients with giant-cell pneumonia after measles. *New Engl. J. Med.*, **261**, 882.,

MORLEY, D. (1969). Severe measles in the Tropics. *Brit. med. J.*, **1**, 297 and 363.

MEDICAL RESEARCH COUNCIL, SECOND REPORT BY THE MEASLES VACCINES COMMITTEE (1968). Vaccination against measles: clinical trial of live measles vaccine. *Brit. med. J.*, **1**, 449.

SCHWARZ, A. J. F. (1962). Preliminary tests of a highly attenuated measles vaccine. *Amer. J. Dis. Child.*, **103**, 386.

SWANSON, B. E. (1956). Measles meningoencephalitis. *Amer. J. Dis. Child.*, **92**, 273.

TORONTO, DEPARTMENT OF PUBLIC HEALTH: Monthly reports 1959–66.

RUBELLA

Clinical and Laboratory Features

Clinical recognition of rubella in a child or adult depends upon the development of a fine, intense macular ("peach bloom") rash over the face and trunk, accompanied regularly by mild fever and enlargement of the post-auricular or suboccipital lymph nodes (Young and Ramsay, 1963). The rash usually persists for two to three days, and not longer than five days (Brody et al., 1965). No skin staining is observed following disappearance of the rash. The eyes may appear suffused, and occasionally photophobia is experienced. Petechiae have rarely been observed. In an Alaskan outbreak of serologically confirmed rubella 110 persons developed rashes together with post-auricular lymphadenopathy, but another 56 subjects showed swelling of post-auricular nodes only (Brody et al., 1965). Rubella without rash occurred in 60 per cent of subjects aged less than 10 years old and in 88 per cent of those aged 15 to 19 years, but rubella virus was recovered from throats of patients in both categories (Sever et al., 1965).

Complications of rubella include arthritis and encephalitis.

During a rubella outbreak in Texas, rubella virus was isolated from the throat of an adult who developed rash, conjunctivitis and swelling of the joints of the ankles, knees and fingers (Phillips et al., 1965), and child household contacts of another virologically confirmed case of rubella developed arthritis in addition to exanthem and post-auricular lymphadenopathy. In a Pittsburgh outbreak of rubella, one in 5000 cases developed encephalitis two to four days after onset of rash, and three of six cases of encephalitis died (Sherman et al., 1965). Rubella virus was recovered from the throat of a non-fatal case and from the lung of a fatal case of encephalitis.

Rubella virus was first isolated from throats of military recruits and children who developed clinical rubella by inoculation of primary monolayer tissue cultures of African green (Cercopithecus sp.) monkey kidney (Parkman et al., 1962; Sever et al., 1962) or human amnion (Weller and Neva, 1962). In monkey kidney cell cultures, these agents interfered with the multiplication of echovirus 11 or coxsackievirus A9 following challenge approximately one week subsequently. Direct microscopic observations of infected human amnion cell cultures revealed cytopathic effects. Rubella virus also multiplies in continuous line cultures of rabbit kidney cells, strain RK13, with the production of a profound cytopathic effect (McCarthy et al., 1963).

Although rubella virus excretion from the throat of infected subjects usually commences five days before onset of the rash and persists regularly for four days after onset (Sever et al., 1965), shedding may sometimes persist for 14 days or longer (Green et al., 1965). Viraemia may be detected during the week preceding onset of the rash, but usually terminates shortly after the rash appears, coinciding with the initial appearance of HI and NT antibodies (Cooper et al., 1969).

Detection of antibody in patients by neutralization tests (NT) in tissue culture was accomplished immediately following the isolation of rubella virus in 1962. Conduct of this technique by inhibition of interference in African green monkey kidney tissue cultures, or by inhibition of cytopathic effects in RK13 cells, elucidated many features of the epidemiology of rubella and the natural history of the rubella syndrome. More than one week was required for completion of the test. Acceleration of conduct of the neutralization test was reported in 1964 through the demonstration of immunofluorescence by the indirect technique (Brown *et al.*, 1964). Coverslips of continuous cultures of rhesus monkey kidney cells strain LLC-MK2, which were persistently infected with rubella virus, were immersed in patient's serum, after which fluorescein-labelled goat antihuman serum was applied. Bright immunofluorescence indicated the presence of rubella NT antibody in the patient's serum.

Development of the complement fixation (CF) test in 1965 resulted from the preparation of cell-associated antigen from infected continuous cultures of rabbit (RK13) (Sever *et al.*, 1965) or hamster (BHK21/13S) kidney cells (Halonen *et al.*, 1967a). The haemagglutination inhibition (HI) test was developed in 1967 using antigen prepared from supernatant fluids (Stewart *et al.*, 1957) or alkaline extracts of suspended cell cultures (Halonen *et al.*, 1967b) of infected continuous cultures of baby hamster kidney cells. The HI test requires only two hours for completion. The HI test appears to be the most accurate of all four antibody tests for diagnosis of rubella, and the most sensitive and reliable for detection of serological evidence of past infection (Herrmann, *et al.*, 1969).

Rubella HI antibodies usually appear in patients' sera one to two days after onset of the rash (Herrmann *et al.*, 1969; Cooper and Krugman, 1967; Rawls *et al.*, 1968). They attain maximum titres at two to four weeks, and persist for at least five years after falling two- to fourfold below peak levels (Halonen *et al.*, 1967b). Neutralizing antibodies are usually first detected about four days after onset of the rash, and CF antibodies appear one to two days later (Halonen *et al.*, 1967a; Rawls *et al.*, 1968; Sever *et al.*, 1965). Neutralizing antibodies usually persist for more than five years, but CF antibodies usually become undetectable within three years.

During the first week after onset of rash, HI antibody will be detected in the macroglobulin (IgM) fraction of the plasma globulins which appear in about 50 per cent of patients who develop rubella (Vesikari and Vaheri, 1968), and rubella HI antibody has persisted as long as 22 days in the IgM component (Best *et al.*, 1969). Since IgM globulins are readily depolymerized by 0·1 M 2-mercaptoethanol which is a sulphydryl-reducing substance, fourfold or greater reduction of the HI antibody titre in sera collected during the first week after onset of rash may provide a convenient and rapid means of serological diagnosis of rubella on a single blood sample (Banatvala *et al.*, 1967; Cooper *et al.*, 1969). Complement-fixing antibody, which is conveyed exclusively in the IgG fraction of plasma globulins (Best *et al.*, 1969) does not normally appear until the second week after onset of rash, at which time the concentration of IgG increases substantially, concomitant with a twofold decline of IgM concentration.

Rubella Syndrome

Following the world-wide massive upsurge of rubella virus activity during 1964 and 1965, several new features in addition to the classical triad of cardiac anomalies, deafness and cataracts were observed among babies born to mothers who contracted rubella during the first trimester.

The term "rubella syndrome" is used to describe the clinical features of newborn infants which result from intra-uterine infections usually during the first trimester of pregnancy (Table 1.4). From virologically confirmed cases

TABLE 1.4

Clinical features of the rubella syndrome in four centres during 1964–65

Sign	Percentage involvement			
	Houston 25 cases[1]	Memphis 17 cases[2]	Philadelphia 21 cases[3]	Toronto 7 cases[4]
Ocular defects	50	72	76	86
Cardiac anomalies	70	100	67	86
Thrombocytopenic purpura	80	42	43	57
Birthweight below 2500 gm	80	72	57	71
Hepatomegaly	70	24	33	43
Bone changes	70	6	33	43
Rubella in first trimester	76	68	—	86
Rubella exposure	8	12	—	14*
Rubella virus in throat	63	96	95	71

[1] RUDOLPH et al. (1965). *J.A.M.A.*, **191**, 843.
[2] KORONES et al. (1965). *J. Pediat.*, **67**, 166.
[3] PLOTKIN et al. (1965). *J. Pediat.*, **67**, 182.
[4] McLEAN et al. (1966). *Canad. med. Ass. J.*, **95**, 1174.
* The mother of this patient received gammaglobulin within 24 hours after her husband developed rubella.

in Houston (Rudolph *et al.*, 1965), Memphis (Korones *et al.*, 1965), Philadelphia (Plotkin *et al.*, 1965) and Toronto (McLean *et al.*, 1966), the stigmata of the rubella syndrome comprise: (1) *ocular defects*, principally cataracts in 50 to 80 per cent of cases, which may occur either unilaterally or bilaterally. In some series (Pitt and Keir, 1965a) embryonic pigmentary retinopathy is observed frequently; (2) *deafness* affected 26 per cent of infants in an Australian study conducted before virological tests were developed, but the incidence increased to 37 per cent when these children attained four to eight years of age (Pitt and Keir, 1965a); (3) *thrombocytopenic purpura* in 42 to 80 per cent of cases giving the appearance of a spotted muffin, with a platelet count depressed to between 10,000 and 30,000 per c.mm, returning to normal spontaneously after two to three weeks; (4) *birth weight below 2500 grams* in 57 to 80 per cent of cases, despite a normal gestational age of 38 to 41 weeks; (5) *hepatomegaly* in 24 to 70 per cent of cases, sometimes accompanied by splenomegaly; (6) *radiological changes* in the metaphyses of the long bones in 6 to 70 per cent of cases, giving the appearance of a celery stalk (Reed, 1969). Although mental retardation (McLean *et al.*, 1966) was noted in 14 per cent of cases, and delay in development of motor activity was observed in 4 per cent of infants (Pitt and Keir, 1965a), the distribution of intelligence quotients among children who contracted intra-uterine rubella infections paralleled that observed in offspring of mothers who had no clinical evidence of rubella during pregnancy (Sheridan, 1964).

An exanthem typical of rubella was noted during the first trimester of pregnancy in 68 to 86 per cent of mothers, but in 8 to 14 per cent of pregnant women who were contacts of clinical cases, no exanthem was observed. In some instances where human gammaglobulin had been administered to mothers following exposure to rubella cases, babies were born with the rubella syndrome (Avery *et al.*, 1965; McLean *et al.*, 1966; Plotkin *et al.*, 1967). Rubella virus was detected in the throat of 63 to 96 per cent of cases.

Prospective studies in London, England (Sheridan, 1964), Nassau County, New York (Tartakow, 1965) and Melbourne, Australia (Pitt and Keir 1965a, b), have shown that maternal rubella in the first trimester was followed by major congenital anomalies in 15 to 19·4 per cent of live off-spring, and a further 8 to 16·5 per cent had one or more minor anomalies. These incidences can be compared with the 3·3 per cent of infants with major anomalies and 1·7 per cent with minor anomalies in those whose mothers did not contract rubella during pregnancy (Tartakow, 1965). Offspring from mothers who developed rubella during the second trimester showed 3·3 per cent with major anomalies and 13·4 per cent with minor defects. When rubella affected mothers during the third trimester, no major anomalies were noted in offspring, but 14·3 per cent showed minor anomalies (Tartakow, 1965).

The risk of development of anomalies in offspring was found in prospective studies to be 50 per cent when rubella affected mothers from the first to the fourth week of gestation, 25 per cent following rubella at five to eight weeks, 17 per cent at nine to 12 weeks, 11 per cent at 13 to 16 weeks, 6 per cent at 17 to 24 weeks and none at later stages of pregnancy (Hill *et al.*, 1958).

Among 225 antenatal patients of a downtown Toronto hospital, 63 per cent of subjects aged 11 to 15 years and 70 per cent or more of those aged 16 to 29 years had rubella neutralizing antibody. This increased to 80 per cent or more among those aged 30 to 44 years (McLean *et al.*, 1966). At an outer suburban hospital, 75 per cent or more of antenatal patients aged 16 to 44 years had rubella antibodies. A survey of female residents of metro-

COOPER, L. Z., MATTERS, B., ROSENBLUM, J. K. & KRUGMAN, S. (1969). Experience with a modified rubella haemagglutination inhibition (HI) antibody test. *J.A.M.A.*, **207**, 89.

DUDGEON, J. A., BUTLER, N. R. & PLOTKIN, S. A. (1964). Further serological studies on the rubella syndrome. *Brit. med. J.*, **2**, 155.

DUDGEON, J. A., MARSHALL, W. C., PECKHAM, C. S. & HAWKINS, G. T. (1969). Clinical and laboratory studies with rubella vaccines in adults. *Brit. med. J.*, **1**, 271.

GIVAN, K. F., ROZEE, K. R. & RHODES, A. J. (1965). Incidence of rubella antibodies in female subjects *Canad. med. Ass. J.*, **92**, 126.

GRAYSTON, J. T., DETELS, R., CHEN, K. P., GUTMAN, L., KIM, K. S. W., GALE, J. L. & BEASLEY, R. P. (1969). Field trial of live attenuated rubella virus vaccine during an epidemic in Taiwan. *J.A.M.A.*, **207**, 1107.

GREEN, R. H., BALSAMO, M. R., GILES, J. P., KRUGMAN, S. & MIRICK, G. S. (1965). Studies of the natural history and prevention of rubella. *Amer. J. Dis. Child.*, **110**, 348.

HALONEN, P. E., CASEY, H. L., STEWART, J. A. & HALL, A. D. (1967a). Rubella complement-fixing antigen prepared by alkaline extraction of virus grown in suspension culture of BHK-21 cells. *Proc. Soc. exp. Biol. Med.*, **125**, 167.

HALONEN, P. E., RYAN, J. M. & Stewart, J. A. (1967b). Rubella haemagglutinin prepared with alkaline extraction of virus grown in suspension culture of BHK-21 cells. *Proc. Soc. exp. Biol. Med.*, **125**, 162.

HERRMANN, K. L., HALONEN, P. E., STEWART, J. A., CASEY, H. L., RYAN, J. M., HALL, A. D. & CASWELL, K. E. (1969). Evaluation of serological techniques for titration of rubella antibody. *Amer. J. Publ. Hlth.*, **59**, 296.

HILL, A. B., DOLL, R., GALLOWAY, T. McL. & HUGHES, J. P. W. (1958). Virus diseases in pregnancy and congenital defects. *Brit. J. prev. soc. Med.*, **12**, 1.

HILLARY, I. B., MEENAN, P. N., GRIFFITH, A. H., DRAPER, C. C. & LAWRENCE, G. D. (1969). Rubella vaccine trials in children. *Brit. med. J.*, **1**, 531.

HUYGELEN, C. & PEETERMANS, J. (1967). Attenuation of rubella virus by serial passage in primary rabbit kidney cell cultures. II. Experiments in animals. *Arch. ges. Virusforsch.*, **21**, 357.

JACK, I. & Grutzner, J. (1969). Cellular viraemia in babies infected with rubella virus before birth. *Brit. med. J.*, **1**, 289.

KORONES, S. B., AINGER, L. E., MONIF, G. R. G., ROANE, J., SEVER, J. L. & FUSTE, F. (1965). Congenital rubella syndrome: new clinical aspects with recovery of virus from affected tissues. *J. Pediat.*, **67**, 166.

MCCARTHY, K., TAYLOR-ROBINSON, C. H. & PILLINGER, S. E. (1963). Isolation of rubella virus from cases in Britain. *Lancet*, **2**, 593.

MCLEAN, D. M., MCNAUGHTON, G. A., GIVAN, K. F., BEST, J. M., SMITH, P. A. & COLEMAN, M. A. (1966). Rubella virus infections during pregnancy, Toronto, 1963–66. *Canad. med. Ass. J.*, **95**, 1174.

MONIF, G. R. G., AVERY, G. B., KORONES, S. B. & SEVER, J. L. (1965). Postmortem isolation of rubella virus from three children with rubella-syndrome defects. *Lancet*, **1**, 723.

PARKMAN, P. D., BUESCHER, E. L. & ARTENSTEIN, M. S. (1962). Recovery of rubella virus from army recruits. *Proc. Soc. exp. Biol. (N.Y.).*, **111**, 225.

PARKMAN, P. D., MEYER, H. M., KIRSCHSTEIN, R. L. & HOPPS, H. E. (1966). Attenuated rubella virus. I. Development and laboratory characteristics. *New Engl. J. Med.*, **275**, 569.

PHILLIPS, C. A., BEHBEHANI, A. M., JOHNSON, L. W. & MELNICK, J. L. (1965). Isolation of rubella virus. An epidemic characterized by rash and arthritis *J.A.M.A.*, **191**, 615.

PITT, D. & KEIR, E. H. (1965a). Results of rubella in pregnancy. *I. med. J. Austral.*, **2**, 647.

PITT, D. & KEIR, E. H. (1965b). Results of rubella in pregnancy, III. *Med. J. Aust.*, **2**, 739.

PLOTKIN, S. A., ASKI, F. A., HARNETT, E. M., HERVADA, A. R., FRIEDMAN, S. & GOWING, J. (1965). Some recently recognized manifestations of the rubella syndrome. *J. Pediat.*, **67**, 182.

PLOTKIN, S. A., COCHRAN, W., LINDQUIST, J. M., COCHRAN, G. G., SCHAFFER, D. B., SCHEIE, H. G. & FURUKAWA, T. (1967). Congenital rubella syndrome in late infancy. *J.A.M.A.*, **200**, 435.

PLOTKIN, S. A., FARQUHAR, J. F., KATZ, M. & INGALLS, T. H. (1967). Immunization against rubella with living virus. II. Trials of a strain adapted to human fibroblasts. *Amer. J. Epidem.*, **86**, 468.

RAWLS, W. E., DESMYTER, J. & MELNICK, J. L. (1968). Serological diagnosis and fatal involvement in maternal rubella. *J.A.M.A.*, **203**, 627.

REED, G. B. (1969). Rubella bone lesions. *J. Pediat.*, **74**, 208.

RUDOLPH, A. J., YOW, M. D., PHILLIPS, A. C., DESMOND, M. M., BLATTNER, R. J. & MELNICK, J. L. (1965). Transplacental rubella infection in newly born infants. *J.A.M.A.*, **191**, 843.

SEVER, J. L., SCHIFF, G. M. & TRAUB, R. G. (1962). Rubella virus. *J.A.M.A.*, **182**, 663.

SEVER, J. L., BRODY, J. A., SCHIFF, G. M., MCALISTER, R. & CUTTING, R. (1965). Rubella epidemic on St. Paul Island in the Pribilofs, 1963. II. Clinical and laboratory findings for the intensive study population. *J.A.M.A.*, **191**, 624.,

SEVER, J. L., HEUBNER, R. J., CASTELLANO, G. A., SARMA, P. S., FABIYI, A., SCHIFF, G. M. & CUSUMANO, C. L. (1965). Rubella complement fixation test. *Science*, **148**, 385.

SHERMAN, F. E., MICHAELS, R. H. & KENNY, F. M. (1965). Acute encephalopathy (encephalitis) complicating rubella. *J.A.M.A.*, **192**, 675.

SHERIDAN, M. D. (1964). Final report of a prospective study of children whose mothers had rubella in early pregnancy. *Brit. med. J.*, **2**, 536.

STEWART, G. L., PARKMAN, P. D., HOPPS, H. E., DOUGLAS, R. D., HAMILTON, J. P. & MEYER, H. M. (1967). Rubella-virus haemagglutination-inhibition test. *New Engl. J. Med.*, **276**, 554.

TARTAKOW, I. J. (1965). The teratogenicity of maternal rubella. *J. Pediat.* **66**, 380.

VESIKARI, T. & VAHERI, A. (1968). Rubella: a method for rapid diagnosis of a recent infection by demonstration of the IgM antibodies. *Brit. med. J.*, **1**, 221.

WELLER, T. H. & NEVA, F. A. (1962). Propagation in tissue culture of cytopathic agents from patients with rubella-like illnesses. *Proc. Soc. exp. Brit. Med.*, **111**, 215.

YOUNG, S. E. J. & RAMSAY, A. M. (1963). The diagnosis of rubella. *Brit. med. J.*, **2**, 1295.

MUMPS

Clinical and Epidemiological Features

Epidemics of mumps affect many established communities within the Temperate Zones at intervals of approximately three years, the majority of cases occurring during winter and spring (Toronto, 1959–66). Concurrent with the upsurge of incidence of mumps, a proportionate increase occurs in the number of complications, especially meningitis (McLean *et al.*, 1967).

Typical mumps induces bilateral parotitis in 70 per cent of patients and unilateral parotitis in 30 per cent. Submandibular glands are involved in 10 per cent of cases, and the sublingual glands are involved occasionally. Orchitis, which is the commonest complication, occurs in 18 per cent of post-pubertal males (Wesselhoeft, 1951). In a mumps epidemic on St George Island, Alaska, during 1965, which had been free of mumps since 1907, clinical attacks involved 56 per cent of 212 native residents, but 27 of these had a past history of mumps contracted elsewhere (Reed *et al.*, 1967). The clinical attack rate amongst this "mumps virgin" population was 65 per cent and an additional 24 per cent developed subclinical infections with production of antibody in the absence of symptoms.

In Erie County, New York, including the city of Buffalo where mumps is endemic, during a survey in April 1967, 53 per cent or more of residents aged 15 to 39 years reported having suffered from a past attack of mumps, in contrast to 10 per cent of those aged four years or less (Harris *et al.*, 1968). Of those who had developed clinical mumps, 20 per cent were affected by the age of five and 74 per cent by the age of 10, but only 5 per cent contracted mumps after 20 years of age. In Alaska where mumps is not endemic, the clinical attack rate increased from 32 per cent of those aged four years or less to 74 per cent of those aged four to nine years and 91 per cent between 10 and 14 years of age. In households within Erie County, 44 per cent of children aged one to nine years developed clinical mumps 14 to 30 days after the initial case occurred in the household, but only 11 per cent of those aged 10 to 19 years contracted mumps. When susceptible children escaped clinical mumps following one household introduction of it, 33 to 45 per cent developed mumps after a second household exposure. When an older sibling was in the household, clinical mumps appeared at a somewhat earlier age.

Complications in addition to orchitis or oophoritis include meningitis which may involve 0·5 to 10 per cent of subjects, pancreatitis in 7 per cent and the thyroid, breast or pre-sternal subcutaneous tissue occasionally (Wesselhoeft, 1951). Sometimes, laparotomy may be required for acute necrotizing pancreatitis (Witte and Schanzer, 1968). In Erie County, N.Y., 12 per cent of post-pubertal males and 0·4 per cent of pre-pubertal males developed orchitis, but four of seven males with a history of mumps orchitis, including one with bilateral involvement, have fathered children. In the same survey, only two of 1598 mumps cases developed meningitis but no other complications were reported. On St George Island, 25 per cent of 60 males aged three to 44 years with mumps developed orchitis, including 20 per cent of those who received hyperimmune gammaglobulin and 27 per cent of those without immunoprophylaxis (Reed *et al.*, 1967). Oophoritis occurred in

7 per cent of 59 female mumps cases. Meningitis affected 6 per cent of 119 cases belonging to both sexes, including 8 per cent of those who received gammaglobulin and 5 per cent unimmunized cases. Delayed involvement of another parenchymatous organ such as the testis, thyroid or breast two to five weeks after onset of parotitis was observed in 8 per cent of cases. Among 279 schoolchildren in Baltimore, Maryland who developed mumps during 1960, 2·5 per cent developed meningitis and 1·4 per cent developed pancreatitis (Meyer, 1962).

Less common complications of mumps infection include weakness of the muscles of the neck, back, hamstrings and abdomen, which persisted less than two months after attacks of serologically confirmed mumps meningitis in 11 Californian patients (Lenette et al., 1960). Arthritis comprising pain, tenderness and swelling of the ankle in a child and an adult, and the hip in another child, occurred in three patients two weeks after onset of parotitis (Lass and Shepard, 1961). An adolescent developed arthritis affecting the right wrist, right elbow, shoulder, hip, knee and ankle 11 days after onset of parotitis (Caranosos and Felker, 1967). Meningoencephalitis was accompanied by polyneuritis and severe hypertension in a woman with serologically suggestive evidence of mumps infection some two weeks previously (Porter and Pallis, 1960). Perivascular demyelinating leucoencephalitis may occur one to two weeks after mumps in 1 : 6000 cases, and 22 fatal cases have been reported (Donohue et al., 1955). Skin hypersensitivity to formalinized mumps antigen in a high proportion of infants with endocardial fibroelastosis, but not other congenital heart lesions (Vosburgh et al., 1965), who were born to mothers with previous history of mumps (including some who were exposed to mumps during the first trimester) suggested that intra-uterine encounters with mumps virus may have evoked this cardiac anomaly (St Geme et al., 1966). However, the absence of mumps antibody from virtually all patients with endocardial fibroelastosis, except those who had contracted clinical mumps (Shone et al., 1966), casts doubt on the possibility that intra-uterine mumps virus infection stimulated the development of endocardial fibroelastosis.

Mumps meningitis

Clinical features of mumps meningitis (McLean et al., 1960) which include headache, vomiting, fever, neck stiffness and lymphocytosis of the CSF may occur one week before and up to two weeks after onset of parotitis. However, mumps meningitis may occur frequently in the absence of swelling of the parotid or submandibular glands. For example, in Toronto during 1966 (McLean et al., 1967), mumps virus infection was demonstrated by virus isolation from CSF and/or increments of mumps antihaemagglutinin titre during convalescence in 16 paediatric patients with mumps meningitis in the absence of parotitis among 39 who had laboratory evidence of mumps infection. In Columbus, Ohio, from 1964 to 1967, 27 of 51 patients with laboratory-confirmed mumps meningitis showed no parotitis (Azimi et al., 1969). The incidence amongst boys was two to three times higher than the prevalence amongst girls. In Toronto (McLean et al., 1967), Northern Ireland (Murray et al., 1960), Pennsylvania (Ritter, 1958) and Melbourne, Australia (Forbes, 1968), mumps meningitis occurred more frequently during winter and spring. In Toronto, peaks of incidence of mumps meningitis during 1960, 1963 and 1966 corresponded to substantially increased numbers of cases of mumps which were reported in the City (Toronto, 1959–66).

In Toronto between May 1959 and April 1967, mumps virus was isolated from CSF of 89 of 254 (35 per cent) of patients from a total of 287 who had clinical and/or laboratory evidence of mumps infection in association with the aseptic meningitis syndrome (Table 1.5) (McLean et al., 1960, 1963,

TABLE 1.5

Isolations of mumps virus from CSF of children with mumps meningitis, Toronto, 1959–67

Month	1959	1960	1961	1962	1963	1964	1965	1966	1967	Totals CSF	Totals cases
Jan.	—	1/4	—	—	5/9	0/7	0/3	0/1	3/7	9/31	35
Feb.	—	2/4	0/1	0/1	2/5	0/1	0/1	1/4	3/5	8/22	24
Mar.	—	1/3	—	—	7/12	0/1	0/3	0/2	4/10	12/31	36
Apr.	—	6/10	—	0/1	4/5	0/2	0/1	0/1	1/5	11/25	30
May	0/1	3/7	0/3	—	0/6	0/1	1/1	1/4	—	5/23	31
June	0/2	3/5	—	0/1	0/3	0/2	2/2	2/4	—	7/19	21
July	1/3	3/5	—	—	2/3	0/1	—	1/6	—	7/18	20
Aug.	0/2	2/2	—	0/2	2/4	0/1	—	1/5	—	5/16	17
Sept.	2/3	1/1	—	0/1	0/1	—	—	1/2	—	4/8	9
Oct.	0/1	—	—	0/2	2/6	—	—	3/6	—	5/15	15
Nov.	1/5	0/2	—	1/3	0/3	—	1/4	2/5	—	5/22	25
Dec.	3/4	1/2	—	1/5	1/2	—	0/1	5/10	—	11/24	24
Total CSF	7/21	23/45	0/4	2/16	25/59	0/16	4/16	17/50	11/27	89/254	—
Total cases	25	58	5	17	67	18	16	52	29	—	287

1967). In 1966, mumps virus was isolated from CSF more frequently when the sample was collected within an average of less than 24 hours after onset of meningitis, but virus was not isolated from CSF when the mean time of collection exceeded one day (McLean et al., 1967). In one case where meningeal signs persisted for eight days, mumps virus was recovered from

CSF 11 days after onset of meningitis, but in the majority of cases, fever and meningeal signs persisted for four days or less. Conversion of HI antibody status from negative to positive, or demonstration of a fourfold increment of anti-haemagglutinin, was regularly detected within one to two days after defervescence. Interferon was found in CSF collected from two of eight patients one to five days after onset of meningitis and virus was recovered from CSF of these two patients also.

An extremely rapid technique for the presumptive diagnosis of meningitis due to mumps virus was illustrated in a Toronto child by observation of paramyxovirus virions in CSF following treatment with phosphotungstic acid and examination with an EM200 (Philips) electron microscope (Doane et al., 1967). The virions were confirmed as mumps in a microhaemagglutination inhibition test employing the patient's CSF as antigen. This procedure, which occupied approximately 15 minutes, contrasted sharply with the standard technique, which involves inoculation of CSF into monolayer cultures of monkey kidney cells, when syncytia characteristic of mumps virus infection are observed after incubation at 35 to 37°C for three to seven days.

Mumps Vaccines

Licensing of the Jeryl Lynn (B level) strain (Buynak and Hilleman, 1966) of live mumps virus vaccine throughout North America during 1968 and 1969 has now provided the physician and health officer with a convenient, effective and long-lasting means of prophylaxis against mumps. This strain was isolated from the throat of a patient who developed clinical mumps on 30th March 1963 by amniotic inoculation of leukosis-free chick embryos. After 17 passages through chick embryo and chick embryo cell culture, a trial group of seronegative children in an institution who received the vaccine subcutaneously produced NT and HI antibodies 28 days later but none developed parotitis nor excreted mumps virus from the throat (Stokes et al., 1967). The neutralization test was a more sensitive indicator of the presence of mumps antibody than the haemagglutination inhibition test. Among 225 initially seronegative children in classrooms who received Jeryl Lynn vaccine, 99·6 per cent showed antibody conversions, and 97 per cent of 177 children in families developed mumps antibody after vaccination (Weibel et al., 1967). The lowest rate of antibody conversion (83 per cent) occurred in children aged less than two years. However, the geometric mean NT titres of nine and HI titre of five in vaccinees were lower than the mean NT titre of 60 and HI titre of nine in children who contracted natural mumps. Absence of antibody conversions among classroom or family contacts of vaccinees demonstrated lack of communicability of the Jeryl Lynn strain. Significant febrile responses were extremely uncommon among vaccinees, who exhibited symptoms less frequently than non-vaccinated controls.

Although mumps was endemic at the time of vaccination, an epidemic of natural mumps occurred four months later. Throughout the observation period, two of 86 (2 per cent) vaccinees in classrooms developed clinical mumps in contrast to 39 of 76 (51 per cent) unvaccinated controls. Within families where mumps was prevalent, clinical cases occurred in none of 14 vaccinees six days to six months after vaccination, but 22 of 24 (92 per cent) unvaccinated controls developed mumps. Within families four to eight months after vaccination, one of 13 (8 per cent) of vaccinees and 19 of 29 (66 per cent) developed clinical mumps. Thus for all the groups of children the attack rate of 62 per cent for unvaccinated subjects was reduced to 3 per cent for vaccinees, giving a protective efficacy of 95 per cent (Hilleman et al., 1967). Protection against natural mumps infection has persisted at least 20 months through two epidemic waves of infection, providing a protective efficacy of 95·1 per cent (Hilleman et al., 1968). No decline of mumps NT antibody titres were observed two years after vaccination. Since no antibody response was observed in infants who possessed maternal antibody, it was recommended that vaccination of all infants be delayed until 13 to 16 months of age. Although most subjects received 5000 tissue culture infective doses (TCD_{50}) of vaccine, antibody responses occurred regularly following injection of as small a quantity of virus as 317 TCD_{50}. Simultaneous administration of 0·05 ml/kg mumps human immune gamma-globulin, with an antibody titre of 500 per 0·1 ml at another injection site, did not interfere with the production of antibody after injection of mumps vaccine. Satisfactory antibody responses to both viruses were observed after injection of a combined live mumps and measles vaccine. Mumps antibody responses have been obtained following vaccine administration by a jet injector (Hilleman et al., 1968).

Formalin-inactivated mumps vaccine has been used for many years for mumps prophylaxis. Among Finnish military personnel between 1954 and 1959 when no vaccine was offered, the attack rate of mumps was 3·1 per cent but this declined to 0·19 per cent when two doses of inactivated vaccine were administered regularly to each person between 1961 and 1966 (Penttinen et al., 1968). The incidence of mumps in the civilian population remained the same as that in military personnel before vaccination was instituted. Although orchitis developed in 35 of 411 men during the vaccination period, the incidence of orchitis, which was 25 per 10,000 in unvaccinated personnel, declined to 12 per 10,000 after one dose of vaccine, and to one per 10,000 after two doses of vaccine.

A common problem in family practice concerns prophylaxis against clinical mumps in a parent when a child in the household develops mumps. In Baltimore during 1960, the attack rate among parents who received inactivated mumps vaccine shortly after a child in the household contracted clinical mumps was reduced to three of 25 (12 per cent) from 18 of 52

(34 per cent) of unvaccinated parents without a previous history of mumps (Meyer, 1962). Subsequent experience in Baltimore during 1963 and 1964, however, showed that 8·0 per cent of 173 parents who received vaccine following household exposure developed clinical mumps, in contrast to an attack rate of 4·5 per cent among 153 unvaccinated parents (Meyer *et al.*, 1966). Among susceptible adults with mumps NT titres less than 2, 12 per cent of fathers and 20 per cent of mothers developed clinical mumps following household exposure. However among all adults without previous histories of mumps, 4 per cent of fathers and 11 per cent of mothers developed mumps after houshold contact with mumps. In Toronto during 1963, administration of one dose of inactivated mumps vaccine to 82 parents without previous histories of mumps, 38 (46 per cent) of whom had mumps HI antibodies before vaccination, was followed by clinical mumps in four parents, three of whom were devoid of pre-vaccination antibody (McLean, 1967). Antibody conversions from negative to positive HI status were observed in 20 of 25 (80 per cent) of vaccinees three to five weeks later, and 18 of 24 (75 per cent) of parents who had HI antibody initially showed fourfold or greater increments of titre. It was demonstrated elsewhere that only 10 per cent of seronegative children developed NT antibodies one week after injection with inactivated mumps vaccine (Friedman *et al.*, 1963). In view of this conflicting evidence regarding the prophylactic efficacy of inactivated mumps vaccine for family contacts after exposure to mumps, it seems justifiable to recommend that live mumps vaccine, rather than inactivated vaccine, be administered to susceptible parents immediately after their children contract mumps.

REFERENCES

AZIMI, P. H., CRAMBLETT, H. G. & HAYNES, R. E. (1969). Mumps meningoencephalitis in children. *J.A.M.A.*, **297**, 509.

BUYNAK, E. B. & HILLEMAN, M. R. (1966). Live attenuated mumps virus vaccine. I. Vaccine development. *Proc. Soc. exp. Biol. Med.*, **123**, 768.

CARANOSOS, G. J. & FELKER, J. R. (1967). Mumps arthritis. *Arch. int. Med.*, **119**, 394.

DOANE, F. W., ANDERSON, N., CHATIYANONDA, K., BANNATYNE, R. M., MCLEAN, D. M. & RHODES, A. J. (1967). Rapid laboratory diagnosis of paramyxovirus infections by electron microscopy. *Lancet*, **2**, 751.

DONOHUE, W. L., PLAYFAIR, F. D. & WHITAKER, L. (1955). Mumps encephalitis. *J. Pediat.*, **47**, 395.

FORBES, J. A. (1968). In Fairfield Hospital, Melbourne, Australia: Medical Superintendent's Reports 1961 through 1968.

FRIEDMAN, R. M., HOLTZ, A. I., BARON, S., SILBERGELD, S. & BUCKLER, C. E. (1963). Studies on rapid immunization with mumps vaccine. *Amer. J. Hyg.*, **78**, 269.

HARRIS, R. W., TURNBULL, C. D., ISACSON, P., KARZON, D. T. & WINKELSTEIN, W. (1968). Mumps in a North-east metropolitan community. I. Epidemiology of clinical mumps. *Amer. J. Epidem.*, **88**, 224.

HILLEMAN, M. R., BUYNAK, E. B., WEIBEL, R. E. & STOKES, J. (1968). Live attenuated mumps virus vaccine. *New Engl. J. Med.*, **278**, 227.

HILLEMAN, M. R., WEIBEL, R. E., BUYNAK, E. B., STOKES, J. & WHITMAN, J. E. (1967). Live attenuated mumps virus vaccine. IV. Protective efficacy as measured in a field evaluation. *New Engl. J. Med.*, **276**, 252.

LASS, R. & SHEPARD, E. (1961). Mumps arthritis. *Brit. med. J.*, **2**, 1613.

LENETTE, E. H., CAPLAN, G. E. & MAGOFFIN, R. L. (1960). Mumps virus infection simulating paralytic poliomyelitis. A report of 11 cases. *Pediatrics*, **25**, 788.

MCLEAN, D. M. (1967). *Aseptic Meningitis. Recent Advances in Medical Microbiology*, ed. A. P. Waterson. London: Churchill, p. 76.

MCLEAN, D. M., BACH, R. D., LARKE, R. P. B. & MCNAUGHTON, G. A. (1963). Mumps meningoencephalitis, Toronto. *Canad. med. Ass. J.*, **90**, 458.

MCLEAN, D. M., LARKE, R. P. B., COBB, C., GRIFFIS, E. D. & HACKETT, S. M. R. (1967). Mumps and enteroviral meningitis in Toronto, 1966. *Canad. med. Ass. J.*, **96**, 1355.

MCLEAN, D. M., WALKER, S. J. & MCNAUGHTON, G. A. (1960). Mumps meningoencephalitis: a virological and clinical study. *Canad. med. Ass. J.*, **83**, 148.

MEYER, M. B. (1962). An epidemiologic study of mumps: its spread in schools and families. *Amer. J. Hyg.*, **75**, 259.

MEYER, M. B., STIFLER, W. C. & JOSEPH, J. M. (1966). Evaluation of mumps vaccine given after exposure to mumps with special reference to the exposed adult. *Pediatrics*, **37**, 304.

MURRAY, H. G. S., FIELD, C. M. B. & MCLEOD, W. J. (1960). Mumps meningoencephalitis. *Brit. med. J.*, **1**, 1850.

PENTTINEN, K., CANTELL, K., SOMER, P. & POIKOLSINEN, A. (1968). Mumps vaccination in the Finnish defence forces. *Amer. J. Epidem.*, **88**, 234.

PORTER, J. H. & PALLIS, C. (1960). Polyneuritis and central hypertension due to non-parotitic mumps. *Lancet*, **1**, 362.

REED, D., BROWN, G., MERRICK, R., SEVER, J. & FELTZ, E. (1967). A mumps epidemic on St. George Island, Alaska, *J.A.M.A.*, **199**, 113.

RITTER, B. S. (1958). Mumps meningoencephalitis in children. *J. Pediat.*, **52**, 424.

ST GEME, J. W., NOREN, G. R. & ADAMS, P. (1966). Relation between mumps virus and primary endocardial fibroelastosis. *New Engl. J. Med.*, **275**, 339.

SHONE, J. D., ARMAS, S. M., MANNING, J. A. & KEITH, J. D. (1966). Mumps antigen skin test in endocardial fibroelastosis. *Pediatrics*, **37**, 423.

STOKES, J., WEIBEL, R. E., BUYNAK, E. B. & HILLEMAN, M. R. (1967). Live attenuated mumps virus vaccine. II. Early clinical studies. *Pediatrics*, **39**, 363.

TORONTO, MEDICAL OFFICER OF HEALTH. *Monthly Reports, Toronto. January 1959–December 1966.*

VOSBURGH, J. B., DIEHL, A. M., LIU, C., LAUER, R. M. & FABIYI, A. (1965). Relationship of mumps to endocardial fibroelastosis. *Amer. J. Dis. Child.*, **109**, 69.

WEIBEL, R. E., STOKES, J., BUYNAK, E. B., WHITMAN, J. E. & HILLEMAN, M. R. (1967). Live, attenuated mumps virus vaccine. III. Clinical and serologic aspects in a field evaluation. *New Engl. J. Med.*, **276**, 245.

WESSELHOEFT, C. (1951). *Modern Practice in Infectious Fevers. Vol. II.* ed. H. Stanley Banks. London: Butterworth, p. 557.

WITTE, C. L. & SCHANZER, B. (1968). Pancreatitis due to mumps. *J.A.M.A.*, **203**, 1068.

2 Immunity, Autoimmunity and Immunosuppression

M. H. LESSOF AND A. S. RUSSELL

MECHANISMS OF IMMUNITY. IMMUNITY IN EARLY LIFE.
IMMUNE DEFICIENCY STATES. DISORDERS OF IMMUNITY IN
ANIMALS. IMMUNE DISORDERS IN MAN. DISEASES AFFECTING
VARIOUS SYSTEMS. IMMUNOSUPPRESSION

MECHANISMS OF IMMUNITY

WHEN an antigen is introduced into the body an immune response leads
to the synthesis of a specific antibody. This antibody either circulates as free
protein in the blood or is bound to cells of the lymphocyte series. A hapten
can also stimulate antibody formation, but only when linked to a larger,
carrier antigen.

Basically, there are two types of immune reactions, humoral and cell-
mediated. Humoral antibodies are formed when the stimulating antigen is
in a soluble form in which it can be carried to the lymph nodes or
spleen, where it is ingested by macrophages. These macrophages stimulate the
plasma cell precursors to proliferate in the germinal centres of the lymph
nodes and the red pulp of the spleen. In the resulting lymph follicles the
antibody is produced.

If the antigen is in the skin or other peripheral tissues, the response may
be mainly cellular, and less circulating antibody is produced. Small lymphocytes migrate into the skin and are sensitized by the antigen. They then
reach the paracortical areas of local lymph nodes and the white pulp of the
spleen and grow to form large cells which proliferate. Some of the new
generations of lymphocytes are immunologically active and pass into the
peripheral blood and into other tissues where antigen may be present. These
sensitized lymphocytes, together with the macrophages, can now react with
antigen wherever it may be present, initiating inflammatory and other
destructive processes.

The initial response to an antigen is relatively slow and weak. Once the subject has been sensitized, further stimulation produces a secondary response which is much more brisk and sustained.

Immunoglobulins

The humoral antibodies constitute the various classes of immunoglobulin. Each antibody molecule contains two heavy (or H) chains, which are specific for each class, and two short, light (or L) chains. In the case of IgM, five of these molecules are combined together. The different classes of antibody are: IgG, which is present in the highest concentration; IgM, the macroglobulin antibody, which is confined within the blood vessels because of its large molecular weight (900,000); IgA, which is concentrated in mucous secretions, joined to another protein known as the secretor or transport piece; and IgE, the reaginic antibody, which fixes at tissue surfaces and takes part in various allergic and anaphylactic reactions. IgD has also been identified. It has the structural characteristics of an immunoglobulin, but as yet little antibody activity can be ascribed to it.

Complement

An important part of the immune response depends on complement, an enzyme system consisting of nine protein components, the first of which contains three separate fractions. In man, the components of complement together contribute nearly 10 per cent of the serum globulin fraction (Kohler and Müller-Eberhard, 1967). The third component (C′3, also known as β_{ic}) is easily measured, and it alone has a serum concentration of 120–200 mg/100 ml. When complement is fixed, the first component to take part in the reaction consists of three separate enzymes, C′1q, C′1r and C′1s. The remaining components are numbered C′2 to C′9 and take part, one after the other, in a cascade reaction reminiscent of the clotting sequence. When they are activated, many small peptides are formed which are important in the initiation of an inflammatory response. A system of inhibitors is also present, which prevents spontaneous activation of the enzyme system.

Complement fixes locally at the site of certain antigen-antibody reactions involving IgG or IgM. The role of antibody is to direct the action of complement towards a specific target. This adds to the local consequences of the antigen-antibody reaction; for example, it generates anaphylatoxin which increases vascular permeability as well as stimulating local histamine release (Dias de Silva and Lepow, 1967). It also promotes the migration of polymorphonuclear leucocytes by means of chemotactic factors. It opsonizes particles and so promotes their phagocytosis, and it disrupts bacterial or other cell membranes by the process of immune cytolysis (Müller-Eberhard, 1968).

Effects of antibody

The combination of antigen and antibody does not always fix complement, and in its absence the neutralization of bacterial exotoxins or viruses may still occur. *In vitro* these can be seen as agglutination or precipitation reactions. These reactions can in theory be mediated by IgG, IgM, or IgA antibodies.

In general IgM and IgG antibodies fix complement, and when they react with an antigenic site on the surface of red cells, bacteria or viruses, they tend to kill or lyse the cell. IgM antibodies are more efficient in this respect than IgG. IgA appears to be incapable of fixing complement, and is ineffective in this situation.

When there is a high concentration of antibody and antigen, they interact to form immune complexes. For example, when antigen is injected into the tissues of an immunized animal, a reaction occurs in and around the small blood vessels. Where the antibody and antigen meet, immune complexes are deposited and provoke a severe inflammatory *Arthus reaction.* Complement is fixed, vaso-active amines liberated, and chemotactic factors are released. Vasodilatation and a very marked polymorphonuclear infiltration produce the histological picture of a vasculitis (Ward and Cochrane, 1965). The reaction takes two to eight hours to develop, and persists from 12 to 24 hours. This is in contrast to the delayed type of reaction, which is mediated by sensitized cells. This takes 24 to 48 hours to develop and several days to subside.

IgE, the reaginic antibody, does not fix complement and so cannot cause inflammation in the same way as IgG and IgM. It is present in the circulation in minute amounts, and its importance lies in its ability to fix to tissues, where it reacts with antigen and induces the local release of vaso-active amines including histamine, 5-hydroxytryptamine and slow reacting substance (SRS-A). IgE is responsible for anaphylaxis, both systemic and local, as can be demonstrated by the passive transfer of sensitivity by means of serum. In the passive transfer of sensitivity, serum from a sensitized individual is injected into the skin of a second healthy subject. Twenty-four to 48 hours later the antigen responsible for the sensitivity is pricked into the site of the previous injection. In cases in which the transfer has been successful, a typical wheal and flare reaction ensues in 15 to 30 minutes. This is the basis of the Prausnitz-Küstner reaction. In the original case Küstner was allergic to fish.

Cellular immunity

When a previously sensitized subject reacts to an intradermal injection of tuberculin there is a proliferation of sensitized cells, and a local area of inflammation slowly arises. In proliferating, the local cells release substances which attract or recruit other unsensitized cells, which are chiefly of bone marrow origin (Spector and Willoughby, 1968). There is a factor which is chemotactic for mononuclear cells, and a factor which inhibits the migration of macrophages and retains them locally, allowing further tissue damage to occur (Ward *et al.*, 1969). Tissue damage will release further peptides which are chemotactic for polymorphonuclear leucocytes, and vasodilatation, by increasing the blood flow, will magnify both the cellular and the humoral attack. Only a very small proportion of the cells that are present are in fact specifically sensitized to react against the irritant antigen.

Whether it is to foreign proteins, bacteria, or tissue grafts, the type of reaction is the same. Mononuclear cells accumulate around the small blood vessels, and some of these cells transform into macrophages, a prominent feature of the lesion. The macrophages have abundant lysosomes, which contain many hydrolytic enzymes, and play a considerable part in the tissue destruction which occurs. Polymorphonuclear leucocytes are also seen but are a minor component, in contrast to the Arthus reaction, where this cell predominates.

Tolerance, Enhancement and Prevention of the Immune Response

The young foetus cannot mount an immune response. Antigen that is present from this time onwards will be recognized as the foetus matures as part of "self", and will not ordinarily induce an immune response (Burnet and Fenner, 1949). This state of tolerance probably results from direct contact between "self" components and cells of the antibody-producing system. If an antigen is presented before immune maturation occurs this may induce a specific tolerance to the antigen. Even after this period of maturation has begun, the immune mechanism can still be temporarily overwhelmed by a larger dose of antigen. In the fully mature subject, however, tolerance to particulate antigens can only be induced at present by using large doses of immunosuppressive drugs or whole body irradiation.

In animal experiments, tolerance to a selected antigen may be induced in other ways. One is to use a soluble antigen which does not contain any aggregates capable of initiating phagocytosis. Another is to give a minute dose of antigen repeatedly over a short period ("low dose tolerance"). The effectiveness of these methods in preventing an immune reaction is puzzling, but a common factor is probably an unusual presentation of the antigen, possibly by-passing the stage of phagocytosis by macrophages (Brown *et al.*, 1969).

The failure of an effective immune reaction does not always imply that a tolerant state exists. The condition known as immunological enhancement was first noted in animals that had received transplanted tumours (see review by Kaliss, 1958). These tumours had their growth rate *enhanced* by previous attempts at immunization with tumour cells or by a prior infusion of anti-body directed against the same tumour. In these circumstances, circulating antibody combines with the antigenic material of the tumour. The antigenic sites are covered up, and so fail to provoke a lymphocytic reaction. Although the host is not tolerant in the immunological sense, the cellular response which leads to rejection of the grafted tumour does not occur. This may have practical implications. For example, attempts to immunize patients against certain tumours are not free of the risk that the rate of tumour growth may be accelerated.

There are other situations where the combination of antibody with anti-genic sites may help to prevent further immunological stimulation, and so enhance the survival of a graft. It has been suggested (see Lessof, 1969) that the deposition of antibody on the endothelium of a grafted kidney may prolong its survival in the recipient, and the survival of a homograft may actually be enhanced by giving an antiserum directed against it (French and Batchelor, 1969). In the same way the deposition of host protein on the surface of some parasites may protect them from attack by the host.

These are not the only circumstances in which an effective immune reaction fails to occur. Some areas, such as the brain, have no lymphatic drainage and appear to be privileged sites where foreign antigen can be transplanted in experimental situations without sensitizing the immune mechanism. The placental barrier can even more strikingly prevent the immunization of the mother by the partly foreign foetus. Currie and colleagues (1968) have suggested that this depends on sialic acid, which coats the trophoblastic cells and prevents contact with cells of the lymphatic system which might initiate immune sensitization.

These mechanisms represent an interference with the afferent side of the immune response by preventing antigenic stimulation. The efferent side of an immune response may also be impaired, for example by imposing a barrier which the effector cells cannot cross. A homograft will survive if it is enclosed in a millipore chamber with holes too small to allow passage of cells. A parallel to this is the survival of corneal homografts, provided that they are not vascularized (Barker and Billingham, 1967).

The graft-versus-host phenomenon

If live cells from one foetus are given to another while both are immuno-logically immature, a situation occurs in which cells of both strains persist and grow alongside each other: the animal becomes a chimaera. This experimental procedure has its counterpart in nature. Most dizygotic cattle twins are chimaeras, having shared their circulation in foetal life through a synchorial placenta. Subsequently, in adult life, there is complete inter-changeability of skin and tissue grafts from one twin to the other.

When living cells from an adult animal are transplanted to a foetus a different situation arises. The foetus, being immature, will accept cells from a donor of another strain, but these grafted cells are immunologically mature and therefore produce a *graft-versus-host* reaction. This results in *homologous disease*, and the foetal host develops into a runted, wasted animal with a poor coat and an enlarged spleen. These animals develop gastro-intestinal and other infections because they cannot muster a normal immuno-logical response.

REFERENCES

BARKER, C. G. & BILLINGHAM, R. E. (1967). The role of regional lymphatics in the homograft response. *Transplantation*, 5, 962.

BATCHELOR, J. C. (1969). *Lancet*, 2, 1103. Immunological enhancement of rat kidney grafts.

BROWN, J. C., SCHWAB, J. & HOLBOROW, E. J. H. (1969). Personal Communication.

BURNET, F. M. & FENNER, F. (1949). In *The Production of Antibodies*. Melbourne: MacMillan.

CURRIE, G. A., VAN DOORNICK, W. & BAGSHAWE, K. D. (1968). Effect of Neura-minidase on the immunogenicity of early mouse trophoblast. *Nature (Lond.)*, 219, 191.

DIAS DE SILVA, W. & LEPOW, I. H. (1967). Biological properties of anaphylatoxin prepared with purified components of human complement. *J. exp. Med.*, 125, 921.

FRENCH, M. E. & KALISS, N. (1958). Immunological enhancement of tumour grafts in mice. *Rev. Cancer Res.*, 18, 992.

KOHLER, P. F. & MÜLLER-EBERHARD, H. J. (1967). Complement component quantitation: immunoassay of C′3, C′4 and C′5. *Clin. Res.*, 15, 296.

LESSOF, M. H. (1969). Medical aspects of transplantation. In *Lectures in Medicine* C. W. H. Havard; Staples Press, 2nd edn. p. 331.

MÜLLER-EBERHARD, H. J. (1968). The serum complement system. In *Textbook of Immunopathology, vol. 1.* ed. P. A. Miescher and H. J. Müller-Eberhard. New York: Grune and Stratton, p. 33.

SPECTOR, W. G. & WILLOUGHBY, D. A. (1968). The origin of mononuclear cells in chronic inflammation and tuberculin reactions in the rat. *J. Path. Bact.*, 96, 389.

WARD, P. A. & COCHRANE, C. G. (1965). Bound complement and immunologic injury of blood vessels. *J. exp. Med.*, 121, 215.

WARD, P. A., RENOLD, H. G. & DAVID, J. R. (1969). Leukotactic factor produced by sensitized lymphocytes. *Science*, 163, 1079.

IMMUNITY IN EARLY LIFE

The development of cellular immune reactions in the foetus

Above the cloaca of the chicken there is a lymphoid mass known as the bursa of Fabricius (Mueller *et al.*, 1962). It influences the production of circulating antibody by plasma cells and their precursors. In neonatal chicks, removal of the bursa interferes with antibody production by suppressing the development of plasma cells and lymphocytes in the splenic red pulp and in the medullary areas of lymph nodes. These are the *bursal dependant areas*. Cooper *et al.* (1966) have produced evidence that lymphoid tissue in the gastro-intestinal tract of the rabbit may have the same function as the chick bursa, and they suggest that a similar situation may exist in other mammals. This type of lymphoid tissue appears to have little or no effect on the cellular immune response, which seems to be largely under the influence of the thymus.

It is generally agreed that in the embryological development of mammals lymphocytes are first seen in the thymus. These cells may originate as mesenchymal cells in the bone marrow or elsewhere, and bone marrow cells have been shown to migrate into the thymus in a number of experimental situations (Ford and Micklem, 1963). It has been suggested that when they reach the thymus these migrating cells differentiate into lymphocytes.

The thymus contains a higher proportion of primitive actively dividing lymphocytes than any other lymphoid tissue. Its cortex contains closely packed masses of lymphocytes surrounded by epithelial and reticular cells. It contains neither germinal centres nor plasma cells, however, and its function remained unclear until Miller (1961) showed the importance of the thymus in the normal development of the cellular immune responses that are mediated by lymphocytes. Miller showed that in mice, after thymectomy in neonatal life, there is a circulating lymphopenia and a poor development of lymphoid tissue. At six weeks of age these mice cannot produce the reactions of delayed hypersensitivity. They fail to reject skin grafts and even fail to reject second grafts from the same donor.

It is now recognized that the paracortical areas of lymph nodes and the splenic white pulp are *thymus-dependent areas*, where the cell-mediated types of immune response evolve. These areas are specifically depleted by early thymectomy but not by thymectomy in adult animals (unless it is accompanied by sub-lethal irradiation—Miller, 1965).

The formation of serum proteins in the foetus

It is well known that all types of immunological function are poorly developed in newborn mice and rats and that cellular immune reactions are severely impaired by neonatal thymectomy. In the dog, on the other hand, some degree of immunological competence is achieved about two-thirds of the way through foetal life, both for cellular and humoral reactions.

In the human foetus the traditional view is that immunological function develops late, that the normal foetus does not synthesize immunoglobin, and that the neonate is almost completely dependent on maternal antibodies in coping with infection. IgG, which is known to cross the placenta, is present in roughly equivalent concentration in both maternal and cord blood, while IgA and the large molecules of IgM do not seem to cross the placenta, and are usually difficult to detect in cord blood. The well-known decline in globulin levels in the two or three months after birth suggests not only that this globulin is derived from the mother, but also that the infant fails to replace it as it is slowly broken down. However, the blood volume is expanding rapidly at this age, and Trevorrow (1959) showed that the total circulating globulin does not often fall. This implies that, as the maternal protein is broken down, even the newborn infant must synthesize some globulin.

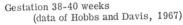

7 MOTHERS WITH HYPOGAMMAGLOBULINAEMIA

Gestation 38-40 weeks
(data of Hobbs and Davis, 1967)

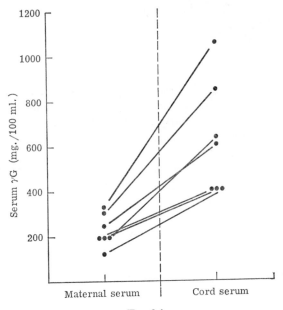

Fig. 2.1

There is also evidence that mothers with hypogammaglobulinaemia may have IgG levels in their plasma considerably below the cord blood level (Fig. 2.1). Hobbs and Davis (1967) have suggested that this may indicate active transport from mother to baby, but it seems more probable that the foetus has synthesized IgG in these cases. However, the plasma immunoglobin levels vary considerably in these infants. If the foetus does respond to intra-uterine infection these variations may depend both on the antigenic stimulation received and on the briskness of the individual foetal response.

The immunological competence of the foetus depends on its ability to recognize antigen and to produce the appropriate cellular response, as well as on the synthesis of immunoglobins and of complement. Adinolfi and his colleagues (1968) have shown that by 14 weeks, human foetal liver can synthesize at least two components of complement. Thorbecke showed in 1965 that human spleen cells can synthesize IgG and IgM globulins by about 25 weeks of gestation. In the developing chick, cells which produce IgM are the first to differentiate, IgG is produced next, and IgA after that (Cain et al., 1969). This order may also apply to man, but it does not follow that an immune response can occur at the stage at which these globulins are first made.

As Silverstein (1962) has noted, by six months the human foetus can respond to antigenic stimulation with the production of plasma cells, and this occurs not only in syphilis but also in toxoplasmosis. Circulating anti-bodies are commonly found in these conditions in later foetal life, and the older literature contains several references to the finding of high Wassermann titres in the blood of the newborn when the mother's blood gives a weak or a negative reaction.

An infected foetus does not develop the changes of congenital syphilis before about the sixth month, and Silverstein has suggested that immuno-logical immaturity prevents the early foetus from producing an immune response to the spirochaete. Early infection, in these circumstances, may not cause sufficient embarrassment to cause death or expulsion of the foetus, though it might still interfere with parenchymal cells such as those of the liver. In fact, very young foetuses may have positive stains for the treponema in the complete absence of an inflammatory response. Silverstein postulates that the infected foetus might still develop an inflammatory response at a later stage as its immune reactions mature. There may be an analogy with the congenital rubella syndrome. In this case specific IgM antibody is found in cord blood, although this antibody is unlikely to be derived from the mother because it cannot ordinarily cross the placenta. Paradoxically, the infant may have a relative deficiency of other antibody globulin (Soothill et al., 1966) and of cellular immunological function (Dent et al., 1968).

The level of IgM and IgA in cord blood may, in general, provide a good index of whether intra-uterine infection has occurred (Alford et al., 1967). Raised levels have been found in the newborn with cytomegalic inclusion disease, rubella, congenital toxoplasmosis and the intra-uterine herpes simplex infection; in some of these the viruses may also be found. The implication, therefore, is that the amounts of IgM found in normal cord blood are low, mainly because of the protected environment of foetal life and the lack of a specific stimulus. The low number of plasma cells in the normal foetus, as van Furth points out, may reflect a protected environment rather than immunological incompetence.

The most important practical relevance of these observations is in connec-tion with immunization procedures in neonatal life. Even premature infants appear to produce antibodies to typhoid-paratyphoid antigens, and

Koprowski (1965) found that premature babies respond to live polio vaccine. Attemps to start immunization procedures on the first day of life, however, have been claimed to be inconstant in their effects, and also to be capable of inducing tolerance in the occasional child. Moreover, the presence of anti-bodies of maternal origin may diminish the neonatal response. Immunization in neonatal life also has the disadvantage that contraindications such as the presence of an immune deficiency state or an allergic disorder may not be recognized at this age. For all these reasons immunization should not normally be carried out in neonatal life.

REFERENCES

ADINOLFI, M., GARDNER, B. & WOOD, C. B. S. (1968). Ontogenesis of two components of human complement: β_{IE} and β_{IC-IA} globulins. *Nature*, **219**, 189.

ALFORD, C. A., SCHAEFER, J., BLANKENSHIP, W. J., STRAUMFJORD, J. V. & CASSADY, G. (1967). A correlative immunologic and clinical diagnosis of infection in newborn infants. *New Engl. J. Med.*, **277**, 437.

CAIN, W. A., COOPER, M. D., VAN ALKEN, P. J. & GOOD, R. A. (1969). Development and function of the immunoglobulin producing system. *J. Immunol.*, **102**, 671.

COOPER, M. D., PERCY, D. Y., McKNEALLY, M. F., FABRIELSON, A. E., SUTHERLAND, D. E. R. & GOOD, R. A. (1966). A mammalian equivalent of the avian bursa of Fabricius. *Lancet*, **1**, 1388.

DENT, P. B., OLSON, G. B., GOOD, R. A., RAWLS, W. E., SOUTH, M. A. & MELNICK, J. L. (1968). Rubella-virus/leucocyte interaction and its role in the congenital rubella syndrome. *Lancet*, **1**, 291.

FORD, C. E. & MICKLEM, H. S. (1963). The thymus and lymph nodes in radiation chimaeras. *Lancet*, **1**, 359.

HOBBS, J. R. & DAVIS, J. (1967). Serum, γG-globulin levels and gestational age in premature babies. *Lancet*, **1**, 757.

KOPROWSKI, H. (1965). Immunization of infants with living attenuated poliomyelitis virus; laboratory investigations of alimentary infection and antibody response in infants under 6 months of age with congenitally acquired antibodies. *J. Amer. med. Ass.*, **162**, 1281.

MILLER, J. F. A. P. (1961). Immunological function of the thymus. *Lancet*, **2**, 748.

MILLER, J. F. A. P. (1965). The thymus and transplantation immunity. *Brit. med. Bull.*, **21**, 111.

MUELLER, A. P., WOLFE, H. R. & MEYER, R. K. (1962). Further studies on the role of the bursa of Fabricius in antibody production. *J. Immunol.*, **88**, 354.

SILVERSTEIN, A. M. (1962). Congenital syphilis and the timing of immunogenesis in the human foetus. *Nature*, **194**, 196.

SOOTHILL, J. F., HAYES, K. & DUDGEON, J. A. (1966). The immunoglobulins in congenital rubella. *Lancet*, **1**, 1385.

THORBECKE, G. J., HOCHWALD, G. M., VAN FURTH, R., MÜLLER-EBERHARD, H. J. & JACOBSON, E. B. (1965). Problems in determining the sites of synthesis of complement components in "complement". ed. G. E. W. Wolstenholm, J. Knight. London: Churchill, p. 99.

TREVORROW, V. E. (1959). Concentration of gamma-globulin in the serum of infants during the first 3 months of life. *Pediatrics*, **24**, 746.

IMMUNE DEFICIENCY STATES

Investigations of immunological deficiency states in man originated with Bruton's report (1952) on agammaglobulinaemia, and have led to recognition of the many different forms of immune deficiency syndromes. A defective resistance to bacterial invasion may be suggested by recurrent infections of the skin, ear, respiratory tract, intestine or urinary tract, or of more than one of these systems on different occasions. Some of these infections are caused by organisms of low virulence, and cases which occur in infancy often go unrecognized.

A number of infants with progressive vaccinia, very florid chicken pox, *pneumocystis carinii* pneumonia, or widespread candidiasis and other skin infections have an underlying immunological deficiency. So have a significant proportion of patients who have persistent diarrhoea in infancy, and many of the infant deaths analysed by Berry and Thompson (1968) have been associated not only with candidiasis and other infections, but also with maldevelopment of the lymphatic system. The infecting organism is often relatively non-virulent, or may be entirely saprophytic in ordinary circumstances. It is only in association with immunological deficiency that such organisms develop invasive properties and give rise to what are now known as opportunistic infections. A similar situation may occur in patients on immunosuppressive drugs.

The immune deficiency syndromes are, as far as possible, best grouped according to whether the defect is chiefly of the humoral antibody response (the bursal mechanisms) or in the cellular response (dependent on the thymus). Many naturally occurring diseases, however, are a mixture of both.

Antibody deficiency syndromes

Bruton's original report concerned a sex-linked recessive condition of male infants characterized by repeated pyogenic infections and absent gammaglobulin on serum electrophoresis. Bacterial infections tend to occur a few months after birth, when the level of maternal antibodies has fallen. These patients have deficient antibody responses but a normal ability to produce the skin reactions of delayed hypersensitivity, and often a normal response to viral infection. There are no plasma cells or germinal centres in lymph nodes, and this is the prototype of the antibody deficient states. In keeping with this, tonsillar tissue is absent and X-rays of the nasopharynx are sometimes diagnostic. It has recently been demonstrated that IgE is lacking in these conditions, as well as IgG, IgM, and IgA. However, it is recognized that total absence of immunoglobins is rare, and in most cases hypogammaglobulinaemia is a more accurate term. The total IgG level is nearly always less than 200 mg/100 ml (Medical Research Council criteria).

The inherited forms are relatively rare, and many causes of hypogamma-globulinaemia are now recognized (Hobbs, 1966). These are:

1. Primary: (a) Physiological, in premature infants
                 (b) Inherited (i) sex-linked
                                   (ii) autosomal recessive, or
                                   (iii) more complicated modes of inheritance
                 (c) Normal levels of immunoglobulins that function abnormally (dysimmunoglobulinaemia)
2. Secondary: (a) Protein deficiency states.
                 (b) Reticuloendothelial diseases—myelomatosis, lymphatic leukaemia, thymoma, marrow aplasia
                 (c) Drug-induced; e.g. cytotoxic drugs.

As in the chick, cells which produce IgA probably differentiate quite late in the human foetus, and an isolated deficiency of IgA is not very uncommon (Bachmann, 1965). In these subjects, IgA levels are low both in mucous secretions and in blood, and while a few are asymptomatic, there is a high incidence of sinusitis, broncho-pulmonary infections and steatorrhoea (South et al., 1968). Interestingly, transfusion reactions have been reported in these patients due to the development of precipitating antibodies which react with the IgA present in the donor plasma (Schmidt et al., 1969). Isolated deficiencies of IgM have also been reported, for example in patients with meningococcal septicaemia (Hobbs, 1967). Low levels of IgA tend to be associated with other deficiencies. The same subject may be deficient in IgM (Giedion and Scheidegger, 1957) and often there also appears to be some functional abnormality of the IgG, since antibody responses are deficient and infection frequent. A combined deficiency of IgA and IgG may also be associated with what seems to be a functional abnormality of IgM (Rosen et al., 1963). The relatives of many patients are themselves subject to immuno-globulin abnormalities, and some have high globulin levels, while others have abnormal antibodies such as rheumatoid factor (Fudenberg et al., 1961). Familial immunoglobulin abnormalities are also found in patients with "primary acquired" hypogammaglobulinaemia (Wollheim et al., 1964) so that there may be no clear-cut genetic distinction between these and the more obviously congenital cases.

It should be added that patients who have normal globulin levels may nevertheless have abnormalities of antibody production. Tests for the production of specific antibodies after immunization with selected antigens are particularly important for evaluating such cases.

Paradoxically, immune deficiency states are associated with striking allergic reactions. There is a high incidence of arthritis resembling rheumatoid arthritis clinically, but without circulating rheumatoid factor. Haemolytic anaemias may be associated with a circulating antibody which coats the red cells and give rise to a positive Coombs test (Fudenberg and Solomon, 1961). Atopic eczema is frequent. So too are lymphomas, and thymoma is not rare. Amyloid disease may also occur. It is not known whether these features are related to the increased susceptibility to infection.

The lymphopaenic immune deficiency states

These have been classified by Seligman *et al.* (1968) on the basis of their inherited features, which almost always include some depression of humoral antibody production.

1. Alymphocytic agammaglobulinaemia (the Swiss type). This disease is inherited as an autosomal recessive. It is characterized by an almost complete lack of lymphocytes and plasma cells, and death from infection is inevitable. A less severe condition (the Boston type) is inherited as an autosomal or sex-linked recessive, and is associated with a less complete depression of peripheral lymphoid development.

2. Inherited lymphopaenia, as described by Nezelof, is an autosomal recessive condition in which there is an almost pure dysfunction of cellular immunity alone. The immunoglobins are normal.

3. Thymic aplasia—Di George's syndrome. This is an abnormality of development of the third and fourth pharyngeal pouches, and is associated with absent parathyroid glands and with anomalies of the aortic arch. Here, too, the immunoglobin levels are normal, and the deficiencies in humoral response which are present are probably the result of multiple infections which, in turn, are due to a failure of lymphocyte function and of the cellular immune response. There is no evidence of a genetic mechanism in this condition.

4. Reticular dysgenesis. In this condition there is an absence of all types of immune response and, in addition, an absence of polymorphonuclear leucocytes (Gitlin and Craig, 1963). It is usually fatal within days.

Patients with severe disorders of cellular immunity are especially prone to fungal, viral and parasitic infections, and it is rare for them to survive more than a year or so. There are also diseases which feature a combined deficiency of cellular and humoral responses together with other genetically transmitted anomalies, and these are usually considered separately.

Wiskott-Aldrich syndrome

This is a sex-linked recessive condition characterized by thrombocytopaenia and purpura (due to the synthesis of abnormal platelets), eczema, recurrent infections, and abnormalities of the immunoglobins which sometimes include raised IgA and diminished IgM levels. Responses to virus infections including vaccinations are normal in early life but become abnormal later (Cooper *et al.*, 1968). There is also lymphocyte depletion in the circulation and a cellular depletion of the paracortical areas of lymph nodes, which tends to increase with age and is associated with deficiencies of the cellular immune response. The humoral antibody response is normal, except to certain polysaccharide-containing antigens (for example, blood group antigens). This suggests a defect of recognition or of the afferent side of the immune response. It is possible that damage to the lymphoid system accounts for the increasing immunological defect with time. There is also a marked increase of lympho-reticular neoplasms.

Ataxia telangiectasia (Peterson et al., 1966)

This is an autosomal recessive condition, which features progressive cerebellar ataxia, widespread telangiectasia and a variety of immunological abnormalities. There appears to be a mesenchymal defect which causes a malformation of blood vessels and leads to ischaemic defects of the brain, thymus and other organs. IgA is often deficient and so, in some cases, are the cellular immune reactions. The abnormally low IgA is associated with recurrent infections of the sinuses and lungs, and here too there is a high incidence of lympho-reticular cancer.

Many of these defects have a congenital background, but other factors may contribute that are not genetic in nature. For example, children with congenital rubella tend to have a diminished IgG level or a raised IgM level during the period in which the virus is being excreted, and in some a persistent hypogammaglobulinaemia has been noted by Soothill and his colleagues. Moreover, there is also an abnormality in the circulating lymphocytes, and they can be shown in vitro to have a markedly diminished response to non-specific lymphocyte stimulants such as phytohaemagglutinin. Cultures of lymphocytes with phytohaemagglutinin show very little blast cell transformation in these patients, in contrast to the high rate of transformation which is obtained with lymphocytes from healthy subjects.

Although the inborn errors of immunity are the easiest to analyse, disorders of the immune response are much more commonly acquired in adult life. Various causes of hypogammaglobulinaemia have been mentioned above, and defects of cellular immunity may also occur as the result of other diseases such as sarcoidosis, lepromatous leprosy, or Hodgkin's disease (Aisenberg, 1964). Such defects may also follow treatment with corticosteroids or with cytotoxic drugs. Skin tests which depend on cellular immunity, such as the Mantoux reaction, may become negative (as they may after a virus infection such as measles—see Starr and Berkovitch, 1964). In addition to an impairment of skin hypersensitivity reactions, there is an abnormal depression of the lymphocyte's reactions in vitro. In sarcoidosis there may be evidence of an impaired reaction to tuberculin (PPD), candida and mumps, both on skin testing and as judged by lymphocyte transformation tests in vitro, yet there is a positive reaction to a suspension of Kveim antigen (Hirschorn et al., 1964). While an increased incidence of virus infections has occasionally been reported in these conditions, the immunological defects are very much milder than those found in the congenital disorders, and may not threaten survival.

In almost all the above conditions the defect is most apparent on the effector side of the immune response, and is secondary to a failure of differentiation of the cells mediating cellular and humoral immune responses. A rational form of treatment is therefore replacement therapy by means of lymphatic tissue transplants. This is still at the experimental stage but has been tried on many occasions, until recently with a total lack of success. One of the dangers of this form of therapy is that of graft-versus-host disease, which has been diagnosed in a child with alymphocytic agammaglobulinaemia after receipt of a blood transfusion from the mother (Hathaway, 1967) Although the child itself was known to be incapable of producing immune reactions, the surviving lymphocytes in the transfused blood appeared to react against the recipient of the transfusion. The same effect has been noted in leukaemic patients who have received marrow infusions from a donor after their own marrow and immune mechanisms have been heavily irradiated and destroyed. In view of these experiences, it is now accepted that either foetal tissue or histocompatible material should be used. There have been two reports of the treatment of Di George's syndrome with an implant of foetal thymus tissue which resulted in a remarkably rapid return of circulating host lymphocytes and of delayed hypersensitivity responses, although a lymph node biopsy showed no changes (August et al., 1968; Cleveland et al., 1968). There has also been a dramatic improvement in two boys with the Swiss type of disease who received bone marrow cells from their histocompatible sisters, and who also received foetal thymus (Gatti et al., 1968; de Koning et al., 1969). Where bone marrow cells are given, graft-versus-host reactions will remain a problem, however incompetent the recipient's own reactions may be. Paradoxically, immunosuppressive drugs may be needed as part of the patient's therapy to prevent an immune reaction by the graft against the host.

At the moment, less dramatic forms of therapy are the rule. It is often said that the oldest patients with the Bruton type of hypogammaglobulinaemia are the same age as penicillin. Antibiotic treatment is life-saving, and without it these children do not survive infections with some of the pyogenic organisms. However, even massive antibiotic therapy is of little help in patients who have combined deficiencies of humoral and cellular immunity. These infants are susceptible, not only to bacteria, but also to fungal, viral and protozoal infections. These infections are usually fatal within months.

Replacement therapy with gammaglobulin offers some protection to the hypogammaglobulinaemic patients. Intramuscular injections of 0·05 g/kg are usually given every three to four weeks, but intravenous plasma obviates the pain of intramuscular injections, and also replaces IgA and IgM as well as IgG (Stickner *et al.*, 1966). The serious danger of infectious hepatitis can be avoided only if a certified panel of donors is used, but it seems possible that the use of tests for detecting the Australia antigen of serum hepatitis will allow this method to become more widespread.

Resistance to infection does not depend only on circulating antibodies and lymphocytes. It is also impaired, for example, in defects of the poly-morphonuclear leucocytes. The Chediak-Higashi syndrome (Barkve, 1967) is probably an inherited enzyme defect. In this disease there is a major lyso-somal abnormality, and giant lysosomes can be seen as red or purple granules in the lymphocytes and especially in the polymorphonuclear leucocytes of the blood. The patient is usually an albino and develops an obvious lympha-denopathy, often associated with photophobia and jaundice as well as with multiple infections. The lymphadenopathy frequently progresses to a malig-nancy of the lympho-reticular tissues (Dent *et al.*, 1966).

Chronic granulomatous disease of childhood is a related condition in which the polymorphonuclear leucocytes can ingest bacteria normally but, because of a defect in oxidase activity, cannot destroy them once they have been ingested, so that they may proliferate inside the phagocytic cell. The child presents with granulomata of the skin or of lung, bone or lymph nodes, sometimes with fistula formation and discharging sinuses.

A further type of deficiency state which may involve one aspect of the effector limb of the cellular response has recently been described by Chilgren *et al.* (1969). Patients with chronic mucocutaneous candidiasis were shown to have negative skin tests to candida and other antigens, and yet positive evi-dence of sensitivity to candida could be obtained *in vitro* in lymphocyte transformation tests. It was postulated that the defect lay in one of the factors responsible for the recruitment of unsensitized inflammatory cells to the site of the lesion.

Congenital deficiencies involving several components of the complement system have been described, but it is notable that they do not lead to increased infections. Deficiencies of C'1 (Kohler and Müller-Eberhard, 1969), C'2, C'3 and of an inhibitor of C'1 (Donaldson and Evans, 1963) have all been reported. The latter is of interest since in this condition an excess of the activated form of C'1 is associated with hereditary angioneurotic oedema, Since the active form of C'1 is an esterase, treatment has been proposed with synthetic esterase inhibitors such as ε-aminocaproic acid (Lundh *et al.*, 1968).

REFERENCES

AISENBERG, A. C. (1964). Hodgkin's disease—prognosis, treatment and etiologic and immunologic considerations. *New Engl. J. Med.*, **270**, 508 and 565.

AUGUST, C. S., ROSEN, F. S., FILLER, R. M., JANEWAY, C. A., MARKOWSKI, B. & KAY, H. E. M. (1968). Implantation of a foetal thymus restoring immunological competence in a patient with thymic aplasia (Di George's Syndrome.) *Lancet*, 2, 1210.

BACHMANN, R. (1965). Studies on the serum gamma-A globulin level III. The frequency of agamma-A globulinaemia. *Scand. J. clin. Lab. Invest.*, 17, 316.

BARKVE, H. (1967). Chediak-Higashi-Steinbrinck syndrome. *Acta paediat. Scand.*, 56, 105.

BERRY, C. L. & THOMPSON, E. N. (1968). Clinico-pathological study of thymic dysplasia. *Arch. Dis. Childh.*, 43, 579.

BRUTON, O. C. (1952). Agammaglobulinaemia. *Pediatrics*, 9, 722.

CHILGREN, R. A., MEVWISSEN, H. J., CLUIE, P. G., GOOD, R. A. & HONG, R. (1969). The cellular immune defect in chronic mucocutaneous candidosis. *Lancet*, 1, 1286.

CLEVELAND, W. W., FOGEL, B. J., BROWN, W. T. & KAY, H. E. M. (1968). Foetal thymic transplant in a case of Di George's Syndrome. *Lancet*, 2, 1211.

COOPER, M. D., CHASE, H. P., VOWMAN, J. T., KRIVIT, W. & GOOD, R. A. (1968). Wiskott Aldrich Syndrome: an immunologic deficiency involving the afferent limb of immunity. *Amer. J. Med.*, 44, 499.

DENT, P. B., FISH, L. A., WHITE, J. G. & GOOD, R. A. (1966). Chediak-Higashi Syndrome. Observations on the nature of the associated malignancy. *Lab. Invest.*, 151, 1634.

DONALDSON, V. H. & EVANS, R. R. (1963). A biochemical abnormality in hereditary angioneurotic oedema. *Amer. J. Med.*, 35, 37.

FUDENBERG, H. & SOLOMON, A. (1961). Acquired agammaglobulinaemia with autoimmune haemolytic disease. *Vox Sang.*, 6, 68.

GATTI, R. A., MEUWISSEN, H. J., ALLEN, H. D., HONG, R. & GOOD, R. A. (1968). Immunological reconstitution of sex-linked lymphopenic immunological deficiency. *Lancet*, 2, 1366.

GIEDION, A. & SCHEIDEGGER, J. J. (1957). Kongenitale Immunparese bei Fehlen Spezifischer beta 2-globuline und quantitativ normalen gammaglobulinen. *Helv. pediat. Acta.*, 12, 12.

GITLIN, D. & CRAIG, J. M. (1963). The thymus and other lymphoid tissues in congenital agammaglobulinaemia. *Pediatrics*, 32, 517.

HATHAWAY, W. E. (1967). Graft versus host reaction following a single blood transfusion. *J. Amer. med. Ass.*, 201, 1015.

HIRSCHORN, K., SCHREIBMAN, R. R., BACH, F. H. & SILTZBACH, L. E. (1964). *In vitro* studies of lymphocytes from patients with sarcoidosis and lymphoproliferative diseases. *Lancet*, 2, 842.

HOBBS, J. R. (1966). Disturbances of the immunoglobulins. In *The Scientific Basis of Medicine Annual Reviews*, p. 106. British Postgraduate Medical Federation. London: Athlone Press.

HOBBS, J. R. (1967). IgM deficiency predisposing to meningococcal septicaemia. *Brit. med. J.*, 2, 583.

KOHLER, P. F. & MÜLLER-EBERHARD, H. J. (1969). Complement immunoglobulin relative deficiency of C'1Q associated with impaired immuno-globulin synthesis. *Science*, 163, 474.

DE KONING, J., DOOREN, L. J., VAN BEKKUM, D. W., VAN ROOD, J. J., DICKE, K. A. & RADL, J. (1969). Transplantation of bone marrow cells and foetal thymus in an infant with lymphopenic immunological deficiency. *Lancet*, 1, 1225.

LUNDH, B., LAURELL, A. B., WETTERQUIST, H., WHITE, T. & GRANERUS, G. (1968). Case of hereditary angioneurotic oedema successfully treated with ε-amino caproic acid. *Clin. exp. Immun.*, 3, 733.

PETERSON, R. D. S., COOPER, D. & GOOD, R. A. (1966). The lymphoid tissue abnormalities associated with ataxia telangiectasia. *Amer. J. Med.*, 41, 342.

ROSEN, F., KEVY, S., MERLER, E., JANEWAY, C. & GITLIN, D. (1963). Recurrent bacterial infections and dysgammaglobulinaemia. Deficiency of 7S gamma-globulins in the presence of elevated 19S gammaglobulins. *Pediatrics*, 28, 182.

SCHMIDT, A. P., TASWELL, H. F. & GLICK, G. J. (1969). Anaphylactic transfusion reactions associated with anti IgA antibody. *New Engl. J. Med.*, 280, 189.

SELIGMAN, M., FUDENBERG, H. H. & GOOD, R. A. (1968). A proposed classification of primary immunologic deficiencies. *Amer. J. Med.*, 45, 817.

SOUTH, M. A., COOPER, M. D., WOLLHEIM, F. A. & GOOD, R. A. (1968). The IgA system. *Amer. J. Med.*, 44, 168.

STARR, S. & BERKOVITCH, S. (1964). Effects of measles, gammaglobulin, modified measles and vaccine measles on the tuberculin test. *New Engl. J. Med.*, 270, 886.

STICKNER, E. R., VAERMAN, J. & FUDENBERG, H. H. (1966). Plasma infusions in immunologic deficiency states; metabolic and therapeutic studies. *Blood*, 28, 918.

WOLLHEIM, F. A., BELFRAGE, S., COSTER, C. & LUNDHOLM, H. (1964). Primary "acquired" hypogammaglobulinaemia. Clinical and genetic aspects of nine cases. *Acta med. scand.*, 176, 1.

DISORDERS OF IMMUNITY IN ANIMALS

Models of human disease

Some of the connective tissue disorders of man have been mimicked in animal experiments. Stasny *et al.* (1963) gave large numbers of foreign lymphocytes to rats in order to induce a graft-versus-host reaction. These animals developed a variety of lesions of the skin, joints, heart, kidney and lymphoid tissue. There was also anaemia and leucopenia associated with a positive Coombs test. During the disease the rats were shown to accept skin grafts from the animals of the original lymphocyte donor strain but to reject grafts of its own skin which were applied at the same time. There was thus evidence of rejection of the host's own skin. A resemblance to human disease was seen in the acute dermatitis, which showed hyperkeratosis, follicular plugging, and a cellular infiltration similar to that seen in systemic lupus in man. Some of the animals with a more chronic dermatitis and hair loss had histological features of scleroderma. Histologically, the other lesions encountered in this condition also showed striking similarities to various human connective tissue disorders.

It is difficult to know how much these findings represent common aetiological factors in experimental and human disease, and some of the similarities may reflect the limited types of response that are available to any given tissue. The same reservations must apply to autoimmune reactions, both in animals and man.

It is now well established that self-damaging immune reactions, (i.e. auto-immune reactions) are produced when animals are injected with homogenates of various organs, especially if these homogenates are emulsified with an adjuvant of mineral oil containing tubercle bacilli; i.e. Freund's complete adjuvant. Histologically the affected tissues show similar changes to those seen in some of the human diseases associated with autoimmune phenomena. For example thyroiditis resembling Hashimoto's disease, with a marked mononuclear cell infiltration of the gland, is readily produced in rabbits by an injection of thyroid tissue from another animal, emulsified in Freund's complete adjuvant. In experimental allergic encephalomyelitis, caused by injecting animals with brain extract, there are areas of perivascular demyelination and inflammation reminiscent of the post-infectious encephalomyelitis that follows virus infections or rabies vaccination in man. Diseases of the adrenals, parathyroids, uveal tract, muscles, testes and kidneys can be similarly induced by injections of the appropriate homogenate, and are accompanied by the release of autoantibodies, that is, of antibodies which react with the subject's own tissues. Glomerulonephritis is the one experimental disease of this kind that can be passed from one animal to another by transferring serum which contains antibody. Experimental allergic encephalomyelitis and thyroiditis, on the other hand, can be transferred to another animal of the same inbred strain by cells alone. In the case of autoallergic disease of the testis it has been claimed that both sensitized cells and humoral antibody are required (Brown et al., 1967).

Many of these immune disorders of experimental animals have been studied in great detail in the past (see review by Batchelor and Lessof, 1964). It is the authors' intention to consider the aetiology of experimental renal disease and of abnormal immune reactions provoked by infection, since some recent work on these disorders appears to provide new analogies with human disease, especially of the kidneys.

Immune complexes and renal disease

It is often assumed that a normal immune response directed towards the elimination of a foreign antigen should be beneficial, but this is not always so. Von Pirquet, in trying to explain serum sickness, was the first to suggest that antigens might combine with antibodies in the circulation to form toxic compounds. A simple model of this process is seen in experimental "one-shot" serum sickness in the rabbit (Dixon et al., 1958). Animals which are injected with large quantities of a foreign protein develop a high incidence of abnormalities of the heart, blood vessels and joints. This is associated with nephritis in virtually all cases. However, there is a latent period of over a week before tissue damage occurs, although the foreign protein antigen is in the circulation all the time. Furthermore, by the time free antibody can be found—after 14 to 16 days—the disease is resolving. If the foreign protein—such as bovine serum albumin—is first labelled with I^{125} it can be shown that the appearance of serum sickness correlates with the rapid disappearance of free antigen and the appearance of labelled antigen-antibody complexes in the blood.

If small daily injections of bovine albumin are given instead of a single massive dose, the type of reaction may be altered and a chronic progressive glomerular nephritis occurs; but this is inconstant, and depends on the individual animal's antibody response and on the nature of the complexes which are formed (Pincus et al., 1968).

The only property of antigen-antibody complexes which is known to affect their localization in blood vessels is their size. Small complexes, which are formed when there is an inadequate antibody response, tend to remain in the circulation. Frank precipitates formed in the presence of antibody excess may however be rapidly taken up by phagocytes. The intermediate-sized soluble complexes are likely to be trapped in vessel walls and induce focal areas of inflammation. Animals that are given repeated small injections of antigen and have only a moderate antibody production tend to produce complexes of this last type. These are the animals that develop the more chronic forms of nephritis. Histological examination of the kidneys in such cases can show either proliferative or membranous lesions or a mixture of the two. Gammaglobulin and components of the complement system (C'3 and C'4) can be demonstrated in the glomeruli by immunofluorescent methods (reviewed by Unanue and Dixon, 1967).

The pathological effect of immune complexes has been shown to be mediated by platelets and possibly other sources of vasoactive amines which release such agents as histamine, serotonin and slow-reacting substance (Kniker and Cochrane, 1968). These in turn alter vascular permeability so that, in the glomeruli and elsewhere, these complexes are deposited in the capillary walls, where they become foci of an inflammatory response.

Activation of the complement system plays an important part in this sequence of events. This, together with polymorphonuclear leucocytes, may cause considerable damage to the glomerular basement membrane, releasing large, identifiable membrane fragments.

Circulating complexes may also arise if the host develops antibodies that combine with its own native proteins. In animals immunized against thyroglobulin there may be circulating antibodies which react with the trace amounts of thyroglobulin normally present in the circulation (Weigle and Nakamura, 1969).

Alternatively, external infective agents may enter the circulation and stimulate antibody formation, as in mice infected with the virus of lymphocytic choriomeningitis (Oldstone and Dixon, 1967). In both cases the appropriate antigen (thyroglobulin or virus) can be demonstrated in the glomeruli by immunofluorescence in addition to gamma globulin and complement.

The same mechanism probably operates in the renal disease of NZB mice (see below). Whether any of these conditions can or should be termed "autoimmune" is something of a semantic question, and does not help in understanding their pathogenesis or treatment.

Nephrotoxic serum nephritis

A second quite distinct mechanism for the development of glomerulonephritis depends on antibodies that react directly with the glomerular basement membrane. This causes complement fixation and membrane damage just as the presence of antigen-antibody complexes does. An experimental example is the nephrotoxic serum nephritis described by Masugi.

First of all, rats are immunized with glomerular basement membrane derived from rabbit kidney. The antiserum produced in the rats is then administered to rabbits and results in the development of a progressive glomerulonephritis. The urine contains protein and casts. Rats used to raise nephrotoxic antisera may themselves develop glomerulonephritis since the antibody can cross-react with the glomerular membranes of many species.

A similar glomerulonephritis may also be produced when a rabbit is given nephrotoxic antiserum which is raised in the duck. In this case, however, there is often a five-day latent period before protein and casts appear in the urine (Masugi, 1934). Although there is an immediate fixation of duck globulin on to the basement membrane of the rabbit's kidney, this reaction does not fix complement. It is only when the host develops antibodies against the duck globulin that marked damage occurs, complement is fixed on the basement membrane, chemotactic factors are released, and white cells also arrive on the scene. Rabbits given injections of duck globulin in neonatal life are tolerant to this protein and do not develop this type of nephrotoxic nephritis. On the other hand, rabbits pre-immunized with duck globulin have a magnified response to nephrotoxic serum (Unanue and Dixon, 1965).

As in the nephritis induced by immune complexes, the kidney in Masugi nephritis (both in recipient and in the animals used to raise the antiserum) contains deposits of gammaglobulin and complement (C'3 and C'4). However, the distribution is different from immune complex disease, and does not show the uneven deposits seen in the glomerulus in that condition. Instead there is a uniform linear pattern along the inner endothelial aspect of the basement membrane (Hammer and Dixon, 1963). The globulin that can be eluted from the glomeruli can be shown to fix to other kidneys both *in vitro* and *in vivo*, reproducing the original nephritis (Unanue and Dixon, 1967). Immunization with lung homogenate produces a very similar glomerulonephritis (Rudovsky and Steblay, 1965), possibly because of similarities between the structure of the capillaries in these two organs. This relationship between nephrotoxic antibody and the lung appears to have its human counterpart in Goodpasture's syndrome (see Immune Disorders of Man) where there are vascular lesions of the lung and a diffuse globulin deposition in the kidney. These globulin deposits have the linear pattern seen in animals after they have been given antibody directed against glomerular basement membrane. In Goodpasture's syndrome the lung lesions are also associated with the deposition of gammaglobulin and C′3 (Koffler *et al.*, 1969). This is one of the few diseases where an auto-antibody has been shown to contribute directly to the disease process. In contrast to the situation in the kidney itself, relatively little antibody is found in the serum, although the circulating antibody level may rise after nephrectomy (Lerner and Dixon, 1966; Lerner *et al.*, 1967).

The role of infection in provoking autoimmune reactions

The immune response to an infecting organism can sometimes be more harmful to the host than the infection itself. Infection with the virus of lymphocytic choriomeningitis is a good example. It is fatal in adult mice if the infecting dose is high, and in the mouse there is major lymphocytic infiltration of most tissues similar to that seen in the meninges in human infection. If given to neonatal animals the virus becomes widely distributed throughout the body, but at this age an immune response may fail to occur, and in 75 per cent there is no evidence of disease—at least in the first few months (Oldstone and Dixon, 1967). The usual pattern of the disease in the adult is prevented by any treatment which abrogates the immune response—such as neonatal thymectomy, amethopterin, irradiation or anti-lymphocytic globulin (Hirsch and Murphy, 1968). It appears that a widespread immune response, occurring in all the tissues, is so damaging to the host that it may be fatal. When the immune response is suppressed, however, the virus may persist in the circulation for many months, and eventually circulating antibody develops. Complexes of virus and antibody then deposit in the kidney, and fatal renal disease develops in an increasing proportion of animals as the months pass.

There are two other well-studied spontaneously occurring diseases of animals closely associated with infection which have even more striking immunological features. Both have a similarity to human systemic lupus and both are associated with a nephritis produced by immune complexes.

Inbred mice of the New Zealand Black (NZB) strain develop a haemolytic anaemia with a positive Coombs test, starting at about the age of five months and increasing until virtually all mice are affected by nine months. About half of them also have circulating antinuclear factors, and they also have a progressive increase of IgM globulin from birth, a high incidence of renal disease, and an increased incidence of neoplasms of the reticulo-endothelial system in old age (reviewed by Howie and Hellyer, 1968).

The first generation offspring of a cross between NZB and a related New Zealand White strain (the F_1 hybrid) also have circulating antinuclear factors

C

and develop glomerulonephritis in all cases by the age of eight to nine months. Males develop the disease somewhat later in life than females. Using immunofluorescence or electron microscopy (with ferritin-labelled antibody), the affected glomeruli can be shown to contain gammaglobulin and complement in the uneven distribution of immune complex nephritis. Further analysis shows that DNA and antibody against DNA are deposited together (Dixon *et al.*, 1967). Also, those mice that have renal disease usually have antibodies against DNA in their serum (Steinberg *et al.*, 1969), and their serum complement level is low (Friou *et al.*, 1968). Thus complexes of DNA and anti-DNA may play a large part in the genesis of the renal disease, as they also appear to do in systemic lupus in man and probably do in the "Aleutian disease" of mink.

The tendency to produce antibodies was thought at first to be a genetic effect. However, electron microscopy demonstrated a virus of the murine leukaemia group in New Zealand mice of all ages, both Black and hybrid. This virus is even present in the foetus, and appears to be transmitted from one generation to the next. The ability to react in the direct Coombs test can be conferred upon young mice by transferring spleen cells from old mice of the same strain (Holmes *et al.*, 1961). The disease has now been transmitted to mice of other strains, either by cells of the NZB mouse spleen (Denman *et al.*, 1969) or, less successfully, by a homogenate of spleen that is free of cells (Mellors and Huang, 1967).

The precise nature and pathogenic effects of this virus are still being studied, and some evidence concerning the Gross leukaemia virus may be relevant. A specific "G"-antigen is found in all mice that harbour the Gross leukaemia virus. This antigen has now been found in the blood and tissues of NZB mice by the age at which they develop a positive Coombs test. By the age of nine months the mouse begins to eliminate this antigen, and the corresponding specific antibody appears in the circulation. There follows a stage of antigen-antibody balance as in serum sickness, and there is progressive renal damage and an increasing mortality. In a very few cases deposits of a virus of the murine leukaemia group have been seen in the mesangium of the glomerulus (Mellors *et al.*, 1969).

Like lymphocytic choriomeningitis, this is a disease in which both an infective agent and its antibody are present, together with an immune complex nephritis. Malaria may provide a comparable example in man (Allison *et al.*, 1969). There is the very intriguing possibility that human diseases such as systemic lupus erythematosus may be an exact counterpart of the renal disease of the New Zealand hybrid (NZB/W) mice, and this adds its own stimulus to further research now proceeding.

Aleutian disease of mink (see Karstad, 1967) is a similar disorder to the disease of New Zealand mice, and is transmissible by an infectious agent that is so contagious that it may infect not only the mink, but also other species such as wild ferrets and possibly man. It is characterized by a glomerulonephritis with uneven deposits of IgG and complement (Henson et al., 1969), and in addition there is fibrinoid degeneration of arteries, thrombocytopenia, haemolytic anaemia and hypergammaglobulinaemia. The hypergammaglobulinaemia progresses to myelomatosis in 10 per cent of cases (Porter et al., 1965). As in the NZB and hybrid mice antinuclear factor is present, and the Coombs test is positive. The infectious agent contains DNA and has been shown to circulate in the plasma together with its antibody (Porter and Larsen, 1967). As in the disease of NZB/W mice, this may provide the basis for immune complex formation and for the renal disease which follows. Recently, Tsai and his colleagues (1969) have demonstrated viral aggregates in the endothelial cells of the glomeruli on electron microscopy.

Therapy of renal disease in experimental animals

The effects of various forms of therapy in the renal disease of NZB/W mice may have implications for the treatment of human disease. Howie and Hellyer (1966) reported that after thymectomy at birth the disease was more rapid in onset. Corticosteroids given in enormous dosage prevented a positive Coombs test from developing or rendered it negative. However, many animals died of haemorrhage into the gastro-intestinal tract or from secondary infection. Administration of cyclophosphamide proved to be very effective in preventing the onset or progression of renal disease in the NZB/W mice (Russell et al., 1966). Azathioprine was much less effective and its use was associated with a high incidence of malignant lymphoma (Casey, 1968). This has raised the possibility that long-term immunosuppressive treatment may also increase the incidence of lymphomas in man, a point which may be of clinical importance when long term immunosuppression is given to transplant recipients (Lancet, 1969).

Antilymphocyte globulin (ALG) has also been used. It is itself a strong antigen and can induce serum sickness and nephritis by provoking immune complex formation. However, NZB/W mice can be made tolerant to ALG of rabbit origin if they receive injections of rabbit protein in neonatal life. These tolerant mice can then receive ALG of rabbit origin without incurring renal damage. This treatment (Denman, Russell and Denman, unpublished) delayed the onset of disease but had no effect after the serological abnormalities were once established.

REFERENCES

ALLISON, A. C., HENDRICKSE, R. G., EDINGTON, G. M., HOUBA, V., DE PETRIS, S. & ADENIYI, A. (1969). Immune complexes in the nephrotic syndrome of African children. Lancet, 1, 1232.

BATCHELOR, J. C. & LESSOF, M. H. (1964). Immunological function and auto-immune disease. In *Recent Advances in Clinical Medicine*. ed. D. N. Baron, N. Compston, A. M. Dawson. London: Churchill.

BROWN, P. C., GLYNN, L. E. & HOLBOROW, E. J. (1967). The dual necessity for delayed hypersensitivity and circulating antibody in the pathogenesis of experimental allergic orchitis in guinea pigs. *Immunology*, **13**, 307.

CASEY, T. (1968). Azathioprine administration and development of malignant lymphomas in NZB mice. *Clin. exp. Immun.*, **3**, 305.

DENMAN, E. J., RUSSELL, A. S. & DENMAN, A. M. (1969). Unpublished results.

DIXON, F., VAZQUEZ, J. J., WEIGLE, W. O. & COCHRANE C. G. (1958). Pathogenesis of serum sickness. *Arch. Path.*, **65**, 18.

DIXON, F. J., EDGINGTON, T. S. & LAMBERT, P. H. (1967). Non-glomerular antigen-antibody complex nephritis. In *Immunopathology V. International Symposium*. P. A. Miescher, P. Graber. Basle: Schwake.

FRIOU, G., NEWCOM, R. & EKHN, M. (1968). Serum complement and anti-DNA antibodies in NZB-NZW mice. *Fed. Proc.*, **27**, 621.

HAMMER, D. J. & DIXON, F. J. (1963). Experimental glomerulonephritis. *J. exp. Med.*, **117**, 1019.

HENSON, J. B., GORHAM, J. R., PADGETT, G. A. & DAVIS, W. C. (1969). Patho-genesis of the glomerular lesions in Aleutian disease in mink. *Arch. Path.*, **87**, 21.

HIRSCH, M. S. & MURPHY, F. A. (1968). Effects of antilymphoid sera on viral infections. *Lancet*, **2**, 37.

HOLMES, M. C., GORRIE, J. & BURNETT, F. M. (1961). Transmission by splenic cells of an autoimmune disease occurring spontaneously in mice. *Lancet*, **2**, 638.

HOWIE, J. B. & HELYER, B. J. (1966). In *Ciba Found. Symp. Thymus: Exptl. Clin. Studies*, p. 360.

HOWIE, J. B. & HELYER, B. J. (1968). The immunology and immunopathology of NZB mice. *Adv. Immun.*, **9**, 215.

KARSTAD, L. (1967). Aleutian disease. A slowly progressive viral infection of mink. In *Current Topics in Microbiology and Immunology*, **40**. Berlin: Springer Verlag.

KNIKER, W. T. & COCHRANE, C. G. (1968). Localisation of circulating immune complexes in experimental animals. *J. exp. Med.*, **127**, 119.

KOFFLER, D., SANDSON, J., CARR, R. & KUNKEL, H. G. (1969). Immunological studies concerning the pulmonary lesions of Goodpasture's syndrome. *Amer. J. Path.*, **54**, 293.

LANCET (1969). Immunosuppression and cancer. **1**, 505 (editorial).

LERNER, R. A. & DIXON, F. J. (1966). Transfer of ovine experimental allergic glomerulonephritis with serum. *J. exp. Med.*, **124**, 431.

LERNER, R. A., DIXON, F. J., YOUNG, F. E. & GLASSOCK, R. J. (1967). Isolation and characterisation of soluble human glomerular basement membrane antigens and the demonstration of pathogenic anti-glomerular antibody in man. *Fed. Proc.*, **26**, 743.

MASUGI, M. (1934). Uber die experimentelle glomerulonephritis durch das speci-fische antinierenserum. Ein beitrag zur pathogenese der diffusen glomerulo-nephritis. *Beitr. path. Anat.*, **92**, 429.

MELLORS, R. C., AOKI, T. & HUEBNER, R. J. (1969). Further implications of murine leukaemia virus in the disorders of NZB mice. *J. exp. Med.*, **129**, 1045.

MELLORS, R. C. & HUANG, C. Y. (1967). Immunopathology of the NZB/BL mice. *J. exp. Med.*, **126**, 53.

OLDSTONE, M. G. A. & DIXON, F. J. (1967). Lymphocytic choriomeningitis: Production of antibody by tolerant infected mice. *Science*, **158**, 1193.

PINCUS, T., HABERKERN, R. & CHRISTIAN, C. (1968). Experimental chronic glomerulitis. *J. exp. Med.*, **127**, 819.

PORTER, D. D., DIXON, F. J. & LARSEN, A. E. (1965). Development of a myeloma-like condition in mink with Aleutian disease. *Blood*, **25**, 736.

PORTER, D. D. & LARSEN, A. E. (1967). Aleutian disease of mink; complexes in serum. *Proc. Soc. exp. Biol. (N.Y.)*, **126**, 680.

RUDOVSKY, V. & STEBLAY, R. W. (1965). Glomerulonephritis induced in sheep by injection of human lung and Freund's adjuvant. *Fedn. Proc.*, **24**, 1963.

RUSSELL, P. J., HICKS, J. D. & BURNET, F. M. (1966). Cyclophosphamide treatment of kidney disease in (NZB/NZW) F_1 mice. *Lancet*, **1**, 1280.

STASNY, P., STEMBRIDGE, V. A. & ZIFF, M. (1963). Homologous disease in the adult rat, a model for autoimmune disease. *J. exp. Med.*, **118**, 635.

STEINBERG, A. D., PINCUS, T. & TALAL, N. (1969). DNA/binding assay for detection of anti DNA antibodies in NZB/NZW mice. *J. Immunol.*, **102**, 788.

TSAI, K. S., GRINYER, I., PAN, K. & KARSTAD, L. (1969). Electron microscopic observation of crystalline arrays of virus-like particles in tissues of mink with Aleutian disease. *Canad. J. Microbiol.*, **15**, 138.

UNANUE, E. R. & DIXON, F. J. (1965). Experimental glomerulonephritis. VI. The autologous phase of nephrotoxic serum nephritis. *J. exp. Med.*, **121**, 715.

UNANUE, E. R. & DIXON, F. J. (1967). Experimental allergic glomerulonephritis induced in the rabbit with heterologous renal antigens. *J. exp. Med.*, **125**, 149.

UNANUE, E. R. & DIXON, F. J. (1967). Experimental glomerulonephritis. Immunological events and pathogenetic mechanisms. In Advances in Immunology, 6. *J. exp. Med.*, **127**, 819.

WEIGLE, W. O. & NAKAMURA, R. M. (1969). Perpetuation of autoimmune thyroiditis and production of secondary renal lesions following periodic injections of aqueous preparations of altered thyroglobulin. *Clin. exp. Immunol.*, **4**, 645.

IMMUNE DISORDERS IN MAN

As in animals, so in man, there are several ways in which the immune response may give rise to hypersensitivity or allergic reactions. The reactions seen in animals often provide an almost identical model for clinical purposes. Coombs has classified these into four types, of which three depend on antibody and the fourth on sensitized cells.

(i) **Reactions depending on sensitizing antibody.** IgE, the reaginic antibody, becomes attached to cells, especially of the skin or mucosa. Reactions with circulating antigen then lead to the release of vasoactive substances which cause an inflammatory reaction in the tissues. This group includes various types of atopic or allergic dermatitis, hay fever, allergic lung diseases including asthma, and anaphylactic reactions.

(ii) **Direct attack on the target cell.** If the antigen is present on the surface of cells and the antibody is free in solution, a reaction between the two leads to the fixing of complement which can cause cell lysis. Transfusion reactions and haemolytic anaemia are of this type.

(iii) **Immune-complex reactions.** When both the antigen and antibody are free in the circulation their interaction leads to the formation of complexes, and complement is fixed in the process. This may cause either serum sickness or the Arthus type of local vascular lesion, depending on the relative concentration, size, and distribution of the antigen-antibody complexes which are formed. It is possible, but not certain, that examples occur in the acute vasculitis occasionally seen in rheumatoid arthritis, and perhaps in polyarteritis nodosa. A more definite example is seen in some of the forms of nephritis characterized by the uneven deposition of gammaglobulin and complement already discussed.

(iv) **Cell-mediated immune reactions.** These involve small lymphocytes which have been specifically sensitized. This is illustrated by delayed hypersensitivity skin reactions of the tuberculin type, by contact dermatitis, various auto-allergic reactions, the rejection of homografts, and the reaction occurring in certain infected tissues, including the lung in pulmonary tuberculosis.

This classification is concerned with the functional anatomy of the allergic response and not with the cause. In any clinical disease, more than one of these mechanisms may be implicated and not all the pathological changes fit obviously into these categories.

Methods of Investigation

A number of laboratory methods are used for the investigation of immune disorders. At their simplest these range from the assessment of the blood levels of serum proteins, complement or immunoglobulins to the analysis of the peripheral blood cells or the histological features of the lesion. There are also a number of specific challenging tests. These assess the response to an antigenic stimulus *in vitro*, in the lymphocyte transformation tests, or *in vivo*, after an appropriate allergen is injected or inhaled. Although some of these are now commonplace their technique deserves a brief description.

The LE cell test

To prepare for this test white blood cells are damaged by mechanical means—for example, by shaking in the presence of glass beads. In the presence of an antinuclear antibody known as LE cell factor the nucleus of a damaged cell swells and becomes susceptible to phagocytosis. The LE cell recognized on a blood smear is a polymorphonuclear leucocyte containing a large, ingested, homogeneous nuclear mass, which stains brightly with haemotoxylin and is derived from dead or damaged leucocytes. This is essentially a laboratory phenomenon. Only on rare occasions has it been reported on direct examination of marrow or body fluids.

Immunofluorescent techniques

When these methods are used to test for circulating autoantibodies the serum under examination is layered on to a tissue section. Autoantibodies in the serum become attached to various parts of the tissue, and remain attached when the section is washed. Antinuclear antibody, for example, becomes fixed to the cell nuclei, and this can be detected in the second stage of the test by adding a specific antiserum which reacts with deposits of antibody globulin. As this antiserum is linked to a fluorescent compound the nuclei to which it becomes attached will be visible under ultra-violet light. By applying serum to appropriate tissues, a whole range of autoantibodies can be detected by this method. Another way in which the method can be used is in the examination of sections of diseased tissue. Where deposited globulin or complement is present in this tissue it can be "stained" by the same type of fluorescent antiserum. Other applications of the method are possible, and it can be adapted to stain for any protein in any tissue.

Coombs test

This is a test of red cells for the presence of immunoglobulin or complement on their surface, and the reagent used is an antiserum which reacts with human serum proteins. This antiserum is mixed with washed red cells, and any cells which are coated with antibody or complement become agglutinated. More specific antisera can be used to analyse whether the protein which coats the red cells is IgG or a component of complement.

In the indirect test, serum which is suspected of containing red cell antibodies is incubated together with red cells. As in the direct test which is described above, a Coombs antiserum is then added to the red cells. This agglutinates any red cells which are coated with globulin.

Tests for rheumatoid factor

These are tests for antibodies which are capable of reacting with gammaglobulin or its denatured products. The gammaglobulin used is of (1) human or (2) rabbit origin.

1. A suspension of latex particles coated with human gamma globulin is obtainable commercially. If mixed with serum which contains rheumatoid factor, the particles will be agglutinated within minutes and give a fine granular appearance visible to the naked eye. This is a sensitive test and, apart from rheumatoid arthritis itself, it gives positive results in other conditions associated with an increased production of gammaglobulin, including bacterial endocarditis, chronic tuberculosis and cirrhosis of the liver.

2. The Rose-Waaler test is based on a similar principle. Sheep red cells are treated with an anti-sheep-cell serum raised in rabbits. The dose used is just sufficient to coat the sheep cells with rabbit gammaglobulin, so that they will be agglutinated by any serum which contains an antibody reacting with rabbit gammaglobulin. They will also be agglutinated if the serum reacts with ordinary sheep cells, and it is customary to test serum both with coated and with uncoated sheep cells at the same time. A comparison of the results in these two tests may be expressed as the Differential Agglutination Titre.

Drug Allergies

Many drugs combine with serum proteins or may be metabolized into substances with this affinity. As a hapten group attached to a protein, the drug may then be strongly antigenic—although the drug alone (or the metabolite) may not be so at all. The immune response can be mediated either by cells or by circulating antibody or both. The clinical features of drug allergy will vary accordingly, from a contact sensitivity in the first case to anaphylaxis or serum sickness in the second, depending on the main type of antibody produced. Not all the drug reactions fit easily, however, into well-defined categories.

Some of the best-studied drug allergies are those affecting the formed elements of the blood. These are of three types:

(i) Reactions against the drug determinants of a drug-protein complex

The first to be described was Sedormid-induced purpura (Ackroyd, 1954). The serum of patients with this condition contains an antibody that will agglutinate platelets or lyse them in the presence of complement, but only if Sedormid is present. The drug is thought to combine with the platelet to form a loose hapten-protein complex which is antigenic to some patients and stimulates antibody formation. It is the drug that is the antigenic determinant and the antibody will not react with platelets in the absence of the drug (Ackroyd and Rook, 1968).

There are other instances where drugs combine with cells of the blood and provoke a reaction. Red cells may be affected, and this probably accounts for the Coombs-positive haemolytic anaemia found with high doses of penicillin (Swanson *et al.*, 1966) or with cephalothin therapy. It is not known whether most drug-induced thrombocytopenias arise in a similar way or even whether they are caused by a true hypersensitivity, an idiosyncrasy, or a toxic effect. Gold thrombocytopenia is often said to be toxic in origin, but there is evidence of an immunological abnormality since gold has now been shown to stimulate lymphocyte transformation in this condition (Denman and Denman, 1968).

(ii) Reactions against a drug, causing indirect effects on blood cells

Some patients who are taking quinine develop antibodies and a positive direct Coombs test, though usually without anaemia. Here—in the words of Damashek—the red blood cells and often the platelets too are "innocent bystanders". The combination of quinine and antibody in the serum fixes complement and the C'3 component attaches to the red cell. Therefore, in this case the antibody has no direct effect on the red cell. The positive Coombs test is given because the Coombs antiserum reacts with complement which has coated the red cell non-specifically (Croft *et al.*, 1968).

(iii) Reactions provoked by a drug but directed against cells of the blood or tissues

Twenty per cent of patients who have taken methyl dopa for periods of six months develop a positive Coombs test (Breckenridge *et al.*, 1967). A small proportion have a frank haemolytic anaemia. About 20 per cent of patients (not necessarily the same 20 per cent) also develop antinuclear antibodies. Antibodies can be eluted from the red blood cells and these antibodies are able to react with the red cells of many healthy people even in the absence of the drug. They are almost always directed against rhesus factors—commonly c or e—but antibodies of several specificities may be present in one patient (Lo Buglio and Jandl, 1967; Bakemeier and Leddy, 1968). The antibody does not react with the drug nor with any of its known metabolites, so there is no question of a mere cross-reaction with rhesus antigens, caused by an antibody which is really directed against the drug. The Coombs test reverts to negative some months after the drug is stopped but, even then, stored antibody eluted during the active phase of the disease can still be shown to react vigorously with the patient's red cells. The drug appears to have provoked the formation of a "warm" antibody directed against the normal red cell, similar to that seen in spontaneous haemolytic anaemia.

Recently, the use of a related drug, L-dopa, in the treatment of Parkinsonism has been associated with similar abnormalities (Lo Buglio *et al.*, 1969). This group of drugs may therefore have a particular tendency to cause this type of haemolytic anaemia. Three similar cases have also been reported with mefenamic acid therapy (Scott *et al.*, 1968).

Drug-induced Systemic Lupus

Many drugs and therapeutic agents have been blamed for the development of antinuclear factor and a lupus-like syndrome, some with more validity than others. There have been occasional reports of cases which follow the administration of penicillin, typhoid vaccine, phenylbutazone or anti-tetanus serum, but it is sometimes difficult to be sure that the symptoms for which the treatment was given were not in fact the presenting features of true systemic lupus. Hydrallazine (Condemi *et al.*, 1967) and procainamide (Fakhro *et al.*, 1967) have consistently provoked a syndrome resembling systemic lupus, i.e. arthritis, pleurisy, pericarditis, skin rashes, fever and leucopaenia. This occurs in about 20 per cent of patients taking these drugs for more than six months. A positive antinuclear factor test is found even more frequently and occurs in 80 per cent of cases when procainamide has been given for only two months (Russell and Ziff, 1968). Isoniazid, the hydantoins, trimethadione and the oral contraceptives also seem to be able to induce this reaction occasionally. The main distinction between the drug-induced disease and systemic lupus is that a complete remission of symptoms usually occurs shortly after the drug is stopped—often within 24 to 48 hours (Fakhro *et al.*, 1967). Antinuclear antibody or LE cells may take rather longer to disappear and sometimes persist for very long periods (Alarcon-Segovia *et al.*, 1967). It is because this disease is so eminently curable when the precipitating drug is stopped that the search for possible cases is so rewarding.

One further distinction between the drug-induced syndrome and spontaneous systemic lupus is that, with the possible exception of hydrallazine lupus, renal involvement has not been reported. As hydrallazine is in any case given for hypertension, it is often difficult to sort out how much of the renal involvement is due to the hypertension and how much to persisting drug-induced lupus.

A study from a rheumatology unit reported that seven out of 167 patients taking oral contraceptives had positive antinuclear factor tests (six had LE cells). These tests became negative—and the patients' symptoms remitted —when oral contraceptives were stopped (Bole *et al.*, 1969). However, screening a different group of patients at a contraceptive clinic failed to show an increased incidence of serological abnormality (McKenna *et al.*, 1969).

The frequency with which therapy with any of the above drugs has resulted in symptoms suggestive of lupus indicates a causal relationship. The evidence becomes most suggestive when the cessation of therapy is followed by a remission. When therapy has been resumed, usually by accident, symptoms often recur after a relatively short period (Ladd, 1962).

The mechanism of this drug-induced disease, as with the haemolytic anaemia provoked by methyl dopa, is unknown. The suggestion has been made that either a virus infection or else true systemic lupus may have been precipitated in predisposed subjects. In the case of patients receiving procainamide, this can only imply that at least 80 per cent of the population are predisposed to this disease—or, at least, to the production of antinuclear factor. However, some patients may indeed have spontaneous systemic lupus and it may be these who show persistence of their symptoms after therapy has stopped.

It is possible that a mechanism similar to that of drug-induced lupus may account for the patient with systemic lupus and dysgerminoma whose lupus went into complete remission after the removal of the tumour (Kahn *et al.*, 1966). However, there is as yet very little information on the occurrence of lupus-like syndromes in malignant diseases.

Agranulocytosis

In studies of many abnormal reactions to drugs it is difficult to distinguish between idiosyncrasy and hypersensitivity. This is especially true here. A very few cases have been reported where an antibody has been found in the serum which, in the presence of the offending drug, can cause agglutination or lysis of compatible leucocytes. The drugs involved have included sulpha-pyridine, chlorpromazine, and salicylazo-sulphapyridine (Ackroyd, 1963). In a few cases of agranulocytosis caused by chlorpromazine, Pisciotta (1965) cultured marrow cells during the recovery phase and claimed that the drug inhibited the granulocyte precursors.

In the case of other manifestations which may be related to drug allergy, such as fever, various types of skin rash, jaundice or retroperitoneal fibrosis, the mechanism is totally unknown.

REFERENCES

ACKROYD, J. F. (1954). The role of sedormid in the immunological reaction that results in platelet lysis in sedormid purpura. *Clin. Sci.*, **13**, 409.

ACKROYD, J. F. (1963). The diagnosis of disorders of the blood due to drug hypersensitivity caused by an immune mechanism. In *Immunological Methods*. ed. J. F. Ackroyd. Oxford: Blackwell.

ACKROYD, J. F. & ROOK, A. (1968). Drug Reactions. In *Clinical Aspects of Immunology*. ed. P. G. H. Gell and D. R. A. Coombs. Oxford: Blackwells, p. 693.

ALARCON-SEGOVIA, D., WAKIM, K. G., WORTHINGTON, J. D. & WARD, L. E. (1967). Clinical and experimental studies on the hydrallazine syndrome and its relationship to systemic lupus erythematosus. *Medicine (Baltimore)*, **46**, 1.

BAKEMEIER, R. F. & LEDDY, J. P. (1968). Erythrocyte autoantibody associated with alpha methyl dopa. Heterogeneity of structure and specificity. *Blood*, **32**, 1.

BOLE, C. G., FRIEDLANDER, M. H. & SMITH, C. K. (1969). Rheumatic symptoms and serological abnormalities induced by oral contraceptives. *Lancet*, **1**, 323.

BRECKENRIDGE, A., DOLLERY, C. T., WORLLEDGE, S. M., HOLBOROW, E. J. & JOHNSON, G. D. (1967). Positive direct Coombs test and antinuclear factor in patients treated with methyl dopa. *Lancet*, **2**, 1265.

CONDEMI, J. J., MOORE-JONES, D., VAUGHAN, J. H. & MITCHELL, P. H. (1967). Antinuclear antibodies following hydrallazine toxicity. *New Engl. J. Med.* **276**, 586.

CROFT, J. D., SWISHER, S. N., GILLILAND, B. C., BAHEMILLER, R. F., LEDDY, J. P. & WEED, R. I. (1968). Coombs test positivity induced by drugs. *Ann. intern. Med.*, **68**, 176.

DENMAN, E. J. & DENMAN, A. M. (1968). The lymphocyte transformation test and gold hypersensitivity. *Ann. rheum. Dis.*, **27**, 581.

FAKHRO, A. M., RITCHIE, R. F. & LOWN, B. (1967). Lupus-like syndrome induced by procainamide. *Amer. J. Cardiol.*, **20**, 367.

KAHN, M. F., RYCKEWAERT, A., CANNAT, A., SOLNICA, J. & DESIZE, S. (1966). Systemic lupus erythematosus and ovarian dysgerminoma: Remission of the systemic lupus erythematosus after extirpation of the tumour. *Clin. exp. Immunol.*, **1**, 355.

LADD, A. G. (1962). Procainamide-induced lupus erythematosus. *New Engl. J. Med.*, **267**, 1357.

LO BUGLIO, A. F. & JANDL, J. H. (1967). The nature of the alpha methyl dopa red-cell antibody. *New Engl. J. Med.*, **276**, 658.

LO BUGLIO, A. F., MASOVEREDIS, S. P., PISCIOTTA, A. V., PAPAVASILIOU, P. S. & COTZIAS, G. C. (1969). Immunoglobulin coating of red cells following L-dopa therapy. *Fed. Proc.*, **28**, 315.

MCKENNA, C. H., WIEMAN, K. C. & SHULMAN, L. E. (1969). Oral contraceptives, rheumatoid disease and autoantibodies. *Arthr. and Rheum.*, **12**, 313.

PISCIOTTA, A. V. (1965). Studies on agranulocytosis. *J. Lab. clin. Med.*, **65**, 240.

RUSSELL, A. S. & ZIFF, M. (1968). Natural antibodies to procainamide. *Clin. exp. Immunol.*, **3**, 901.

SCOTT, G. L., MYLES, A. B. & BACON, P. A. (1968). Autoimmune haemolytic anaemia and mefenamic acid therapy. *Brit. med. J.*, **3**, 534.

SWANSON, M. A., CHANMOUGAN, D. & SCHWARTZ, R. A. (1966). Immunohaemolytic anaemia due to antipenicillin antibodies. *New Engl. J. Med.*, **274**, 178.

IMMUNOLOGICAL DISORDERS PROVOKED BY INFECTION

Immune disorders are closely associated with infection, for example, in the lymphocytic choriomeningitis infections of mice, in Aleutian disease of mink, and in the syndrome of New Zealand mice that resembles systemic lupus. In man, although there are a number of conditions showing auto-immune phenomena which are associated with an infection, there are others in which there is as yet no evidence of an association with a drug, a virus or any other provocative agent.

An immune response directed against an infecting micro-organism has been shown to be responsible for the thrombocytopenic purpura that occasionally follows rubella. In this case it is an immune reaction that damages the host cells (i.e. the platelets) which carry the virus. Damage caused by an immune reaction is also largely responsible for the widespread tissue destruction which can be seen in tuberculosis and syphilis. Similarly, post-infectious encephalomyelitis also seems to be due largely to the host's immune response, and not to the direct effects of a virus (Waksman, 1959).

Some infections in man can provoke hypersensitivity reactions, as well as the formation of classical autoantibodies that react with components of the patient's own body. For example, an infection with *Mycoplasma pneumoniae* may give rise to haemolytic anaemia with cold agglutinins directed against the "I" antigen of red cells (Feizi, 1967). Cold agglutinins may also be present in syphilis (Dacie, 1965) and the Wassermann reaction itself is an autoimmune response. Waldenström shrewdly pointed out that had the spirochaete not been discovered, syphilis would be an ideal model of "an autoimmune disease"; widespread lymphocytic tissue damage, vasculitis and abnormal autoantibodies are all prominent features. Another example is glandular fever which, despite the epidemiological and clinical features of an infectious illness (and the close association with Epstein-Barr virus), is marked by the frequent presence of unexplained antibodies to sheep red cells and of antinuclear factor, rheumatoid factor and cold agglutinins (Kaplan, 1968).

It is not known whether autoantibodies are provoked by the increased breakdown of infected cells in these various infections. In theory, there are several other mechanisms which could be involved in these disorders, but little evidence as to which of the following may be most significant.

Direct antibody attack

This is provoked by an antigenic infectious agent which cross-reacts with similar antigens in the host's tissues; for example, the antibodies against the Group A β-haemolytic streptococcus which cross-react with heart muscle in rheumatic fever (Kaplan and Meyeserian, 1962). Antibodies have also been demonstrated in ulcerative colitis which react both with the O14 strain of *E. coli* and with colonic mucosal cells (Perlmann *et al.*, 1967).

Modifications of host cells by enzyme action

Myxoviruses, which contain neuraminidase, can digest off part of a red blood cell to reveal a previously hidden "T" antigen, to which most people already have antibodies (Springer, 1963). This can cause agglutination of the cells and is responsible for the Thomsen-Friedenreich phenomenon, in which the agglutination of old infected cells interferes with the cross-matching of blood.

Release of a sequestered antigen

Thyroglobulin was previously regarded as a classical example of a sequestered antigen, which provoked an immune response when spilled into the blood stream. However, these ideas of inaccessibility have had to be revised. Traces of thyroglobulin are frequently present in the circulation in health, and an autoimmune mopping-up reaction to tissue breakdown, so far from being pathological, is probably normal. It is possible that the release of normally sequestered antigen may contribute to the reaction seen in sympathetic ophthalmia, but this is exceptional.

Development of antiglobulins

Chronic infections of almost any type may be associated with the presence of an antiglobulin antibody known as "rheumatoid" factor, which may possibly be provoked by the increased turnover and breakdown of gamma-globulins. Bacterial endocarditis is especially important in this respect (Messner and Williams, 1968), and so are leprosy, trypanosomiasis and kala-azar (Houba and Allison, 1966). Rheumatoid factors have also been reported in infectious hepatitis, glandular fever and tuberculosis, and have even been noted after vaccination (Aho et al., 1967). Christian attempted to mimic the underlying mechanism by the repeated immunization of rabbits with heat-killed E. coli. Macroglobulin rheumatoid factors were found in these rabbits, and a few also developed antinuclear factor (Christian et al., 1965).

REFERENCES

AHO, K., SOMER, T. & SALO, O. P. (1967). Rheumatoid factors in S.B.E. Ann. intern. Med., 68, 746.

CHRISTIAN, C. C., DESIMONE, A. R. & Abruzzo, J. L. (1965). Anti-DNA antibodies in hyperimmunised rabbits. J. exp. Med., 121, 309.

DACIE, J. V. (1965). Hemolytic anaemia. Ann. N.Y. Acad. Sci., 124, part II, 415.

FEIZI, T. (1967). Cold agglutinins, direct Coombs test and immunoglobulins in mycoplasma pneumoniae infections. Ann. N.Y. Acad. Sci., 143, 801.

HOUBA, V. & ALLISON, A. C. (1966). M. antiglobulins (rheumatoid factor-like globulins) and other gammaglobulins in relation to tropical parasitic infections. Lancet, 1, 848.

KAPLAN, M. H. (1968). Cryoglobulinaemia in infectious mononucleosis. J. Lab. clin. Med., 71, 754.

KAPLAN, M. H. & MEYESERIAN, M. (1962). An immunological cross-reaction between Group A streptococcal cells and human heart tissue. Lancet, 1, 706.

MESSNER, P. & WILLIAMS, J. C. (1968). Rheumatoid factors in S.B.E. Ann. intern. Med., 68, 746.

PERLMANN, P., HAMMERSTROM, S., LAGERCRANTZ, R. & CAMPBELL, D. (1967). Antibodies to colon in rats and human ulcerative colitis. Cross-reactivity with Escherichia coli O-14 antigen. Proc. Soc. exp. Biol. (N.Y.), 125, 975.

SPRINGER, G. F. (1963). Enzymatic and non-enzymatic alterations of erythrocyte surface antigens. Bact. Rev., 27, 191.

WAKSMAN, B. H. (1959). In Experimental Allergic Encephalomyelitis and the Auto-allergic Diseases. Basel: Karger.

DISEASES OF THE RESPIRATORY SYSTEM

Bronchial Asthma

The presence in the blood of specific reaginic antibodies (IgE) has been shown to correlate very well with clinical evidence of allergy, both in the case of castor bean sensitivity (Coombs *et al.*, 1968) and in a recent American study of allergy to ragweed pollen (Sadan *et al.*, 1969). Some individuals are especially prone to develop reaginic antibody in response to a variety of antigenic stimuli. Therefore many different types of allergic reaction may be present in the same patient, including asthma and eczema. These are the "atopic individuals" of the older medical literature. As in hay fever, so in allergic asthma, skin testing is the only practical method of assessing the antigens to which the patient is sensitive and an immediate wheal reaction indicates a positive test. Pollens, moulds, feathers and dander are all important allergens, and a species of mite—*Dermatophagoides Pteronyssinus*—is also a potent sensitizing agent present in house dust.

It has recently been shown that the serum IgE level is markedly elevated in asthma, eczema and, to a lesser extent, in hay fever. In some countries high levels may be found in the population at large, and this is so in Ethiopia, where the high levels may be related to worm infestations (Johansson *et al.*, 1968).

For clinical purposes, "desensitization" to an allergen may be achieved by giving repeated injections of small but increasing doses of antigen or by using a depot preparation in oil. In effect "desensitization" overshadows the reaginic reaction by provoking an immune response of a different type, which is associated with the so-called *blocking antibodies*. In a recent controlled trial Sadan and his colleagues (1968) showed that effective clinical desensitization to ragweed pollen was associated with blocking antibodies of the IgG type. The implication is that when ragweed pollen enters the body it encounters an excess of the harmless blocking antibodies, which prevent the allergic response which would otherwise follow.

The syndrome of bronchial asthma, transient pulmonary shadows, and eosinophilia may have a number of causes. In some cases allergy to *Aspergillus fumigatus* appears to be implicated. Skin testing demonstrates the immediate wheal response of reaginic antibody but also, after about four hours, an area of oedema and a typical Arthus reaction develop, which fades after 24 hours or so. In these patients there is therefore evidence of two kinds of reaction. The presence of reaginic antibody is the distinguishing feature of the asthmatic, and it is this antibody which produces the immediate wheal reaction in the skin. There are, in addition, circulating precipitating antibodies to the antigens of *Aspergillus fumigatus*. These are responsible for the formation of immune complexes leading to the Arthus reaction, and can also be demonstrated in patients with an aspergilloma who do not suffer from asthma.

Other causes of the pulmonary eosinophilic syndrome include infestations with migrating parasites such as ascaris and liver fluke, though in these cases asthma is uncommon. In some patients with tropical eosinophilia, microfilariae are the probable cause. Drugs such as nitrofurantoin have also been implicated in a few cases, and pulmonary eosinophilia with asthma may also be the presenting feature of polyarteritis nodosa.

Extrinsic Allergic Alveolitis

This is a group of diseases which are all characterized by cough, weight loss, severe dyspnoea, fever, chills, malaise and fine crepitant rales. These features occur in association with an allergic alveolitis, and when this is due to external irritants the symptoms begin some three to six hours after exposure to the relevant antigen. A chronic syndrome may develop after prolonged or recurrent exposure, leading to pulmonary fibrosis.

"Farmer's lung" was the first syndrome of this type to be studied in detail. It results from the inhalation of the dust of mouldy hay and other vegetable materials. The clinical features are due to a reaction in the alveoli rather than the bronchioles, and radiologically there is reticular shadowing. Eosinophilia is rare. The syndrome is associated with a positive skin test of immune complex (Arthus) type, which occurs four to eight hours after prick-testing with mouldy hay extracts and is due to the presence of circulating antibodies to *Micropolyspora faeni* (Pepys *et al.*, 1964). Antibodies may also be found occasionally in asymptomatic farmers who have been exposed to the mouldy hay fungus, and serum samples from many areas of the world react with the same fungal antigens.

There are a large number of analogous diseases. In many, the antigen has been demonstrated by inhalation tests if not by more specific immunological techniques.

Disease	Dust exposure	Specific antigen
Farmer's lung	Mouldy hay	Micropolyspora faeni
Bagassosis	Mouldy bagasse	Thermoactinomyces vulgaris
Suberosis	Cork dust	
Pituitary snuff taker's lung	Porcine and bovine pituitary powder	Serum protein and pituitary antigens
Bird-breeder's lung	Pigeon and budgerigar droppings	Pigeon or budgerigar proteins
Elephant allergy	Elephant skin and hair	? elephant proteins
Mushroom picker's lung	Mushroom dust	Micromonospora vulgaris or Micropolyspora faeni
Wheat weevil disease	Wheat flour	Sitophilus granarius
New Guinea lung	Roof thatch	
Cheese worker's lung	Cheese	Penicillin spores
Malt worker's lung	Malt	Aspergillus fumigatus and clavatus
Maple bark stripper's lung	Maple bark	Cryptostroma corticale
Sequoiosis	Redwood dust	Aerobasidium pullulans and graphium
Smallpox handler's lung	Smallpox scabs	
Paprika splitter's lung	Paprika	
Washing-powder worker's lung	Enzyme dust	Enzymes from B. subtilis

Modified from Parish and Pepys (1968).

In some of the above diseases reagins are present in addition to the precipitating antibodies, and asthma may be a feature together with an eosinophilia. This may occur, for example, in suberosis.

Byssinosis is not one of this group of diseases and is probably due to a primary irritant, rather than an allergen, resulting in asthmatic symptoms (Bouheys *et al.*, 1967).

REFERENCES

BOUHEYS, A., HEAPHY, L. J., SCHILLING, R. S. F. & WELBORD, J. W. (1967). Byssinosis in the United States. *New Engl. J. Med.*, **280**, 623.

COOMBS, R. R. A., HUNTER, A., JONAS, W. E., BERNICH, H., JOHANSSON, S. G. O. & PANZANI, R. (1968). Detection of IgE (IgND) specific antibody (probably reagin) to Castor-bean allergen by the red-cell-linked antigen-antiglobulin reaction. *Lancet*, **1**, 1115.

JOHANSSON, S. G. O., MELLBIN, T. & VAHLQUIST, B. (1968). Immunoglobulin levels in Ethiopian pre-school children with special reference to high concentrations of immunoglobulin E (IgND). *Lancet*, **1**, 1118.

PARISH, W. E. & PEPYS, J. (1968). The lung in allergic disease. In *Clinical Aspects of Immunology*. eds. P. G. H. Gell and R. R. A. Coombs, 2nd edition. Oxford: Blackwell.

PEPYS, J., LONGBOTTOM, J. L. & JENKINS, P. A. (1964). Vegetable dust pneumoconioses. Immunologic responses to vegetable dusts and their flora. *Amer. Rev. resp. Dis.*, **89**, 842.

SADAN, N., RHYME, M. B., MELLITS, E. D., GOLDSTEIN, E. O., LEVY, D. A. & LICHTENSTEIN, L. M. (1969). Immunotherapy of pollinosis in children: immunological basis of improvement. *New Engl. J. Med.*, **280**, 623.

DISEASES AFFECTING THE KIDNEY

In man, as in animals, glomerulonephritis is not a disease but a syndrome with many causes. Most cases can, at least in theory, be fitted into two main groups:

1. Immune complex nephritis
The deposition of antibody complexed with antigens, which may be derived from streptococci (in post-streptococcal glomerulonephritis) from the infective agents of bacterial endocarditis or *Plasmodium malariae*, or even from the damaged cell-nuclei of the host (in systemic lupus).

2. Direct antibody attack
The deposition of antibody direct on to the basement membrane in Goodpasture's syndrome or in some cases of chronic, progressive glomerulonephritis or renal vein thrombosis (Muerhke, 1968). This group is analogous to nephrotoxic serum nephritis in animals.

Some forms of glomerulonephritis and of the nephrotic syndrome cannot yet be fitted into this schema because no antigen is known to be responsible or because an underlying vasculitis or polyarteritis has been identified without any obvious cause. In Henoch-Schönlein purpura, for example, there are discrete deposits of IgG and of complement (Urizar et al., 1968), but it is not known whether this is the cause or the result of the inflammatory changes around the capillaries which are present in this disease.

Systemic lupus and nephritis

Although neurological lesions, cardiac failure, or secondary infection may cause death in systemic lupus, the major, lethal effects of the disease are due to renal involvement. As in the renal disease of NZB/W mice, anti-DNA antibodies are probably intimately concerned in causing the renal lesion. There are deposits of IgG and complement in the glomeruli and a low level of complement in the serum. The deposited IgG has been shown, in some cases, to be an antinuclear factor which is deposited together with DNA (Koffler et al., 1967). The antibodies most important in causing lupus nephritis are complement-fixing, antinuclear antibodies which react with DNA, and patients with a low titre of these antibodies do not usually have renal involvement. In diseases associated with other types of antinuclear antibody (Tojo and Friou, 1968)—e.g., rheumatoid arthritis, or drug-induced lupus—immune complex nephritis is not found. Histologically, there may be a mild glomerulitis or a proliferative or membranous glomerulonephritis, and proteinuria relates to histological severity but not to the activity or the disease (Pollak et al., 1964). Disappointingly, there is little correlation between clinical or serological features and the histological type.

Antinuclear antibodies are not pathogenic in all circumstances, and intact cells may be cultured and even multiply in their presence. Also, infants born to affected mothers may have antinuclear antibodies in their serum without ill effects. Other autoantibodies found in systemic lupus react with cell fractions such as mitochondria or ribosomes, and may react with red cells giving a positive Coombs test. Rheumatoid factor is present in about one case in three, leucopenia is frequent, and thrombocytopenia is an occasional accompaniment, but the pathogenesis of these complications is uncertain (Miescher et al., 1966). The Wassermann reaction is positive in 10 to 20 per cent of patients, and of 81 patients who had persistent biological false positive reactions for syphilis 30 per cent developed probable or definite systemic lupus during a follow-up period which averaged five years (Putkonen et al., 1967).

Discoid lupus erythematosus

Although this may have similar skin manifestations, it is not associated with the systemic disease and is thought to be a distinct entity (Swanson-

Beck *et al.*, 1966). Only one in twenty develop overt systemic lupus, although a third of patients have antinuclear antibodies.

Post-streptococcal glomerulonephritis

On biopsy there are characteristic discrete subepithelial deposits of IgG and complement ($C'3$), and there is now evidence that streptococcal antigens are present too (Andres *et al.*, 1966). The finding of a low complement level in the serum is another characteristic feature of immune complex nephritis. A rise in this level usually heralds the phase of resolution.

Nephrotic syndrome of childhood

In the most common type there is no thickening of the glomerular basement membrane and no deposition of IgG or complement. The serum complement level remains within normal limits. Paradoxically it is this type of renal disease that responds best to therapy with corticosteroids or cytotoxic drugs (Drummond *et al.*, 1966).

In adults with the nephrotic syndrome, the most common cause is a glomerulonephritis and most patients have demonstrable deposits of IgG and complement. Eventually the glomeruli become completely hyalinized and at this stage the deposits are no longer found. The serum complement level may be low or normal (Lange *et al.*, 1965).

Since it has become the practice to carry out nephrectomy prior to renal transplantation, it has been noted that after removal of the kidneys an antibody may appear in the serum of a few patients that can react with glomerular basement membrane. A similar antibody can be eluted from the removed kidneys (Lerner *et al.*, 1967). Although these antibodies may be a secondary result of chronic renal damage, it is of interest that they are usually absent from the circulation so long as the kidneys are intact. Only when the kidneys are removed does this antibody appear free in the blood stream.

One of the features of an immune complex nephritis is a low serum complement level, and this is seen in systemic lupus, in post-streptococcal glomerulonephritis, and in serum sickness. However, if the levels of the individual components of complement are examined, some differences emerge. Serum sickness has very low levels of all factors. In systemic lupus the early factors are reduced, but the later factors (from $C'5$ onwards) are normal. In acute post-streptococcal glomerulonephritis $C'1$ is relatively normal and the reduction is chiefly of $C'2$, 3 and 4.

As the serum level of complement depends on the rate at which it is destroyed and also on the rate of synthesis, it is conceivable that these differences may reflect merely the rate of formation. However, they have been shown to have some value in the diagnostic assessment of glomerulonephritis

(Kohler and Ten Bensel, 1969). A favourable response to therapy is often preceded by a rise in serum complement levels, and it has been claimed that this is a useful clue to prognosis.

Bacterial endocarditis

Focal glomerulonephritis is occasionally found in association with sub-acute bacterial endocarditis; it used to be thought of as embolic, but it is as frequent with right-sided heart lesions as with lesions of the left side of the heart. Here too, discrete deposits of IgG and complement are found, in association with a lowered level of complement in the serum. By inference this may therefore be another form of immune complex disease.

Goodpasture's syndrome

Just as lupus nephritis has features suggesting that it is a human counter-part of immune complex disease in animals, so Goodpasture's syndrome resembles another animal disease, in this case caused by the deposition of antibody directly upon the glomerular basement membrane, i.e. nephrotoxic serum nephritis. Goodpasture's syndrome usually presents in young males who develop a cough with pulmonary infiltration and haemorrhage. It terminates fatally in almost every case, because of a rapidly progressive membranous or proliferative nephritis. At necropsy, it can be demonstrated that IgG can be eluted from the kidney. The IgG is capable of attaching itself, specifically, to glomerular basement membrane in a uniform linear pattern. It is also capable of attachment to lung capillary membranes, and if it is infused into a monkey, as little as 4 mg has been shown to cause a severe glomerulonephritis (Koffler et al., 1969). The same properties are true for the gammaglobulin eluted from the lung lesions. It is of interest that a membranous glomerulonephritis of similar appearance may follow renal vein thrombosis. Here, too, there is the deposition of IgG and complement, but the mechanism of these secondary changes is unknown.

REFERENCES

ANDRES, G. A., ACCINI, L., HSU, K. C., ZABRISKIE, J. B. & SEEGAL, B. C. (1966). Electron microscopic studies of human glomerulonephritis with ferritin conjugated antibody. J. exp. Med., 123, 399.

DRUMMOND, K. N., MICHAEL, A. F., GOOD, R. A. & VERNIER, R. L. (1966). The nephrotic syndrome of childhood. Immunologic, clinical and pathologic considerations. J. clin. Invest., 45, 620.

KOFFLER, D., SCHUR, P. H. & KUNKEL, H. G. (1967). Immunological studies concerning the nephritis of systemic lupus erythematosus. J. exp. Med., 126, 607.

KOFFLER, D., SANDERSON, J., CARR, R. & KUNKEL, H. J. (1969). Immunological studies concerning the pulmonary lesions of Goodpasture's syndrome. Amer. J. Path., 54, 293.

KOHLER, P. F. & TEN BENSEL, R. (1969). Serial complement component alterations in acute glomerulonephritis and systemic lupus erythematosus. *Clin. exp. Immunol.*, **4**, 191.

LANGE, K., TRESER, G., TY, ANTONIA & WASSERMAN, E. (1965). The histologic and immunologic features of acute, subacute and chronic glomerulonephritis. *Trans. Ass. Amer. Phycns.*, **78**, 117.

LERNER, R. A., GLASSOCK, R. J. & DIXON, F. J. (1967). Antiglomerular antibody in human nephritis. *J. exp. Med.*, **126**, 989.

MIESCHER, P. A., ROTHFIELD, D. & MIESCHER A. (1966). Immunologic phenomena in patients with systemic lupus erythematosus. In *Lupus Erythematosus*. ed. E. L. Dubois. McGraw Hill.

MUERHKE, R. (1968). Membranous glomerulonephritis secondary to renal vein thrombosis. *Ann. intern. Med.*, **68**, 1179.

POLLAK, V. E., SCHWARTZ, F. D. & PIRANI, C. L. (1964). Systemic lupus erythematosus: the failure of renal tests to predict reliably the underlying renal pathology. *Med. Bull. Presb. St Luke's Hosp.*, **3**, 94.

PUTKONEN, T., JOKINEN, E. J., LASSUS, A. & MUSTAKALLIO, K. K. (1967). Chronic biologic false positive seroreactions for syphilis as a harbinger of systemic lupus erythematosus. *Acta derm. venerol.*, **47**, 83.

SWANSON-BECK, J. & ROWELL, N. R. (1966). Discoid lupus erythematosus. *Quart. J. Med.*, **35**, 119.

TOJO, T. & FRIOU, G. J. (1968). Lupus nephritis: varying complement-fixing properties of IgG antibodies to antigens of cell nuclei. *Science*, **161**, 904.

URIZAR, R. E., MICHAEL, A., SISSON, S. & VERNIER, R. L. (1968). Anaphylactoid purpura. II. Immunofluorescent and electron microscopical studies of the glomerular lesion. *Lab. Invest.*, **19**, 437.

RHEUMATOID ARTHRITIS

This is a chronic yet episodic polyarthritis in its most usual form, involving especially the peripheral joints, usually in a symmetrical distribution. However, it is not solely a disease of joints, and there may be marked associated systemic disturbances including fever and weight loss, pleurisy, nodular and fibrotic forms of lung disease, pericarditis, neuropathy and vasculitis. It may be difficult on some occasions to distinguish between the more complicated forms of the disease and systemic lupus, and even LE cells and antinuclear antibody are occasionally found in the blood of a patient who appears to have classical rheumatoid arthritis. The disease affects approximately 3 per cent of the population, and females are affected about twice as commonly as males. The incidence rises steeply with age, and at the age of 80 15 per cent of females and 5 per cent of males are affected.

One of the characteristics of rheumatoid arthritis is the presence of a macroglobulin antibody, rheumatoid factor, which reacts with IgG or with its breakdown products. Rheumatoid factor is most commonly found in long-standing rheumatoid arthritis, expecially when nodules are present. Nevertheless, it is found in only 60 to 90 per cent of patients with otherwise typical rheumatoid arthritis. Its absence does not therefore rule out the diagnosis, but when a negative test is found, it is especially important to rule out other disease, such as psoriasis or ankylosing spondylitis.

Rheumatoid factor is not pathogenic in itself, and transfusions of blood with a high titre of rheumatoid factor do no harm. Nevertheless, patients with a positive test have a worse prognosis and fewer remissions than those whose rheumatoid test remains negative. The presence of nodules and such systemic complications as vasculitis occur only in seropositive patients. If the test for rheumatoid factor remains negative at the end of the first year of disease, the likelihood that a patient will ever develop a positive test for rheumatoid factor is less than one in ten, a point of some prognostic value.

The incidence of rheumatoid arthritis as measured on population surveys is not, contrary to popular belief, affected by climate. Nor is there any factual support for the suggestion that it is familial. In a set of identical twins only one had rheumatoid arthritis and rheumatoid factor, so that environmental influences may be important (O'Brien et al., 1967).

There have been large numbers of epidemiological surveys in different areas of the world; in the U.K. from 1·1 to 5·2 per cent of different population samples had positive tests for rheumatoid factor. About a quarter of those with positive tests had clinical rheumatoid arthritis at the time, but there is also an increased likelihood that those who do not have rheumatoid arthritis will develop it in the future (Ball and Lawrence, 1963).

In contrast to patients who have clinical disease, people who have a positive test for rheumatoid factor are not predominantly females. The incidence tends to rise with age, but this relationship is irregular and there is an increased prevalence in urban as compared with rural areas, again suggesting an environmental influence (Bennett and Burch, 1968).

Lung involvement

There are several pulmonary syndromes that show a significant association with rheumatoid arthritis.

1. Pleurisy

Walker and Wright (1968) found radiological evidence of pleural effusions, occasionally in association with pericarditis, in 8 per cent of males with rheumatoid arthritis. The effusion was often unilateral and the average age 52 years. Open pleural biopsy usually revealed the presence of nodules on the pleura. In some cases there is an unexplained block to the transport of glucose across the pleura, so that the glucose level in the effusion is low compared with that in the serum.

2. Nodules

Intra-pulmonary nodules that are not pneumoconiotic may rarely occur in the lung, usually in association with subcutaneous nodules. However, the radiological appearances are not diagnostic.

3. Caplan's syndrome

This was originally described during an epidemiological study of rheumatoid arthritis in a Welsh mining community (Miall, 1955). On enquiry among miners who had massive pulmonary fibrosis, especially of the nodular type, a significant number of cases of rheumatoid arthritis were found.

4. Diffuse interstitial fibrosis

There is also an increased incidence of this type of lung disease in patients with rheumatoid arthritis. Nevertheless, the total incidence of cases is still low, and it is interesting that patients with this disease who do not have clinical rheumatoid arthritis may nevertheless have rheumatoid factor in their blood in 50 to 80 per cent of cases (Ward and Stalker, 1965).

REFERENCES

BALL, J. & LAWRENCE, J. S. (1963). The relationship of rheumatoid serum factor to rheumatoid arthritis. A 5-year follow-up of a population sample. *Ann. rheum. Dis.*, **22**, 311.

BENNETT, P. H. & BURCH, T. A. (1968). The epidemiology of rheumatoid arthritis. *Med. clin. N. Amer.*, **52**, 479.

MIALL, W. E. (1955). Rheumatoid arthritis in males. *Ann. rheum. Dis.*, **14**, 150.

O'BRIEN, W. M., BENNETT, P. H., BURCH, T. A. & BUMIN, J. J. (1967). A genetic study of rheumatoid arthritis and rheumatoid factors in the Blackfeet and Pima Indians. *Arthr. and Rheum.*, **10**, 163.

WALKER, W. C. & WRIGHT, V. (1968). Pulmonary lesions and rheumatoid arthritis. *Medicine (Baltimore)*, **47**, 501.

WARD, R. & STALKER, R. (1965). Sheep cell agglutination test in chronic interstitial pulmonary fibrosis. *Ann. rheum. Dis.*, **24**, 246.

HEART DISEASE

The relationship between antigens of group A streptococci and those of heart muscle was first demonstrated by Kaplan and Meyeserian (1962). About 50 per cent of patients with active rheumatic fever, and between 10 and 20 per cent of patients with inactive rheumatic heart disease have circulating antibodies that react not only with the streptococcus, but also with cardiac antigens localized in the sarcolemmal and subsarcolemmal region of the muscle fibre (Kaplan and Svec, 1964). This led to suggestions that these antibodies may play some part in the pathogenesis of the disease. There is some circumstantial evidence that this is so, in the finding of deposits of gammaglobulin and complement in the hearts of patients who have had rheumatic carditis or rheumatic heart disease. It is clear that, in addition to the close clinical relationship, there is a close antigenic relationship between the heart and group A streptococci which may be responsible for a cross-reacting immune response (reviewed by Kaplan, 1968).

This evidence does not prove that the antibodies detected are themselves pathogenic. Similar antibodies have been demonstrated in endomyocardial fibrosis, and bound gammaglobulin has been demonstrated here too (Shaper et al., 1967). A slightly lower incidence of these antibodies has also been found in the serum of normal subjects coming to live in a malarial zone (Shaper et al., 1968). The significance of these findings is not yet known.

Post-cardiotomy and Post-myocardial Infarction Syndromes

This syndrome consists of fever, pleurisy, pericarditis and a raised sedimentation rate occurring within weeks of cardiac surgery or myocardial infarction. It has been diagnosed in about 10 per cent of patients operated on for cardiac disease (both congenital and rheumatic) and about 3 per cent of cases of myocardial infarction (Wood, 1968). After a myocardial infarction the disease tends to appear within the first two weeks, but whatever the precipitating cause there is a strong tendency for the clinical features to subside and recur two or three times before finally remitting. It was felt at one time that the common factor in all cases was the presence of blood in the pericardium. In keeping with this is the report by Segal and Tabatznik (1960) that the syndrome may follow the type of penetrating injury of the heart that may be caused by a bicycle spoke. In addition, haemorrhagic effusions are certainly frequent in the post-infarction syndrome. After cardiotomy a similar syndrome may arise, and Van der Geld (1964) has shown cardiac reactive antibodies in about 80 per cent of these patients, compared with an incidence of 15 per cent in post-operative patients without this syndrome. This finding is of value both as a diagnostic tool and as an illustration of an immunological abnormality which may well play a part in the aetiology of the condition. As might be expected, corticosteroid therapy produces dramatic improvement.

REFERENCES

Kaplan, M. H. (1968). Autoimmunity to heart and its relation to heart disease. In *Allergology*. eds. B. Rose, M. Rickter, A. Sehou, A. W. Frankland. *Excerpta Med. Foundation.*

Kaplan, M. H. & Meyeserian, M. (1962). Immunologic studies of heart tissue. V. Antigens related to heart tissue revealed by cross-reaction of rabbit antisera to heterologous heart. *J. Immunol.*, **88**, 450.

KAPLAN, M. H. & SVEC, K. H. (1964). Immunologic relation of streptococcal and tissue antigens. III. Presence in human sera of streptococcal antibody cross-reactive with heart tissue. Association with streptococcal infections, rheumatic fever and glomerulonephritis. *J. exp. Med.*, **119**, 651.

SEGAL, F. & TABATZNIK, B. (1960). Post-pericardiotomy syndrome following penetrating stab wounds of the chest: comparison with the post-commissurotomy syndrome. *Amer. Heart J.*, **59**, 175.

SHAPER, A. G., KAPLAN, M. H., FOSTER, W. D., MACINTOSH, D. M. & WILKS, N. E. (1967). Immunological studies in endomyocardial fibrosis and other forms of heart disease in the tropics. *Lancet*, **1**, 598.

SHAPER, A. G., KAPLAN, M. H., MODY, N. J. & MCINTYRE, P. A. (1968). Malarial antibodies and autoantibodies to heart and other tissues in the immigrant and indigenous peoples of Uganda. *Lancet*, **1**, 1342.

VAN DER GELD, H. (1964). Anti-heart antibodies in the post-pericardiotomy and the post-myocardial infarction syndrome. *Lancet*, **2**, 617

WOOD, P. H. (1968). In *Diseases of the Heart and Circulation*. 3rd Edition. London: Eyre and Spottiswoode, pp. 657 and 858.

DISEASES OF MUSCLE

Myasthenia gravis

The weakness in this disease develops in the affected voluntary muscles during sustained or repeated contraction. There is a blockage of neuro-muscular conduction (Whipple, 1966) and histologically the motor end-plates appear abnormal (Grob, 1961). Neuromuscular block may possibly be induced, at least in part, by a circulating agent, and it is consistent with this suggestion that about 20 per cent of infants born of affected mothers develop a transient myasthenia which may persist for up to six weeks (Osserman, 1969).

The myasthenic syndrome may have no obvious cause, or it may be second-ary to various types of cancer. Its most notable association is with a thymoma, which is present in 10 per cent of cases. It may also be associated with poly-myositis or with thyrotoxicosis, and has occasionally been reported in cases of systemic lupus erythematosus. Apart from cases secondary to other diseases, myasthenia gravis is most common in young subjects. Even in the absence of a thymoma, such a patient frequently has an abnormal thymus with unusually prominent germinal centres.

Antibodies that react with striated muscle were first demonstrated in this disease by Strauss *et al.* (1961) and are found in about 50 per cent of patients. This finding has been confirmed several times, but the exact incidence varies with the technique used. Using immunofluorescent techniques the antibodies appear to react with the A and I bands of muscle fibres (Lang *et al.*, 1969).

Goldstein and Whittingham (1966) have produced a syndrome resembling myasthenia gravis in guinea-pigs by immunizing them with calf thymus or muscle mixed with Freund's adjuvant. About a quarter of these animals developed weakness and neuromuscular block, but previously thymecto-mized animals did not develop this disorder. Thus it appeared that the presence of an intact thymus was required. These authors suggested that a damaged thymus could release an agent that affected the motor end-plates. Since then, Goldstein has shown that administration of a thymic extract ("thymin") can induce myasthenic features. Large amounts of this extract induced a full-blown myositis (Goldstein, 1968).

There is another possible explanation for the influence of the thymus on muscular function. There are antigenic similarities between thymic cells and muscle, first reported by Van der Geld and Strauss (1966). Myoid cells of the thymic medulla, which resemble muscle cells ultrastructurally and on light microscopy, have been identified in man and in many other species (Feltkamp-Vroom, 1966). It has been suggested that when myasthenia gravis is associated with a thymoma, the neoplasm virtually always involves large epithelioid cells that originate in the myoid cells of the medulla. An immune reaction to cancerous thymic cells might therefore cross-react with cells of striated muscle; at least 95 per cent of myasthenic patients with thymoma have muscle reactive antibodies. The incidence is much lower (30 per cent) in myasthenics who do not have a thymoma, and these antibodies are never found in healthy controls. This relationship is so reliable that in a myasthenic the absence of antibodies virtually excludes a thymoma (Osserman *et al.*, 1967). A *positive* result with serum diluted to 1 : 60 indicates primary myasthenia gravis, with or without a thymoma. Cases secondary to an oat-cell carcinoma of the bronchus or occurring as part of a myopathy give a negative result at this dilution. It has been pointed out that myasthenia gravis may occasionally first appear after the removal of a thymoma. Such cases are nearly always fatal, and at necropsy some remaining tumour or hyperplastic thymus has invariably been found.

Aberrant antibody production is also a feature of this disease. The antinuclear factor test is positive in about one-third of patients, a similar proportion have antithyroid antibodies, and about 5 per cent have macroglobulin "rheumatoid" factor. The serum complement level is reduced in acute attacks (Nastuk *et al.*, 1960) and this provides further evidence of an immunological disorder.

Treatment of myasthenia gravis

The place of thymectomy remains a source of controversy but it is certainly of value in young females with severe disease who have no thymoma (Perlo *et al.*, 1966). In these patients there is usually post-operative clinical improvement that may continue for many months, and also a gradual disappearance of any antibodies that may have been present. Attempts at treatment with corticosteroids, ACTH, or 6-mercapto-purine have on the whole been unsuccessful, and are indicated only in refractory cases (Osserman, 1969). Myasthenia gravis, as a clinical syndrome, may comprise many different varieties. This may in part explain the variations in behaviour and in response to treatment.

Polymyositis

It is uncommon to find any of the more usual hallmarks of an altered immunological response in polymyositis or dermatomyositis. It is exceptional to find antinuclear factor or muscle-reactive antibodies. On the other hand, there is marked infiltration of the muscle with mononuclear cells and in children there is often a prominent vasculitis. These changes often settle, even if only temporarily, when corticosteroids are given and cyclophosphamide has been reported as beneficial in a few cases. This poses, once again, the question of the significance of immunological reactions in causing the pattern of disease, and underlines the need to continue a search for an underlying cause or causes. Myxovirus particles have been seen in the muscles with electron microscopy (Chou, 1967), but the significance of this observation is still uncertain. In a different type of case—that of dermatomyositis associated with carcinoma of the bronchus—Curtis *et al.* (1961) showed that there was skin hypersensitivity of the cellular type to extracts of bronchial carcinoma cells.

REFERENCES

CHOU, S. H. (1967). Myxovirus-like structures in human chronic polymyositis. *Science*, **158**, 1453.

CURTIS, A. C., HECKAMAN, J. H. & WHEELER, A. H. (1961). Study of the autoimmune reaction in dermatomyositis. *J. Amer. Med. Ass.*, **178**, 571.

FELTKAMP-VROOM, T. (1966). Myoid cells in human thymus. *Lancet*, **2**, 1320.

GOLDSTEIN, G. (1968). The thymus and neuromuscular function. A substance in thymus which causes myositis and myasthenic neuromuscular block in guinea-pigs. *Lancet*, **2**, 119.

GOLDSTEIN, G. & WHITTINGHAM, G. (1966). Experimental autoimmune thymitis. An animal model of myasthenia gravis. *Lancet*, **2**, 315.

GROB, D. (1961). Myasthenia gravis; a review of pathogenesis and treatment. *Arch. intern. Med.*, **108**, 615.

LANG, R. W., KORNFELD, P., WEINER, L. B. & OSSERMAN, K. B. (1969). Studies in myasthenia gravis. Incidence of muscle precipitating antibodies correlated with immunofluorescence. *Amer. J. clin. Path.*, **51**, 238.

NASTUK, W. L., PLESCIA, O. J. & OSSERMANN, K. E. (1960). Changes in serum complement activity in patients with myasthenia gravis. *Proc. Soc. exp. Biol. (N.Y.)*, **105**, 177.

OSSERMANN, K. E. (1969). Muscles (Myasthenia gravis). In *Textbook of Immunopathology, vol. 2.* eds. P. A. Miescher, H. J. Müller-Eberhard. New York: Grune and Stratton, p. 607.

OSSERMANN, K. E., TSAIRIS, P. & WEINER, L. B. (1967). Myasthenia gravis and thyroid disease: clinical and immunologic correlation. *J. Mt. Sinai Hosp.*, **24**, 469.

PERLO, V. P., POSKANZER, D. C., SCHWAB, R. S., VIETS, H. R., OSSERMANN, K. E. & GENKINS, G. (1966). Myasthenia gravis: evaluation of treatment in 1,355 patients. *Neurology*, **16**, 43.

STRAUSS, A. J. L., SEEGAL, B. C., HSU, K. C., BURKHOLDER, P. M. NASTUK, W. L. & OSSERMANN, K. E. (1961). Immunofluorescence demonstration of a muscle-binding complement-fixing serum globulin fraction in myasthenia gravis. *Fed. Proc.*, **20**, 38.

VAN DER GELD, H. W. R. & STRAUSS, A. J. L. (1966). Myasthenia gravis. Immunological relationship between striated muscle and the thymus. *Lancet*, **1**, 57.

WHIPPLE, H. E. (1966). Myasthenia gravis. *Ann. N.Y. Acad. Sci.*, **135**. Part 1.

ENDOCRINE DISORDERS

The Thyroid

The histological similarity between the thyroid of Hashimoto's disease and that of experimentally induced allergic thyroiditis is now well known. There is a high incidence of antibodies to a variety of thyroid constituents both in this disorder and in primary myxoedema arising in adult life. Thyroid antibody tests are chiefly of value in establishing the endocrine origin of unilateral exophthalmos, and in differentiating Hashimoto's disease from other goitres including virus thyroiditis and from anxiety states. However, a positive test (and even a positive biopsy showing lymphocytic thyroiditis) cannot rule out the possibility of a neoplasm, since the association of Hashimoto's disease and lymphosarcoma is not very rare.

Many reports indicate that a high proportion of normal individuals have antithyroid antibodies detectable by one of the many tests available. However, complement-fixing (microsomal) antibodies are present only in immune disorders of the thyroid, and if this is borne in mind the results are rarely confusing. Patients with Hashimoto's disease or myxoedema may also have other autoantibodies, and gastric parietal cell antibodies are found among the relatives of patients with Hashimoto's disease as well as among the patients themselves. The discovery of Long Acting Thyroid Stimulator (LATS) in about 80 per cent of patients with Graves' disease (Carneiro *et al.*, 1966) has cast a new light on the aetiology of this disease. Long Acting Thyroid Stimulator is an immunoglobulin (IgG) which reacts with thyroid microsomes. It is still not clear why the highest LATS levels are found in middle-aged patients with pre-tibial myxoedema, or sometimes in patients with progressive exophthalmos. The mechanism of thyroid stimulation by LATS is unknown but its combination with thyroid microsomes is presumably relevant. It has the characteristics of an autoantibody and is unusual in having a stimulating effect on the end-organ. An effect that is thought to mimic that of LATS has been reproduced by immunizing rabbits with human thyroid microsomal fractions and Freund's adjuvant. The rabbits develop a series of antithyroid antibodies including an immunoglobulin (IgG) which has some of the biological characteristics of LATS and which increases the uptake of radio-iodine when it is injected into mice (Beall and Solomon, 1968). It is curious, however, that the animals do not themselves become thyrotoxic; and histologically their thyroids are normal.

Adrenal Disease

The evidence for an immune aetiology in Addison's disease is very similar to that for Hashimoto's disease. The histology of the gland shows lymphocytic infiltration, and circulating antibodies to adrenal cortex are present in some 60 per cent of cases (Blizzard and Kyle, 1963). These antibodies do not develop as a consequence of non-specific adrenal damage, for they are absent in tuberculosis or amyloidosis of the adrenal, or in adrenal failure secondary to pituitary disease. There is a known clinical association of primary disease of the adrenal with thyroid disease (Schmidt's syndrome) and also with chronic lymphocytic gastritis. Patients with Addison's disease also have an increased incidence of antibodies to gastric mucosa and to parathyroid tissue (Blizzard, 1969). Recently patients have also been found to have antibodies which react with the *theca interna* of the ovary and the interstitial cells of the testis (Irvine, 1968); all these patients had an early menopause.

The Parathyroids

Idiopathic hypoparathyroidism may occur in association with Addison's disease, hypothyroidism and pernicious anaemia. In all of these associated diseases, autoantibodies are frequently found which react with the affected organ. Therefore, it seemed reasonable to look for antibodies to parathyroid tissue in idiopathic hypoparathyroidism. These have been found in about one-third of the patients examined by Blizzard *et al.* (1966). Antibodies against oxyphil cells have been found by Irvine and Scarth (1969). The actual parathyroid component which reacts with these antibodies has not been fully investigated but it is not parathormone itself.

This disease is more common among females, but, unlike the other endocrine disorders considered here, it is very much more common in children than adults. About one case in four is associated with mucocutaneous candidiasis which may itself be associated with an abnormality of the immune response.

Immune Reactions to Sperm

While it is known that a small proportion of women have antibodies reactive with sperms, the part played by these in inducing female infertility is still under dispute. Rare cases have been reported in which a woman has had mild anaphylactic reactions regularly after coitus (Halpern *et al.*, 1964). In these cases skin testing with diluted semen from the husband showed a typical, immediate wheal and flare response.

More important, there appears to be an association between autoantibodies to sperm and relative infertility in the male (Rühmke, 1965). These antibodies are agglutinins which are especially likely to develop if there is any obstruction to the seminal passages. There is no evidence that previous mumps orchitis is in any way responsible for these changes.

REFERENCES

BEALL, G. & SOLOMON, D. (1968). Thyroid stimulating factor in the serum of immunised rabbits. *Proc. roy. Soc. Med.*, **61**, 1302.

BLIZZARD, R. M. (1969). Idiopathic hypoparathyroidism. A probable autoimmune disease. In *Textbook of Immunopathology, vol. 2*, ed. P. Miescher and P. Graber.

BLIZZARD, R. M., CHEE, D. & DAVIS, W. (1966). The incidence of parathyroid and other antibodies in the serum of patients with idiopathic hypoparathyroidism. *Clin. exp. Immunol.*, **1**, 119.

BLIZZARD, R. M. & KYLE, M. (1963). Studies of the adrenal antigens and antibodies in Addison's disease. *J. clin. Invest.*, **42**, 1653.

CARNEIRO, L., DONNINGTON, K. J. & MUNRO, D. S. (1966). Recovery of the long-acting thyroid stimulator from serum of patients with thyrotoxicosis by concentration of immunoglobulin. *Clin. Sci.*, **31**, 215.

HALPERN, B., NGUYEN, K. & ROBERT, B. (1964). Etudie immunologique d'un cas exceptionnel de sensibilisation spontanée au semen humain. *C.R. Acad. Sci., Paris*, **259**, 2025.

IRVINE, W. J. (1968). Immunological aspects of ovarian failure with Addison's disease. *Lancet*, **2**, 883.

IRVINE, W. J. & SCARTH, L. (1969). Antibody to the oxyphil cells of the human parathyroid in idiopathic hypoparathyroidism. *Clin. exp. Immunol.*, **4**, 505.

RÜHMKE, PH. (1965). Autospermagglutinins: A cause of infertility in men. *Ann. N.Y. Acad. Sci.*, **124**, 696.

THE GASTRO-INTESTINAL TRACT

The Stomach

Three types of antibody are found in pernicious anaemia.

1. Intrinsic-factor blocking antibody. This prevents the combination of intrinsic factor with vitamin B_{12} and may be detected in 50 to 60 per cent of cases.

2. Intrinsic-factor binding antibody. This is less common and binds on to a different part of the intrinsic-factor molecule. It does not prevent the combination of intrinsic-factor with B_{12} but prevents its uptake by the intestinal mucosa.

3. Antibody reactive with the microsomes of the gastric parietal cells. This is most easily detected by immunofluorescent methods, and is present in 90 per cent of adults with pernicious anaemia and in other situations where atrophic gastritis is present, though in this case intrinsic-factor antibodies are absent.

The rare juvenile subjects with atrophic gastritis and megaloblastic anaemia all have intrinsic-factor antibodies but do not as rule have parietal cell antibodies. Thus the finding of intrinsic-factor antibodies is of diagnostic value, and although they are not present in every case of pernicious anaemia there are no false positives. Although parietal cell antibodies occur almost invariably in pernicious anaemia, they may also be found in atrophic gastritis.

Steroid administration has been shown to lead to a restoration of gastric cells and a reversal of the changes of atrophic gastritis as shown by biopsy. There is also a recovery of the ability to secrete acid (Ardeman and Chanarin, 1965). The duration of this effect is unknown, and it is of theoretical interest only, since the complications of corticosteroid treatment are so much greater than those of simple replacement therapy. They do, however, suggest that most, if not all, the features of the disease are secondary to the lymphocytic gastritis and the other associated immunological changes.

Ulcerative Colitis and Crohn's Disease

These diseases are associated with other disorders of a possible allergic nature, e.g. iritis, erythema nodosum, arthritis and aphthous ulcers of the mouth. Many patients with Crohn's disease (Deodhar et al., 1969) or with ulcerative colitis have antibodies that react with the duct cells present in human and animal colon. In many cases these antibodies cross-react with an antigen in O14 strain of E. coli. The implication is that an immune reaction provoked by an E. coli infection may be self-damaging. There is also evidence that lymphocytes from patients with ulcerative colitis may be cytotoxic for human colon cells in tissue culture, and this may be of some importance in the aetiology of the disease (Perlmann and Broberger, 1963). The response to corticosteroid or immunosuppressive treatment is certainly consistent with the view that cell-mediated immune damage plays an aetiological role in these diseases. Recently (Brooke et al., 1969) azathioprine has been shown to be effective even in advanced cases of Crohn's disease with fistulae.

Gluten Induced Enteropathy

High titres of antibody to gliadin—a fraction of gluten—have been found in patients with this disease but not in tropical sprue (Kivel et al., 1964). In patients maintained on a gluten-free diet the rapid development of a lymphocytic inflammatory reaction in the mucosa after the introduction of gluten into the ileum also indicated a possible allergic aetiology for this disease (Rubin *et al.*, 1960). The immunological basis of gluten enteropathy is thus a little more clearly defined, though some problems remain. There is a deficiency of circulating IgM in 37 per cent of patients (Hobbs and Hepner, 1968) and this is remedied by a gluten-free diet. The significance of this finding is not clear.

Diseases of the Liver

Increased serum immunoglobulin levels are found in both acute and chronic liver disease. The blood level of IgA is elevated, especially in portal cirrhosis, in which it contributes to the apparent merging of the beta- and gammaglobulin peaks on electrophoresis. The IgM level is raised, especially in primary biliary cirrhosis, and so is the level of IgG in chronic active hepatitis, in which it may reach 4–6 g/100 ml. Another indication of altered immune reaction is the high incidence of biologically false positive serological tests for syphilis and the finding of positive tests for rheumatoid factor and other autoantibodies. These autoantibodies may react with the nuclei or mitochondria of cells, with smooth muscle, and with bile ductules. Auto-antibodies are especially liable to be present in three chronic liver diseases—chronic active hepatitis (also known as lupoid hepatitis, or juvenile cirrhosis), primary biliary cirrhosis, and cryptogenic cirrhosis (Berg *et al.*, 1967). They are not found in cirrhosis secondary to a metabolic disorder such as Wilson's disease or haemochromatosis. Nor are they present in jaundice due to extra-hepatic obstruction or in secondary biliary cirrhosis.

Although many of the clinical features of chronic active hepatitis are like systemic lupus—hence the term lupoid hepatitis—the two diseases are distinct, and liver involvement is very uncommon in true systemic lupus.

Antinuclear antibodies are found in 80 per cent of cases of chronic active hepatitis and smooth muscle antibodies in 60 per cent. Mitochondrial antibodies, though less common in this disease, are found in 90 per cent of cases of primary biliary cirrhosis. Nevertheless, there is a strong serological and clinical overlap between these diseases. Doniach and Walker (1969) have recently put forward a unifying hypothesis and suggest that auto-immune hepatitis, whatever its actual cause, may present with the clinical features of either chronic hepatitis or biliary cirrhosis, depending on whether hepatic parenchymal cells or biliary ductules are the main targets of immune aggression. Cryptogenic cirrhosis may in many cases represent the end stage of either condition. The proof for this suggestion must await evidence that cell-mediated immune injury occurs in the liver, for the autoantibodies are not themselves pathogenic and may occur occasionally as a secondary phenomenon in various forms of liver injury, acute and chronic, infectious or toxic.

Whatever their relationship to the aetiological process, autoantibodies are useful pointers in the differential diagnosis of hepatic diseases. It is of interest that there is a marked histological similarity between chronic active hepatitis and a homologous liver transplant undergoing rejection (Popper et al., 1965).

REFERENCES

ARDEMAN, S. & CHANARIN, I. (1965). Steroids and Addisonian pernicious anaemia. New Engl. J. Med., 273, 1352.

BERG, P. A., DONIACH, D. & ROITT, I. M. (1967). Mitochondrial antibodies in primary biliary cirrhosis. J. esp. Med., 126, 277.

BROOKE, B. N., HOFFMANN, D. C. & SWARBRICK, E. T. (1969). Azathioprine for Crohn's Disease. Lancet, 2, 612.

DEODHAR, S. D., MICKENER, W. M. & FARMER, R. G. (1969). A study of the immunological aspects of chronic ulcerative colitis and transmural colitis. Amer. J. clin. Path., 51, 591.

DONIACH, D. & WALKER, J. G. (1969). A unified concept of autoimmune hepatitis. Lancet, 1, 813.

HOBBS, J. R. & HEPNER, G. (1968). Deficiency of gamma M. globulin in coeliac disease. Lancet, 1, 217.

KIVEL, R. M., KEARNS, D. H. & LIEBOWITZ, D. (1964). Significance of antibodies to dietary proteins in the serum of patients with non-tropical sprue. New Engl. J. Med., 271, 769.

PERLMANN, P. & BROBERGER, O. (1963). In vitro studies of ulcerative colitis. II. Cytotoxic action of white blood cells from patients on human foetal colon cells. J. exp. Med., 117, 717.

POPPER, H., PARONETTO, F. & SCHAFFNER, F. (1965). Immune processes in the pathogenesis of liver disease. Ann. N.Y. Acad. Sci., 124, 781.

RUBIN, C. E., BRANDBORG, L. L., FLICK, A. L., PHELPS, P., PARMENTIER, C. & VAN NIEL, S. (1960). Effect of wheat installation into the proximal ileum of patients on a gluten-free diet, in celiac sprue. Gastroenterology, 43, 621.

IMMUNE DISORDERS OF THE EYES

There are two diseases in which an abnormal immune response may be involved.

Phacogenic uveitis follows injury to the lens, and may sometimes follow a cataract operation. In this condition, a sterile inflammatory reaction results from the liberation of lens material into the eye. It is typically uniocular, and in one study seven out of twelve patients had anti-lens antibodies as compared with two out of 75 control subjects (Luntz, 1964).

Sympathetic ophthalmia is a rare condition which occasionally follows a perforating wound of the eye involving the ciliary body or root of the iris. After a period of weeks uveitis develops in the uninjured eye and both eyes form granulation tissue with progressive damage, leading in most untreated

D

cases to permanent blindness. Early removal of the injured eye may reverse this condition, and large doses of corticosteroids have a suppressive effect. The condition is associated with cellular hypersensitivity to proteins of the uveal tract, and with a positive skin test when these proteins are injected.

Tests for the presence of circulating antibodies against uveal proteins may be of some diagnostic value after an eye wound. It is normal for these antibodies to develop during healing reactions following uveal injury, but circulating antibodies are absent in sympathetic ophthalmia. On the other hand, the skin reaction to uveal extracts in sympathetic ophthalmia indicates a state of cellular hypersensitivity. This delayed hypersensitivity is in fact the basis of the disease.

DISORDERS OF THE NERVOUS SYSTEM

Autoimmune allergic encephalomyelitis can be produced in experimental animals by injections of brain tissue and Freund's adjuvant. An allergic basis has also been attributed to various human neurological disorders, such as the rare form of allergic encephalomyelitis that follows vaccination with rabies virus, when the virus has been grown on rabbit spinal cord. More important than this rare disease are the immunological reactions which affect the nervous system during very common virus infections. There is an analogy with lymphocytic choriomeningitis in mice, which is most lethal in those animals which develop a brisk immune response of the delayed hypersensitivity type. In man, when neurological symptoms develop during the course of measles, rubella, mumps, or after vaccination, immunological mechanisms are probably as important in determining the pattern of the disease as is the virus itself. There is usually a delay of a week or more after the febrile stage of the infection before the neurological disorder manifests itself. Perivascular lymphocytic infiltration and areas of demyelination occur, and these are reminiscent of those seen in experimental allergic encephalomyelitis.

Idiopathic polyneuritis of the type described by Guillain and Barré may also represent an infective condition with immunological overtones. This condition has been observed to follow 1 to 30 days after a non-specific infection, and is associated with perivascular lymphocytic infiltration of spinal roots and nerves (Asbury et al., 1969). This is reminiscent of the allergic neuritis which follows when experimental animals are injected with peripheral nerve and Freund's adjuvant.

It is tempting to look for other analogous situations in which an immune response may influence or cause neurological disease. In multiple sclerosis a number of patients have been shown to have humoral antibodies against brain antigens. However, evidence of cellular hypersensitivity is lacking in these patients, and skin tests for hypersensitivity give negative results. Also, similar antibodies against brain antigens have been found in other neurological disorders, including occasional cases of cerebral arterial disease. These antibodies may well be a secondary reaction to brain damage, and the underlying cause of the brain damage in multiple sclerosis remains as uncertain as ever. One current theory is that a slow virus may be present, similar to the agent which causes scrapie in sheep. A fresh interest in this theory has been aroused by the discovery that another insidious neurological disorder, subacute sclerosing panencephalitis, is associated with the presence of measles antibodies in the blood and electron microscopic evidence of a virus infection (Legg, 1967). Although the histological features are not comparable with those of multiple sclerosis, much further research is needed. Even a clear demonstration of some type of autoimmune reaction in multiple sclerosis cannot exclude the possibility of an important, underlying virus infection.

REFERENCES

ASBURY, A. K., ARNASON, B. G. & ADAMS, R. D. (1969). The inflammatory lesion in idiopathic polyneuritis: its role in pathogenesis. *Medicine, Baltimore*, **48**, 173.

LEGG, N. G. (1967). Virus antibodies in subacute sclerosing panencephalitis: a study of 22 patients. *Brit. med. J.*, **3**, 350.

LUNTZ, M. H. (1964). Autoimmune responses to lens and uveal protein. *S. Afr. med. J.*, **38**, 130.

IMMUNOSUPPRESSION

For the purpose of treatment, immune reactions may be suppressed by a variety of agents which damage lymphocytes. If this can be achieved by methods which do not affect the production of circulating antibodies, this has the advantage of leaving an important defence mechanism intact and allows the subject to respond to bacterial infections.

Lymphoid cells are rapidly destroyed by irradiation and by a variety of drugs which include the corticosteroids, colchicine, certain antibiotics, and the nitrogen mustards. These agents interfere at specific points in the metabolic pathways which synthesize DNA, RNA, proteins or other materials necessary for cell division. However, immunosuppressive drugs which act by interfering with cell division are likely to damage the rapidly proliferating cells of the bone marrow and the gut. There is also the risk that a suppression of cellular immunity may cause some increase in the susceptibility to bacterial infections and a markedly increased susceptibility to viral or fungal infections. It may also impair the body's resistance to the origin and spread of cancer.

A depression of cell proliferation is the basis of the chemotherapy of cancer, and antimitotic agents developed for this purpose are often toxic to lymphoid cells. The same applies to antibiotics employed to interfere with bacterial proliferation or cell wall synthesis. It is no accident that X-ray therapy and the cytotoxic anti-cancer drugs are also potent immuno-suppressive agents, and chloramphenicol is an example of an antibiotic which is immunosuppressive, at least in animals, and interferes with protein synthesis.

In searching for more effective immunosuppressive agents, it is unfor-tunate that experimental results cannot always be transferred to another species. For example, 6-mercaptopurine is an effective immunosuppressive drug in rabbits but not in mice. Methotrexate, on the other hand, is rapidly destroyed by the high levels of aldehyde oxidase in rabbit liver and is useless in this species (Redetzki et al., 1966). In the modest doses used in treating renal or connective tissue diseases in man neither of these drugs is a very effective immunosuppressive agent, but the clinical effect may be satisfactory. The most dramatic effect of methotrexate is seen in psoriasis, where no immunological abnormality has been described. In the empirical situation in which drugs are given to treat human diseases of unknown origin some of the most successful agents may not act entirely in the manner intended. Some of the drugs used have not only immunosuppressive but also anti-inflammatory, anti-viral and anti-bacterial effects, each of which may con-tribute to the effect of the drug in a particular situation.

Anti-lymphocyte globulin (ALG) is the product of a search for more selective agents, and will be considered in detail below. A current aim is the specific suppression of reactions to individual antigens or of reactions involving one specific type of immune response.

The possible ways in which an inflammatory immune reaction may be suppressed are various:

1. Removal of the provoking antigen or the induction of specific tolerance to it

An example is the dramatically successful use of Rhesus antiserum in preventing Rhesus disease (Clarke, 1967). Protection is achieved by giving anti-D serum to the Rhesus-negative mother following parturition or an abortion. At these times a transplacental bleed of foetal cells commonly occurs. However, any Rhesus-positive cells that reach the mother's blood stream are rapidly coated with antibody and removed once antiserum has been given. The mother cannot produce an immune response to these coated cells and so avoids being sensitized against a subsequent pregnancy.

2. The general suppression of the immune response, both cellular and humoral

Any agent which damages lymphoid tissue sufficiently will cause immuno-suppression. This applies to X-ray therapy and to other agents which damage cells or interfere with the division of cell nuclei.

The precise mode of action of many of these agents is now known. For example, X-rays are responsible for scission or fragmentation of the DNA chain. 6-mercaptopurine and its derivative azathioprine prevent the metabolism of the purine inosinic acid along the pathway which leads to DNA and RNA synthesis. The chief effect of folic acid antagonists is to inhibit the formation of tetrahydrofolic acid, which has several functions and is of importance in the synthesis of thymidylate, a component of DNA. A number of other antimetabolites, such as fluouracil, introduce bogus substance into an incomplete or abnormally functioning nucleic acid. Alkylating agents, including chlorambucil, melphalan, cyclophosphamide, and other nitrogen mustards, form cross-links which interfere with the separation of the two strands of DNA in the course of cell reproduction. Corticosteroids and antilymphocyte globulin appear to cause lymphocyte destruction but the mechanism is not entirely clear. Actinomycin interferes with the synthesis of the RNA template.

3. Inhibition of the inflammatory response

Many drugs introduced as immunosuppressive agents depend on an anti-inflammatory action for much of their effect: 6-mercaptopurine was introduced by Schwartz et al. (1959) because it was shown to prevent a primary immune response to foreign serum protein injected into rabbits. It has been used in several diseases, including systemic lupus, glomerulonephritis, and rheumatoid arthritis, and appears to be effective in the "minimal change" type of glomerulonephritis in which no abnormal immune reaction has been demonstrated. This anomaly may in part be explained by its potent anti-inflammatory effect (Page et al., 1962; Hurd and Ziff, 1968). In the case of azathioprine, this anti-inflammatory effect may be of considerable value in the management of patients with systemic lupus or other severe collagen disorders who are dependent on large doses of corticosteroids. Used for its steroid-sparing action, azathioprine may be continued in a dosage of 3 mg/kg/day for many months in combination with a reduced dose of corticosteroids. In view of its ability to suppress the bone marrow, its use should be monitored by a weekly total white cell count and examination of the platelets. The dose should be reduced or stopped if the count falls to dangerous levels.

Much of the dramatic effectiveness of corticosteroids or ACTH depends on an anti-inflammatory action, perhaps associated with the decreased permeability of cell membranes which these substances cause. The action of corticosteroids is not simple, and they also have a toxic effect on lymphocytes. The results of long-term corticosteroid treatment are often disappointing, and these drugs have hazards and side-effects which make it preferable to limit their use to potentially fatal disorders such as status asthmaticus or fulminating rheumatic fever. Despite these disadvantages, many allergic or immune disorders are treated with corticosteroids for want of a better drug. It must be accepted that with doses of 50 mg cortisone daily (or the equivalent) side-effects become inevitable.

It is possible to reduce the side-effects of corticosteroids by giving either corticotrophin or a corticosteroid on alternate days. It is not always possible to follow this regime because of increased activity of the disease on the days without corticosteroids, but it has been used successfully in the nephrotic syndrome, in juvenile rheumatoid arthritis, and in systemic lupus (Martin et al., 1968).

The mode of action of a number of other drugs depends on an anti-inflammatory effect. Antihistamines and drugs which antagonize the action of serotonin are widely used in allergic disorders and are of particular value in reactions which involve reaginic antibody. In disorders which involve the lungs, inhalations of disodium cromoglycate (Intal) inhibit the release of histamine and of vasoactive substances. This can prevent asthmatic attacks provoked by an inhaled allergen and can also inhibit both the asthmatic and late systemic reactions seen in the extrinsic alveolitis of bird-fancier's lung.

The use of other anti-inflammatory agents plays some part in most of the connective tissue diseases, and in one of the most common, rheumatoid arthritis, aspirin is the major and often the only drug used. The main anti-inflammatory effects of salicylates, like those of corticosteroids, may depend on an effect on cell membrane permeability. They may help to maintain the integrity of the vascular endothelium (Willoughby and Walters, 1965) and of the ground substance between the cells.

Anti-lymphocyte globulin. A preparation which is unique in its effects is the IgG fraction of anti-lymphocyte serum. This serum is raised by immunizing an animal with lymphocytes of a foreign species. It acts by coating or eliminating the circulating small lymphocytes which mediate the cellular immune reactions, and it may itself act as a distracting ineffective antigenic stimulus. As humoral antibodies are much less affected than the cellular response the subject's resistance to bacterial infections is left almost intact, although other types of infection may be potentiated. Although there have been no controlled trials of its use in man, its widespread use in transplant surgery is based on its very striking effect in prolonging the survival of homografts in animals.

The doses in which anti-lymphocyte globulin has been used in animals have been very much higher than the doses used in man, and non-specific stress may account for some of its effects. Nevertheless, it is encouraging that in the experimental animal it can not only prevent the development of allergic encephalomyelitis (Waksman et al., 1961), but also has some effect on the disease once it has developed (Leibowitz et al., 1968). It can also prevent the development of experimental "adjuvant" arthritis (Currey and Ziff, 1966).

For these reasons its use has been proposed, in combination with various immunosuppressive drugs, in other immune disorders in man. Before its effectiveness can be assessed, less toxic preparations are needed. Even if local pain and thrombocytopenia can be avoided, there may be troublesome complications of serum therapy to contend with, such as anaphylaxis and the kidney damage which immune complexes can cause. As in animals, it may eventually prove possible to prevent these complications by first making the patient tolerant to the animal protein used.

Complications of immunosuppressive therapy

The possible risks of infection, the potentiation of tumours, the hazards of marrow suppression, and the specific complications of the use of anti-lymphocyte globulin have already been touched on. Thrombocytopenia may be first suspected with the development of purpura, bruising, or a spontaneous bleeding tendency. With this complication, as with peptic ulceration, it is difficult to apportion the blame between the different immunosuppressive agents which a patient often receives in combination. The risk of cancer is equally difficult to analyse, and although there is a significantly high incidence of lymphosarcoma and other lymphoreticular tumours in patients receiving immunosuppressive treatment it is not yet known whether the hazard is higher with particular drugs such as azathioprine or anti-lymphocyte globulin. Infection is now the main cause of death in patients who have had renal homografts and are receiving immunosuppressive drugs. This includes infection with normally harmless organisms from the patient's own skin or mucous membrane. These opportunistic infections include *Herpes simplex*, *Candida albicans*, cryptococci, and *Pneumocystis carinii*. There is also a high incidence of infections with Gram-negative organisms of relatively low virulence, which often have a high resistance to the antibiotics given in the early stages of the patient's infection.

The individual immunosuppressive drugs may have other characteristic toxic effects of their own. Since methotrexate and cyclophosphamide are largely excreted in the urine, their toxic effects as well as their clinical effectiveness are strikingly increased in patients with renal failure. The dose of 6-mercaptopurine or azathioprine must also be reduced if renal failure develops. Various methods of reducing toxicity have been attempted, and methotrexate is characteristically given in a weekly intravenous dose; 30 mg given weekly in this way has been found to cause less oral ulceration and less nausea than 3 mg given daily. Alternatively, methotrexate may be given for periods of one month, followed by intervals of one month, and when used in this way it has produced impressive results in the treatment of severe psoriasis.

Oral ulcers, nausea and vomiting are possibly the most troublesome of the toxic effects caused by methotrexate. As with many other cytotoxic agents, a dangerous degree of marrow depression is occasionally seen with this drug, and a megaloblastic anaemia can also occur. Hepatic dysfunction is a less frequent complication. The toxic effects of methotrexate are sometimes reversible by folinic acid.

Marrow depression, thrombocytopenia, nausea and vomiting are also seen with the use of 6-mercaptopurine, and so are cholestatic jaundice and skin pigmentation. Cyclophosphamide is less liable to cause a serious degree of marrow depression, and even if a severe leucopaenia appears the recovery rate is high. On the other hand, alopecia is a frequent complication and, although it is always reversible it is often intensely disliked by patients. Cyclophosphamide may also induce a chemical cystitis.

Other occasional complications of immunosuppressive drugs include gross muscular wasting. This is seen in patients on azathioprine, but is much more common in patients who are receiving corticosteroids, and who may have other features of florid Cushing's syndrome.

There are a few conditions in which immunosuppression is an end in itself. This is so in transplantation surgery and in allergic reactions due to a drug or to some other transient stimulus. In most of the situations in which they are used, however, immunosuppressive drugs are of palliative and symptomatic value only. These agents damage the body's defences, are toxic in other ways and, in general, do nothing to control the underlying cause of a disease. More specific methods of immunosuppression are therefore needed, as in the prevention of Rhesus disease with Rhesus antiserum. French and Batchelor (1969) have used a specific "enhancing" antiserum to prolong the life of homografts in dogs; presumably the antibody in this serum covers the vascular endothelium and other areas where an immune reaction might be initiated. Another approach has been suggested by Calne et al. (1969) who induced tolerance to transplantation antigens with cellular extracts derived from the liver. Until methods such as these are more generally applicable, the toxicity of immunosuppressive treatment will continue to limit its usefulness.

REFERENCES

CALNE, R. Y., SELLS, R. A., PENA, J. R., DAVIS, D. R., MILLARD, P. R., HERBERTSON, B. M., BINNS, R. M. & DAVIES, D. A. L. (1969). Induction of immune tolerance by porcine liver allograft. *Nature, Lond.*, **223**, 472.

CLARKE, C. A. (1967). Prevention of Rh-haemolytic disease. *Brit. med. J.*, **4**, 7.

CURREY, H. L. F. & ZIFF, M. (1966). Suppression of experimentally induced polyarthritis in the rat by heterologous A. L. S. *Lancet*, **2**, 889.

FRENCH, M. F. & BATCHELOR, J. R. (1969). Immunological enhancement of rat kidney grafts. *Lancet*, **2**, 1103.

HURD, E. R. & ZIFF, M. (1968). Studies on the anti-inflammatory action of 6-mercaptopurine. *J. exp. Med.*, **128**, 785.

LEIBOWITZ, S., LESSOF, M. H. & KENNEDY, L. (1968). The effect of anti-lymphocyte serum on experimental allergic encephalomyelitis in the guinea pig. *Clin. exp. Immunol.*, **3**, 753.

MARTIN, M. M., GABOARDI, F., PODOLSKY, S., RAITI, S. & CALCAGNO, P. L. (1968). Intermittent steroid therapy. *New Engl. J. Med.*, **279**, 273.

PAGE, A. R., CONDIE, R. M. & GOOD, R. A. (1962). Effect of 6-mercaptopurine on inflammation. *Amer. J. Path.*, **40**, 519.

REDETZKI, H. M., REDETZKI, J. E. & ELIAS, A. L. (1966). Resistance of the rabbit to methotrexate: isolation of a drug metabolite with decreased cytotoxicity. *Biochem. Pharmacol.*, **15**, 425.

SCHWARTZ, R., EISNER, A. & DAMASHEK, W. (1959). The effect of 6-MP on the primary and secondary immune response. *J. clin. Invest.*, **13**, 1394.

WAKSMAN, B. H., ARBOUYS, S. & ARNASON, B. G. (1961). The use of specific lymphocyte antisera to inhibit hypersensitive reactions of the "delayed type". *J. exp. Med.*, **114**, 997.

WILLOUGHBY, D. A. & WALTERS, M. N.-I. (1965). The effect of ribonucleic acid on vascular permeability and its possible relationship to LNPF. *J. Path. Bact.*, **90**, 193.

3 Gastroenterology

BRIAN CREAMER

BILE SALTS. INTESTINAL BACTERIA. SMALL INTESTINE
RESECTIONS. THE IMMUNE SYSTEM IN GUT DISEASE

OVER the past few years, progress in three fields, namely bile salts, intestinal
bacteria and the effects of resection of the small intestine, have been spectacular. Furthermore, much of this advance has integrated so that knowledge
has become comprehensive rather than fragmentary, with the satisfactory
sensation of a jig-saw puzzle clicking into place. In the first half of this chapter,
these stories are woven together to make a running narrative.

BILE SALTS

While a considerable amount of knowledge has accumulated about bile
salts in a hundred years, it is the recent application of the concepts of detergent chemistry, particularly by Borgstrom and Hofmann, that has suddenly
produced an understanding of their role in fat absorption.* Bile salts are
ubiquitous among vertebrates, though there is a remarkable range of chemical
structure seeming to imply an evolutionary process. In man at least six
different bile salts are found, but the reason for this diversity is unknown.

Bile salts act as detergents to solubilize fat. In structure they are part fat,
part amino-acid, being formed in the liver from cholesterol to the intermediary
bile acid and then conjugated with glycerine or taurine. The whole molecule
is water-soluble, but the affinity to fat gives it the distinctive detergent property; such substances are called amphipaths. If a solution of bile salts
reaches a certain concentration, the molecules aggregate into patterns
called *micelles*. The bile salts are oriented with the fat-soluble part opposed
and the water-soluble pole on the outside. Micelles are usually pictured as
spheres, and this is probably the common form, but with increasing concentration of bile salts, rods, helices and lamellar structures are found,

* A number of key articles and reviews are listed in the references.

although this is probably outside the physiological range. Micelles are not permanent structures, and are constantly breaking down and reforming, the bile salts changing with those in the surrounding liquid. The interior of a micelle is a fat solution the consistency of petrol. Within this, other fatty substances can be dissolved; indeed, a large amount of cholesterol is excreted in bile and this is suspended in micellar form.

The ability of micelles to dissolve fat in their interior is modified by their incorporating monoglycerides formed by the pancreatic lipolysis of tri-glyceride. Monoglycerides are also molecules with a water-soluble end— glycerol, and a fat-soluble part—fatty acid, and they arrange themselves alongside bile salts in the micelle wall. The resultant interior has an improved fat solubilizing property so that fatty acids, fat-soluble vitamins and other substances are taken up. Such a solution of fat-laden micelles appears water-clear.

To complete the picture it should be remembered that bile salts also facili-tate the dispersion of globular fat into a fine emulsion with a large surface area for pancreatic lipase, and may even facilitate the action of lipase. Micelles pass to the brush border of the intestinal epithelial cells and in some way discharge their burden, but this part of the process is obscure. Bile salts are poorly absorbed by the proximal small intestine, and return to the lumen to repeat the micellar transport. This poor absorption of bile is clearly crucial to the maintenance of a critical concentration to form micelles.

Enterohepatic circulation

While little bile salt is absorbed in the upper small intestine only a small amount reaches the colon. It is established that most of the bile salts are reabsorbed in the ileum by an active transport process that can be blocked by inhibitors such as ouabain. From this site the bile salts travel up the portal circulation in a protein-bound form. In the liver they are avidly extracted and re-excreted in bile, so that a constant recirculation takes place. Of the small amount of bile salt that reaches the colon, much is deconjugated by bacterial action to bile acids, and some of these are absorbed. The liver reconstitutes them to bile salts and they add to the enterohepatic circulation.

In healthy persons the bile salt pool is of the order of 3 g, but about 18 g of bile salts is excreted daily into the intestine. This means six cycles daily or twice each meal. About 600 mg is lost in the stool each day, and hepatic synthesis exactly balances this to keep the pool size constant.

Bile salts in disease

The crucial parts of this system, the necessity for a critical concentration of bile salts and the conservation of the enterohepatic circulation, are vividly demonstrated in disease states. Clearly if bile-salt production fails, as it may do in liver disease, or if bile excretion is blocked, steatorrhoea will result.

However, interruption of the enterohepatic circulation by the stagnant loop syndrome and in ileal disease or resection is not so immediately obvious.

Stagnant loop syndrome

This title (preferred to the blind loop syndrome) covers a whole range of anatomical and function conditions—diverticulosis, surgically created cul-de-sacs, internal fistulae and strictures, afferent loops of gastrectomies, and scleroderma—which are united by the common factor of an increased and abnormal small bowel flora. This flourishes in the stagnant backwaters of poorly emptying diverticulae and loops, in feebly mobile and dilated bowel, and through jejuno-colic and ileo-colic fistulae. The clinical picture is of diarrhoea, steatorrhoea and vitamin B_{12} malabsorption.

BACTERIOLOGY OF THE SMALL INTESTINE

The concept that the healthy small intestine is sterile is untrue. Previous studies have been hindered by doubts about the validity of using simple open-ended tubes for collecting intestinal juice (shown to be groundless), and even more by difficulty in culturing all the organisms. Recent work has revealed a substantial flora in health. The duodenum and jejunum usually has a population of 10^3 to 10^4 bacteria per ml of fluid. The common organisms are *streptococci, staphylococci* and *lactobacilli,* while fungi may also be present. These organisms are similar to the oropharyngeal flora and probably come from this area. There is little doubt that gastric acidity is normally a barrier to many organisms and in achlorhydria an increased flora may be found. By contrast the ileum has more colonic-type bacteria, coliforms, bacteroides and bifobacteria. In the upper small intestine the flora may fluctuate with meals and increase after eating. Some of the bacteria are intimately associated with the mucous layer, and cannot be cleared by washing.

The function of the small bowel flora in health is unknown, and germ-free animals show no obvious deficiency. However, the bacteria certainly dictate the structure and turnover of the intestinal epithelium. In the germ-free animal villi are slender, with few lymphocytes and plasma cells, while the life of the epithelial cells is twice the normal span.

Bacteria in the stagnant loop syndrome

The population of organisms in the small intestine is increased, and cultures show concentrations of 10^4 to 10^9 per ml. Cultures from multiple sites show that the greatest increase in organisms is related to the level and type of lesion. Therefore, in a stricture of the terminal ileum only, the ileal flora may be increased, while in jejunal diverticulosis the whole small intestine shows the change. In localized proximal lesions such as duodenal diverticulum, the greatest change may be confined to the duodenum and upper jejunum. The organisms are more commonly colonic in type, with many anaerobes such as bacteroides and bifobacteria, though it has been estimated that as many as twenty different organisms may be present.

Steatorrhoea in the stagnant loop syndrome

Steatorrhoea is not found in every case, but where it is present the upper small bowel has an abnormal flora. Mucosal damage has been reported, but in most instances the biopsy findings, including electron microscopy, have been quite normal, so it is most unlikely that the steatorrhoea is mucosal in origin. In these cases the luminal fluid contains free bile acids, and there is now ample evidence that bacteria cause the deconjugation. The anaerobe *bacteroides* is almost certainly the chief offender and can be shown to split bile salts *in vitro*. With deconjugation, the concentration of bile salts falls below the critical micellar level of 5 m/moles per litre. Below this concentration, micelles are not formed and fat absorption is impaired.

Confirmation of this mechanism has come from the dramatic reversal of steatorrhoea by antibiotics and by the improvement on giving bile salts orally. However, this improvement of fat absorption with bile salts may be accompanied by a worsening diarrhoea, as bile salts and acids in excess have a purgative action. The ordinary commercial preparations of bile salts now available are without this beneficial effect, and a simple therapeutic detergent has not yet emerged.

Other causes of bile salt inactivity

Steatorrhoea is frequently present in the Zollinger-Ellison syndrome, and has been known for years to accompany the administration of neomycin. Bile salts not only have an optimum pH from 6 to 8, but outside this range they become inactive. Thus in the Zollinger-Ellison syndrome the large volumes of acid that flood into the small intestine may lower jejunal pH to 2, with the effect of causing a subcritical concentration of bile salts.

Neomycin has the property of precipitating bile salts in insoluble complexes, and once again producing a subcritical concentration. However, its effects may be more complex, and there is evidence that pancreatic lipase is inhibited.

Bacteria and amino-acids

An abnormal small intestinal flora does not only alter the bile salts. The full effect of their metabolism on all substances of the luminal contents is unknown, but there is good evidence that amino-acids are implicated. An excess of indican in the urine is known to be a measure of bacterial activity in the small intestine. Indican (Indoxyl sulphate) is the bacterial metabolite of tryptophan, and it is absorbed and excreted unchanged in the urine. Several other amino-acids are metabolized; phenylalanine and tyrosine are changed into volatile phenols, while ornithine, argenine, lysine and glycine are changed into piperidine, pyrrolidine and other amines. Indican can be conveniently measured and is expressed as a 24-hour urinary output, the normal range being from 23 to 92 mg per day. Patients with the stagnant loop syndrome have levels from 150 to 350 mg per day. However, some increase may occur in other malabsorptions such as the coeliac syndrome or in intestinal resections. By contrast, pancreatic steatorrhoea is accompanied by a normal or low indican excretion.

This abnormal metabolism of amino-acids may also deplete the intake, and can be a source of protein depletion in the case of essential amino-acids: the urinary excretion of indican may amount to two-thirds of the dietary intake of tryptophan.

Bacteria and anaemia

Megaloblastic anaemia frequently complicates stagnant loops and is caused by vitamin B_{12} deficiency. Absorption of vitamin B_{12} is diminished, but the exact mechanism by which bacteria influence this has not yet been settled. Evidence has been produced that *E. coli* can sequestrate vitamin B_{12}, and may utilize the vitamin for its own metabolism. However, there has also been some work suggesting that the site of vitamin B_{12} absorption in the distal ileum may be affected by bacterial products so that the transport receptors are blocked. Whatever the mechanism, the abnormality can be swiftly reversed by antibiotics.

An interesting observation is that some patients with the stagnant loop syndrome have high levels of serum folate. The inference is that the abnormal flora may synthesize a folic acid derivative which is absorbed, but whether this is haematologically active and significant is uncertain.

SMALL INTESTINE RESECTIONS

It has been recognized for some time that extensive resections of the small intestine can be compatible with reasonable health; even with only one or two feet remaining, a few patients have remarkably survived. Clearly there is considerable reserve in the normal small intestine, but there is now growing evidence that compensatory hypertrophy takes place. Clinical improvement may occur following resection, in that diarrhoea lessens and absorption tests improve. This compensation is both anatomical and functional.

Anatomical hypertrophy undoubtedly occurs. This is usually negligible in the jejunum if the ileum is removed, but marked in the ileum following resection of the jejunum. Villi increase in size, individual epithelial cells are larger than before, and even cell turnover may be speeded up. Functional hypertrophy follows the same pattern, being greatest in the ileum following jejunal resection. The mechanism of these compensatory changes is uncertain, but the striking response of the ileum suggests that so-called "topical nutrition" may be responsible. This depends on the fact that the small bowel nearest the stomach normally has the greatest concentration of nutrients in the lumen, consequently, if the jejunum is removed the ileum changes from an under-privileged position to one of nutritional affluence.

In spite of this hypertrophy, specialized absorption areas, particularly for vitamin B_{12} and bile salts in the distal ileum, do not reappear if they are resected. This fact explains why jejunal resection is better tolerated than loss of the ileum. Although anatomical and functional hypertrophy is more marked in the ileum if the jejunum is resected than *vice versa*, the failure to reabsorb bile salts is probably the crucial factor.

Resection and bile salts

If the distal small intestine is resected (and in man this probably means at least three to four feet) bile salts are not reabsorbed. There are two con-sequences of this, the first being a swift depletion of the body's pool of bile salts. The reserve capacity of the liver to increase the synthesis of new bile salts is limited, and it is probable that about 3 g daily is the upper limit that can be achieved. This means that the daily output of bile salt is cut to 20 per cent or less of normal, with the consequence that the concentration in the upper small bowel is below the critical level necessary to form micelles. This is the mechanism of steatorrhoea in ileal resection.

The second consequence is that more bile salts than usual enter the colon, even allowing for the depletion. These have a purgative action and are responsible for the diarrhoea that many of these patients suffer. Explosive watery diarrhoea, particularly after meals, frequently follows ileal resection or may accompany Crohn's disease where the ileal function is destroyed. This syndrome has been called *cholerheic enteropathy* by Hofman (1967). A bile-salt binding resin, cholestyramine, sometimes causes a dramatic improve-ment in the diarrhoea, even though the steatorrhoea may be increased.

Gallstones and the liver and bile salts

Clinical observation suggests that gallstones are more common following ileal resection than in the ordinary population. The failure of biliary detergent probably allows cholesterol to come out of solution and may be one of the factors involved. Furthermore, samples of bile from gallstone patients and animals prone to stone formation show that the bile salt : cholesterol ratio lies close to the zone of cholesterol crystallization; in normal bile it lies in the micellar zone, so that there may be a predisposition to this in some people.

Another suggestion comes from the fact that colonic bacteria change the primary bile acids cholate and chenodeoxyoholate to deoxycholate and lithocholate. Lithocholate will produce gallstones if fed to experimental animals.

The enterohepatic circulation may have a special significance for the liver. To quote Hofman; "Thus, the liver is continuously washed with a special detergent, bile salt. This washing transfers substances from the liver to the small intestinal lumen, which are reabsorbed or excreted. Therefore the enterohepatic circulation is analogous to a Soxhlet extraction". Once again, not only may depletion of detergent be a possible factor in disease, but the presence of an abnormal concentration of the secondary bile acid lithocholate might be toxic. Certainly lithocholate in the experimental animal has produced cholestasis and liver damage. It is speculative but tempting to think that the liver disease accompanying Crohn's disease and colitis may be due to the increased formation or increased absorption of lithocholic acid through a damaged colonic mucosa.

REFERENCES

Bile salts

BADLEY, B. W. D., MURPHY, G. M. & BOUCHIER, I. A. D. (1969). Intraluminal bile-salt deficiency in the pathogenesis of steatorrhoea. *Lancet*, 1, 400.

BORGSTRÖM, B., DAHLQUIST, G., LUNDH, G. & SJOVALL, J. (1957). Studies of intestinal digestion and absorption in the human. *J. clin. Invest.*, 36, 1521.

BORGSTRÖM, B., LUNDH, G. & HOFMANN, A. F. (1963). The site of absorption of conjugated bile salts in man. *Gastroenterology*, 45, 229.

DAWSON, A. M. (1968). Fat absorption from the small intestine; the luminal phase. *Fourth Symposium on Advanced Medicine. Pitman Medical.*, p. 235.

HOFMANN, A. F. (1965). Clinical implications of physiochemical studies on bile salts. *Gastroenterology*, 48, 484.

HOFMANN, A. F. (1966). A physiochemical approach to the intraluminal phase of fat absorption. *Gastroenterology*, 50, 56.

HOFMANN, A. F. & BORGSTRÖM, B. (1964). The intraluminal phase of fat digestion in man. *J. clin. Invest.*, 43, 247.

HOFMANN, A. F. & Small, D. M. (1967). Detergent properties of bile salts: correlation with physiological function. *Ann. Rev. Med.*, 18, 333.

WEINER, I. M. & LACK, L. (1968). Bile-salt absorption: enterohepatic circulation. *Handbook of Physiology. Section 6, Vol. 4.* p. 1439.

Small intestinal bacteriology

DONALDSON, R. M. Jr., DOLCINE, H. A. & GRAY, S. J. (1961). Urinary excretion of indolic compounds in rats with intestinal pouches. *Amer. J. Physiol.*, 200, 794.

DRASER, B. S. & SHINER, M. (1969). Studies on the intestinal flora: bacterial flora of the small intestine in patients with gastrointestinal disorders. *Gut*, 10, 812.

DRASER, B. S., SHINTER, M. & McLEOD, G. M. (1969). Studies on the intestinal flora: the bacterial flora of the gastrointestinal tract in healthy and achlorhydric persons. *Gastroenterology*, 56, 71.

NEAL, G. (1968). Protein malabsorption. *Fourth Symposium on Advanced Medicine. Pitman Medical*, p. 260.

TABAQCHALI, S. & BOOTH, C. C. (1966). Jejunal bacteriology and bile-salt metabolism in patients with intestinal malabsorption. *Lancet*, 2, 12.

TABAQCHALI, S. & BOOTH, C. C. (1967). Relationship of the intestinal bacterial flora to absorption. *Brit. med. Bull.*, 23, 285.

TABAQCHALI, S., HATZIOANNOU, J. & BOOTH, C. C. (1968). Bile salts deconjugation and steatorrhoea in patients with the stagnant loop syndrome. *Lancet*, 12, 16.

Small intestinal resection

DOWLING, R. H. (1967). Compensatory changes in intestinal absorption. *Brit. med. Bull.*, 23, 275.

DOWLING, R. H. & BOOTH, C. C. (1966). Functional compensation after small bowel resection in man. *Lancet*, 2, 146.

HEATON, K. W. & READ, A. E. (1969). Gallstones in patients with disorders of the terminal ileum and disturbed bile salt metabolism. *Brit. med. J.*, 2, 494.

HOFMANN, A. F. (1967). The syndrome of ileal disease and the broken enterohepatic circulation: cholerheic enteropathy. *Gastroenterology*, 52, 752.

ROWE, G. G. (1967). Control of tenesmus and diarrhoea by cholestyramine administration. *Gastroenterology*, 53, 1006.

THE IMMUNE SYSTEM IN GUT DISEASE

The gut, as well as being a tube of immunologically active tissue, is a tube of epithelium or muscle. Recent advances in immunology have been reflected in gastroenterology, but in this connection the gut shows certain differences from other organs. This account attempts to review current thinking, but it is important to remember that progress in this area is rapid, and little of the following can be regarded as a final statement.

Immunocytes of the gut

The whole gut is richly endowed with an immunological system; the *lamina propria*, once looked upon as "histological stuffing", has been revealed as an exciting array of immunocytes, mainly lymphocytes, and plasma cells. While these vary from immunocytes elsewhere in the body in the type of immunoglobulin produced, there seems no reason to suppose that they are different from the lymphocytes and plasma cells of other organs.

The immunological cells are present in localized areas and diffused throughout the mucosae. The upper gut is guarded by the tonsils and adenoids; focal collections are also present in the ileum in Peyer's patches, the appendix, and about the anus. In the *lamina propria* of the stomach, small intestine and colon lymphocytes and plasma cells are present between the basement membrane of the epithelium and the *muscularis mucosae*. Furthermore, lymphocytes are frequently seen in the epithelium, where electron micro-scopy shows them to be present between the cells. It is not known whether lymphocytes actually enter the lumen and return again. This mucosal system together with the lymph nodes of the gastro-intestinal tract make up a con-siderable part of the body's immune system, and point to the importance of the gut as a portal of entry for antigens.

Crabbé and Heremans (1966) have delineated the types of immunocytes by identifying the immunoglobulin produced within cells, using specific fluorescent antisera. In lymph nodes from the rest of the body, IgG-producing plasma cells predominate, reflecting the plasma concentrations of immuno-globulin. By contrast, the cells of the lamina propria of the stomach, small intestine and colon show a predominance of IgA-producing cells. The ratio of IgA to IgG cells is 20 to 1, with IgM producing cells in the middle. IgD cells are rarely found in the gut. It is of interest that typical plasma cells are sometimes found in the gut which do not react to any of the known immuno-globulins. The adenoids and appendix have a slightly different pattern, with almost equal numbers of IgA- and IgG-producing cells.

REFERENCES

CRABBÉ, P. A. & HEREMANS, J. F. (1966). The distribution of immunoglobulin-containing cells along the human gastrointestinal tract. *Gastroenterology*, **51**, 305.
CRABBÉ, P. A. & HEREMANS, J. F. (1968). Normal and defective production of immunoglobulins in the intestinal tract. In *Intestinal Absorption and Mal-absorption*. Basel, p. 161.

Immunoglobulins of the gut

As more than 80 per cent of the plasma cells of the gut produce IgA, it is not unexpected that the major immunoglobulin in gastro-intestinal secretions is IgA, and the same holds for other secretory fluids from epithelial surfaces in the body. There are certain important differences between serum IgA and IgA secreted in gastro-intestinal juice. Secretory IgA is heavier; 11S sedimentation in the ultracentrifuge compared with serum IgA which is 7S, and they have different complement-fixing properties. The concept is that IgA is produced in the subepithelial plasma cells and passes through the mucosal cells. Here, two molecules are bound together by a polypeptide, so that a large complex molecule passes out into the lumen as secretory IgA. Some IgA from the subepithelial plasma cells may diffuse into the blood and contribute to serum IgA, and indeed secretory IgA has even been detected in the blood. Secretory IgA is an exocrine immune defence working within the gastro-intestinal lumen, and in support of this it has been shown that the rice-water stools of cholera contain a considerable amount of IgA.

REFERENCES

PLAUT, A. G. & KEONIL, P. (1969). Immunoglobulins in human small intestinal fluids. *Gastroenterology*, **56**, 522.

TOMASI, T. (1968). Current concepts: human immunoglobulins. *New Engl. J. Med.*, **279**, 1327.

Pathological Reactions

The reactions seen in disease range from the appearance of true auto-immune disease to non-specific responses. The disorders and disintegration of the immune system accompanying the coeliac syndrome in the phase when malignancy becomes a common complication are of particular interest.

The coeliac syndrome

This term is synonymous with childhood and adult coeliac disease and idiopathic steatorrhoea. There is no direct evidence that this condition is due to an immune disorder or even to an immune response to gluten. However, histologically there is an intense chronic inflammatory reaction in the *lamina propria* which would appear to be the response to antigens leaking through the abnormal mucosa. It has been shown by immunofluorescent studies that most of the plasma cells are producing IgA as in health. By contrast, the serum immunoglobulins show a mild depletion of IgM in about 61 per cent of adult cases, which returns to normal with successful treatment by gluten withdrawal. There is some evidence that IgM-producing cells are relatively increased in number in the small intestine, but turnover studies are conflicting, some showing a normal catabolism but a diminished synthesis of IgM, others a normal synthesis but increased intestinal loss. Some workers have shown a similar diminution of serum IgG. IgA may be moderately elevated, but this happens in many diseases, and is probably non-specific.

A number of cases of the coeliac syndrome with selective IgA deficiency in the serum have been reported. In the normal population this deficiency turns up about once in every 700 adults. The incidence in the coeliac syndrome is unknown but probably more frequent than this, being two out of 75 in one series (Hobbs and Hepner, 1968). The deficiency is reflected in the small intestine, there being few IgA-secreting cells in these cases. Furthermore, the deficiency persists in spite of treatment. It is difficult to assess the situation, but it looks as though IgA-deficient subjects may be susceptible to, or share a linkage with, the coeliac syndrome.

REFERENCES

ASQUITH, P., THOMPSON, R. A. & COOKE, W. T. (1969). Serum-immunoglobulins in adult coeliac disease. *Lancet*, **2**, 129.

BROWN, D. L., COOPER, A. G. & HEPNER, G. W. (1969). IgM metabolism in coeliac disease. *Lancet*, 1, 858.
HOBBS, J. R. & HEPNER, G. W. (1968). Deficiency of 8-M-globulin in coeliac disease. *Lancet*, 1, 217.
RUBIN, W., FARREI, A. S., SLEISENGER, M. H. & JEFFRIES, G. H. (1965). Immuno-fluorescent studies in adult coeliac disease. *J. clin. Invest.*, 44, 475.

Steatorrhoea and hypogammaglobulinaemia

There is an undoubted association between these variables, but the meaning of the relationship is obscure. It is known that primary or secondary hypogammaglobulinaemia is sometimes accompanied by diarrhoea or steatorrhoea. Most of these cases have a normal jejunal biopsy; the few reported instances with a flat mucosa have not usually responded to gluten withdrawal.

Hermans has described a small group of patients with severe deficiency of serum IgA and IgM, but only a moderate deficiency of IgG, all of whom had steatorrhoea. These patients had nodular lymphoid hyperplasia of the small intestine detected by biopsy but also visible on X-ray, and all were infested with *giardia lamblia*. This syndrome does not appear to be common outside the United States.

REFERENCES

CRABBÉ, P. A. & HERMANS, J. F. (1967). Selctive IgA deficiency with steatorrhoea. *Amer. J. Med.*, 42, 319.
HERMANS, P. E., HUIZENGA, K. A., HOFFMAN, H. N., BROWN, A. L. & MARKOWITZ, H. (1966). Dysgammaglobulinaemia associated with nodular hyperplasia of the small intestine. *Amer. J. Med.*, 40, 78.

Malignancy and the Coeliac Syndrome

It is now well established that the coeliac syndrome is a pre-malignant condition. After the age of 40, many cases develop a lymphoma of the small intestine, almost invariably a reticulum cell sarcoma. Furthermore, there is an increased incidence of carcinoma in the rest of the gastro-intestinal tract, particularly in the oesophagus, and perhaps elsewhere. Extreme interest has developed over the mechanism of this complication. Read and his colleagues have drawn attention to an atrophy and disruption of the lympho-reticular system in long-standing coeliacs that seems to precede the malignant change. Splenic atrophy occurs, and may be recognized by the presence of Howell-Jolly bodies, while node biopsy has shown similar lymphoid atrophy. Peripheral blood lymphocytes show a failure to transform *in vitro*. Such a recession of normal lymphoid activity may well allow malignant clones to develop, as is seen with immunosuppressive drugs. Three cases have been reported where a progressive rise in serum IgA has heralded a lymphoma, and this may well prove to be a useful test to predict malignant change.

REFERENCES

ASQUITH, P., THOMPSON, R. A. & COOKE, W. T. (1969). Serum-immunoglobulins in adult coeliac disease. *Lancet*, **2**, 129.

GOUGH, K. R., READ, A. E. & NAISH, J. M. (1962). Intestinal reticulosis as a complication of idiopathic steatorrhoea. *Gut*, **3**, 232.

HARRIS, O. D., COOKE, W. T., THOMPSON, H. & WATERHOUSE, J. A. H. (1967). Malignancy in adult coeliac disease and idiopathic steatorrhoea. *Amer. J. Med.*, **42**, 899.

MacCARTHY, C. F., FRASER, I. D., EVANS, K. T. & READ, W. (1966). Lympho-reticular dysfunction in idiopathic steatorrhoea. *Gut*, **7**, 140.

Atrophic Gastritis and Pernicious Anaemia

Serum antibodies against a microsomal component of parietal cells can be demonstrated in many cases of atrophic gastritis and pernicious anaemia; these are both in the IgG and IgA. Furthermore, the loss of parietal cells is accompanied by a heavy infiltrate of immunocytes. This has led to the suggestion that the gastric atrophy of these two conditions is an autoimmune process; the evidence is moderately firm, proof in autoimmune disease being notoriously hard to produce. Histological atrophy and the acid response to stimulation correlates well with the level of parietal cell antibodies. Furthermore, there is a link with thyroid disease where evidence for autoimmunity is impressive.

However, the presence of pernicious anaemia as characterized by malabsorption of vitamin B_{12} does not correlate so well with parietal cell antibodies. The deciding factor appears to be antibodies to intrinsic-factor (I.F.). There is a better correlation between intrinsic-factor antibodies and vitamin B_{12} malabsorption. There are two types of antibody, both in the IgG fraction. The first is a blocking antibody (Type I, combining site antibody) which inhibits the combination of vitamin B_{12} with intrinsic-factor, while the second is a binding antibody (Type II, complex antibody, precipitating antibody) which combines with the B_{12}-I.F. complex or I.F. alone, but does not prevent the binding of B_{12} by I.F. It is suggested that these serum antibodies get into the gastric lumen, and so bring about vitamin B_{12} malabsorption. However, there are a few anomalies. Some 30 per cent of patients with pernicious anaemia do not have I.F. antibodies, and indeed the condition can occur in the presence of hypogammaglobulinaemia. Furthermore these antibodies are IgG and not IgA as might be predicted.

REFERENCES

IRVINE, W. J. (1965). Immunologic aspects of pernicious anaemia. *New Engl. J. Med.*, **273**, 432.

TAYLOR, K. B. & FISHER, J. M. (1968). *Gastritis in Progress in Gastroenterology.* New York: Grune and Stratton, pp. 1–21.

Crohn's Disease

Although the affected gut is heavily infiltrated by lymphocytes, and serum IgA is frequently elevated, the evidence that Crohn's disease is either auto-immune or is even accompanied by a disturbance of immunity is slight. Because of the granulomatous nature of the histology and inevitable comparisons with sarcoid, delayed skin sensitivity has been repeatedly investigated and reports have been produced showing both decreased and normal responses to tuberculin and other substances. However, it has recently been shown that the Kveim test is positive in about half the cases of Crohn's disease.

REFERENCES

FLETCHER, J. & HILTON, J. M. (1967). Tuberculin sensitivity in Crohn's disease, a controlled study. *Lancet*, **2**, 753.

MITCHELL, D. N., CANNON, P., DYER, N. H., HIRISON, K. F. W. & WILLOUGHBY, J. M. T. (1969). Kveim test in Crohn's disease. *Lancet*, **2**, 571.

ULCERATIVE COLITIS

Histologically, this disease is even less suggestive of autoimmunity than Crohn's disease, and conventional immunological abnormalities have not been prominent. Other lines of thought have been pursued. It has been shown that some strains of *E. coli* share antigenicity with both animal and human colonic cells. However, there is no direct proof that antibodies against these organisms will cause colitis. Another approach has shown a cytotoxic effect of lymphocytes from patients with ulcerative colitis for colon epithelial cells. A similar abnormality has been shown in Crohn's disease. At the moment the relevance of both these observations to the aetiology of ulcerative colitis is speculative. However, immunosuppressive drugs have been tried in both Crohn's diseases and ulcerative colitis. No controlled trial has yet been published, and the status of this therapy must be regarded as non-proven.

REFERENCES

STEFANI, S. & FINK, S. (1967). Effect of *E. coli* antigens, tuberculin and phyo-haemaglutinin upon ulcerative colitis lymphocytes. *Gut*, **8**, 249.

WATSON, D. W., QUIGLEY, A. & BOLT, R. J. (1966). Effect of lymphocytes from patients with ulcerative colitis on human adult colon epithelial cells. *Gastroenterology*, **51**, 985.

IMMUNITY AND LIVER DISEASE

This topic has exploded with new observations and ideas, making for excitement in the field but hampering critical assessment.

The outstanding achievement has been the discovery of a virus-like particle in some forms of hepatitis which can not only be detected immunologically but seen under the electronmicroscope either by itself or complexed with antibody. Because it was originally discovered in a precipitin reaction with serum from an Australian aborigine, it is called the Australian antigen (Au). That this may be the actual virus causing hepatitis has been widely canvassed, but results are not uniform and show some geographic variation. In one recent series from America, 49 per cent of cases of serum hepatitis were positive for Au antigen, but it was found in only 25 per cent of cases of classical acute infective hepatitis.

The antigen may appear and disappear with relapse and remission of the disease. However there can be no doubt that it is the causal agent in some outbreaks, and in particular it has been found in dialysis units where hepatitis is common (see p. 84).

The next question is whether the Au antigen is ever found in relation to chronic liver disease. Laennec cirrhosis and primary biliary cirrhosis have not shown it, but in one series, 25 per cent of cases with chronic active hepatitis had the antigen. Chronic active hepatitis has been known for some time to show many features of an overactive or perverted immune response; elevated IgG, antinuclear factor positive in about 50 per cent of cases, smooth muscle antibodies positive in about 50 per cent and LE cells found in about 15 per cent. It is of interest that the Au antigen was seen in the blood of a patient with chronic active hepatitis both free and complexed with antibody, suggesting that the virus was present in excess of a fully extended but perhaps abnormal antibody response. Thus chronic active hepatitis appears to be a situation where continued viraemia overwhelms the immune system and causes recurrent liver damage.

Primary biliary cirrhosis also has distinguishing immunological features. In the serum, IgM is increased and this can also be demonstrated in a deposition about the abnormal bile ducts. However, the diagnostic reaction is an antibody to mitochondria that can be demonstrated by immunofluorescence in 98 per cent of cases. This is in serum IgG, and does not appear to be involved in the reaction about the bile ductules. Reliance on this test has certainly helped in the difficult diagnostic problem of obstructive jaundice in a middle-aged woman.

REFERENCES

ALMEIDA, J. D. & WATERSON, A. P. (1969). Immune complexes in hepatitis. *Lancet*, **2**, 983.

TURNER, G. C. & BRUCE WHITE, G. B. S. H. (1969). Antigen in haemodialysis-associated hepatitis. *Lancet*, **2**, 121.

WALKER, J. G., DONIACH, D., ROITT, I. M. & SHERLOCK, S. (1967). Immune studies in liver disease. In *The Liver*. Butterworths, p. 83.

WRIGHT, R., McCOLLUM, R. W. & KLATSKIN, G. (1969). Australia antigen in acute and chronic liver disease. *Lancet*, **2**, 117.

4 Renal Diseases

D. N. S. KERR

URINARY INFECTION. RENAL SCARRING AND CHRONIC PYELONEPHRITIS. ANALGESIC NEPHROPATHY. ACUTE RENAL FAILURE. LESIONS OF THE MAIN RENAL ARTERIES. RENAL VEIN THROMBOSIS. HAEMOLYTIC URAEMIC SYNDROMES. OTHER FORMS OF MICROANGIOPATHY. TREATMENT OF NEPHROTIC SYNDROME AND ITS MAIN CAUSES. DIALYSIS FOR CHRONIC RENAL FAILURE. THE PATHOLOGY ASSOCIATED WITH REGULAR HAEMODIALYSIS

URINARY INFECTION

BACTERIAL infection is much the commonest disease of the urinary tract, but it was neglected by clinicians until the late 1950s when Kass (1956) showed that midstream urine could be used for bacteriological diagnosis if cultured quantitatively, and Beeson (1958) published his editorial "The case against the catheter". The revulsion against catheterization that followed was entirely justified at the time. Catheters were passed not only for all bacteriological samples but even to test for proteinuria in antenatal clinics. The procedure was left to junior nurses ignorant of female anatomy who contaminated the catheter with vaginal secretions while groping for the urethral orifice. Asepsis was limited to a perfunctory wash at the ward sink and the brief immersion of an old rubber catheter in an inefficient ward sterilizer. Indwelling catheters were drained into open bottles and it was accepted that infection would inevitably result within a few days. The circumspect use of the catheter and the higher standards of asepsis that have emerged after a decade of campaigning are wholly beneficial, but evangelical zeal is in danger of overtaking the facts. Catheterization still has its uses, and midstream culture its limitations.

The impressive volume of research into urinary infection up to 1967 has been summarized in two major symposia (Kass, 1965; O'Grady and Brumfitt,

1968). Much of the evidence for the following account is contained in these two volumes, and text references are given predominantly to subsequent work.

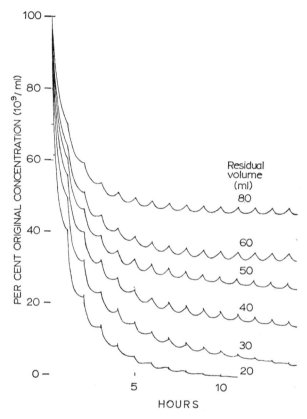

FIG. 4.1. Effect of residual urine volume on the elimination of urinary bacteria by hourly micturition in the presence of a urinary flow rate of 1 ml/minute; predicted from an analogue computer model. (From O'Grady and Brumfitt, 1968; Figure 10.4. Reproduced by permission of Professor O'Grady.)

Normal Defence Mechanisms

Urine at 37°C is an excellent culture medium, but multiplication of bacteria in the bladder is opposed by two protective mechanisms: (1) dilution with sterile urine from the kidneys followed by micturition and (2) an ill-understood bactericidal action of bladder mucosa which is not apparently dependent on plasma antibodies. The first process can be simulated *in vitro*, and a computer model has confirmed that bacterial counts fall if the bladder is emptied frequently and the residual bladder volume is small (Fig. 4.1).

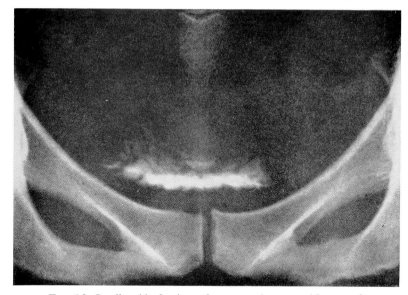

Fig. 4.2. Small residual urine volume spread over a wide area of bladder mucosa at the end of a micturating cystogram. (From Kass, 1956, p. 575. Reproduced by permission of Dr Hinman.)

The fast replication rate of *Escherichia coli* enables it to withstand this flushing action of the urinary tract better than other bacteria, and may explain its predominance in spontaneous infection of the normal urinary tract. The second process has been demonstrated by instilling bacteria into the bladders of normal subjects and comparing their growth rate *in vivo* with that of a control population in the subject's urine *in vitro*. The bactericidal effect of bladder mucosa is most effective after micturition when a small volume of urine is spread over a wide area of bladder mucosa (Fig. 4.2). Both of these mechanisms are vitiated by a high residual urine volume due to bladder neck obstruction or reflux into dilated ureters and pelvis. They are at their weakest during the long gap between acts of micturition at night, and in those subjects who void infrequently with a large bladder volume (Lapides *et al.*, 1968).

There is therefore a tendency for small inocula of bacteria to be eliminated rapidly from a normal urinary tract. If bacteria persist in the bladder they usually do so at a high and fairly constant concentration (Fig. 4.1) between 100,000 and 10^9 bacteria per ml.

Diagnosis of Urinary Infection

The high bacterial counts in persistent bacteriuria contrast with low counts (usually below 10,000 bacteria per ml) found in midstream urine from contamination, and led Kass to introduce quantitative culture as a method of distinguishing between them. Midstream urine from an adult male with retracted prepuce is virtually sterile. Female urine can be collected with little contamination if a thorough vulval wash is followed by collection, with the labia parted by an attendant nurse (Lemieux and St Martin, 1968) or through a sterile funnel placed over the urethral orifice. These methods are too time-consuming and embarrassing to the patient for routine use, but they can replace catheterization in the investigation of patients with equivocal counts after less meticulous collection. Samples must be plated out within two hours of collection unless stored in a refrigerator or ice-box, in which case they can be used up to 24 hours after collection.

For routine use, simpler methods of collection have proved sufficiently accurate (Linton and Gillespie, 1969). The patient collects her own sample into a wide-mouthed container such as a disposable sputum carton while sitting on the toilet with thighs widely abducted. The carton can be held by the patient or placed at the front of a suitably designed lavatory pan. No vulval wash is employed unless there is a vaginal discharge or during menstruation, in which case a vaginal tampon is inserted after the wash before collection.

Heavy contamination from vulval skin is fairly common when these methods are used. It is indicated by the presence of numerous squames in the deposit, by a mixed culture including skin commensals or by an equivocal count (10,000–100,000 per ml). The procedure should be repeated at least once, after an interval of at least one day, and the same organism should be found in high count on both occasions before infection is diagnosed in an asymptomatic patient. This gives about 95 per cent accuracy in diagnosis compared with catheter urine; the number of repeat samples required to meet more exacting demands are shown in the nomogram of Cohen and Kass (1967). Antiseptics should be avoided during vulval washing; some laboratories check the urine routinely for bactericidal activity to detect contamination with antiseptics or with antibiotics and other drugs (such as some barbiturates) which inhibit bacterial growth.

Bacterial counts below 100,000 per ml may indicate infection in patients receiving antibacterial drugs or undergoing a brisk diuresis. They are also found in the early stages of infection, e.g. during recrudescence after treatment or soon after catheterization.

If these limitations are acknowledged, midstream urine can be employed for the great majority of ambulant females. It is of less value in children too young to void on request, in women with prolapse, in the very obese or the bedridden. In countries where female circumcision is still practised the distortion of the vulva makes skin contamination almost inevitable.

For these special circumstances suprapubic aspiration of bladder urine through a fine (22 SWG) needle offers a reasonable alternative. The first syringe-full may contain a few skin bacteria and should be discarded. Subsequent samples are usually sterile so that even low bacterial counts are significant. Samples can be sent through the post to a central laboratory (Bailey and Little, 1969) and the method has therefore been recommended for routine use in domiciliary practice. However, there are less uncomfortable ways of bringing urine culture into general practice. Midstream urine samples which cannot be sent immediately to a laboratory can be transported in an ice-box or in containers with a small content of boric acid (Porter and Brodie, 1969). A quicker result can be obtained by plating urine on the spot by a semi-quantitative technique such as the dipslide (Guttmann and Naylor, 1967), or the filter paper inoculating strip (Layman et al., 1968; Seligman et al., 1968), and the inoculated medium is posted to the laboratory. Guttmann has taught his patients to inoculate their own urine and avoid unnecessary trips to hospital during follow-up.

Between the clinical suspicion of urinary infection and receipt of the report on culture and sensitivity lies a gap of 24 to 72 hours. Confirmation of infection at the time of consultation has traditionally rested on the detection of pyuria. Ten years ago many hospital laboratories refused to culture urine if pyuria was absent on an insensitive qualitative test. Examination of the urinary deposit is still the most widely used immediate test for urinary infection, but faith in its diagnostic significance has diminished. The rate of white cell excretion in patients with chronic pyelonephritis is so close to the normal range that careful quantitative counts on timed urine samples are required to distinguish between them (Hutt *et al.*, 1961). Moreover, these tests were originally performed on catheter urine and are vitiated by contamination of non-catheter whole urine samples. False positive results are therefore common in women and young children (Newman *et al.*, 1967; Meadow, 1969). The morphology of white cells varies with the osmolality of urine (Gadeholt, 1968a) making distinction from tubular epithelial cells difficult, and unpredictable errors are introduced by changes in urine flow (Gadeholt, 1968b) and pH. The main contributions of urine microscopy are the confirmation of acute symptomatic infection and the detection of casts indicating renal damage.

There have therefore been many attempts to develop an immediate test for the presence of bacteria in urine. Examination of stained deposit is surprisingly accurate; the presence of more than five bacteria per oil immersion field correlates well with a significant count (Sacks and Abramson, 1967) but it is hardly an "office procedure". The Griess test for nitrites in urine produced by bacteria has been developed into a dipstick test, but it fails to detect about a quarter of bacteriurics because they excrete insufficient nitrate substrate for the bacteria. The value of the test is improved if the urine is tested simultaneously with diphenylamine to detect nitrites-plus-nitrates; this replaces the false negatives by a group of "don't knows" who must be tested by other means (Finnerty and Johnson, 1968). The triphenyl tetrazolium chloride test (Simmons and Williams, 1967) detects about 85 per cent of bacteriurics and has enjoyed some popularity for population screening, but the need to incubate the urine for four hours reduces its attraction to the clinician. A promising test recently introduced is the use of a sensitive test paper for urinary dextrose (Schertsen *et al.*, 1968) which gives a positive reaction with normal urine and a negative reaction with urine containing a significant number of bacteria which metabolize glucose; it awaits full evaluation.

Prevalence of Urinary Infection

The introduction of midstream culture gave Kass (1960) the opportunity to conduct large population surveys for bacteriuria. At the end of the first trimester of pregnancy he found a prevalence of about 6 per cent, and many subsequent surveys in antenatal clinics have revealed prevalence rates in the range 4 to 10 per cent (Kunin, 1966; Beard and Roberts, 1968; Gruneberg *et al.*, 1969). Kass at first assumed that this high prevalence began in the first few weeks of pregnancy, and reflected an enhanced susceptibility of the pregnant female to bacterial invasion of the urinary tract. It has been pointed out that in pregnancy, urine pH rises, osmolality falls and the urinary concentrations of dextrose and amino-acids increase—all factors favouring bacterial growth. However it has not been shown that bacteriuria is any commoner in pregnant women than in non-pregnant married women of the same age, and an equally high prevalence has been found in infertility clinics (Williams *et al.*, 1969). It is now generally believed that bacteriuria becomes common with the onset of regular sexual activity rather than at the start of pregnancy. Evidence for this view has come from the studies of Turner (1961), who found a prevalence of only 1 per cent in unmarried young women in Aberdeen, and of Kunin and McCormack (1968) who found that bacteriuria was more than twelve times as common in young working women as in a matched series of nuns.

Some authorities feel that first urinary infections in adolescent girls are so often associated with sexual activity that they call for gratuitous advice on contraception. Emerson (1969) states "the presence of a urinary infection in any girl over the age of 12 immediately raises my suspicions, and direct questioning usually reveals that intercourse has been occurring". However, bacteriuria is quite common in schoolgirls, long before puberty. Kunin is following a large cohort of American schoolgirls through childhood. He has found a prevalence of bacteriuria of about 1·5 per cent in the youngest girls (aged six to seven years) falling to less than 1 per cent as they reach age eight to nine (Kunin *et al.*, 1964). A survey of five-year-old girls entering school in Dundee revealed bacteriuria in 2·1 per cent and a study of primary schoolgirls in Newcastle upon Tyne a prevalence of 2·4 per cent (Selkon, 1969).

Prevalence studies in infancy are impeded by the problem of contamination, but criteria for the diagnosis of infection on "clean catch urine" have been established (Braude *et al.*, 1967a, b). O'Doherty (1968), using pyuria as a screening test and suprapubic aspiration for bacteriological confirmation, has confirmed previous reports that infection is fairly common in the first month of life, affecting 1 to 2 per cent of infants, and almost entirely confined to males. Only a minority of these boys have demonstrable abnormalities of the urinary tract, and the formerly grave prognosis has been abolished by chemotherapy. Neonatal girls with pyuria usually have sterile bladder urine, but are liable to develop bacteriuria in the first few months of life. Their initial pyuria is presumably due to vulvitis or urethritis. In pre-school girls, Randolph and Greenfield (1964) found 2 per cent prevalence of bacteriuria. After the first few months of life bacteriuria is rare in boys— about 0·1 per cent in Kunin's study and in the Newcastle survey of school children.

At the other end of life, urinary infection becomes increasingly common in old age, reaching about 30 per cent in admissions to geriatric hospitals (Walkey *et al.*, 1967). This rising prevalence is attributed to prolapse and prostatism. Bacteriuria in middle life has received less attention. A study of female hospital visitors in Wales showed a 3 per cent prevalence in non-pregnant non-diabetic women aged 20 to 65, but the total prevalence must have been higher since patients with symptoms of urinary infection at the time were excluded from the screening programme (Asscher *et al.*, 1969; Sussman *et al.*, 1969). In the white working women studied by Kunin and McCormack (1968) the prevalence rate was between 3 and 5 per cent in all age groups. Infection in middle-aged men is commonly associated with calculous disease (Steensberg *et al.*, 1969).

The changing prevalence of urinary infection throughout life in the two sexes is shown diagrammatically in Figure 4.3.

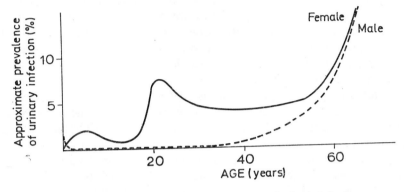

FIG. 4.3. Diagram of the changing prevalence of urinary infection throughout life

Incidence of Urinary Infection

Most of the surveys quoted in the preceding section were carried out at a single point in time. Repeated surveys at close intervals are required to discover the attack rate and the cure rate due to spontaneous recovery and to treatment with antibacterial drugs either for urinary symptoms or for unrelated illness. At Charlottesville, two surveys two years apart on the school population suggested that the incidence of new cases of bacteriuria was 0·5 per cent per two years for girls under 15, and 1·2 per cent for those aged 15 to 19 (Kunin *et al.*, 1964). The figure would presumably have been higher if urine cultures had been performed at shorter intervals. Even on this conservative estimate, about one girl in 10 will have had an episode of urinary infection by the time she leaves school.

This high incidence rate must be balanced by a similar rate of resolution except perhaps in old age. Sussman and his colleagues (1969) placed half their bacteriuric non-pregnant women on placebos and found that 20 per cent had reverted to sterile urine six months later. Whalley, Martin and Peters (1965) followed up 111 patients with bacteriuria in pregnancy eight to 12 months after delivery, and found that 21 had lost their bacteria. Spontaneous cure rates from 20 to 50 per cent between first antenatal visit and delivery have been reported by others (LeBlanc and McGanity, 1964; Low *et al.*, 1964; Gold *et al.*, 1966).

Natural History of Urinary Infection

The majority of patients with bacteriuria found in population surveys are unaware that they have a urinary infection. Direct questioning reveals that most of them have mild symptoms of urgency and frequency (Savage *et al.*, 1969), but these symptoms are common in the general female population, and in pregnancy they are found as commonly in the patients with sterile urine as in those with bacteriuria (Condie *et al.*, 1968). Indeed, half of the patients presenting in general practice with more definite symptoms suggesting urinary infection turn out to have sterile urine (Steensberg *et al.*, 1969). It is therefore reasonable to describe most bacteriurics as asymptomatic. Symptomatic cystitis or pyelonephritis may develop in the course of chronic bacteriuria, or may appear suddenly in women whose urine is sterile until 24 hours before the attack. The former sequence is probably the commoner at all ages and is certainly so in pregnancy. Between 30 per cent and 60 per cent of all cases of pyelonephritis of pregnancy occur in the 5 per cent or so of women with bacteriuria at the first antenatal visit. If untreated, these women carry a risk of developing pyelonephritis during that pregnancy of about 25 per cent (Little, 1966; Dixon and Brant, 1967; Beard-Roberts, 1968; Williams, Campbell and Davies, 1969). In non-pregnant women, 36 per cent of those with bacteriuria at the start developed symptoms of cystitis within one year compared with 7 per cent of those with initially sterile urine (Asscher *et al.*, 1969).

These findings raised the hope that both acute and chronic pyelonephritis could be prevented by the screening of adult women and the treatment of their asymptomatic bacteriuria. Some success has been achieved in the prevention of acute pyelonephritis in pregnancy, but the prevention of chronic pyelonephritis is proving more difficult. An appreciable proportion of the adult women found in population surveys already have renal scarring. Fairley and his colleagues (1966) found infection of ureteric urine, associated with renal scarring, in 44 per cent of their patients with bacteriuria in pregnancy. Pyelograms in 163 English patients followed up after pregnancy showed acquired defects, such as scarring in 13 per cent (Gower *et al.*, 1968), and a similar post-partum survey in Wales showed renal scarring in 17 per cent (Williams *et al.*, 1968). The latter study included micturating cystography, which revealed vesico-ureteric reflux in 21 per cent. During pregnancy, bacteriurics produce urine of subnormal osmolality, suggesting established medullary damage (Williams, Campbell and Davies, 1969). In asymptomatic non-pregnant women Sussman and his colleagues (1969) found radiological evidence of chronic pyelonephritis in 17 per cent while

Murdoch *et al.* (1966), found such evidence in one-third of all symptomatic patients referred to their pyelonephritis clinic. Even asymptomatic bacteriurics have higher blood ureas and blood pressures on average than control patients, but the differences are small (Sussman *et al.*, 1969). These findings should encourage therapeutic enthusiasm, since the renal function of women with bacteriuria is usually close to normal, and well worth preserving at this level.

However, the high prevalence of renal scarring suggests that detection and treatment should begin before adult life. Renal scarring can develop following acute pyelonephritis in adults (Bailey *et al.*, 1969) but it is uncommon. Gross renal distortion almost invariably results from damage to the growing kidney.

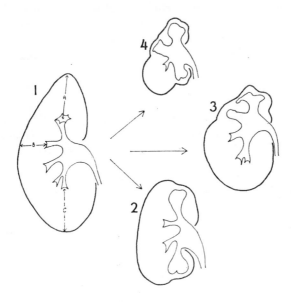

FIG. 4.4. Patterns of renal scarring. (1) Normal kidney; A and C represent the thickness of medulla plus cortex in the two polar regions; they are usually equal and always greater than B. (2) Bipolar scarring. (3) Upper half scarring. (4) Generalized scarring except for one remaining hypertrophied region. These are common patterns of scarring peculiar to "childhood" pyelonephritis. (From Hodson, 1969. Reproduced by permission of Dr Hodson.)

Hodson (1967, 1969) has illustrated the different patterns of scarring that produce grotesque deformity of the kidney in childhood (Fig. 4.4) and distinguished them from the uniform atrophy that follows obstruction. Even severe scarring can be halted, and growth of the child's kidney permitted, if chronic infection is controlled by chemotherapy (Edwards *et al.*, 1968). There should therefore be a gratifying therapeutic yield from the screening

E

of schoolgirls, and adequate investigation and follow-up of the bacteriurics. The cost of detecting one child with chronic pyelonephritis is about £100 (Selkon, 1969)—roughly the price of two weeks' hospital admission or one month on regular dialysis. However, the scarring found even in school entrants is sometimes gross, and prevention of all chronic pyelonephritis would require an even earlier approach, possibly in the local authority clinics, where urine collection is particularly difficult.

Ecology of Urinary Infection

Escherichia coli remains the commonest pathogen in the urinary tract, particularly in first infections acquired outside hospital (Table 4.1). The organism is probably derived from the gut, and earlier suggestions that particular strains were "nephropathic" have not been confirmed. The strain causing urinary infection is usually that which is commonest in the faecal

TABLE 4.1

Bacteria isolated from 2500 urinary infections by Dr J. C. Gould
of the Central Microbioligical Laboratories, Edinburgh
(From O'Grady and Brumfitt, 1968, p. 43.)

PRIMARY (800 patients)		SECONDARY (1,700 patients)		
Organism isolated	%	Organism isolated	Sole species %	Mixed flora %
Esch. coli	91	*Esch. coli*	38	47
		Coliform bacilli	21	28
Strept. faecalis	2	*Klebsiella*	4	7
Other streptococci	2	*Proteus mirabilis*	18	25
Klebsiella		*Proteus spp.*	2	3
Proteus	<5	*Pseudomonas*	8	13
Coliform bacilli		*Achromobacter*	2	—
Myco. tuberculosis	—	*Strept. faecalis*	4	17
		Staphylococcus	2	—

flora and on the perineum (Gruneberg, 1969). Antibiotics which sterilize the urinary tract do not eliminate the organism from the gut and carrier sites. Antibiotic resistance is becoming more common even in infections arising outside hospital (Robertson, 1968); the resistant strains may be ingested within the hospital or home, and while in the gut they can transfer genetic material determining antibiotic resistance ("R factors") to other Gram-negative bacteria (Smith and Armour, 1966). Resistance to sulphonamides has already displaced them from first choice in some areas of the United Kingdom, and no future statements about the most suitable drug for initial treatment, pending sensitivity reports, will have more than local and temporary interest.

Chemotherapy of Urinary Infection

Bacteria are rapidly eliminated from a urinary tract without gross abnormality by any effective antibacterial drug to which they are sensitive *in vitro*, whether it gives high levels in urine and renal medulla and low levels in blood and renal cortex or *vice versa*. Some antibiotics work more effectively if the urine pH is adjusted by the administration of acids or alkalis (Tallgren and von Bonsdorff, 1965), and on theoretical grounds they should sometimes be given just after micturition and with water administration or restriction depending on the drug. However, the immediate success rate is usually over 80 per cent without these additional manoeuvres, and they are rarely employed in practice. The choice of drug is dictated more by cost and side-effects than by its renal pharmacology, provided renal function is close to normal. Sulphonamides alone are waning in popularity—more rapidly than the facts justify (Editorial, 1968)—but a combination of a sulphonamide with trimethoprim ("Bactrim", "Septrin") is highly effective, and probably the most popular therapy at the time of writing. The choice of drug when renal function is severely compromised is much more critical; dosage must be adjusted to the glomerular filtration rate (Douglas and Kerr, 1968). The duration of therapy required in uncomplicated patients is unknown but probably shorter than the orthodox 10 to 14 days. Gruneberg and Brumfitt (1967) achieved a success rate of 88 per cent with two drug regimes effective for one week.

The immediate success is followed by a high rate of relapse, whatever the initial treatment. Relapse is due to at least two phenomena—reinfection from an uneradicated focus in the urinary tract, usually in the kidney, and recurrent reinfection from below. The former is indicated by the reappearance of the same serotype of the organism after a short interval (Turck *et al.*, 1968). The presence of renal infection is usually signalled by the appearance in the blood of "O" antibodies to the particular serotype of *E. Coli* in the urinary tract (Bremner *et al.*, 1969). Proteus infections produce no antibody response. Patients with elevated antibody titres have a lower initial cure rate, as well as a higher relapse rate, than those with normal titres (Reeves and Brumfitt, 1968); they probably respond better to high dose antibacterial therapy than to the conventional treatment of urinary infection (Gruneberg *et al.*, 1968), though the evidence supporting this statement is still slender.

Following treatment with drugs such as the penicillins which interfere with bacterial cell wall synthesis, "L forms" or spheroplasts (i.e. bacteria without normal cell walls) may survive in the kidney and be excreted in the urine (Gutman *et al.*, 1967; Conner *et al.*, 1968). They require special culture methods for detection and are lysed in dilute urine. Their sensitivity pattern may differ from that of the organisms from which they are derived. They probably play a significant role in relapse after a period of apparent sterility of the urine.

Reinfection from below is usually produced by a new serotype or species of organism. It commonly occurs in the first few months after treatment of an infection, the peak incidence being at four months. Since many symptomatic reinfections are preceded by a period of asymptomatic bacteriuria, routine midstream culture at monthly intervals for six months after apparent cure will permit the treatment of most reinfections at a pre-symptomatic phase. Long-term therapy with suppressive doses of sulphonamides, nitrofurantoin, cycloserine and other drugs has significantly reduced the reinfection rate (Murdoch *et al.*, 1966; Freeman *et al.*, 1968). In childhood this effect is well worth achieving during the period of renal growth, but in the adult it has yet to be shown whether long-term chemotherapy abolishes or merely postpones the relapses, and whether renal function is better preserved with a policy of regular urine culture and treatment of each relapse in turn.

Whatever scheme of chemotherapy is adopted, the patient with renal scarring or other anatomical abnormalities in the urinary tract requires life-long follow-up, of which urine culture and blood-pressure measurement are the most important facets.

The Role of Structural and Functional Abnormalities in the Urinary Tract

Major abnormalities such as neurogenic bladder, calculi, prostatism and cystocoele produce undoubted susceptibility to infection and resistance to cure. A search for these and other defects in the appropriate age groups, and for congenital anomalies in male infants, is mandatory. A good case can also be made for full investigation, including pyelography and micturating cystography, in all children who have a single episode of infection or who are found on population surveys to have asymptomatic bacteriuria. Much the commonest abnormality discovered in this group is vesico-ureteric reflux which was present in 55 per cent of 201 children who were investigated in hospital by Scott and Stansfeld (1968a). It is almost exclusively in the group with reflux that urinary infection is followed by renal scarring (Smellie and Normand, 1968). In the less selected series found by population study, the proportion with reflux will no doubt be lower, but preliminary results from the Newcastle study suggest that it will be high enough to justify routine investigation (Selkon, 1969).

Surgical correction of reflux is remarkably successful in skilled hands; Scott (1969) restored the competence of the uretero-vesical valves in 85 of 87 children. In a controlled trial (Scott and Stansfeld, 1968b) elimination of reflux resulted in fewer infections and faster renal growth than conservative treatment. However, spontaneous cure of reflux sometimes follows treatment of infection and is common at puberty; meticulous follow-up and antibiotic therapy will permit renal growth even in the presence of reflux if the infection is controlled (Smellie and Normand, 1968). On current evidence, surgical correction of all but the mildest examples of reflux should be undertaken if specialist skill of sufficiently high standard is available, but all patients, operated on or not, require life-long close follow-up.

The cause of recurrent urinary infection in girls without reflux is still in dispute. Many were subjected to bladder neck resection before the range of normal appearances on micturating cystography was realized. "Bladder neck obstruction" has recently been replaced in the diagnostic index of some paediatric departments by "distal urethral stenosis" (Brannan et al., 1968). This diagnosis is based on an arbitrary definition of the normal distensibility of the immature female urethra. It has not yet been placed on a sufficiently scientific basis to justify the current vogue for urethral meatotomy (Burke and Kelalis, 1969). However, there does appear to be a correlation between recurrent infection and a high residual urine volume for a variety of reasons, apart from reflux (McGregor and Wynne Williams, 1966). The practice of "triple micturition" to empty the bladder completely has been recommended, but its efficacy has not been proven.

The full radiological investigation of every adolescent and young woman with a urinary infection would be a formidable task, and it is doubtful if sufficient treatable abnormalities would be found to justify the effort and the radiation exposure. A common practice is to request an intravenous pyelogram only in those with proteinuria (after the first few days), impaired excretory function, a recurrence after adequate antibiotic therapy, or a history of infection in childhood. The last group includes most of the few adults who have reflux and severely scarred kidneys (McGovern and Marshall, 1968). If the infection is diagnosed in pregnancy, pyelography is postponed until after delivery. It is most likely to reveal abnormalities in those patients who relapse after a short course of an appropriate antibiotic (Leigh et al., 1968).

Effect of Urinary Infection on the Course of Pregnancy

Early studies of bacteriuria in pregnancy suggested that it predisposed to premature delivery and to maternal anaemia, but since all three conditions are social-class related the conclusion was regarded with some scepticism. Subsequent studies have confirmed that bacteriuria does predispose to prematurity, but the effect is small and treatment of bacteriuria will have little effect on the total prematurity rate (Kunin, 1966; Beard and Roberts, 1968; Gruneberg *et al.*, 1969).

Infection Following Catheterization and Instrumentation

Many of the infections associated with these procedures are due to contamination of instruments (Moore and Forman, 1966) or irrigating fluids (Mitchell and Hayward, 1966) including antiseptics. Improved methods of sterilization, closed drainage, and protection of the urethral orifice produce a dramatic fall in the infection from bladder drainage after urological or gynaecological surgery (Gillespie *et al.*, 1964). Failure to employ pre-sterilized catheters and closed drainage bags which can be emptied without disconnection (Gonzales, 1966) now verges on malpractice. However, the fear that catheter infection would lead to a high incidence of chronic pyelonephritis was exaggerated. Over 90 per cent of patients with unobstructed urinary tracts are free of infection, and have no evidence of permanent renal damage, when followed up several years after operation (Slade *et al.*, 1965).

REFERENCES

ASSCHER, A. W., SUSSMAN, M., WATERS, W. E., EVANS, J. A. S., CAMPBELL, H., EVANS, K. T. & EDMUND WILLIAMS, J. (1969). The clinical significance of asymptomatic bacteriuria in the non-pregnant woman. *J. infect. Dis.*, **120**, 17.

BAILEY, R. R. & LITTLE, P. J. (1969). Suprapubic bladder aspiration in diagnosis of urinary tract infection. *Brit. med. J.*, **1**, 293.

BAILEY, R. R., LITTLE, P. J. & ROLLESTON, G. I. (1969). Renal damage after acute pyelonephritis. *Brit. med. J.*, **1**, 550.

BEARD, R. W. & ROBERTS, A. P. (1968). Asymptomatic bacteriuria during pregnancy. *Brit. med. Bull.*, **24**, 44.

BEESON, P. B. (1958). The case against the catheter. *Amer. J. Med.*, **24**, 1.

BRANNAN, W., OCHSNER, M. G., KITTREDGE, W. E., BURNS, E. & MEDEIROS, A. (1969). Significance of distal urethral stenosis in young girls: experience with 241 cases. *J. Urol.*, **101**, 570.

BRAUDE, H., FORFAR, J. O., GOULD, J. C. & McLEOD J. W., (1967a). Cell and bacterial counts in the urine of normal infants and children. *Brit. med. J.*, **4**, 697.

BRAUDE, H., FORFAR, J. O., GOULD, J. C. & McLEOD, J. W. (1967b). Diagnosis of urinary tract infection in childhood based on examination of paired non-catheter and catheter specimens of urine. *Brit. med. J.*, **4**, 702.

BREMNER, D. A., FAIRLEY, K. F. & KINCAID-SMITH, P. (1969). The serum antibody response in renal and bladder infections. *Med. J. Austral.*, **1**, 1069.

BURKE, E. C. & KELALIS, P. P. (1969). Recurrent urinary tract infections in children: clinical approach to diagnosis and treatment. *Mayo Clin. Proc.*, **44**, 489.

COHEN, S. C. & KASS, E. H. (1967). A simple method for quantitative urine culture. *New Engl. J. med.*, **277**, 176.

CONDIE, A. P., WILLIAMS, J. D., REEVES, D. S. & BRUMFITT, W. (1968). Complications of bacteriuria in pregnancy. In *Urinary Tract Infection*. ed. F. O'Grady, and W. Brumfitt. London: Oxford University Press, p. 148.

CONNER, J. F., COLEMAN, S. E., DAVIS, J. L. & McGAUGHEY, F. S. (1968). Bacterial L-forms from urinary-tract infections in a veteran's hospital population. *J. Amer. Geriat. Soc.*, **16**, 893.

DIXON, H. G. & BRANT, H. A. (1967). The significance of bacteriuria in pregnancy. *Lancet*, **1**, 19.

DOUGLAS, A. P. & KERR, D. N. S. (1968). *A Short Textbook of Renal Disease*. London: Pitman, p. 70.

EDITORIAL (1969). Urinary infection. *Scot. med. J.*, **14**, 69.

EMERSON, M. S. (1969). Changes in sexual behaviour. *Newcastle med. J.*, **31**, 251.

FAIRLEY, K. F., BOND, A. G. & ADEY, F. D. (1966). The site of infection in pregnancy bacteriuria. *Lancet*, **1**, 939.

FINNERTY, F. A. & JOHNSON, A. C. (1968). A simplified accurate method for detecting bacteriuria. *Amer. J. Obstet. Gynec.*, **101**, 238.

FREEMAN, R. B., BROMER, L., BRANCATO, F., COHEN, S. I., GARFIELD, C. F., GRIEP, R. J., HINMAN, E. J., RICHARDSON, J. A., THURM, R. H., URNER, C. & SMITH, W. M. (1968). Prevention of recurrent bacteriuria with continuous chemotherapy. *Ann. intern. Med.*, **69**, 655.

GADEHOLT, H. (1968a). Erythrocytes and leucocytes in urine. Variability of shape and size. Acta Universitatis Bergensis. Series medica. Bergen: Norwegian Universities Press.

GADEHOLT, H. (1968b). Quantitative estimation of cells in urine. *Acta med. scand.*, **183**, 369.

GILLESPIE, W. A., LENNON, G. G., LINTON, K. B. & SLADE, N. (1964). Prevention of urinary infection in gynaecology. *Brit. med. J.*, **4**, 243.

GOLD, E. M., TRAUB, F. B., DAICHMAN, I. & TERRIS, M. (1966). Asymptomatic bacteriuria during pregnancy. *Obstet. and Gynec.*, **27**, No. 2, p. 206.

GONZALES, E. B. (1966). Control of infection after prostatectomy. *Brit. med. J.*, **1**, 24.

GOWER, P. E., HASWELL, B., SIDAWAY, M. E. & DE WARDENER, H. E. (1968). Follow-up of 164 patients with bacteriuria of pregnancy. *Lancet*, **1**, 990.

GRUNEBERG, R. N. (1969). Relationship of infecting urinary organisms to the faecal flora in patients with symptomatic urinary infection. *Lancet*, **2**, 766.

GRUNEBERG, R. N. & BRUMFITT, W. (1967). Single-dose treatment of acute urinary tract infection: a controlled trial. *Brit. med. J.*, **3**, 649.

GRUNEBERG, R. N., LEIGH, D. A. & BRUMFITT, W. (1968). *Escherichia coli* serotypes in urinary tract infection. In *Urinary Tract Infection*. ed. F. O'Grady and W. Brumfitt. London: Oxford University Press, p. 68.

GRUNEBERG, R. N., LEIGH, D. A. & BRUMFITT, W. (1969). Relationship of bacteriuria in pregnancy to acute pyelonephritis, prematurity and fetal mortality. *Lancet*, **2**, 1.

GUTMAN, L. T., SCHALLER, J. & WEDGWOOD, R. J. (1967). Bacterial L-forms in relapsing urinary-tract infections. *Lancet*, **1**, 464.

GUTTMANN, D. & NAYLOR, G. R. E. (1967). Dip-slide: an aid to quantitative urine culture in general practice. *Brit. med. J.*, **3**, 343.

HODSON, C. J. (1967). The radiological contribution toward the diagnosis of chronic pyelonephritis. *Radiology*, **88**, 857.

HODSON, C. J. (1969). The effects of disturbance of flow on the kidney. *J. infect. Dis.*, **120**, 54.

HUTT, M. S. R., CHALMERS, J. A., MACDONALD, J. S. & DE WARDENER (1961). Pyelonephritis. Observations on the relation between various diagnostic procedures. *Lancet*, **1**, 351.

KASS, E. H. (1956). Asymptomatic infections of the urinary tract. *Trans. Ass. Amer. Physns.*, **69**, 56.

KASS, E. H. (1960). Bacteriuria and pyelonephritis of pregnancy. *Arch. intern. Med.*, **105**, 194.

KASS, E. H. (1965). *Progress in Pyelonephritis*. Philadelphia: Davis.

KUNIN, C. M. (1966). Asymptomatic bacteriuria. *Ann. Rev. Med.*, **17**, 383.

KUNIN, C. M., DUETSCHER, R. & PAQUIN, A. (1964). Urinary tract infection in school children: an epidemiologic, clinical and laboratory study. *Medicine*, **43**, 91.

KUNIN, C. M. & McCORMACK, R. C. (1968). An epidemiologic study of bacteriuria and blood pressure among nuns and working women. *New Engl. J. Med.*, **278**, 635.

LAPIDES, J., COSTELLO, R. T., ZIERDT, D. K. & STONE, T. E. (1968). Primary cause and treatment of recurrent urinary infection in women; preliminary report. *J. Urol.*, **100**, 552.

LAYMAN, H. D., WAGNER, M. K. & MENDELOW, H. (1968). Comparative study of three methods for detecting significant bacteriuria. *Amer. J. clin. Path.*, **50**, 710.

LEBLANC, A. L. & McGANITY (1964). The impact of bacteriuria in pregnancy—a survey of 1300 pregnant women. *Tex. Rep. Biol. Med.*, **22**, 336.

LEIGH, D. A., GRUNEBERG, R. N. & BRUMFITT, W. (1968). Long-term follow-up of bacteriuria in pregnancy. *Lancet*, **2**, 604.

LEMIEUX, G. & ST MARTIN, M. (1968). Reliability of clean-voided midstream urine specimens for the diagnosis of significant bacteriuria in the female patient. *Canad. med. Ass. J.*, **98**, 241.

LINTON, K. B. & GILLESPIE, W. A. (1969). Collection of urine from women for bacteriological examination. *J. clin. Path.*, **22**, 376.

LITTLE, P. J. (1966). The incidence of urinary infection in 5000 pregnant women. *Lancet*, **2**, 925.

LOW, J. A., JOHNSTON, E. E., McBRIDE, R. I. & TUFFNELL, P. G. (1964). The significance of asymptomatic bacteriuria in the normal obstetric patient. *Amer. J. Obstet. Gynec.*, **90**, 897.

McGOVERN, J. H. & MARSHALL, V. F. (1968). Reflux and pyelonephritis in 35 adults. *J. Urol.*, **101**, 668.

MACGREGOR, M. E. & WYNNE WILLIAMS, C. J. E. (1966). Relation of residual urine to persistent urinary infection in childhood. *Lancet*, **1**, 893.

MEADOW, S. R. (1969). Prevalence of symptomless urinary tract disease in Birmingham schoolchildren. I—Pyuria and bacteriuria. *Brit. med. J.*, **3**, 81.

MITCHELL, R. G. & HAYWARD, A. C. (1966). Postoperative urinary tract infections caused by contaminated irrigating fluid. *Lancet*, **1**, 793.

MOORE, B. & FORMAN, A. (1966). An outbreak of urinary *Pseudomonas aeruginosa* infection acquired during urological operations. *Lancet*, **2**, 929.

MURDOCH, J. McC., GEDDES, A. M., TULLOCH, W. S., NEWSAM, J. E., THOMSON, W. N., BIDWELL, D. & WALLACE, E. T. (1966). The problem of pyelonephritis. *Practitioner*, **196**, 800.

NEWMAN, C. G. H., O'NEILL, P. & PARKER, A. (1967). Pyuria in infancy, and the role of suprapubic aspiration of urine in diagnosis of infection of urinary tract. *Brit. med. J.*, **2**, 277.

O'DOHERTY, N. (1968). Urinary tract infection in the neonatal period and later infancy. In *Urinary Tract Infection*. ed. F. O'Grady and W. Brumfitt. London: Oxford Medical Publications.

O'GRADY, F. & BRUMFITT, W. (1968). *Urinary Tract Infection*. London: Oxford University Press.

PORTER, I. A. & BRODIE, J. (1969). Boric acid preservation of urine samples. *Brit. med. J.*, **2**, 353.

RANDOLPH, M. F. & GREENFIELD, M. (1964). The incidence of asymptomatic bacteriuria and pyuria in infancy. *J. Pediat.*, **65**, 57.

REEVES, D. S. & BRUMFITT, W. (1968). Localization of urinary tract infection. In *Urinary Tract Infection*. ed. F. O'Grady and W. Brumfitt. London: Oxford University Press, p. 53.

ROBERTSON, M. H. (1968). Antibiotic resistance patterns of organisms causing acute urinary tract infections occurring in general practice. *Brit. J. clin. Pract.*, **22**.

SACKS, T. G. & ABRAMSON, J. H. (1967). Screening tests for bacteriuria. *J. Amer. med. Ass.*, **201**, 1.

SAVAGE, D. C. L. WILSON, M. I., ROSS, E. M. & FEE, W. M. (1969). Asymptomatic bacteriuria in girl entrants to Dundee primary schools. *Brit. med. J.*, **3**, 75.

SCHERTSEN, B., DAHLQUIST, A., FRITZ, H., KOHLER, L. & WESTLUND, L. (1968). Screening for bacteriuria with a test paper for glucose. *J. Amer. med. Ass.*, **204**, 205.

SCOTT, J. E. S. (1969). Results of anti-reflux surgery. *Lancet*, **2**, 68.

SCOTT, J. E. S. & STANSFELD, J. M. (1968a). Ureteric reflux and kidney scarring in children. *Arch. Dis. Childh.*, **43**, 468.

SCOTT, J. E. S. & STANSFELD, J. M. (1968b). Treatment of vesico-ureteric reflux in children. *Arch. Dis. Childh.*, **43**, 323.

SELIGMAN, S. J., DEIGH, R. A. & HEWITT, W. L. (1968). Detection of bacteriuria by a filter paper inoculating strip. *Amer. J. Obstet. Gynec.*, **102**, 890.

SELKON, J. (1969). Personal communication.

SIMMONS, N. A. & WILLIAMS, J. D. (1967). Use of a solid reagent in the triphenyl tetrazolium chloride test for bacteriuria. *J. clin. Path.*, **20**, 767.

SLADE, N., MATHER, H. G., LINTON, K. B., LEATHER, H. M. & POWELL, D. E. B. (1965). Sequela of post-operative urinary infection in women. *Brit. med. J.*, **1**, 1278.

SMELLIE, J. M. & NORMAND, K. S. (1968). Experience of follow-up of children with urinary tract infection. In *Urinary Tract Infection*. ed. F. O'Grady and W. Brumfitt. London: Oxford University Press.

SMITH, D. H. & ARMOUR, S. E. (1966). Transferable R factors in enteric bacteria causing infection of the genitourinary tract. *Lancet*, **2**, 15.

STEENSBERG, J., BARTELS, E. D., BAY-NIELSEN, H., FANØE, E. & HEDE, T. (1969). Epidemiology of urinary tract disease in general practice. *Brit. med. J.*, **4**, 390.

SUSSMAN, M., ASSCHER, A. W., WATERS, W. E., EVANS, J. A. S., CAMPBELL, H., EVANS, K. T. & EDMUND WILLIAMS, J. (1969). Asymptomatic significant bacteriuria in the non-pregnant woman. I. Description of a population. *Brit. med. J.*, **1**, 799.

TALLGREN, L. G. & VON BONSDORFF, C.-H. (1965). The effect of varying the pH level upon the sensitivity of urinary bacteria to antibiotics. *Acta med. scand.*, **178**, 543.

TURCK, M., RONALD, A. R. & PETERSDORF, R. G. (1968). Relapse and reinfection in chronic bacteriuria. II. The correlation between site of infection and pattern of recurrence in chronic bacteriuria. *New Engl. J. Med.*, **278**, 422.

TURNER, G. C. (1961). Bacilluria in pregnancy. *Lancet*, **2**, 1062.

WALKEY, F. A., JUDGE, T. G., THOMPSON, J. & SARKARI, N. B. S. (1967). Incidence of urinary infection in the elderly. *Scot. med. J.*, **12**, 411.

WHALLEY, P. J., MARTIN, F. G. & PETERS, P. C. (1965). Significance of bacteriuria detected during pregnancy. *J. Amer. med. Ass.*, **193**, 897.

WILLIAMS, G. L., CAMPBELL, H. & DAVIES, K. J. (1969). Urinary concentrating ability in women with asymptomatic bacteriuria in pregnancy. *Brit. med. J.*, **3**, 212.

WILLIAMS, G. L., DAVIES, D. K. L., EVANS, K. T. & EDMUND WILLIAMS, J. (1968). Vesico-ureteric reflux in patients with bacteriuria in pregnancy. *Lancet*, **2**, 1202.

WILLIAMS, J. D., THOMLINSON, J. L., COLE, J. G. L. & COPE, E. (1969). Asymptomatic urinary infection in gynaecological outpatients. *Brit. med. J.*, **1**, 29.

RENAL SCARRING AND CHRONIC PYELONEPHRITIS

From the picture of urinary tract infection presented in the preceding section, one would anticipate encountering chronic non-obstructive pyelonephritis predominantly in two sections of the population: (1) adolescents and young adults of both sexes, but with a female preponderance, who had contracted the disease in early childhood and (2) middle-aged women whose infection dated from the period of peak incidence in early married life. It is agreed that the disease does appear in these situations, and the young adults provide about one-fifth of the intake to regular haemodialysis and transplant centres (Drukker *et al.*, 1969). However, some descriptions based on autopsy evidence have presented chronic pyelonephritis as a much commoner disease affecting both sexes equally and spread over a wide age-range. The reasons for this discrepancy are discussed by Kimmelsteil *et al.* (1961), Beeson (1967) and Heptinstall (1967). It stems mainly from a tendency to attribute all focal scarring in the kidney to bacterial infection if no other cause is obvious. One of the slow advances of the last two decades has been the gradual definition of other diseases that cause chronic interstitial nephritis and focal scarring. A major cause in the older male is atheroma and atheroembolism (see below). Other causes are discussed by Beeson (1967), Heptinstall (1967) and Kerr (1970). One of the most important and controversial is analgesic nephropathy.

REFERENCES

BEESON, P. B. (1967). Urinary tract infection and pyelonephritis. In *Renal Disease*. ed. D. A. K. Black. 2nd edition. Oxford: Blackwell, p. 382.

DRUKKER, W., HAAGSMA-SCHOUTEN, W. A. C., ALBERTS, CHR. & SPOEK, M. G. (1969). Report on regular dialysis treatment in Europe V, 1969. *Proc. Eur. Dial. Transpl. Assoc.*, **6**, 99.

HEPTINSTALL, R. H. (1967). The limitations of the pathological diagnosis of chronic pyelonephritis. In *Renal Disease*. ed. D. A. K. Black. 2nd edition. Oxford: Blackwell, p. 350.

KERR, D. N. S. (1970). Differential diagnosis of chronic renal failure. In *Cecil-Loeb Textbook of Medicine*. 13th edition. ed. P. B. Beeson and W. McDermott.

KIMMELSTEIL, P., KIM, O. J., BERES, J. A. & WELLMAN, K. (1961). Chronic pyelonephritis. *Amer. J. Med.*, **30**, 589.

ANALGESIC NEPHROPATHY

In an article on interstitial nephritis in 1953, Spuhler and Zollinger suggested that some cases might be due to excessive consumption of analgesics containing phenacetin; analgesic mixtures are freely consumed in Switzerland where some watchmakers spread them in their sandwiches to prevent headache from eyestrain. Many of the subsequent reports have come from Scandinavia and Australia where abuse of analgesic mixtures is common and where they are often taken "for kicks" or to relieve depression rather than for their original purpose. The condition has been described as quite common in North-east and South-west Scotland (Prescott, 1966; McMillan et al., 1968) but less so in North-east England (Bell et al., 1969).

Controversy raged for several years on three issues: (1) is there a real association between consumption of analgesics and renal damage? (2) if so, is phenacetin the sole or main culprit? (3) does drug consumption damage the kidney directly, or by predisposing it to infection?

1. A real association has been difficult to prove. Sørensen (1966) who studied renal function in a large group of patients taking analgesics for rheumatic complaints concluded that even heavy consumption (more than 1 g phenacetin a day for over ten years) was not associated with any decline in the mean creatinine clearance of the group. However, he did note a significantly higher incidence of papillary necrosis in the absence of renal obstruction in phenacetin consumers. Although no similar prospective study has been produced to refute Sørensen, the world-wide accumulation of experience of an increasingly distinct disease associated with phenacetin abuse has convinced nearly all nephrologists that the entity exists, but that only a minority of all patients taking drugs develop renal damage. Studies of the metabolism of phenacetin have shown considerable variation in plasma level after an oral dose, and the appearance of numerous unidentified metabolites in the urine (Prescott et al., 1968); about four-fifths of the dose is recovered as paracetamol or its conjugates. Previous consumption of barbiturates alters the pattern of excretion, presumably by inducing enzymes in the liver;

there is an increased output of 2-hydroxy-4-ethoxyaniline which may be carcinogenic. No correlation has been found between these variations in the handling of phenacetin and its effect on the excretion of renal tubular cells, but it is uncertain whether the latter bears any relationship to chronic renal damage. Aspirin causes a more dramatic output of renal cells in the urine after acute administration than phenacetin (Prescott, 1965). Individual susceptibility to the effects of analgesics may be genetically determined since the disease has appeared in members of the same family (Frithz, 1967), but the environment may also be important; experimental renal damage is produced much more readily if the animal is deprived of fluid overnight and if the drug is given on an empty stomach (Kincaid-Smith, 1968); the hot climate of Queensland has been blamed for the very high incidence of analgesic nephropathy there.

2. The suggestion that phenacetin is the main offender has been hotly contended, particularly by Gilman (1964). Certainly phenacetin alone has rarely produced renal damage, but the drug is rarely consumed alone. The evidence incriminating phenacetin is largely epidemiological. It is the only ingredient common to nearly all the mixtures that have been held responsible for renal damage. Aspirin, which must be viewed with suspicion because of its acute effects on the renal tubule and because it may produce acute renal failure in overdosage (Campbell and McLaurin, 1958) is not contained in the phenacetin-phenazone-caffeine mixture which is the main offender in Sweden; nor in the analgesic hypnotic mixture (Saridone) often blamed for renal damage on the continent of Europe. Aspirin is consumed alone in very large quantities but "pure aspirin nephropathy" has only occasionally been reported (Prescott, 1969). Paracetamol, as a metabolite of phenacetin, must also be suspect, but only one case of "paracetamol nephropathy" has so far been reported (Krikler, 1967), although the drug is widely consumed in this country. This epidemiological evidence has been marshalled by Bengtsson (1969), whose advocacy of the view that phenacetin is the important ingredient has led to a ban on its over-the-counter sale in Sweden which has been followed by a decline in the incidence of the disease.

One factor that has prolonged the controversy over the role of phenacetin is the difficulty that has been experienced in reproducing the human lesion in animals with doses of phenacetin in any way comparable to those taken by patients. A mixture of aspirin, phenacetin and caffeine is a more potent nephrotoxin in rats than phenacetin alone (Saker and Kincaid-Smith, 1969), and it is at least possible that other ingredients in analgesic mixtures act synergistically with phenacetin in man as well as the rat.

3. Many early reports suggested that analgesic nephropathy was essentially chronic pyelonephritis due to an increased susceptibility to infection produced by the drugs. However, a convincing history of long-standing infection is seldom obtained (Nordenfelt and Ringertz, 1961; Young et al.,

1965; McMillan *et al.*, 1968; Bell *et al.*, 1969), and the fairly high incidence of infection and the susceptibility to fulminant pyelonephritis which characterize established papillary necrosis are probably late features of the disease. Dawborn, Kincaid-Smith and McLaren (1964) could not demonstrate any enhanced susceptibility to ascending infection in rats treated with aspirin, phenacetin or both.

The earliest lesion is probably the development of papillary necrosis which may be either fulminant, resulting in sloughing of the papilla, or more gradual, with coalescence of localized areas of necrosis (Kincaid-Smith, 1968). The tip of the papilla, supplied by the spiral artery, is sometimes spared. The area of cortex above the necrotic papilla is replaced by a thin scar, but cortical tissue in the renal columns hypertrophies, since the collecting ducts from this area open into the fornix of the calyx. The papillae may calcify and separate, producing a form of renal calculus. The subsequent changes have been described by Burry (1968). A discrete line of demarcation forms above the necrotic papilla, tubules in the adjacent zone show epithelial necrosis, and the overlying cortex is the site of diffuse uniform tubular atrophy and hyalinization of glomeruli. These changes are so characteristic that a pathologist given a nephrectomy or autopsy specimen can make a firm diagnosis which is nearly always substantiated by further probing into the history. Renal biopsy samples, however, do not usually include papillary tissue and cannot consistently distinguish analgesic nephropathy from other causes of severe renal scarring.

The *clinical features* are very similar to those of chronic pyelonephritis and are predictable from the damage to distal tubules. Polyuria, polydypsia and nocturia are usually present for some years before the onset of renal failure. Hypertension is a late feature which affects about half the patients, and is less resistant to treatment than in chronic glomerulonephritis. Accurate renal function studies reveal an acidifying defect and impairment of concentrating power which are more severe for any given reduction in glomerular filtration rate than in other renal diseases, including even pyelonephritis (Bengtsson, 1967; Steele *et al.*, 1969). There is a hyperchloraemic acidosis which is severe for the degree of uraemia and which may contribute to the high incidence of renal bone disease (Bell *et al.*, 1969). Hyperuricaemia is probably commoner than in other forms of renal failure, and impaired excretion of citrate may contribute to the formation of renal calculi.

The separation of sloughed papillae causes attacks of renal colic, and may produce acute renal failure from impaction of the papilla at the ureterovesical valve. Haematuria was present in 23 per cent of the patients described by McMillan and his colleagues (1968). Sterile pyuria is a very common feature (Dawborn *et al.*, 1966; McMillan *et al.*, 1968; Bell *et al.*, 1969) and analgesic nephropathy is now a more common cause of sterile pyuria in this country than renal tuberculosis.

Several associated clinical features have been described, but none is sufficiently constant to be of great value in diagnosis. Peptic ulcer has been common in some series (Dawborn *et al.*, 1966; Prescott, 1966) presumably as a result of the aspirin intake. Anaemia is sometimes out of proportion to uraemia; it may be hypochromic from chronic gastro-intestinal blood loss due to aspirin, or normochromic from haemolysis produced by phenacetin. Sideroblastic anaemia has been described in several patients (Dacie and Mollin, 1966; McMillan *et al.*, 1968). Methaemoglobinaemia is sometimes present. Swiss workers have described a diathesis of straight straggly hair and marked pigmentation but these are not prominent features of British patients.

Intravenous pyelography may show normal appearances even in the presence of papillary necrosis (Fairley and Kincaid-Smith, 1968). As scarring develops—and this may occur over a few months—the renal outline becomes indented and is often described as showing foetal lobulation. At the site of papillary separation calcyces become clubbed, as in chronic pyelonephritis. A diagnostic "ring sign" is occasionally seen on retrograde pyelography; contrast medium enters the line of cleavage proximal to the papilla.

In spite of the many diagnostic clues that have been listed, the diagnosis is often missed during life. A drug consumption history is so seldom volunteered, and is so often initially vague, that the patients are accused of concealing the history. Our own experience however is that they rarely deny analgesic intake when directly questioned and that their vagueness is due to a genuine lack of concern over the intake of what they regard as harmless household remedies. A careful drug history has become part of the essential routine in all patients with renal disease, and particularly careful probing is necessary if they suffer from headache, rheumatic complaints or insomnia. The diagnosis is well worth seeking, since withdrawal of analgesics is followed by stabilization, and sometimes even by improvement of renal function (Young *et al.*, 1965; Bell *et al.*, 1969). Careful follow-up of these patients is essential since they survive for many years in severe renal failure with acidosis, and are liable to develop bone disease and gout. Urinary infections must be eliminated and follow-up cultures continued indefinitely.

An additional hazard that the analgesic abuser runs, at least in Sweden, is the development of transitional cell carcinoma of the renal pelvis (*Lancet*, editorial, 1969). The incidence is high enough to justify routine examination of the urine for malignant cells in the follow-up of these patients.

The *prevention* of analgesic nephropathy is a challenge to the medical profession which has not been met outside Scandinavia. Phenacetin has no special properties that justify its continued use in the face of the evidence against it. However, the minor analgesics play an important role particularly in the treatment of rheumatic diseases, and as an alternative to aspirin is required for those with gastric intolerance. Paracetamol appears safer than phenacetin to date, but it should be regarded with suspicion, and a careful watch kept on patients consuming high doses over long periods. When any of these drugs are prescribed, a high fluid intake should be administered (Kincaid-Smith, 1968). When codeine is recommended, care should be taken to dispel confusion between pure codeine phosphate and Tab. Codeine Co. Consumption of the latter drug for diarrhoea caused renal failure in a Newcastle patient, and in one reported by Dyer and Lee (1967).

REFERENCES

BELL, D., KERR, D. N. S., SWINNEY, J. & YEATES, W. K. (1969). Analgesic nephropathy. Clinical course after withdrawal of phenacetin. *Brit. med. J.*, 3, 378.

BENGTSSON, U. (1967). Analgesic nephropathy—chronic pyelonephritis. In *Proceedings of the Third International Congress of Nephrology.* ed. R. H. Heptinstall. Basle: Karger.

BENGTSSON, U. (1969). Phenacetin. *Lancet*, 1, 264.

BURRY, A. F. (1968). The evolution of analgesic nephropathy. *Nephron*, 5, 185.

CAMPBELL, E. J. M. & MacLAURIN, R. E. (1958). Acute renal failure in salicylate poisoning. *Brit. med. J.*, 1, 503.

DACIE, J. V. & MOLLIN, D. L. (1966). Siderocytes, sideroblasts and sideroblastic anaemia. *Acta med. scand. Suppl.*, 455, 237.

DAWBORN, J. K., FAIRLEY, K. F., KINCAID-SMITH, P. & KING, W. E. (1966). The association of peptic ulceration, chronic renal disease and analgesic abuse. *Quart. J. Med.*, 35, 69.

DAWBORN, J. K., KINCAID-SMITH, P. & McLAREN, J. (1964). The effect of aspirin. and phenacetin on ascending infection in the rat kidney. *Aust. Ann. Med.*, 13, 217.

DYER, N. H. & LEE, F. I. (1967). Phenacetin nephropathy in a patient with an ileostomy. *Postgrad. med. J.*, 43, 791.

FAIRLEY, K. F., KINCAID-SMITH, P. (1968). Renal papillary necrosis with a normal pyelogram. *Brit. med. J.*, 1, 156.

FRITHZ, G. (1967). Phenacetin nephropathy in a mother and daughter. *Acta med. scand.*, 181, 529.

GILMAN, A. (1964). Analgesic nephropathy. *Amer. J. Med.*, 36, 167.

KINCAID-SMITH, P. (1968). Analgesic nephropathy and papillary necrosis. *Postgrad. med. J.*, 44, 807.

KRIKLER, D. M. (1967). Paracetamol and the kidney. *Brit. med. J.*, 2, 615.

LANCET EDITORIAL (1969). Analgesic abuse and tumours of the renal pelvis. *Lancet*, 2, 1233.

McMILLAN, J. M., LAWSON, D. H., PATON, A. M. & LINTON, A. L. (1968). The occurrence and clinical features of analgesic abuse in Western Scotland. *Scot. med. J.*, 13, 382.

NORDENFELT, O. & RINGERTZ, N. (1961). Phenacetin takers dead with renal failure. *Acta med. scand.*, 170, 385.

PRESCOTT, L. F. (1965). Effects of acetylsalicylic acid, phenacetin, paracetamol, and caffeine on renal tubular epithelium. *Lancet*, 2, 91.

PRESCOTT, L. F. (1966). Analgesic abuse in North-East Scotland. *Lancet*, 2, 1143.
PRESCOTT, L. F. (1969). Renal papillary necrosis and aspirin. *Scot. med. J.*, 14, 82.
PRESCOTT, L. F., SANSUR, M., LEVIN, W. & CONNEY, A. H. (1968). The comparative metabolism of phenacetin and N-acetyl-p-aminophenol in man with particular reference to effects on the kidney. *Clin. Pharmacol. Ther.*, 9, 605.
SAKER, B. M. & KINCAID-SMITH, P. (1969). Papillary necrosis in experimental analgesic nephropathy. *Brit. med. J.*, 1, 161.
SØRENSEN, A. W. S. (1966). Is the relation between analgesics and renal disease coincidental and not causal? *Nephron*, 3, 366.
SPUHLER, O. & ZOLLINGER, H. U. (1953). Die chronischinterstitielle Nephritis. *Z. klin. Med.*, 151, 1.
STEELE, T. W., GYORY, A. Z. & EDWARDS, K. D. G. (1969). Renal function in analgesic nephropathy. *Brit. med. J.*, 2, 213.
YOUNG, J. V., HAYDON, G. B., GRAY, C. P., HECKER, S. P. & LEE, P. R. (1965). Nephropathy associated with the use of analgesic medications. *Ann. intern. Med.*, 62, 727.

ACUTE RENAL FAILURE

The commonest cause of acute renal failure is the condition described by Shaldon in the last edition of this book as "acute intrinsic renal failure" but still generally known as "acute tubular necrosis". Its management has been reviewed in some detail by Blagg (1967), Gallagher and Polak (1967), Luke and Kennedy (1967), Schreiner (1967), Kerr (1968) and others. The trends predicted by Shaldon have materialized; the more severe cases, following accidental trauma and major surgery, are treated by daily haemo-dialysis and free protein diet with only moderate restriction of water and electrolyte intake (Robson, 1969; Kerr, 1970). This has undoubtedly improved the outlook of acute renal failure, but published series continue to show mortality rates around 50 per cent (see Kerr *et al.*, 1968 for review). This reflects a change in the pattern of disease; the most treatable forms are disappearing. Post-partum renal failure is becoming rare as the incidence of its main precipitants—septic abortion and pre-eclamptic toxaemia—declines. Following accidental trauma, the early cases of acute renal failure are largely prevented by the better management of shock but late cases still occur; they are often precipitated by infection and run a protracted course (Whelton and Donadio, 1969). Post-surgical acute renal failure is increasingly a disease of the elderly following major operations on the abdominal aorta and its main branches (*Lancet*, editorial, 1969).

The intake to an acute renal failure service contains a growing section classified as "medical", and is made up of a host of different syndromes, many of them individually rare, which together recreate general medicine in microcosm in a highly specialized ward. A recent monograph by Muehrcke

(1969) beautifully illustrates the renal histology and clinical course of many of these diseases. Some, which have attracted recent attention, are reviewed below.

REFERENCES

BLAGG, C. R. (1967). The management of acute reversible intrinsic renal failure. *Postgrad. med. J.*, **43**, 290.

GALLAGHER, L. & POLAK, A. (1967). The management of acute renal failure. *Hospital Medicine*, **1**, 287.

KERR, D. N. S. (1968). Renal failure. In *Paediatric Urology*. ed. D. Innes Williams. London: Butterworth.

KERR, D. N. S. (1970). The treatment of acute renal failure. In *Symposium on Intensive Therapy*. Royal College of Physicians, Edinburgh.

KERR, D. N. S., RABINDRANATH, G. & ELLIOTT, R. W. (1968). The treatment of acute renal failure. In *Fourth Symposium on Advanced Medicine*. ed. O. Wrong. London: Pitman.

LANCET EDITORIAL (1969). Abdominal aortic aneurysms. *Lancet*, **1**, 1199.

LUKE, R. G. & KENNEDY, A. C. (1967). Prevention and early management of acute renal failure. *Postgrad. med. J.*, **43**, 280.

MUEHRCKE, R. C. (1969). *Acute Renal Failure; Diagnosis and Management*. Saint Louis: Mosby.

ROBSON, J. S. (1969). Recent advances in renal disease. *Practitioner*, **203**, 483.

SCHREINER, G. E. (1967). Acute renal failure. In *Renal Disease*. ed. D. A. K. Black. Oxford: Blackwell.

WHELTON, A. & DONADIO, J. V. (1969). Post-traumatic acute renal failure in Vietnam. *Johns Hopk. med. J.*, **124**, 95.

LESIONS OF THE MAIN RENAL ARTERIES

Complete avulsion of the renal pedicle or renal artery follows blunt trauma to the abdomen, usually in deceleration injuries such as falls and car crashes. It causes pain and bruising in the loin and is often accompanied by shock, though this is sometimes prevented by rapid thrombosis of the avulsed artery. Acute tubular necrosis in the contralateral kidney has caused acute renal failure (Løkkegaard and Fredens, 1968).

Less severe trauma causes a localized crack in the intima of the artery and *traumatic renal artery thrombosis*. Bilateral thrombosis, which is rare, causes acute renal failure (Steiness and Thaysen, 1965). Unilateral lesions (Baichwal and Walch, 1968) cause pain and swelling with or without shock.

Surgical correction of these severe lesions has not been reported but the surprising success of late embolectomy suggests that reconstruction of the artery might be feasible if the diagnosis were made early enough. If symptoms are confined to the loin, an intravenous pyelogram will be performed in search of evidence for renal rupture (Elkin *et al.*, 1966) and will show a non-functioning kidney if the artery is thrombosed or avulsed. Early aortography is essential for confirmation; it shows a tapered proximal block in the renal artery (Cornell and Culp, 1968). In oliguric subjects, the diagnosis will not usually be suspected until catheterization or cystoscopy have excluded more familiar lesions such as rupture of the bladder and posterior urethra. Early aortography is necessary to distinguish renal artery lesions from the more common condition of acute tubular necrosis, following shock. In the latter, aortography shows thin spidery vessels in swollen kidneys and there is no nephrogram phase (Shaldon and Sheville, 1964).

Renal arterial embolism

This is usually produced by thrombus, vegetation or atheromatous debris. The common sources of thrombus are fibrillating atria and mural thrombi following myocardial infarction. Emboli from these sources, and vegetations from heart valves, usually lodge in several organs simultaneously (Table 4.2). The renal lesion tends to be overshadowed by the primary illness or by the more dramatic results of embolism in the brain and limbs.

TABLE 4.2

Other sites of embolism in 92 patients with clot emboli in the kidney
(from the autopsy data of Peterson and McDonald, 1968)

Lung	25
Brain	21
Spleen	18
Mesenteric	10
Other Viscera	6
Saddle	8
Limbs	4
No other sites	8

Many of the patients diagnosed at autopsy have apparently suffered no characteristic symptoms in life. The diagnosis was made before death in only three out of 348 cases of renal infarction reported by Barney and Mintz (1933) and Hoxie and Coggin (1940). In 18 patients with embolism diagnosed during life at Cornell (Goldsmith et al., 1968) the commonest symptom was pain in the renal angle, sometimes radiating to groin or upper abdomen, and the only common sign was tenderness in the renal angle and upper abdomen; these features were present in only about half the patients. Gross haematuria is uncommon in renal embolism, and proteinuria had been detected in only about one-third of the patients described by Peterson and McDonald (1968). Diagnosis therefore requires a high pitch of clinical awareness, coupled with a readiness to embark on pyelography and aorto-graphy on suspicion, in patients who are often badly disabled by their primary disease.

The justification for a vigorous diagnostic approach is the surprising success of embolectomy. Recovery of renal function has been described when embolectomy was performed five hours after apparently complete occlusion of the renal artery (Goldsmith *et al.*, 1968). Emboli have been removed several days after the episode with similar success, but in most of these the occlusion of the artery was probably incomplete; the arteriogram illustrated by Klinger and Nisnewitz (1968) demonstrated some flow of contrast past the embolus. The fate of kidneys in this precarious state on conservative treatment is largely unknown, but Fergus and his colleagues (1969) have described recovery of function in seven patients, two with acute renal failure from involvement of the sole functioning kidney, with anticoagulation and supportive therapy only. A large partly occlusive embolus in the renal artery may produce malignant hypertension within a few weeks, calling for late embolectomy (Mundth *et al.*, 1969). However this risk has to be weighed against the hazards of surgery in patients with severe cardiac disease, and it seems reasonable to advise conservative management in such patients unless aortography shows a complete block of the main renal artery.

Athero-embolism of the renal arteries

This is an important hazard of operations on the diseased aorta close to the origin of the renal arteries; to avoid it, some surgeons occlude the renal arteries during the critical few minutes of an aortic graft. The soft emboli of lipid and platelets are easily dislodged by the catheters used for aortography (Sieniewicz *et al.*, 1969). Enthusiastic efforts to confirm the diagnosis in patients oliguric after aortic surgery are therefore hazardous and since the emboli reach small renal vessels (Kassirer, 1969) they are unlikely to bring much therapeutic benefit. It is better to assume that post-operative oliguria is due to acute tubular necrosis until time proves the assumption right or wrong. The oliguric phase of tubular necrosis can be unusually long in this situation.

Spontaneous athero-embolism

This produces focal renal scarring in the elderly, leading to chronic renal failure and sometimes to renal hypertension resembling that of renal artery stenosis. Pyelography may show inequality of the kidney shadows and irregular indentations of the renal outline which are likely to elicit a radiological diagnosis of chronic pyelonephritis (Sieniewicz *et al.*, 1969). The correct diagnosis will be suggested by the absence of any history of infection and by the age and sex of the patient—athero-embolism occurs predominantly in males and almost exclusively over the age of 50 (Peterson and McDonald, 1968). There are often features of atheroma or embolism elsewhere—cerebrovascular disease, myocardial infarction, pancreatitis, limb ischaemia, etc. A fulminant form of athero-embolism is described in which renal function declines over a few weeks to fatal uraemia (Kassirer, 1969).

Thrombosis of the renal artery

This commonly occurs on the basis of atheroma and produces renal hypertension. However, acute thrombosis may destroy renal function completely and, in a single functioning kidney, produce anuria (Baird *et al.*, 1965; Smith *et al.*, 1968). These patients can be expected to have some collateral circulation as a result of antecedent partial occlusion, and surgical correction has been successful as late as 42 hours after the onset of anuria.

In the infant, thrombosis of a single renal artery has caused acute renal failure, even when the contralateral artery was intact (Woodward *et al.*, 1967). This resembles the situation in unilateral renal vein thrombosis of infancy; in both situations early removal of the affected kidney has been advised, but the natural history of the condition on conservative treatment is too poorly documented for this advice to be accepted uncritically.

REFERENCES

BAICHWAL, K. S. & WAUGH, D. (1968). Traumatic renal artery thrombosis. *J. Urol.*, **99**, 14.

BAIRD, R. J., YENDT, E. R. & FIROR, W. B. (1965). Anuria due to acute occlusion of the artery to a solitary kidney. *New Engl. J. Med.*, **272**, 1012.

BARNEY, J. D. & MINTZ, E. R. (1933). Infarcts of the kidney. *J. Amer. med. Ass.*, **100**, 1.

CORNELL, S. H. & CULP, D. A. (1968). Acute occlusion of the renal artery demonstrated by renal angiography. *J. Urol.*, **100**, 2.

ELKIN, M., MENG, C. H. & DE PAREDES, R. G. (1966). Correlation of intravenous urography and renal angiography in kidney injury. *Radiology*, **86**, 496.

FERGUS, J. N., JONES, N. F. & LEA THOMAS, M. (1969). Kidney function after renal arterial embolism. *Brit. med. J.*, **4**, 587.

GOLDSMITH, E. L. FULLER, F. W., LAMBREW, C. T. & MARSHALL, V. F. (1968). Embolectomy of the renal artery. *J. Urol.*, **99**, 366.

HOXIE, H. J. & COGGIN, C. B. (1940). Renal infarction: statistical study of 205 cases and detailed report of an unusual case. *Arch. intern. Med.*, **65**, 587.

KASSIRER, J. P. (1969). Athero-embolic renal disease. *New Engl. J. Med.*, **280**, 812.

KLINGER, M. E. & NISNEWITZ (1968). Renal artery embolectomy. *Amer. J. Surg.*, **115**, 669.

LØKKEGAARD, H. & FREDENS, M. (1968). Complete avulsion of the renal pedicle due to non-penetrating trauma. *Acta chir. scand.*, **134**, 79.

MUNDTH, E. D., SHINE, K. & AUSTEN, W. G. (1969). Correction of malignant hypertension and return of renal function following late renal artery embolectomy. *Amer. J. Med.*, **46**, 985.

PETERSON, N. E. & McDONALD, D. F. (1968). Renal embolization. *J. Urol.* **100**, 140.

SHALDON, S. & SHEVILLE, E. (1964). Angiography in acute renal failure. *Clin. Radiol.*, **15**, 123.

SIENIEWICZ, D. J., MOORE, M. D., MOIR, F. D. & DADE, D. F. (1969). Atheromatous emboli to the kidneys. *Radiology*, **92**, 1231.

SMITH, H. T., SHAPIRO, F. L. & MESSNER, R. P. (1968). Anuria secondary to reno-vascular disease. *J. Amer. med. Ass.*, **204**, 928.

STEINESS, I. & THAYSEN, J. H. (1965). Bilateral traumatic renal-artery thrombosis. *Lancet*, **1**, 527.

WOODWARD, J. R., PATTERSON, J. H. & BRINSFIELD, D. (1967). Renal artery thrombosis in newborn infants. *Amer. J. Dis. Child.*, **114**, 191.

RENAL VEIN THROMBOSIS

Thrombosis of renal veins in oedematous patients was described 130 years ago from the autopsy room, but the first reports of diagnosis in life in adults with the nephrotic syndrome did not appear until the 1950s (Harrison *et al.*, 1956; Pollak *et al.*, 1956). The clinical syndromes produced by renal vein thrombosis also include acute and chronic renal failure and renal hyper-tension, depending on the site and extent of the occlusion and the age of the patient. About half of all reported cases have been in young infants, pre-dominantly in the first month of life, in whom the condition is often uni-lateral. The other half are spread over a wide age-range and are usually bilateral. In spite of this, acute renal failure is commoner in the infantile type.

Renal vein thrombosis in infancy (McFarland, 1965)

This is usually precipitated by gastroenteritis, systemic infection or other causes of dehydration. It is possibly a significant association of maternal diabetes (Takenchi and Benirschke, 1961) and it can occur without any obvious precipitant (Haddad *et al.*, 1966). These "primary" cases are some-times detected in the first few hours of life, suggesting that the thrombosis occurred *in utero*.

The onset is characteristically acute with pain and swelling in the loin, haematuria and proteinuria. Fever, vomiting and diarrhoea are often present either from the primary disease or following the renal complication, and haemoconcentration shown by a high haematocrit is usual. Thrombocyto-penia has been reported, and is presumably secondary to the renal damage since it has been cured by nephrectomy (Jones and Reed, 1965). The affected kidney is palpably enlarged and tender. Its large size is confirmed by straight radiographs of the renal tract, and it is usually non-functioning on intra-venous pyelography. Retrograde pyelography may reveal compression of calyces by the swollen kidney, blood clot in the renal pelvis, and extravasation of contrast into the renal parenchyma (Karafin and Stearns, 1964).

Oliguria and acute renal failure are common even when the condition is unilateral. Because the renal failure often progresses rapidly to death, the usual treatment has been emergency nephrectomy. The excised kidney shows extensive haemorrhagic infarction, suggesting that little functioning tissue has been lost as a result of the operation, and rapid recovery from acute renal failure has often followed the removal of the infarcted kidney (Miller and Benjamin, 1962; Karafin and Stearns, 1964). However the prognosis in children treated conservatively for acute renal failure without nephrectomy is uncertain. Three infants who recovered on conservative treatment were described by Stark (1964) but in all of these the renal failure was mild and did not necessitate dialysis. They reviewed 17 further spontaneous recoveries, some with bilateral thrombosis, and advised a more restricted use of surgery, on the grounds that some recovery of funtion may occur following venous infarction. If the damaged kidney is left *in situ*, careful follow-up is necessary to detect the late onset of nephrotic syndrome and renal hypertension. Unrecognized renal vein thrombosis may explain some cases of hypertension with unilateral renal atrophy encountered in later childhood, at present attributed to chronic pyelonephritis or hypoplasia.

Renal vein thrombosis in the adult (Rosemann *et al.*, 1968)

This has many causes. Infection in and around the kidney was often mentioned in early reports but is now rare; septic clot in the renal vein gave rise to septicaemia and pyaemia. Thrombosis may follow invasion of the renal vein by hypernephroma or compression by retroperitoneal tumours or fibrosis. It may spread from the femoral veins *via* the inferior vena cava. It has followed blunt trauma to the abdomen or lumbar region, and violent effort. Dehydration following excessive use of diuretics had been incriminated. A major group of cases complicates other renal diseases including amyloidosis, diabetic nephropathy, glomerulonephritis and nephrosclerosis. It is most commonly described as a complication of nephrotic syndrome with "minimal change" or membranous glomerulonephropathy, though the problem of "which came first?" often arises in these cases. A hypercoagulable state exists in nephrotic patients due to elevation of fibrinogen and factors v, vii, viii, and x, enhanced thromboplastin generation and sometimes elevated platelet count; fibrinolysis is diminished (Menon, 1967). Steroid therapy probably increases the tendency to thrombosis unless it cures the nephrotic syndrome (Lieberman *et al.*, 1968).

An acute onset with severe pain in the renal angle and hypochondrium, radiating to groin and testicle is uncommon in the adult; it occurred in only one of 15 patients studied by Rosemann, Pollak and Pirani (1968). Three other patients in this series had a dull ache in the renal area. The diagnosis must therefore be sought in patients without obvious localizing signs and it is still frequently missed in life. Only one of 16 patients recently reported from San Francisco (Cohn *et al.*, 1968) had been diagnosed before autopsy. Many of the cases recognized after death have suffered from acute or chronic renal failure; nephrotic syndrome is over-represented in patients diagnosed clinically since its more prolonged course allows time for diagnosis; 11 of the 15 patients described by Rosemann and colleagues presented with nephrotic syndrome. The prognosis in the whole group is gloomy—41 of 65 patients reviewed by Kowal, Figur and Kitzig (1963) died within two months of onset and only 14 survived two years. Major causes of death are renal failure and pulmonary embolism.

Hypertension is found in about half the patients with nephrotic syndrome. Haematuria is usually present but seldom macroscopic. A grossly enlarged tender kidney is found in those with an acute onset, and enlargement followed by shrinkage is demonstrable on radiographs in the majority. Fever and leucocytosis occur only with an acute onset or with pulmonary embolism.

The radiological findings have been reviewed by Hipona and Crummy (1966) and Chait and his colleagues (1968). When the occlusion is acute they are similar to those in infancy. Confusion with polycystic disease is possible but the renal outline is smooth. A very late and persistent nephrogram may indicate acute occlusion (Duncan et al., 1970). Slowly developing occlusion may lead to the development of a collateral circulation through the ureteric veins, which is shown as notching of the ureters on pyelography. Transfemoral inferior venocavography in the normal subject shows non-opacified streams of blood emerging from the renal veins. Absence of one or both of these suggests renal vein occlusion, which can be confirmed by failure of the contrast to enter the renal vein during a vigorous valsalva manœuvre or during selective renal venography. If the vena cava is occluded, or if there is a history of embolism, inferior cavography can be performed from above or by injection into the greater trochanter of the femur. Aortography or selective renal arteriography gives valuable information about the state of the parenchyma; it shows displacement of interlobular arteries by oedematous medulla and may outline collateral veins on late films; Chait and his colleagues regarded it as a more valuable investigation than venography.

Renal biopsy may show haemorrhagic infarction if the onset is acute. If it is more gradual, tubular atrophy, vacuolization, and basement membrane thickening and interstitial oedema and fibrosis are usually prominent. A rough quantitative grading of tubular and interstitial damage and of glomerular changes separates renal vein thrombosis from membranous glomerulonephropathy, with which it is most likely to be confused (Rosemann et al., 1968). The glomerular changes include diffuse basement membrane thickening, stasis of leucocytes within glomeruli ("margination of leucocytes") and widening of capillary loops. Thrombi are only occasionally seen in arcuate veins.

The close similarity between the glomerular changes following renal vein thrombosis and those in idiopathic membranous glomerulonephropathy has led to speculation that the membranous change often antedates the thrombosis. This view is particularly attractive in the case of unilateral thrombosis which is usually accompanied by glomerular change in, and heavy proteinuria from, *both* kidneys (Richet *et al.*, 1965; Rosemann *et al.*, 1968; Duncan *et al.*, 1970). However, experimental occlusion of one renal vein in the dog also causes bilateral glomerular change, with deposition of gammaglobulin in the basement membranes, suggesting that an autoimmune reaction is set up by damage to one kidney (Harris *et al.*, 1968). It is uncertain whether this occurs in other species; in the rat, nephrotic syndrome is not produced by renal vein occlusion unless the contralateral kidney is removed (Fisher *et al.*, 1968), and in man ligation of the left renal vein, which is occasionally a surgical necessity, causes remarkably few sequelae (Erlik *et al.*, 1965). Current evidence suggests that the commoner sequence of events is: clinically silent membranous glomerulonephropathy—thrombotic tendency—renal vein thrombosis—clinically obvious nephrotic syndrome (Maltzer *et al.*, 1969), but the possibility that renal vein thrombosis sometimes initiates a membranous glomerulonephropathy cannot be excluded.

Treatment with anticoagulants has sometimes been followed by improvement in renal function and remission of nephrotic syndrome (Pollak *et al.*, 1966). When it fails, surgical removal of the thrombus with the thickened intima should be considered. It has produced some improvement in renal function, though without complete relief of nephrotic syndrome (Cohn *et al.*, 1968; Fein *et al.*, 1968).

REFERENCES

CHAIT, A., STOANE, L., MOSKOWITZ, H. & MELLINS, H. Z. (1968). Renal vein thrombosis. *Radiology*, **90**, 886.

COHN, L. H., LEE, J., HOPPER, J. & NAJARIAN, J. S. (1968). The treatment of bilateral renal vein thrombosis and nephrotic syndrome. *Surgery*, **64**, 387.

DUNCAN, A. W., SCHORR, W., CLARK, F. & KERR, D. N. S. (1970). Unilateral renal vein thrombosis and nephrotic syndrome. *J. Urol.* In press.

ERLIK, D., BARZILAI, A. & SHRAMEK, A. (1965). Renal function after left renal vein ligation. *J. Urol.*, **93**, 540.

FEIN, R. L., CHAIT, A. & LEVITON, A. (1968). Renal vein thrombectomy for the treatment of renal vein thrombosis associated with the nephrotic syndrome. *J. Urol.*, **99**, 1.

FISHER, E. R., SHARKEY, D., PARDO, V. & VUZEVSKI, N. (1968). Experimental renal vein constriction. Its relation to renal lesions observed in human renal vein thrombosis and the nephrotic syndrome. *Lab. Invest.*, **18**, 689.

HADDAD, P., FARAH, M. & HAKIM, Z. (1966). Acute idiopathic renal vein thrombosis in a newborn infant. *J. Pediat.*, **69**, 454.

HARRIS, J. D., EHRENFIELD, W. K. & WYLIE, E. J. (1968). Experimental renal vein occlusion. *Surgery*, **126**, 555.

HARRISON, C. V., MILNE, M. D. & STEINER, R. E. (1956). Clinical aspects of renal vein thrombosis. *Quart. J. Med.*, **25**, 285.

HIPONA, F. A. & CRUMMY, A. B. (1966). The Roentgen diagnosis of renal vein thrombosis; clinical aspects. *Amer. J. Roentgenol.*, **98**, 122.

JONES, J. E. & REED, J. F. (1965). Renal vein thrombosis and thrombocytopoenia in a newborn infant. *J. Pediat.*, **67**, 681.

KARAFIN, L. & STEARNS, T. M. (1964). Renal vein thrombosis in children. *J. Urol.*, **92**, 91.

KOWAL, J., FIGUR, A. & KITZIG, W. M. (1963). Renal vein thrombosis and the nephrotic syndrome with complete remission. *J. Mt Sinai Hosp.*, **30**, 47.

LIEBERMAN, E., HEUSER, E., GILCHRIST, G. S., DONNELL, G. N. & LANDING, B. H. (1968). Thrombosis, nephrosis and corticosteroid therapy. *J. Pediat.*, **73**, 320.

MALTZER, J. I., TANNENBAUM, M., SEEGAL, B. C. & SOMMERS, S. C. (1969). Immunological study of four consecutive patients with renal vein thrombosis and the nephrotic syndrome. *Abstracts of the Fourth International Congress of Nephrology*, **1**, 251.

McFARLAND, J. B. (1965). Renal vein thrombosis in children. *Quart. J. Med.*, **34**, 269.

MENON, I. S. (1967). Pulmonary artery thrombosis and the nephrotic syndrome. *Brit. med. J.*, **2**, 110.

MILLER, H. C. & BENJAMIN, J. A. (1962). Acute idiopathic renal vein thrombosis in infants. *Pediatrics*, **30**, 247.

POLLAK, V. E., KARK, R. M., PIRANI, C. L., SHAFTER, H. A. & MUEHRCKE, R. C. (1956). Renal vein thrombosis and the nephrotic syndrome. *Amer. J. Med.*, **21**, 496.

POLLAK, V. E., PIRANI, C. L., SESKIND, C. & GRIFFEL, B. (1966). Bilateral renal vein thrombosis. Clinical and electron microscopic studies of a case with complete recovery after anticoagulant therapy. *Ann. intern. Med.*, **65**, 1056.

RICHET, G., GILLOT, C., VAYSSE, J. & MEYEROVITCH, A. (1965). La thrombose isolée de la veine rénale. *Presse méd.*, **73**, 2035.

ROSEMANN, E., POLLAK, V. E. & PIRANI, C. L. (1968). Renal vein thrombosis in the adult; a clinical and pathological study based on renal biopsy. *Medicine*, **47**, 269.

STARK, H. (1964). Renal vein thrombosis in infancy; recovery without nephrectomy. *Amer. J. Dis. Child.*, **108**, 430.

TAKENCHI, O. & BENIRSCHKE, K. (1961). Renal vein thrombosis of newborn and its relation to maternal diabetes. *Biol. Neonat.*, **3**, 237.

HAEMOLYTIC URAEMIC SYNDROME

In 1955, Gasser and colleagues described five children with haemolytic anaemia, thrombocytopenia and fatal renal failure under the title "Hämolytisch-urämische Syndrom". With hindsight some cases can now be recognized in earlier literature, but they are very few compared with the flood of reports covering many hundreds of patients in the 14 years since Gasser's description. These have been reviewed by Lieberman and colleagues (1966), Piel and Phibbs (1966), Habib, Mathieu and Royer (1967) and

Hammond *et al.* (1967). The most authoritative personal account is that of Gianantonio, Vitacco and Mendilaharzu (1967) based on 162 patients in Buenos Aires.

The disease affects young children with a peak incidence between six and 18 months. It is common in those of high social class, occurs in minor epidemics (Ruthven and Fyfe, 1968) and is more common in the winter and spring months than in summer and autumn. The prodromal symptoms are usually (about 70 per cent) vomiting and diarrhoea, with soft mucoid and blood-streaked stools, but about 10 to 20 per cent begin with symptoms of an upper respiratory infection. This initial phase lasts two to seven days, and seldom leads to hospital admission. After an interval of up to seven days, during which the prodromal symptoms subside but the child remains pale and irritable, the second phase begins with the onset of oliguria and acute renal failure, severe pallor or convulsions, stupor or coma. A smaller proportion present with "cardiac failure" due to fluid overload, oedema, haematuria or gastro-intestinal haemorrhage.

The *anaemia* is usually severe (average Hb 6·6 g per 100 ml in Buenos Aires) and is accompanied by signs of haemolysis—raised reticulocyte count (usually over 10 per cent) and normoblasts in peripheral blood, raised plasma haemoglobin level and reduced or absent haptoglobins. The most striking and diagnostic feature is the presence of fragmented and misshapen red cells—burr cells, triangular, crescentic, helmet-shaped cells, microspherocytes and fragments. Plasma bilirubin is sometimes elevated but jaundice is unusual. The Coombs test is negative but cold agglutinins have occasionally been found (Habib *et al.*, 1967). Transfused cells have a very short survival. Leucocytosis is considerable, averaging 22,000 in the children described by Habib *et al.* (1967) and immature forms appear in the peripheral blood.

Thrombocytopenia

This is almost universal at some time in the illness; it was present in 81 per cent during hospital admission at Buenos Aires. It is probably due to excessive destruction of platelets and is followed by a rebound thrombocytosis. The platelets are presumably deposited in the thrombotic lesions found predominantly in the kidneys. Fibrin is also deposited in these vessels, and the increased deposition and solution of fibrin is shown by the presence of fibrin degradation products in plasma and urine, and by an increased rate of fibrinogen turnover (Brain *et al.*, 1968). The new fibrinogen formed is abnormal (Rivero and Ritz, 1968), producing loose porous clots (Editorial, 1969) which may be less efficient in haemostasis than normal dense clot. Low plasma levels of fibrinogen have sometimes been detected; circulating levels of other clotting factors such as V and VIII which are presumably consumed are normal or raised (Desmit *et al.*, 1965; Gianantonio *et al.*,

1967) but plasma levels of clotting factors are an insensitive index of their rates of catabolism (Brain *et al.*, 1968).

A bleeding tendency is a common and troublesome feature of the illness. Melaena was present in 60 per cent, haematemesis in 20 per cent and subcutaneous haematomata in 38 per cent of the children described by Gianantonio *et al.* (1967). Abdominal pain is common, presumably as a result of the melaena. Skin rash, hepatosplenomegaly and lymphadenopathy are described in a minority and probably reflect the original infection.

Renal failure

This is the main cause of the high mortality and morbidity. About half the patients reported have been anuric for at least four days, and oliguria is often prolonged even in those who survive (Sharpstone *et al.*, 1968). Uraemia is aggravated by a high catabolic rate. Haematuria is almost invariable, usually heavy and sometimes macroscopic. Proteinuria is heavy, causing a nephrotic syndrome in about one-third (Habib *et al.*, 1967). A small minority have no uraemia but only haematuria, proteinuria and casts in the deposit.

The renal histology ranges from cortical necrosis, sometimes bilateral and symmetrical, sometimes focal, with necrosis of the pyramids, to mild glomerular lesions. Thrombi are found in afferent arterioles and glomerular capillaries but less often in interlobular arteries. There is interstitial oedema and patchy tubular necrosis. The glomeruli show obliteration of capillary lumina by subendothelial deposition of fibrinoid material, hypercellularity, focal tuft necrosis and sometimes crescent formation.

Hypertension is present during the acute illness in about half, and it often remits as the child improves, but there is a progressive increase in the incidence of hypertension at follow-up which reaches about 33 per cent by the fourth year (Gianantonio *et al.*, 1968). Hypertensive retinopathy is found particularly in those with convulsions.

Cerebrovascular symptoms

These have been common in some series. Convulsions occurred in two-thirds of the patients at Buenos Aires, stupor in a quarter and coma in a fifth. Stupor, rigidity and involuntary movement sometimes persisted for several weeks. There is little evidence of vascular damage in other organs even at autopsy.

Treatment

Treatment consists primarily of good management of acute renal failure, including the liberal use of peritoneal dialysis or haemodialysis and adequate diet. On this regime alone the mortality rate in Argentina fell from 47 per cent in 1957–61 to 5 per cent by 1968. In other centres the mortality has remained much higher. Heparin therapy has been widely recommended and some successes reported (Desmit *et al.*, 1965; Brain *et al.*, 1968; Gilchrist *et al.*, 1969). In a few of these cases an immediate rise in plasma fibrinogen or platelet count or a fall in fibrinogen turnover indicated that heparin was doing something of benefit, but in most the results are open to individual interpretation. Continuous heparinization for several weeks in a small infant is a formidable undertaking and more evidence for its value is needed. It is almost certainly useless if given late in the illness. Steroid therapy has been tried on a fairly large scale and discarded as unhelpful, possibly harmful (Piel and Phibbs, 1966; Gianantonio *et al.*, 1967).

Relapse in the first few weeks is quite common, but second attacks are rare. The haemopoietic system returns to normal but the kidneys are often the site of permanent damage. Of 76 survivors followed up at Buenos Aires (Gianantonio *et al.*, 1968), 33 recovered normal excretory function within six months, lost proteinuria and had only minimal scarring on biopsy; 20 recovered more slowly over several years; 16 had declining renal function with continuing activity of the renal lesion and seven were left in critical chronic renal failure, with extensive renal scarring.

The *aetiology* remains uncertain, but it is generally believed that haemolytic uraemic syndrome is a reaction to several different infective agents. In Buenos Aires, two-thirds of the patients show serological evidence of recent infection with an arbovirus, related to that of Argentinian haemorrhagic fever (Gianantonio *et al.*, 1967), but this agent has not been incriminated elsewhere. Gram-negative bacteria including *E. coli* and *salmonellae*, and other viruses including measles vaccine have been suggested as possible precipitants in individual cases (Hammond *et al.*, 1967). A familial predisposition is suggested by its occurrence in siblings (Anthony and Kaplan, 1968).

The pathogenesis is also in dispute. The most popular view is that the original immunological insult triggers the widespread deposition of fibrin and platelet in small vessels, possibly the site of intimal damage, and that red cells are distorted and damaged by contact with the fibrin (Brain, 1968). The typical red cell changes have been reproduced *in vitro* by forcing blood through a loose mesh of fibrin or synthetic fibres (Bull *et al.*, 1967).

REFERENCES

Anthony, P. P. & Kaplan, A. B. (1968). Fatal haemolytic-uraemic syndrome in two sibs. *Arch. Dis. Childh.*, **43**, 316.
Brain, M. C. (1968). Haemolytic-uraemic syndrome. *Lancet*, **2**, 1394.
Brain, M. C., Baker, L. R. I., McBride, J. A., Rubenberg, M. L. & Dacie, J. V. (1968). Treatment of patients with microangiopathic haemolytic anaemia with heparin. *Brit. J. Haemat.*, **15**, 603.

BULL, B. S., RUBENBERG, M. L., DACIE, J. V. & BRAIN, M. C. (1967). Red-blood cell fragmentation in microangiopathic haemolytic anaemia; *in vitro* studies. *Lancet*, 2, 1123.

DESMIT, E. M., HART, H. CH., HELLEMAN, P. W. & TIDDENS, H. A. W. M. (1965). Heparin treatment in a patient with haemolytic uraemic syndrome. *Proc. Eur. dial. transpl. Ass.*, 2, 68.

GASSER, C., GAUTIER, E., STECK, A., SIEBERMANN, R. E. & OESCHLIN, R. (1955). Hämolytisch-urämische Syndrom: bilaterale Nierenrindennekrosen bie akuten erworbenen hamolytisch anamien. *Schweiz. med. Wschr.*, 85, 905.

GIANANTONIO, C. A., VITACCO, M. & MENDILAHARZU, F. (1967). The hemolytic-uremic syndrome. In *Proceedings of the Third International Congress of Nephrology*. Vol. 3, p. 24. ed. E. L. Becker, Basle: Karger.

GIANANTONIO, C. A., VITACCO, M., MENDILAHARZU, F. & GALLO, G. (1968). The hemolytic-uremic syndrome. *J. Pediat.*, 72, 757.

GILCHRIST, G. S., LIEBERMAN, E., EKERT, H., FINE, R. N. & GRUSHKIN, C. (1969). Heparin therapy in the haemolytic-uraemic syndrome. *Lancet*, 1, 1123.

HABIB, R., MATHIEU, H. & ROYER, P. (1967). Le syndrome hémolytique et urémique de l'enfant. Aspects cliniques et anatomiques dans 27 observations. *Nephron*, 4, 139.

HAMMOND, D., LIEBERMAN, E., WRIGHT, H. T., HEUSER, E. T. & RAPAPORT, S. J. (1967). Seminar: Hemolytic-Uremic Syndrome. *Amer. J. Dis. Childh.*, 114, 440.

LIEBERMAN, E., HEUSER, E., DONNELL, G. N., LANDING, B. H. & HAMMOND, G. D. (1966). Hemolytic-uremic syndrome. Clinical and pathological consideration. *New Engl. J. Med.*, 275, 227.

PIEL, C. F. & PHIBBS, R. H. (1966). The hemolytic-uremic syndrome. *Pediat. Clin. N. Amer.*, 13, 295.

RIVERO, I. & RITZ, N. D. (1968). Abnormal fibrinogen in thrombotic thrombocytopenic purpura. *Blood*, 32, 140.

RUTHVEN, I. S. & FYFE, W. M. (1968). The haemolytic-uraemic syndrome—an epidemic disease? *Scot. Med. J.*, 13, 162.

SCOTTISH MEDICAL JOURNAL EDITORIAL (1969). Microangiopathic haemolytic anaemia, 14, 187.

SHARPSTONE, P., EVANS, R. G., O'SHEA, M., ALEXANDER, L. & LEE, H. A. (1968). Haemolytic-uraemic syndrome: survival after prolonged oliguria. *Arch. Dis. Childh.*, 43, 711.

OTHER FORMS OF MICROANGIOPATHY CAUSING RENAL FAILURE

Typical haemolytic uraemic syndrome with gastro-intestinal prodromata and explosive onset is virtually confined to childhood, but many of its features—including damage to small vessels, red-cell fragmentation and disseminated intravascular coagulation—are found in other diseases which occur at all ages. Dacie (1967) suggested a classification of the diseases combining haemolytic anaemia with acute renal failure. This separated two distinct syndromes—haemolytic uraemic syndrome of childhood and "thrombotic thrombocytopoenia" occurring mainly in adults—from the other illnesses such as malignant hypertension, pre-eclampsia and renal failure with hypertension post-partum, in which haemolysis and thrombocytopenia were epiphenomena or occurred only terminally. However, the dividing line is not always distinct.

Thrombotic thrombocytopenia purpura

This was described in 1924 by Moschcowitz and reviewed in detail by Amorosi and Ultmann (1966) and a concise description is given by Hamburger and colleagues (1968). The onset is often acute. The manifestations include abdominal pain, joint pains, fever, jaundice, hepatomegaly and splenomegaly, but the cardinal features are haemolytic anaemia, thrombocytopenia, neurological signs and renal failure. The neurological signs are often focal, and characteristically wax and wane. They include monoplegia, cranial nerve palsies, speech disorder, psychological disturbance, fits and coma. The kidneys are affected in about half the adult cases; afferent arterioles are obliterated by "onion skin" proliferation of the intima and subendothelial deposition of fibrin. Glomerular, tubular and interstitial changes are similar to those in haemolytic uraemic syndrome but cortical necrosis is not a usual feature. Irreversible anuria often develops in those with renal involvement. The vascular lesions are widespread throughout the body and can be demonstrated in biopsies of various organs, of which bone marrow aspirates are the most convenient (Blecher and Raper, 1967). Heparin infusion has achieved about the same success as in haemolytic uraemic syndrome, and presents fewer problems in the adult.

About 20 per cent of all reported cases of thrombotic thrombocytopoenic purpura have been associated with disseminated lupus erythematosus (Amorosi and Ultman, 1966). It also occurs rarely in association with polyarteritis, rheumatoid arthritis (Thomson and Gardner, 1969) and purpura fulminans (Hollingsworth and Mohler, 1968). A similar syndrome occurs with disseminated carcinoma, but here the thrombi also affect large vessels (Tapp and Raltston, 1969).

Malignant hypertension

This is often accompanied by microangiopathic haemolytic anaemia; it was present in 16 of 24 patients with retinal haemorrhage and exudates studied by Linton and colleagues (1969) but was not found in any of 63 patients with benign hypertension, without these fundal changes. The condition usually remits with successful treatment of hypertension, but some of these anuric patients are resistant to conventional therapy, and occasionally success has been achieved only after bilateral nephrectomy (Giromini and Laperrouza, 1969). Pregnancy occasionally triggers a thrombotic thrombocytopoenic purpura which may remit after delivery and recur in subsequent pregnancies (Baker and Brain, 1967; Piver et al., 1968). Whether it arises de novo or complicates pre-eclampsia is uncertain. A progressive illness in the few weeks following delivery has been described by Robson and his colleagues (1968) as *irreversible post-partum renal failure*. Renal failure was caused by severe narrowing of afferent arterioles, leading to focal glomerular infarction and accompanied by endothelial proliferation in the remaining glomeruli. Haemolytic anaemia and thrombocytopoenia affected most of the patients described by Robson *et al.* (1968) and were seen personally at Newcastle. Intractable cardiac failure developed in the absence of usual causes such as uncontrolled hypertension and with ECG changes suggesting a cardiomyopathy.

The *Schwartzman reaction* is a term which, used correctly, describes the production of disseminated intravascular coagulation and cortical necrosis by two injections of staphylococcal endotoxin given 24 hours apart to rabbits. Only a single injection is required if reticuloendothelial function is blocked or fibrinolysis suppressed as in pregnancy. Acute renal failure with haemolytic anaemia, thrombocytopoenia, consumption of clotting factors and response to heparin, exactly mirroring the Schwartzman reaction, has been described following abortion complicated by septicaemia with *E. coli* and *Clostridium perfringens* (Rubenberg *et al.*, 1967; Clarkson *et al.*, 1969). A similar mechanism may play a part in the initiation of acute renal failure complicating other infections and even in different circumstances, when the full-blown Schwartzman reaction cannot be demonstrated (Wardle, 1968). There is at least some evidence that the onset of acute renal failure following transfusion reactions involves intravascular coagulation and is ameliorated by heparin (Rock *et al.*, 1969).

REFERENCES

AMOROSI, E. L. & ULTMANN, J. E. (1966). Thrombotic thrombocytopoenic purpura: report of 16 cases and review of the literature. *Medicine*, **45**, 139.

BAKER, L. R. I. & BRAIN, M. C. (1967). Heparin treatment of haemolytic anaemia and thrombocytopoenia in pre-eclampsia. *Proc. roy. Soc. Med.*, **60**, 477.

BLECHER, T. E. & RAPER, A. B. (1967). Early diagnosis of thrombotic microangiopathy by paraffin sections of aspirated bone-marrow. *Arch. Dis. Childh.*, **42**, 158.

CLARKSON, A. R., SAGE, R. E. & LAWRENCE, J. R. (1969). Consumption coagulopathy and acute renal failure due to Gram-negative septicaemia after abortion and complete recovery with heparin. *Ann. intern. Med.*, **70**, 1191.

DACIE, J. V. (1967). *The Haemolytic Anaemias*, Part 3. London: Churchill.

GIROMINI, M. & LAPERROUZA, C. (1969). Prolonged survival after nephrectomy in an adult with haemolytic-uraemic syndrome. *Lancet*, **2**, 169.

HAMBURGER, J., RICHET, G., CROSNIER, J., FUNCK-BRENTANO, J. L., ANTOINE, B., DUCROT, H., MERY, J. P. & DE MONTERA, H. (1968). *Nephrology*, Vol. 2. Philadelphia: Saunders, p. 928.

HOLLINGSWORTH, J. H. & MOHLER, D. N. (1968). Microangiopathic hemolytic anaemia caused by purpura fulminans. *Ann. intern. Med.*, **68**, 1310.

LINTON, A. L., GAVRAS, H., GLEADLE, R. I., HUTCHISON, H. E., LAWSON, D. H., LEVER, A. F., MACADAM, R. F., McNICHOL, G. P & ROBERTSON, J. I. S. (1969). Microangiopathic haemolytic anaemia and the pathogenesis of malignant hypertension. *Lancet*, **1**, 1277.

MOSCHCOWITZ, E. (1924). Hyaline thrombosis of the terminal arterioles and capillaries: a hitherto undescribed disease. *Proc. N.Y. path. Soc.*, **24**, 21.

PIVER, M. S. M., LISKER, S. A., ROWAN, N., WEBER, L. L., BRODY, J. I. & BEIZER, L. H. (1968). Thrombotic thrombocytopenic purpura during pregnancy. *Amer. J. Obstet. Gynec.*, **100**, 302.

ROBSON, J. S., MARTIN, A. M., RUCKLEY, V. A. & McDONALD, M. (1968). Irreversible post-partum renal failure. *Quart. J. Med.*, **37**, 423.

ROCK, R. C., BOVE, J. R. & NEMERSON, Y. (1969). Heparin treatment of intravascular coagulation accompanying hemolytic transfusion reactions. *Tranfusion*, **9**, 57.

RUBENBERG, M. L., BAKER, L. R. I., McBRIDE, J. A., SEVITT, L. H. & BRAIN, M. C. (1967). Intravascular coagulation in a case of *Clostridium perfringens* septicaemia: treatment by exchange transfusion and heparin. *Brit. med. J.*, **4**, 271.

TAPP, E. & RALSTON, A. (1969). Thrombotic microangiopathy associated with squamous carcinoma. *Brit. med. J.*, **4**, 209.

THOMSON, D. & GARDNER, D. L. (1969). Thrombotic microangiopathy in rheumatoid arthritis. *Scot. med. J.*, **14**, 190.

WARDLE, E. N. (1968). Fibrin breakdown products and fibrinolysis in renal disease. *J. clin. Path.*, **21**, 140.

TREATMENT OF NEPHROTIC SYNDROME AND ITS MAJOR CAUSES

In the fourth edition of this book, de Wardener and Holland defined nephrotic syndrome as "proteinuria, hypoproteinaemia and oedema. irrespective of aetiology and any other additional abnormal clinical feature", and pointed out: "This unification stresses the occasional clinical similarity of many unrelated diseases". The most important contribution of renal biopsy to clinical medicine has been the definition of these diseases and the study of their response to treatment with corticosteroids and other immunosuppressive drugs. The symptomatic treatment of nephrotic syndrome has not significantly altered since de Wardener and Holland's account, except in the addition of the more powerful diuretics frusemide and ethacrynic acid to the armamentarium.

The investigation of a patient with nephrotic syndrome or proteinuria of unknown cause involves a search for the 20 or 30 systemic causes for the syndrome and for a history of contact with drugs (mersalyl, gold, tridione, penicillamine, etc.), or other allergens (bee-sting, poison ivy, etc.). When these have been excluded nephrotic syndrome due to primary renal disease can be subdivided on the basis of renal histology into three main subgroups (Editorial, 1969a).

Minimal change nephropathy (lipoid nephrosis)

This is defined as the absence of glomerular abnormality on light microscopy and the fusion of epithelial foot processes over normal basement membrane on electronmicroscopy. The corresponding clinical syndrome often begins explosively and is characterized by heavy proteinuria which is "selected" (i.e. consists mainly of low molecular weight proteins, notably albumin), slight or absent microscopic haematuria, normal blood pressure and excretory function except in the presence of severe hypovolaemia which occasionally results in reversible acute renal failure (Connolly *et al.*, 1968). Minimal change is much the commonest finding in childhood nephrosis and accounts for 18 to 30 per cent of adult cases (Rogson, 1967; Sharpstone *et al.*, 1969a). It is the usual picture found in association with drug and other allergies and in the cases where nephrotic syndrome coexists with neoplasm (Lee *et al.*, 1966; Cantrell, 1969).

Over 90 per cent of children with minimal change, and about 80 per cent of adults, respond to a short course of corticosteroids, e.g. prednisone 30–60 mg/day with a complete remission (Arneil, 1968; Robson, 1968) but about half of these relapse if steroids are withdrawn after a few weeks. A proportion of the total, variously estimated as 10 to 30 per cent, relapse sufficiently often to suffer from corticosteroid toxicity, notably growth retardation in childhood (Editorial, 1969b). There is some evidence that giving oral steroids on alternate days reduces the side-effects for a given therapeutic result, and the growth retardation can be prevented by changing to corticotrophin (Friedman and Strang, 1966). However, dosage is more difficult to adjust predictably with corticotrophin, and the results of treatment with cyclophosphamide are so encouraging that it is becoming standard practice to change to this drug as soon as steroid toxicity becomes a problem. Of 46 children treated by Moncrieff and colleagues (1969), 33 had a lasting remission after one course of three to four months and five others after a second. Late relapse has so far been rare, in contrast to steroid therapy. Moncrieff's regime involved suppressing the white count to between 1000 and 4000 per cu. mm and this was associated with troublesome side-effects—36 developed temporary alopecia, followed by regrowth of curly, depigmented hair, three had cystitis, two hepatitis and one ulcerative stomatitis. Personal experience suggests that the same benefit can be obtained, albeit more slowly, at a lower dose. The major side-effects of cyclophosphamide and similar drugs are also appreciable, although it is not easy to separate them from those of steroids given concurrently. Two of Moncrieff's patients died of pneumonia, and fatalities have occurred from measles (Meadow *et al.*, 1969) and chickenpox (Scheinman and Stamler, 1969). Children taking the drug must be kept away from likely sources of infection and warned against vaccination. Long-term follow-up should be instituted so that any increased incidence of neoplasia can be detected.

F

Experience with cyclophosphamide in the adult is limited, but suggests that it is just as effective as in children, with similar side-effects, except that alopecia is less common. Patients of any age who are totally resistant to steroids in spite of minimal change histology are uncommon, and the value of cyclophosphamide in this situation is uncertain. None of the three patients treated by Moncrieff and his colleagues responded, but Coldbeck (1963) recorded five successes, and some success was also achieved earlier with nitrogen mustards.*

Patients with minimal change stand pregnancy well (Studd and Blainey, 1969), and the administration of corticosteroids during pregnancy in the minimum dose to control the syndrome has seldom caused stillbirth or congenital anomalies. A rare form of nephrotic syndrome with minimal change is precipitated by pregnancy and recurs in successive pregnancies. It is probable, though difficult to prove, that the same syndrome occurs rarely in women taking contraceptive pills.

In the MRC trial of steroids in adult nephrotic syndromes (Rose and Black, 1970) patients with minimal change in the control group usually underwent spontaneous remission after one to two. Excretory function is usually maintained at normal levels during long-term follow-up after steroid therapy or spontaneous remission (Pollak et al., 1968), and steroids do not prevent the occasional progression of minimal change to chronic sclerosing glomerulonephritis (Hayslett et al., 1969). It is therefore reasonable to withhold these drugs and use symptomatic treatment only, if there is a major contraindication such as active duodenal ulceration.

Membranous glomerulonephropathy (Editorial, 1969c)

This is a distinct disease of unknown aetiology which accounts for 12 to 30 per cent of primary adult nephrotic syndromes (Robson, 1968; Sharpstone et al., 1969a) but is rare in childhood. It is characterized by gradual onset of moderate to heavy proteinuria, considerable microscopic haematuria, late onset of hypertension, and progression to renal failure over a variable period from a few to more than 20 years. The basement membrane is uniformly thickened on light microscopy, but silver stains and electron-microscopy show that the thickening is predominantly due to deposits of material under the endothelial cell and extending into the basement membrane. These "extramembranous deposits" or "spiky projections" stain for gammaglobulin and the C'3 component of complement on fluorescence microscopy, suggesting an immunological origin. Spontaneous remission is rare, and steroids are usually described as totally ineffective (Robson, 1968), but an appreciable minority of early cases respond to steroid therapy with a loss of oedema and diminution or loss of proteinuria, provided it is con-

* An annotated bibliography on earlier trials of immunosuppressive therapy for nephrotic syndrome is available on request from the author.

tinued for at least six months (Rastogi *et al.*, 1969). Other immunosuppressive drugs have so far achieved little success, but two patients have recently been described who underwent complete remission with restoration of the basement membrane to normal on immunosuppressive therapy (Bariety *et al.*, 1969). Since these drug regimes act slowly and benefit only a minority, their toxicity has to be weighed carefully against the chance of success particularly in older patients. The mortality and morbidity of steroids outweighed their benefits up to four years in the whole field of adult nephrotic syndrome in the MRC trial (Rose and Black, 1970).

Proliferative glomerulonephritis

This covers a much more heterogeneous group of cases. Very mild endothelial proliferation is difficult to distinguish from minimal change on light microscopy; there is considerable discrepancy between the opinions of experts. Patients with very mild lesions should therefore be regarded as having minimal change until proved otherwise and given the chance of steroid therapy if it is not contraindicated.

The remaining patients are difficult to subclassify. One distinct but fortunately small group is rapidly progressive ("stormy subacute") nephritis in which all glomeruli are severely affected by epithelial proliferation with widespread crescent formation and often with localized tuft necrosis. This group has a particularly gloomy prognosis with a mean survival well under one year, but prolonged remission is occasionally obtained even after protracted anuria (Richards *et al.*, 1968). Therapeutic benefit has been claimed from high dose steroids (Nakamoto *et al.*, 1965) and from a combination of heparin, dipyridamole and cyclophosphamide, given in the belief that fibrin deposition in response to an immunological insult is important in the genesis of this lesion (Kincaid-Smith *et al.*, 1968). None of these measures, individually or in combination, has been subjected to controlled trial, though an MRC trial is now under way, and all have been uniformly ineffective in my hands.

A less well-defined subgroup is membrano-proliferative (lobular) glomerulonephritis, which is often associated with reduced plasma levels of C′3 component of complement (Ogg *et al.*, 1968). Typical diffuse exudative nephritis following streptococcal infection contributes a few cases to the spectrum, but nephrotic syndrome is only a rare late complication of post-streptococcal nephritis (Jennings and Earle, 1961; Poon-King *et al.*, 1967). The aetiology of the remaining patients whom Cameron (1968) lumped together as "all other proliferative" is unknown. In the tropics they are often associated with quartan malaria (Kikbukamusoke. 1968).

The prognosis of proliferative glomerulonephritis is as variable as its histology, and this has rendered the evaluation of therapy particularly difficult. Steroids were ineffective in the MRC trial in adults (Rose and Black,

1970) except in the group where differentiation from minimal change was difficult. The addition of azathioprine produced no significant change in a regional trial in South-east England (Sharpstone et al., 1969b) and the MRC trial of azathioprine has so far shown no significant benefit. There have been a number of more favourable reports on the response to cyclophosphamide and indomethacin, but no reports of a controlled trial of either drug. Until the results of controlled trials now being conducted by the MRC and on a regional basis in North-east England and elsewhere are available, these "therapies" should be regarded as experimental.

Tests for the selectivity of protein clearance

These and more complex tests for glomerular permeability using dextrans, etc. (Mogensen, 1968) have made a smaller contribution to clinical medicine than expected a few years ago. The overlap in results between different histological categories is considerable (Cameron, 1968; Robson, 1968) so they do not form an adequate substitute for renal biopsy. They give some additional information about the likelihood of a response to steroids (the more selective the proteinuria, the more likely a good response). Their main usefulness is in young children, in whom successful treatment with steroids is so likely, if the proteinuria is selected, that renal biopsy can reasonably be omitted. They also make a useful contribution in those patients with "mild proliferative glomerulonephritis" in whom steroid therapy is contemplated.

Late effects of the plasma lipid changes

In nephrotic syndrome these are receiving increasing attention. Ischaemic heart disease is a definite risk (Berlyne and Mallick, 1969) and presumably atheroma elsewhere also develops at an accelerated rate. Clofibrate has been used to lower plasma lipid levels when the nephrotic syndrome resists specific therapy, but its long-term benefits have yet to be assessed.

REFERENCES

ARNEIL, G. C. (1968). Management of the nephrotic syndrome. Arch. Dis. Childh., 43, 257.

BARIETY, J., SAMARQ, P., LAGRUE, G., FRITEL, D. & MILLIEZ, P. (1968). Presse méd., 76, 2179.

BERLYNE, G. M. & MALLICK, N. P. (1969). Ischaemic heart-disease as a complication of nephrotic syndrome. Lancet, 2, 399.

CAMERON, J. S. (1968). Histology, protein clearances and response to treatment in the nephrotic syndrome. Brit. med., J., 4, 352.

CANTRELL, E. G. (1969). Nephrotic syndrome cured by removal of gastric carcinoma. Brit. med. J., 2, 739.

COLDBECK, J. H. (1963). Experience with alkylating agents in the treatment of children with the nephrotic syndrome. Med. J. Aust., 50, 987.

CONNOLLY, M. E., WRONG, O. M. & JONES, N. F. (1968). Reversible renal failure in idiopathic nephrotic syndrome with minimal glomerular changes. *Lancet*, 1, 665.

EDITORIAL (1969a). Nephrotic syndrome in adults. *Brit. med. J.*, 2, 529.

EDITORIAL (1969b). Corticosteroid therapy and growth. *Brit. med. J.*, 1, 394.

EDITORIAL (1969c). Membranous glomerulonephritis. *Lancet*, 2, 626.

FRIEDMAN, M. & STRANG, L. B. (1966). Effect of long-term corticosteroids and corticotrophin on the growth of children. *Lancet*, 2, 568.

HAYSLETT, J. P., KRASSNER, L. S., BENSCH, K. G., KASHGARIAN, M. & EPSTEIN, R. H. (1969). Progression of lipoid nephrosis to renal insufficiency. *New Engl. J. Med.*, 281, 181.

JENNINGS, R. B. & EARLE, D. P. (1961). Post-streptococcal glomerulonephritis. Histopathological and clinical studies of the acute, subsiding acute and early chronic latent phases. *J. clin. Invest.*, 40, 1525.

KIBUKAMUSOKE, J. W. (1968). Nephrotic syndrome and chronic renal disease in the tropics. *Brit. med. J.*, 2, 33.

KINCAID-SMITH, P. SAKER, B. M. & FAIRLEY, K. F. (1968). Anticoagulants in "irreversible" acute renal failure. *Lancet*, 2, 1360.

LEE, J. C., YAMAUCHI, H. & HOPPER, J. (1966). The association of cancer and the nephrotic syndrome. *Ann. intern. Med.*, 64, 25.

MEADOW, S. R., WELLER, R. O. & ARCHIBALD, R. W. R. (1969). Fatal systemic measles in a child receiving cyclophosphamide for nephrotic syndrome. *Lancet*, 2, 876.

MOGENSEN, C. E. (1968). The glomerular permeability determined by dextran clearance using sephadex gel filtration. *Scand. J. clin. Lab. Invest.*, 21, 77.

MONCRIEFF, M. W., WHITE, R. H. R., OGG, C. S. & CAMERON, J. S. (1969). Cyclophosphamide therapy in nephrotic syndrome in childhood. *Brit. med. J.*, 1, 666.

NAKAMOTO, S., DUNEA, G., KOLFF, W. J. & McCORMACK, L. J. (1965). Treatment of oliguric glomerulonephritis with dialysis and steroids. *Ann. intern. Med.*, 63, 359.

OGG, C. S., CAMERON, J. S. & WHITE, R. H. R. (1968). The $C'3$ component of complement (β_{1C} globulin) in patients with heavy proteinuria. *Lancet*, 2, 78.

POLLAK, V. E., ROSEN, S., PIRANI, C. L., MUEHRCKE, R. C. & KARK, R. M. (1968). Natural history of lipoid nephrosis and of membranous glomerulonephritis. *Ann. intern. Med.*, 69, 1171.

POON-KING, T., MOHAMMED, I., COX, R., POTTER, E. V., SIMON, N. M., SIEGEL, A. C. & EARLER, D. P. (1967). Recurrent epidemic nephritis in South Trinidad. *New Engl. J. Med.*, 277, 728.

RASTOGI, S. P., HART-MERCER, J. & KERR, D. N. S. (1969). Idiopathic membranous glomerulonephritis in adults; remission following steroid therapy. *Quart. J. Med.*, 38, 335.

RICHARDS, P., EVANS, D. J. & WRONG, O. M. (1968). Recovery from acute renal failure due to "irreversible" glomerular disease. *Brit. med. J.*, 2, 459.

ROBSON, J. S. (1967). The nephrotic syndrome. In *Renal Disease*. ed. D. A. K. Black. Oxford: Blackwell, p. 276.

ROBSON, J. S. (1968). The nephrotic syndrome. In *Fourth Symposium on Advanced Medicine*. ed. O. Wrong. London: Pitman.

ROSE, G. A. & BLACK, D. A. K. (1970). Steroid therapy in adult nephrotic syndrome: report of the M.R.C. subcommittee. *Brit. med. J.* In press.

SCHEINMAN, J. I. & STAMLER, F. W. (1969). Cyclophosphamide and fatal varicella. *J. Pediat.*, 74, 117.

SHARPSTONE, P., OGG, C. S. & CAMERON, J. S. (1969a). Nephrotic syndrome due to primary renal disease in adults. 1. Survey of incidence in South-east England. *Brit. med. J.*, **2**, 533.

SHARPSTONE, P., OGG, C. S. & CAMERON, J. S. (1969b). Nephrotic syndrome due to primary renal disease in adults. 2. A controlled trial of prednisone and azathioprine. *Brit. med. J.*, **2**, 535.

STUDD, J. W. W. & BLAINEY, J. D. (1969). Pregnancy and nephrotic syndrome. *Brit. med. J.*, **1**, 276.

DIALYSIS FOR CHRONIC RENAL FAILURE

In the decade since its introduction in Seattle, regular haemodialysis has become the major preoccupation of nephrologists in affluent countries, and its details fill several textbooks (Hampers and Schupak, 1967; Dittrich *et al.*, 1969; Nose, 1969; Kennedy and Kerr, 1970). By the end of 1969, about 700 patients were receiving treatment in Great Britain. The procedure has emerged as one which works extremely well in highly competent, dedicated hands but is disastrously ineffective if performed at a lower standard of enthusiasm and skill. The European results, collated annually by Drukker and his colleagues (1968, 1969), display an extraordinary range of mortality from 8 to 80 per cent of all patients accepted within the last five years. Annual mortality rates can be estimated only roughly from published series, from Drukker's reports and from the figures collected by the Department of Health and Social Security; they range from about 5 per cent per annum in some well-established specialist centres (Scribner, 1967; Baillod *et al.*, 1969; Curtis *et al.*, 1969) through about 15 per cent per annum in Great Britain as a whole, to more than 40 per cent per annum in newly established European centres. The typical centre in Europe sustains this high mortality for the first two years of its operation but achieves a big improvement by the third year.

Success depends on (*a*) a medical team prepared to concentrate effort on this task even at the sacrifice of training, teaching, research and normal social life, (*b*) a well-trained nursing and technical staff with a low turnover rate and (*c*) meticulous attention to the details of treatment outlined below. Physical surroundings are also important; the value of regular haemodialysis was established in medical slums, but the emergence of hepatitis in dialysis units has made hygienic surroundings essential. The difficulty of recruiting medical, nursing and technical staff of the right calibre is a more important brake on this form of treatment than lack of finance.

Access to the Vascular System

The original all-Teflon arteriovenous cannulas which made haemodialysis possible were difficult to insert and handle, and were soon replaced by a Silastic-Teflon shunt (Quinton *et al.*, 1962) which has been progressively simplified since. The metal parts were replaced by silk ties, the outside loop was disconnected at only one point and closed securely with little disturbance of the smooth bore. The subcutaneous U-bend has often been omitted, the cannula being stabilized by Silastic wings or by careful ligation to the vessel. Straight shunts are cheaper and easier to insert, remove and declot than the curved variety, and they probably provide a faster flow of blood (Walls and Kopp, 1968). On the other hand, they are more often slowly extruded and carry a small risk of being avulsed, particularly if infected. A full description of shunts is provided by Quinton and Baillod (1970) in their description of haemodialysis (table 4.3).

TABLE 4.3

Main elements in successful regular haemodialysis

1. Ready access to the vascular system
2. Suitable low-volume dialysers
3. Sufficient blood flow through the dialyser
4. Constant source of dialysis fluid
5. Reliable monitoring
6. Adequate diet conscientiously consumed
7. Appropriate dialysis schedule
8. Economy in the use of blood

The life of these cannulas is limited by thrombosis and infection. Thrombosis nearly always starts in one of the vessels—more commonly the vein—just beyond the Teflon tip, where epithelium is denuded (Glashan and Walker, 1968) and degenerative changes occur in the vessel wall (Papadimitriou *et al.*, 1969). Angiograms, performed by injecting 2 or 3 ml of a suitable buffered contrast medium, show a characteristic narrowing of the vessel due to firmly adherent clot; they may also reveal younger clot proximally and abnormalities of alignment, aneurysm formation and stenosis (Dathan *et al.*, 1969; De Palma *et al.*, 1969).

Arterial clot can often be aspirated by direct suction on the cannula. If saline injection is necessary to dislodge it, only 2 ml at 37°C should be used since cerebrovascular accidents have often followed the forcible injection of cold saline into upper limb arteries. These have usually caused only transient hemianopia, hemiparesis or monoplegia but permanent cerebral damage, fits, coma and death have occurred. The attacks have been attributed to retrograde displacement of clot into the carotid or vertebral artery (Gaan *et al.*, 1969) but some may be due to widespread arterial spasm, which is revealed by extensive patchy pallor of the skin and persistent pain after vigorous declotting.

Venous and resistant arterial clot can be aspirated though a nylon catheter, drawn down by a thin Fogarty's balloon catheter, or dissolved with proteolytic enzymes or their activators. Urokinase is safest but most expensive (Watt *et al.*, 1969); streptokinase, in high local concentration, is often effective (Anderson *et al.*, 1967; Kjellstrand *et al.*, 1967), but should be preceded by intravenous prednisone 20 mg to prevent anaphylactic reactions; Protease 1, a proteolytic enzyme derived from *Aspergillus oryzae*, can be used as a last resort, but is often painful (Bennhold *et al.*, 1968). Recurrent clotting is common after a single episode and presages final occlusion of the shunt. Coumarin anticoagulants or intermittent heparin, self-adminstered through a siliconized rubber segment inserted into the shunt, prolong shunt survival (Wing *et al.*, 1967).

Infection around the cannula is usually caused by staphylococci and is a major problem only in staphylococcal carriers (Martin *et al.*, 1967). It can be prevented or suppressed by long-term administration of cloxacillin, at the risk of breeding cloxacillin-resistant organisms in the renal ward. Treatment of infection with cloxacillin, lincomycin, fucidic acid or vancomycin is often effective, but irreversible thrombosis of the shunt occurs in about half the major episodes.

The mean survival of shunts varies from a few weeks in some hands to one or two years in others (Baillod *et al.*, 1969). They work well when they are inserted with scrupulous attention to alignment, stabilization and asepsis by a few individuals who are also responsible for their after-care. This ideal is difficult to achieve in a large unit where the "shunt load" can fully occupy one surgeon and where most of the operations are performed as semi-emergencies to fit the dialysis timetable. The problems of shunt care therefore rank high among the headaches of nephrologists, and patients continue to die from exhaustion of all shunt sites (Drukker *et al.*, 1969).

An alternative approach is the subcutaneous arteriovenous fistula introduced by Brescia and colleagues (1966). The radial artery is anastomosed side by side with a forearm vein through which a leash of superficial veins fills with arterial blood. Wide-bore needles are inserted percutaneously at two sites in these veins at each dialysis, blood being drawn from the distal and returned to the proximal needle with the aid of a blood pump. Fistulas have a much longer life than shunts and are preferred by most patients who have tried both. Apparently the disadvantages of an external shunt outweigh the discomfort of two venepunctures per dialysis, occasional haematomas and "Dutch boy" exercises to stop the bleeding after withdrawal of the needles. Even in centres using shunts initially, one arm is kept "virgin" so that a fistula can be inserted when cannulation sites are becoming scarce. Blood flow through a fistula is limited by the bore of the artery rather than the surgical technique and is rarely sufficient to cause cardiac embarrassment (Walsh, 1968). A few patients have been taught to insert their own needles so that a fistula can be employed in home dialysis (Shaldon and McKay, 1968).

A suitable low-volume dialyser

The Kiil flat-plate dialyser was adopted by the Seattle team (Cole *et al.*, 1962) because of its low volume, reasonable performance, low resistance to blood flow—eliminating the need for a pump—and because slow dialysis was regarded as essential to avoid disequilibrium. The risk of severe disequilibrium in well-managed patients is in fact negligible, and the blood pump has proved to be so small an inconvenience that it was back in use long before the fistula made it mandatory. However, the Kiil has retained its popularity because of its other advantages and is used in more than half of all European dialyses (Drukker *et al.*, 1969). The basic design is unchanged in 1970, but a host of minor modifications have reduced its priming volume from 400 to 110 ml and increased its urea clearance to 100 ml/min at a blood flow of about 240 ml/min. Its major drawbacks are the need to rebuild it manually and sterilize it chemically, and a rather high leakage rate unless it is built by particularly conscientious staff. These problems have been offset to some extent by the successful re-use of the Kiil two to five times, after thorough washing and resterilization.

Pyrogenic reactions, starting about one hour after the beginning of dialysis and causing angor animi, chest pain, muscle ache, hypotension and extensive facial herpes are a problem virtually confined to hand-built machines like the Kiil. They are usually blamed on the dialysis fluid but are more frequently due to foreign protein within the blood pathway. Inefficient sterilization may permit the growth of saprophytic bacteria (Curtis *et al.*, 1967) and even complete sterilization will not prevent reactions if the membranes have been soaked in solutions contaminated with bacteria.

The Kiil will certainly be discarded as soon as a good disposable dialyser is sold at a price not too far above the realistic cost of Kiil dialysis, including labour. However, new designs need careful scrutiny (Kerr, 1969) since adequate information on all aspects of performance is rarely available when they are marketed, and all the really good long-term results so far published have been achieved with slow dialysis on the Kiil. Several disposable flat-plate dialysers are on the market of which the Alwall-Gambro (Kulatilake *et al.*, 1969; Rastogi *et al.*, 1969) has achieved some success, but the main competitor to the Kiil is the concentric coil which in its recent modifications (Ultraflow-60; Ex-O1) gives a urea clearance about 50 per cent higher than the Kiil at the usual clinical blood flow (around 200 ml/min) with an acceptable priming volume (about 200 ml), high but predictable ultrafiltration (Muth and Wells, 1969) and clean wash-out characteristics. Clinical results with previous coils have been poorer than those with the Kiil (Drukker *et al.*, 1969) mainly because of a false but widespread belief that doubling the urea clearance permits halving the dialysis time. In my experience, if the newer coils are used on a reasonable schedule, they give at least as good results as those of the Kiil.

Sufficient blood flow through the dialyser

When A-V shunts are beginning to fail or needles are inserted at an unfavourable point in a fistula, blood flow through the dialyser falls and the removal of solutes is reduced. Patients should be taught to check blood flow through the dialyser by bubble transit time, and extend the dialysis if flow is poor. If low flow persists in subsequent dialyses it indicates that shunt failure is imminent and angiographic studies are required. Early revision of failing shunts avoids under-dialysis and prevents the disruption of normal life caused by frequent clotting episodes (Baillod et al., 1969) but it is a policy which can only be applied if the average shunt survival is already high.

Constant source of dialysis fluid

The 300 litres of fluid required in one dialysis can be mixed in a tank, and in hospital the composition can be checked before use. The problem of bacterial multiplication in dialysis fluid, which is an excellent culture medium, has led to the gradual displacement of this system by the proportioning machine which mixes the fluid continuously from a concentrate and softened tap water. The correct functioning of the machine is checked by continuous monitoring of electrical conductivity. If there is a human error in mixing the contents of a tank, or if the machine and its monitoring system fail, the patient may be dialysed against fluid with an abnormally high or low ionic concentration.

Hypernatraemia has usually followed the insertion of two lots of concentrate into a tank and has caused severe headache, vomiting, hypertension and death within a few hours from cerebral oedema or intracranial haemorrhage. *Hyponatraemia* of moderate degree occurred when salts were added individually to the tank and one was omitted. It produces severe muscle cramp followed eventually by convulsions. Dialysis against pure water has been the commonest accident with tank systems. It causes severe pain up the vein, followed by generalized muscle aches, hypotension and malaise. The severity of the symptoms and the translucent, port-wine appearance of blood in the venous line usually alert the staff within a few minutes and surprisingly few fatalities have been recorded.

Failure of a water softener causes a rise in calcium and magnesium concentration of the dialysate. A "hard-water syndrome" of headache, vomiting and hypertension results from the rise in serum calcium. Burning sensation, muscle weakness, somnolence and sweating may occur (Drukker, 1968), probably as a result of *hypermagnesaemia* since these symptoms, with visual disturbance, developed when hypermagnesaemia occurred in isolation following an error in composition of the concentrate (Govan et al., 1968). Acute *hypomagnesaemia* has been blamed for cramps which developed during dialysis against fluid with a low magnesium content and were relieved by intravenous magnesium sulphate (Triger and Joekes, 1969), but the evidence is equivocal.

Trace quantities of many other elements are found in tap water. They are unimportant when only a litre or two is drunk every day and the impurities can be excreted through normal kidneys, but can become very important when a patient without renal function is exposed to several hundred litres through his dialyser in a few hours. Many metallic ions are adsorbed on to the membrane and picked up on the other side by carrier proteins in plasma; they are therefore taken up by the patient against a concentration gradient (Maher *et al.*, 1965). Copper piping used in most domestic water supplies becomes coated with a film of insoluble salts and the copper concentration remains a fraction of one part per million (mg/litre). Copper piping beyond a water softener is more easily attacked and the concentration rises slightly if the water stands in the pipes; static water must be run off before the start of dialysis. Lethal copper poisoning, heralded by vomiting, epigastric pain, diarrhoea, headache, haemolysis of red cells, methaemoglobinaemia, acidosis and hypoglycaemia, has occurred when very acid water from a spent de-ionizer attacked copper piping in a proportioning machine (Matter *et al.*, 1969). Some copper overload is inevitable because the Cuprophane membrane used in nearly all dialysers has a significant copper content (Barbour *et al.*, 1969); to avoid any additional risk, new dialysis centres are being equipped with stainless steel, polypropylene or polyethylene pipework.

Iron from pipework is also absorbed by patients, but the quantities involved are small compared with the changes in iron stores that occur during transfusion and blood loss (Lawson *et al.*, 1968). *Arsenic* accumulation has been reported but no correlation with neurological complications has been found (Christoffersen *et al.*, 1969). *Zinc* has been absorbed in considerable amounts from the zinc-oxide plaster used to wrap coils (Blomfield *et al.*, 1969), and it is also released from water softeners if rinsing is inadequate, but typical zinc poisoning has not yet been described from this source. *Fluoride*, occurring naturally in tap water or added by health authorities for its effect on growing teeth, is rapidly absorbed by patients and accumulates in their plasma and bones. It has been blamed for the occurrence of bone disease in dialysed patients, but no convincing correlation between fluoride level in the tap water and the incidence of bone disease has yet been established.

Bacteria in dialysis fluid provide an undesirable pool of infectants in close proximity to the patient. When they reach very high concentrations—a common occurrence when fluid is stored at 37°C—they lower the pH of the dialysis fluid and produce dialysable metabolites (Kidd, 1964) which may be responsible for malaise and fever appearing late in dialysis. Patients on regular haemodialysis develop antibodies to the endotoxin of bacteria which grow in their dialysis fluid (Gazenfield and Eliahou, 1969). Whether the endotoxin diffuses through the membrane in spite of its high molecular weight or reaches the patient by other routes is uncertain.

Reliable Monitoring

One nurse now cares for five to ten patients in a hospital centre; at home the patient sleeps through his night dialysis relying on the machine to wake him if anything goes wrong. Pressure gauges record the positive pressure in the blood circuit and the negative pressure in the dialysis fluid. High and low alarm contacts detect any change outside pre-set limits. A temperature probe with similar high and low alarms detects any malfunction of the thermostat governing the temperature of the dialysis fluid. A flow meter displays the flow rate of dialysis fluid but no alarm system is fitted since a failure is not an immediate danger to the patient. The systems in common use (Fig. 4.5) are not "fail-safe", i.e. failure of a mechanical or electrical component does not result in the machine sounding an alarm and switching itself off; however, they are well tried, robust and reliable.

The measurement of electrical conductivity as a check on the function of the proportioning system gives more trouble than any other monitor. Temperature variations, air on electrodes, and a film of organic slime with calcium salts that is deposited on every surface in contact with infected dialysis fluid all reduce the sensitivity and reliability of the conductivity meter.

A blood leak detector, which sounds an alarm and stops the blood pump when blood-stained dialysis fluid leaving the dialyser interrupts a light pathway to a photoelectric cell, is fitted in most machines. It has been abandoned in some centres because it causes false alarms when air bubbles or turbid fluid containing bacteria reduce the translucency of dialysis fluid and because most blood leaks occur in the first few minutes of dialysis and can be detected by the patient.

Monitors cannot be more reliable than the personnel who install, maintain and operate them. They are a complement to, not a substitute for well-trained staff and patients.

Adequate Diet Conscientiously Consumed

A Kiil artificial kidney provides about the same creatinine clearance as one normal human kidney, for about a fifth of the time. The patient remains in mild chronic renal insufficiency and the success of his treatment is critically dependent on dietary restrictions at least as irksome as those in diabetes or obesity. Co-operation is encouraged by the imminent threat of death, but it is not consistently achieved unless the medical staff know McCance and Widdowson like a muezzin knows the Koran, and teach it with the same

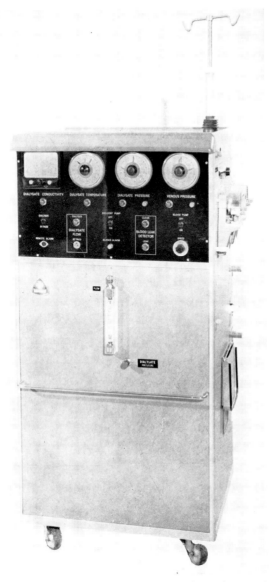

FIG. 4.5. A proportioning system (Lucas A) with patient monitors. The circular dials from left to right monitor dialysis fluid temperature and negative pressure and venous bubble trap pressure. The square dial records electrical conductivity. All of these have high and low alarms. A flow meter with control valves is mounted below the control panel. An alarm light on the panel shows the presence of a blood leak.

religious fervour. Access to a dietitian and the provision of diet books are useful adjuncts, but no substitute for detailed authoritative instruction from the medical staff. The enthusiastic indoctrination of patients about diet is the outstanding characteristic of successful dialysis units.

Sodium restriction to about 500 mg (22 mEq) per day or less is essential in all patients with severe hypertension, at least for the first year. This requires avoidance of all bread, biscuits, cakes and pastry made with ordinary flour, all vegetables cooked with salt, most tinned vegetables, and certain foods such as bacon, sausage, preserved meats, sauces and chocolate. The number of prohititions is so high that eating in canteens, restaurants and the homes of uninstructed friends is virtually impossible. Medicines must be carefully selected to avoid sodium intake; aluminium hydroxide should be used in place of magnesium trisilicate mixture; calcium gluconate in place of Sandocal; ion exchange resins should be in the calcium or aluminium, not the sodium, phase. Some relaxation of sodium intake may be possible when blood pressure has been consistently normal for at least a year.

Water intake in food and drinks must be limited to 800–1000 ml per day unless there is considerable residual urine output. A weight gain of more than 500 g per day between dialyses indicates excessive fluid intake. The removal of more than two litres of fluid during a single dialysis causes muscular cramps, and post-dialysis lethargy and postural hypotension. It may also result in a rise in renin output by the damaged kidneys which increases thirst and perpetuates hypertension (Gleadle *et al.*, 1969).

Potassium intake can often be kept in bounds by quite simple precautions like limited intake of fresh and tinned fruit (oranges, apricots, bananas) and by pre-boiling potatoes, which cuts their potassium content by about half. However, hyperkalaemia was responsible for at least 5 per cent of the deaths on regular dialysis in Europe last year (Drukker *et al.*, 1969) and some patients are particularly prone to this complication. They can be protected by routine administration of 5–15 g of Calcium Resonium daily, but at some risk of developing hypercalcaemia (Papadimitriou *et al.*, 1968).

Protein was originally restricted to 40 g per day, but the daily allowance has gradually crept up to 60 or 80 g without a corresponding increase in dialysis time. Minor uraemic symptoms are less troublesome in patients who stick conscientiously to a 40 g intake of high biological value (Shinaberger and Ginn, 1968) and this probably applies to some more major complications, particularly pericarditis. However, there is real difficulty in maintaining adequate calorie intake with low protein diet, and the advantages of a well-nourished patient probably outweigh the disadvantages of a 60g diet.

Appropriate Dialysis Schedule

Since we are uncertain which substances cause the uraemic syndrome, the time spent on dialysis has been determined by trial and error and by practicability. Long dialysis times increase depletion of amino-acids, water-soluble vitamins and other substances from plasma, but this has not so far proved a problem to patients on well-constructed diets who receive multivitamin supplements including folic acid and pyridoxine, and it would appear that we still err on the side of under-dialysis. Theoretical calculations, based on the assumption that "uraemic toxins" behave in the same way as urea or creatinine suggest that dialysis should be performed at least three times a week (Fig. 4.6), and this accords with practical experience. Successful units

EFFECT OF TREATMENT FREQUENCY ON TOTAL TREATMENT TIME

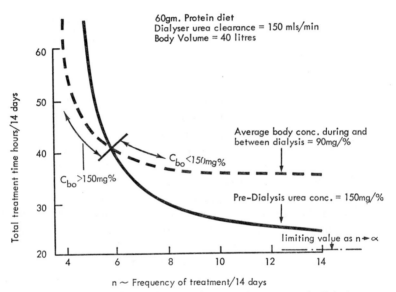

FIG. 4.6. The effect of increasing the frequency of dialysis (expressed in dialyses per fortnight) on the total dialysis time required to achieve a prescribed pre-dialysis blood urea (solid line) or a prescribed mean blood urea, i.e. (pre-post dialysis blood urea) (broken line). Computer predictions are shown for a constant 60 g protein intake. C_{bo} = pre-dialysis blood urea concentration. From Frost, T. (1970) "Theory of dialyser design" in: Kennedy and Kerr (1970).

usually achieve an average pre-dialysis plasma urea of about 150 mg and a plasma creatinine of about 12 mg/100 ml. Some patients remain very well at higher levels than these, but if the average for the unit is higher, dialysis and/or diet is probably inadequate.

The most popular schedule of dialysis at the time of writing is three sessions of 10 hours per week on a good quality Kiil dialyser at a blood flow of more than 120 ml/min. This must be increased, preferably by adding a fourth session per week, during intercurrent infections, periods of high protein feeding, childhood and adolescence (Shaldon *et al.*, 1969; Fine *et al.*, 1969), and in men over 75 kilos.

Economy in the Use of Blood

In the last edition of this book Shaldon estimated the average transfusion requirement of a patient on dialysis as 1000 ml/month—a reduction on the 2000 ml/month used in the early days of the procedure. Subsequently he pioneered a non-transfusion policy. Blood loss in the dialyser was reduced to less than 5 ml per dialysis by better design and adequate wash-back, which usually requires at least 800 ml saline. Blood for chemical analysis was limited to 8 ml per month in the well-stablized patient. Declotting procedures were kept to a minimum by early revision of shunts. Patients were found to tolerate haematocrits down to about 15 without much complaint and even down to 12 with a stiff upper lip. After a few weeks, the haematocrit gradually rose and eventually stabilized at a new level, usually between 20 and 30 (Crockett *et al.*, 1967; Verroust *et al.*, 1967). Iron deficiency sometimes developed in contrast to the iron overload that was an invariable feature of the early regular dialysis patients. Intravenous iron in doses up to several grams appears to raise the haemoglobin even in the absence of demonstrable iron deficiency (Wright *et al.*, 1968). Supplements of folic acid and pyridoxine may also be of benefit (MacKenzie *et al.*, 1968). Anabolic steroids, particularly methyl testosterone, have been given to many of these patients for their erythropoietic effect, and there is some evidence for their efficacy (Eschbach, 1970).

Adequate control of uraemia reduces transfusion requirement or raises haematocrit (Lindholm *et al.*, 1969). Bilateral nephrectomy performed in anticipation of transplant or for control of blood pressure increases the need for transfusion, suggesting that even kidneys with no excretory function may continue to secrete erythropoietin (van Ypersele *et al.*, 1969). Transfusion depresses erythropoiesis, introduces hepatitis and may sensitize the patient against transplant antigens; its routine use has been abandoned in most dialysis units, at least in Britain, but it is still required occasionally for accidents such as clotting in, or leakage from, a dialyser.

THE PATHOLOGY ASSOCIATED WITH REGULAR HAEMODIALYSIS

On starting regular haemodialysis, the patient is spared the more imminent dangers of his original disease but remains exposed to some of its long-term hazards. He also acquires many new sources of pathology (Table 4.4).

TABLE 4.4

Some sources of pathology in patients on regular haemodialysis

Incomplete replacement of renal excretory function
Retention of dietary water, sodium, potassium, magnesium, etc.
Persistent fluctuating azotaemia and acidosis

Renal endocrine abnormalities
Hypersecretion of renin
Impaired erythropoietin output

Effect of oliguria on the renal tract
Susceptibility to infection, calculi
Bladder contraction

Dietary deficiencies
Depletion through the dialyser
Excessive ultrafiltration
Loss of amino acids, vitamins, etc.

Blood losses
External—dialyser residue, leaks, declotting, sampling, menorrhagia, etc.
Internal—post-dialysis bruising, haemolysis

Damage to blood elements in extracorporeal circuit
Effects of blood pumping on red cells
Effects of contact with PVC, cellulose, etc. on red cells, white cells and
platelets

Anticoagulation
Heparin, protamine during dialysis
Coumarins to prevent shunt clotting

Retention of other drugs dependent on renal excretion
Cardiovascular effects and infection from shunts and fistulas
Cross infection with bacteria and viruses in ward and dialysis unit
Absorption of contaminants in tap water
Technical errors during dialysis

The major causes of death and disability in such patients in Europe during 1967–69 are listed in Table 4.5. Numerous overall reviews of the problem have been published in the last four years (Johnson *et al.*, 1966; McLeod *et al.*, 1966; Pendras and Erickson, 1966; Thomson *et al.*, 1967; Schreiner *et al.*, 1967; Bluemle, 1968; Curtis *et al.*, 1969). They paint a bewildering picture of multiple pathology which led Schreiner to describe regular dialysis as "the last remaining form of general practice". Although many of these complications of treatment, or of under-treatment, can be avoided by adherence to the rules set out in the preceding section, they are bound to occur when limited resources are applied to an almost unlimited demand.

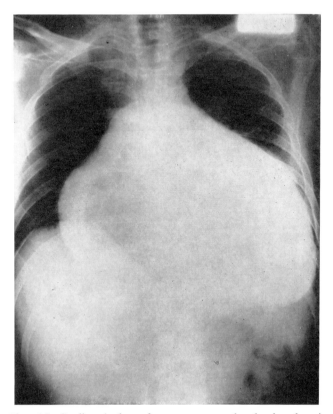

FIG. 4.7. Cardiac shadow of a young man who developed pericarditis in the second year of haemodialysis while receiving three
10-hour dialyses per week on the Kiil dialyser. Contrast medium
has been injected into the pericardial fluid, estimated at about
1 litre. A loud friction rub was audible in spite of the effusion.

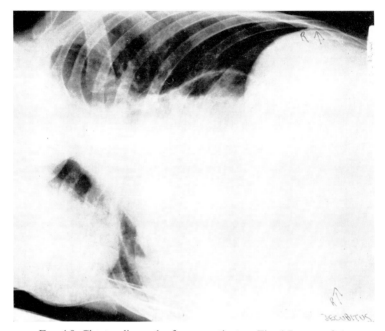

FIG. 4.8. Chest radiograph of same patient as Fig. 4.7; part of the peritoneal fluid has been replaced by air to show the thickness of the pericardial sac.

TABLE 4.5

Major causes of mortality and morbidity during regular
haemodialysis in Europe
(from Drukker *et al.*, 1969)

Cause of death	Percentage of total deaths	
	1967–68	1968–69
Mortality		
Heart failure	32	19
Infections	19	15
Cerebrovascular accidents	12	10
Pericarditis	*	6
Hyperkalaemia	*	4·7
Sudden death	*	3·4
Myocardial infarction	4	3·1
Viral hepatitis	2	3·0
Technical errors	3	2·6
Cachexia	7	2·2
Others	13	31
Morbidity		
Peripheral neuropathy	11	18
Psychosis Hospital	*	11
Home	*	5
Bone disease	4	8·5
Metastatic calcification	4	8
Acute arthritis	3	4

* Not separately classified 1967–68

Hypertension, heart failure and myocardial infarction

These are the most important killers. Hypertension in chronic renal disease is accompanied by an increase in total body sodium, most of the excess being in an expanded extracellular fluid volume (Blumberg *et al.*, 1967; Comty, 1968; Rastogi *et al.*, 1968). Considerable excess of extracellular fluid accumulates before oedema becomes apparent, but this excess conceals the wasting of subcutaneous and muscular tissue which are common in terminal uraemia. Gradual reduction of the extra-cellular fluid by sodium and water restriction combined with gentle ultrafiltration on the artificial kidney controls even malignant hypertension, without drug therapy, within three to six months (Editorial, 1969a). This phenomenon has been observed largely in young adults with hypertension of recent origin. When the vasculature has undergone permanent change from prolonged hypertension the patient remains difficult to control, and even after bilateral nephrectomy he is still much more sensitive to salt and water overload than the patient who has never been hypertensive (Wilkinson *et al.*, 1970). Since older patients with longer histories of inadequate blood pressure control are now being admitted to dialysis programmes, the superb results reported by Comty and colleagues (1965), Curtis and colleagues (1969) and others are unlikely to be maintained.

Even in the most favourable patients success is entirely dependent on co-operation by the patient in the dietary restrictions (see p. 160). There are many reports of failure to control blood pressure in a minority of patients in spite of the prescription of these dietary restraints. In some, blood pressure has remained out of control despite the reduction of total body sodium or extracellular fluid to normal or below. These patients with refractory hypertension usually have high plasma renin levels, in contrast to most hypertensive patients in renal failure before dialysis (Brown *et al.*, 1969; Vertes *et al.*, 1969; Wilkinson *et al.*, 1970); their blood pressure is much more readily controlled after bilateral nephrectomy. It is uncertain how often this refractory state requiring nephrectomy is the result of the original renal disease, and how often it is produced by excessive intake of salt and water followed by too vigorous fluid depletion during dialysis, causing a rise in plasma renin which sets up a vicious spiral (Gleadle *et al.*, 1969).

Severe atherosclerosis is common in hypertensive patients with chronic renal failure; it gives rise to problems during arteriovenous shunting. It also results in a high incidence of myocardial ischaemia. Anginal pain at the start of dialysis, during hypotension and periods of severe anaemia, cardiac irregularities during dialysis, and some of the episodes of sudden death referred to in Table 4.3 are no doubt due to this cause. A contributory factor is the hyperlipaemia which occurs in chronic renal failure and is accentuated by regular haemodialysis (Roodvoets *et al.*, 1967).

Cerebrovascular accidents

Intracranial haemorrhage has been the commonest cause of death at Newcastle-upon-Tyne and ranks third in Europe. Most of the episodes are associated with inadequate control of hypertension, but long-term anti-coagulation for shunt problems, heparinization during dialysis and berry aneurysms in patients with polycystic disease are contributory causes. Most are intracerebral, but a significant minority are subdural haematomata and subarachnoid haemorrhages (Leonard *et al.*, 1969). Temporary hemiplegia, coma and other signs following declotting procedures (p. 339) and episodes of hypotension, rebound hypoglycaemia after dialysis, and disequilibrium syndrome often recover spontaneously. Every such catastrophe should be regarded as potentially reversible until intensive investigation and time have proved the assumption false.

Infections

Untreated uraemia depresses several defence mechanisms against infection including phagocytosis, antibody production and delayed hypersensitivity (Montgomerie *et al.*, 1968). The last of these is not completely corrected by regular haemodialysis (Traeger *et al.*, 1969), and it is a reasonable assumption that the other defects, like most manifestations of uraemia, are reduced but not abolished. The importance of arteriovenous shunts as a portal of infection has been previously stated; it is our impression that they are occasionally colonized like Spitz-Holtzer valves and then require continuous antibiotic therapy until they are replaced. Early fears that arteriovenous fistulas would frequently be the site of endophlebitis have not been substantiated, though Lazorthes (1969) has isolated the organism causing fatal septicaemia from a fistula. Bacterial endocarditis is not uncommon in dialysed patients, in the absence of preceding abnormality of the heart valves; this was attributed by Goodman and colleagues (1969) to the circulatory strain of an arteriovenous fistula.

Pericarditis

Before 1960, pericarditis was the harbinger of death in uraemia. Survival for more than a few months was rare, but the pericarditis was not usually regarded as a major contributory factor in accelerating death. However, since the late 1950s there have been a number of reports of cardiac tamponade, often associated with haemorrhagic effusion, which threatened life unless rapidly relieved by paracentesis (Symons and Wrong, 1964; Marikas *et al.*, 1966; Kalliterakis *et al.*, 1968). This syndrome gained immediate prominence after the introduction of regular haemodialysis; the high incidence in the first few weeks of treatment was blamed on heparinization in the presence of fibrinous pericarditis and many centres adopted reduced heparinization, regional heparinization or peritoneal dialysis for this critical early period, in an attempt, not always successful, to avoid haemorrhagic pericarditis. The onset of pericarditis after the first few weeks usually reflects a period of under-dialysis but it occasionally develops for no obvious reason when dialysis is adequate by present criteria (Fig. 4.7).

Precordial pain is usually a prominent feature but the rub may be obvious before and after the pain. Initially the pain may resemble left-sided pleurisy. Contrary to popular belief, the rub does not disappear when fluid accumulates; we have removed up to a litre of haemorrhagic fluid from patients with severe tamponade who still had a loud rub. *Pulsus paradoxus*—best detected while taking systolic blood pressure—is an early sign, when the paradoxical movement of jugular venous pressure is inconstant. The classical electrocardiographic signs of pericarditis are seldom present. The most serious prognostic signs are a falling systolic pressure and pulse pressure, cyanosis (sometimes central) and cold extremities. Mental confusion is common. Any residual renal function declines and urinary sodium excretion falls dramatically. The syndrome is well described by Alfrey *et al.* (1968).

The presence of constriction—either by fluid or by thickened pericardium —can be confirmed by measurement of the reduced cardiac output and by demonstration of increased right atrial pressure and right ventricular end-diastolic pressure. Cardiac catheterization should be performed by a per-cutaneous "stab" technique or through the external jugular vein to conserve forearm veins. A thick pericardial shadow can be shown by superimposing a photoscan on the chest radiograph (Cohen *et al.*, 1968), or by performing an angiogram through the right heart catheter or by screening with the catheter against the right atrial wall. The only way to determine how much of the extracardiac shadow is fluid and how much thickened pericardium is to aspirate the effusion and replace it with air, having first confirmed that the catheter is in the pericardial sac, and not the atrium (Fig. 4.8). The haemato-crit of the pericardial effusion is often close enough to that of the circulating blood to cause alarm when it is aspirated.

Paracentesis may be required on several occasions, or the catheter may be left *in situ* for a few days while intensive dialysis is carried out. A proportion of the patients so treated later develop subacute constrictive pericarditis, usually without calcification, requiring pericardiectomy (Baudry *et al.*, 1965; Spalding, 1967; Reyman, 1968).

Hyperkalaemia

A typical patient on regular dialysis has a pre-dialysis plasma potassium level of 5–6 mEq/l falling to 3–4 mEq/l during dialysis against fluid with a potassium content of 1–2·5 mEq/l. This see-saw pattern of plasma potassium is accentuated by the acidosis which precedes dialysis and by its correction during the procedure; it is hazardous if the patient is digitalized, but probably has no other deleterious effect providing it stays within these limits. However, it leaves little margin for safety, and dangerous peaks are liable to occur before dialysis following dietary indiscretions, infections and tissue trauma including surgery. To diminish this hazard the potassium content of the dialysis fluid has been gradually lowered. After some months of dialysis against low-potassium fluid total body exchangeable potassium is low (Seedat, 1969) but part of the deficit may be due to loss of muscle mass. The majority opinion at the moment is that serious depletion is unlikely to occur except in the minority of patients who are still losing potassium in the urine and those who take an inadequate diet.

Cachexia

When the uraemic patient is stripped of his excess fluid he is often revealed as severely undernourished and wasted. With proper dialysis and diet he gradually regains his former habitus; the patients of Comty *et al.* (1965)

gained an average of 7·5 kg dry weight over the first year and Curtis *et al.* (1969) described seven patients who gained 5–12 kg. Positive nitrogen balance is maintained in spite of considerable losses into the dialysis fluid (Kaye and Comty, 1968; Kopple *et al.*, 1969; Editorial, 1969c). However, it takes only two or three weeks of inter-current infection or under-dialysis to undo the painstaking work of many months. Most deaths assigned to cachexia occur in patients admitted to the dialysis programme much too late and already *in extremis*. It is the constant plea of the nephrologist that he should be allowed to supervise patients from early in the course of renal failure, and not be regarded as a last-minute alternative to the undertaker.

Viral hepatitis

Sixty-one dialysis centres in Europe reported outbreaks of hepatitis during 1968–69; 16 of 158 affected patients and one of 88 affected staff died (Drukker *et al.*, 1969). Dialysis centres are strangely susceptible to these dangerous epidemics, and the many studies already published (Editorial, 1969d) and those now in progress at Sefton General, Guy's and Royal Free hospitals (Cameron, S., Goldsmith, J. and Moorhead, J. personal communications) have only partially unravelled the problem. Screening of staff and patients for Australia or SH antigen (Editorial, 1970) and a search for the presumed virus particles of infective hepatitis by electronmicroscopy in jaundiced patients (Zuckerman *et al.*, 1970) is now in progress at all British centres, and should throw further light on the problem.

Recent work has supported the theory that serum hepatitis is usually caused by a different virus from infective hepatitis; however, it appears that both viruses can be transmitted both by innoculation and by the faecal-oral route under the right circumstances (Editorial, 1970). In the epidemic at Fulham Hospital the incubation period was short (about six weeks), and the circumstances suggested faecal-oral transmission; the disease was probably modified by the administration of gammaglobulin and was attributed to infective hepatitis (Eastwood *et al.*, 1968). In Stockholm, on the other hand, the incubation period was long (60–100 days), there was a long prodromal period, gammaglobulin was ineffective and the disease was attributed to serum hepatitis (Ringertz *et al.*, 1969). It is therefore probable that virus can enter the Unit either by the infection of a patient or member of staff from outside, or by the administration of blood to the patients; in either case, the patients must be regarded as potentially infectious through their blood, which is teeming with virus, and through their excreta. Modes of transmission which are strongly supported by circumstantial evidence in recent epidemics include skin puncture with needles used on patients, contamination of the hands with blood during surgical operations, and accidental ingestion of serum during mouth pipetting.

Suggested precautions against the spread of viral hepatitis include the wearing of gloves for handling shunts and used dialysers, movement of blood samples to laboratories in sealed and marked containers, use of each dialyser by one patient only, and prohibition of eating, drinking and smoking by staff within the dialysis area (PHLS, 1969). Even the most stringent precautions do not prevent all contact between staff and the blood of patients, and epidemics have occurred in spite of their conscientious use. Gammaglobulin has therefore been given prophylactically in many countries to patients and staff of dialysis units. In other situations this has reduced the incidence or severity of attacks of infective hepatitis (PHLS 1968; Conrad, 1969) although the ideal schedule of administration has still to be determined; a 1·5 g dose every six to 24 weeks has been used in dialysis centres; since the material has a half-life of about three weeks the longer schedule results in blood level falling to about 0·5 per cent of its peak by the time the next injection is due.

It is probable that serum hepatitis is the commoner infectant in dialysis centres; gammaglobulin is effective against this agent when given in large doses intravenously at the time of transfusion (Creuzfeld et al., 1967) but is probably ineffective in spaced smaller doses. Repeated injections of gammaglobulin induce the production of antibodies of unknown long-term significance. The value of the current expensive programme of gammaglobulin cover is therefore in doubt, but it is at least reasonable to inoculate all staff and patients at risk at six-week intervals during an epidemic.

For the future the best hope lies in screening all blood donors for Australia and similar antigens (Gocke and Kavey, 1969), since this would reduce post-transfusion hepatitis by about 75 per cent even with current techniques, and in the economical use of blood. The regular screening of dialysis units has already proved useful in detecting the source of infection; patients carrying virus are isolated and transferred to home dialysis with all possible dispatch. Viraemia persists much longer in patients than in staff, presumably because of impaired immunity in uraemia; virus has been detected up to three years after jaundice in one patient (Editorial, 1970). It is possible that patients with uraemia are more often carriers of virus than the general population (Editorial, 1969d) even before starting dialysis, and they should certainly be examined for Australia antigen before entering the dialysis unit.

Psychosis

A toxic psychosis is not uncommon in uraemia. It is associated with slow wave activity on the electroencephalogram. Both clinical and electro-encephalographic abnormalities clear up within two or three weeks on intensive dialysis. Many of the psychiatric abnormalities recorded by Drukker et al. (1969) were probably due to under-dialysis or increased dialysis requirements during infection.

In well-dialysed patients serious psychiatric illness has been surprisingly uncommon (Curtis *et al.*, 1969), perhaps because any past history of mental illness has excluded patients from the programme. However, the stress of this unnatural form of life takes its toll; the range of interests narrows, the patients become self-centred and sometimes demanding. During the six-day war, patients in Jerusalem continued to read the papers only to find out what was happening to kidney transplantation (Kaplan de Nour and Czaczkes, 1968a). Relaxation therapy (Crammond *et al.*, 1968) and group therapy (De Veber and McDonald, 1969) have been employed to help patients cope with their psychological problems, apparently with some success since they were said often to look back on their time in the dialysis community as "an experience of great support, personal warmth and growth". Newcastle patients clearly view the experience differently; after successful transplant they avoid the dialysis unit like the morgue.

An important contribution to mental ill-health is the accumulation of drugs dependent on renal excretion, particularly antihypertensives and phenothiazines. Professor Richet's favourite dictum is "the best thing you can do for a uraemic is stop all his drugs". The polypharmacy to which these patients are sometimes subjected is illustrated by the investigation of a case of cholestatic jaundice (Stewart and Fleming, 1968) who had been exposed to 40 different drugs in the preceding year.

Stress in the dialysis unit is not confined to the patients. According to Kaplan de Nour and Czaczkes (1968b) the medical staff suffer from "feelings of guilt, possessiveness, over-protectiveness, and withdrawal from patients".

Peripheral neuropathy

Impaired nerve conduction and slight clinical evidence of predominantly sensory neuropathy are common when the plasma creatinine rises above 10 mg/100 ml in chronic renal failure (Jennekens *et al.*, 1969), but disabling paralysis is rare, It affects a small proportion of patients starting regular dialysis and may progress to quadriplegia. It is commoner if dialysis is inadequate but may progress in spite of intensive dialysis. The only patient with troublesome neuropathy at Newcastle has never had less than 30 hours dialysis per week and similar isolated patients are found in other centres. The onset of neuropathy calls for a review of drug therapy; in our experience nitrofurantoin has been the main offender.

Bone disease and myopathy

Virtually all patients requiring regular haemodialysis have enlarged parathyroid glands, raised plasma parathyroid hormone levels, and osteitis fibrosa cystica on bone biopsy. With adequate dialysis radiological evidence of hyperparathyroidism diminishes (Curtis *et al.*, 1968), the parathyroid glands decrease in size, the blood parathyroid hormone level falls, though not to normal, and the histological evidence of osteitis fibrosa decreases but does not disappear (Kerr et al., 1969; O'Riordan et al., 1970).

Against this background of slowly diminishing hyperparathyroidism there may appear a new bone disease peculiar to patients on regular haemo-dialysis. It has a puzzling geographic distribution (Harrison, 1968) and is common in Chicago (Kim et al., 1968), Iowa City and Ottawa but rare in Rochester, Minnesota and Montreal; it affects all patients dialysed for more than three years at Newcastle but very few of those in London (O'Riordan et al., 1970) or Birmingham. Its outstanding features are bone pain, often starting in the feet on exercise, and pathological fractures in ribs, metatarsals, femoral necks and other sites. The plasma alkaline phosphatase rises late in the course of the disease, in contrast to renal osteodystrophy before dialysis. Radiographs show loss of cortex in phalanges and later in major long bones, but subperiosteal erosions are absent. Bone biopsy reveals a progressive osteoporosis with persisting osteomalacia in many, and decreasing evidence of hyperparathyroidism in some.

The aetiology of this disease is still obscure. The patients clearly lose calcium from the skeleton but their renal calcium excretion is close to zero. They have a low dietary calcium intake, poor calcium absorption (Genuth et al., 1969) and negative gut balance for calcium (Verberckmoes, 1969). Large quantities of calcium can be lost or gained by the patient in response to changes in dialysis fluid calcium concentration (Wing, 1968; Kaye et al., 1969), but there is now general agreement that the concentration should be close to 6·0 mg/100 ml; therefore, loss into the dialysis fluid should not occur except in hypercalcaemic patients.

Large doses of Vitamin D (2·5–7·5 mg/day; 50,000–150,000 i.u. per day) will produce positive calcium balance in these patients (Verberckmoes, 1969) but it often precipitates hypercalcaemia, corneal and vascular calcification without benefiting the bone disease.

A *proximal myopathy* commonly accompanies renal osteomalacia in the undialysed uraemic patient; it responds rapidly to high-dose vitamin D therapy. A similar myopathy is common in patients with bone disease complicating regular haemodialysis (Floyd et al., 1969). Like the bone disease, it responds poorly if at all to Vitamin D. Both the myopathy and the bone disease are rapidly improved clinically by successful transplantation. Recalcification of the bones is obvious on radiographs within one year (Kerr et al., 1969) but bone biopsies may remain abnormal, particularly if graft function is imperfect (Carroll et al., 1969).

Arthropathy and metastatic calcification

Attacks of arthritis are now uncommon in well-dialysed patients. They are probably of two types: (1) true secondary gout, responsive to colchicine and other agents effective in acute gout, and prevented by the administration of allopurinol; (2) pseudo-gout, often associated with soft tissue calcification around the joint. The latter type usually responds to increased dialysis, with the oral adminstration of aluminium hydroxide to limit phosphate absorption. In a minority with extensive metastatic calcification parathyroidectomy is justified, and produces a speedy cure. It also relieves pruritus and may benefit the accompanying bone disease (Katz *et al.*, 1968; Johnson *et al.*, 1969).

Haemodialysis or Transplantation?

Two patients have passed their tenth anniversary on regular haemodialysis and many are well past their fifth. Their life is compatible with full-time work, social activity and even successful parenthood (Elstein *et al.*, 1969). Nevertheless, it is beset by the major hazards detailed above and by a host of minor inconveniences. Nearly all these patients live in anticipation of the day when a successful transplant will release them from dependence on the machine and restore them to full activity on a normal diet; they are not discouraged by close association with a transplant unit and familiarity with the risks of surgery. There is now general agreement that these forms of treatment should be provided in an integrated nephrological service run by a team of physicians and surgeons, and that patients should be accepted for both forms of treatment (Hopewell *et al.*, 1969; Sheil *et al.*, 1969; Branch *et al.*, 1970). If they reject a transplant they are guaranteed a return place on dialysis.

Arrangements at Newcastle are typical of those at many large centres in Europe and North America. About five patients, aged up to 55, present each month from a population of three million. On average, one of these has a suitable live donor with a good tissue match and has no contraindication to transplant (vascular disease, lower urinary tract abnormalities, etc.). Of the remaining four, we are able to accept two or three for long-term haemodialysis, predominantly in the home as our hospital dialysis facilties are full and places are created only by transplantation, or death of one of the present incumbents. Nearly all these patients request the chance of a cadaver transplant, and they are therefore tissue-typed and their data is fed into a computer which collects details of patients in Northern England and Southern Scotland. When a donor kidney becomes available locally it is used for any suitable patient in the Newcastle area with whom it is compatible by our current (rather strict) criteria. If no compatible recipient is available it is offered to the neighbouring centre with the closest matching recipient. As we have 80-odd patients on dialysis and receive only about one donor kidney a month, the average waiting time on dialysis is likely to remain long and the recipient pool will grow for the immediate future. This will, however, have the effect of permitting closer matching of donor and recipient, and longer graft survival should compensate for the long weary wait.

REFERENCES

ALFREY, A. C., GOSS, J. E., OGDEN, D. A., VOGEL, J. H. K. & HOLMES, J. H. (1968). Uremic hemopericardium. *Amer. J. Med.*, **45**, 391.

ANDERSON, D. C., MARTIN, A. M., CLUNIE, G. J. A., STEWART, W. K. & ROBSON, J. S. (1967). Eight months' experience in the use of streptokinase locally for declotting arteriovenous cannulae. *Proc. eur. Dial. Transpl. Ass.*, **4**, 55.

BAILLOD, R. A., KNIGHT, A. H., CROCKETT, R. E. & NAISH, P. F. (1969). Comparative assessment of arteriovenous shunts and Cimino-Brescia fistulae. *Proc. eur. Dial. Transpl. Ass.*, **6**, 65.

BARBOUR, B. H., BISCHEL, M. & DUDIO, S. (1969). Copper accumulation in patients undergoing chronic hemodialysis. The role of Cuprophane. *Abstracts of fourth International Congress of Nephrology*, **2**, 415.

BEAUDRY, C., NAKAMOTO, S. & KOLFF, W. J. (1966). Uremic pericarditis and cardiac tamponade in chronic renal failure. *Ann. intern. Med.*, **64**, 990.

BENNHOLD, I., FROESE, P., SCHOLTZ, A. & KESSEL, M. (1968). Shunt declotting with a new locally applied thrombolytic agent. *Proc. eur. Dial Transpl. Ass.*, **5**, 50.

BLOMFIELD, J., McPHERSON, J. & GEORGE, C. R. P. (1969). Active uptake of copper and zinc during haemodialysis. *Brit. med. J.*, **2**, 141.

BLUEMLE, L. W. (1968). Current status of chronic hemodialysis. *Amer. J. Med.*, **44**, 749.

BLUMBERG, A., NELP, W. B., HEGSTROM, R. M. & SCRIBNER, B. H. (1967). Extracellular volume in patients with chronic renal disease treated for hypertension by sodium restriction. *Lancet*, **2**, 69.

BRANCH, R. A., COLES, G. A., CROSBY, D. L., JONES, J. H., SUSSMAN, M. & THOMAS, W. H. C. (1970). Integrated regional haemodialysis and renal transplantation centre. *Brit. med. J.*, **1**, 291.

BRESCIA. M. J., CIMINO, J. E., APPEL, K. & HURWICH, B. J. (1966). Chronic haemodialysis using venipuncture and surgically created arterio-venous fistula. *New Engl. J. Med.*, **275**, 1089.

BROWN, J. J., CURTIS, J. R., LEVER, A. F., ROBERTSON, J. I. S., DE WARDENER, H. E., & WING, A. J. (1969). Plasma renin concentration and the control of blood pressure in patients on maintenance haemodialysis. *Nephron*, **6**, 329.

CARROLL, R. N. P., AUNG, T., WILLIAMS, E. D. & SHACKMAN, R. (1969). Osteodystrophy and renal substitution. *Proc. eur. Dial. Transpl. Ass.*, **6**, 276.

CHRISTOFFERSEN, P., DAMSGAARD, EL., HEYDORN, K., LARSEN, N. A., NIELSEN, B. & PAKKENBERG, H. (1969). Concentration of arsenic, manganese and selenium in peripheral nervous tissue of patients with uraemia and a control group. *Proc. eur. Dial. Transpl. Ass.*, **6**, 198.

COHEN, M. B., GRAL, T., SOKOL, A., RUBINI, M. E. & BLAHD, W. H. (1968). Pericardial effusion in chronic uremia. Detection by photoscanning. *Arch. intern. Med.*, **122**, 404.

COLE, J. J., QUINTON, W. E., WILLIAMS, C., MURRAY, J. S. & SHERRIS, J. C. (1962). The pumpless low temperature hemodialysis system. *Trans. Amer. Soc. Artif. intern. Organs*, **8**, 209.

COMTY, C. M., BAILLOD, R. A. & SHALDON, S. (1965). Two-and-a-half years' experience with a nurse-patient operated chronic dialysis unit. *Proc. eur. Dial. Transpl. Ass.*, **2**, 88.

COMTY, C. M. (1968). A longitudinal study of body composition in terminal uremics treated by regular hemodialysis. I. Body composition before treatment *Canad. med. Ass. J.*, **98**, 482.

CONRAD, M. E. (1969). Infectious hepatitis in military populations: problems encountered with gammaglobulin prophylaxis. *Bull. N.Y. Acad. Sci.*, **45**, 167.

CRAMMOND, W. A., KNIGHT, P. R., LAWRENCE, J. R., HIGGINS, B. A., COURT, J. H., MACNAMARA, F. M., CLARKSON, A. R. & MILLER, C. D. J. (1968). Psychological aspects of the management of chronic renal failure. *Brit. med. J.*, **1**, 539.

CREUZFELD, W., SEVERIDT, H. J., BRACHMANN, H., SCHMIDT, G. & TSCHAEPE, U. (1967). The use of gammaglobulin in the prophylaxis of transfusion hepatitis. *Germ. med. Mth.*, **12**, 101.

CROCKETT, R. E., BAILLOD, R. A., LEE, B. N., MOORHEAD, J. F., STEVENSON, C. M., VARGHESE, Z. & SHALDON, S. (1967). Maintenance of fifty patients on intermittent haemodialysis without blood transfusion. *Proc. eur. Dial. Transpl. Ass.*, **4**, 17.

CURTIS, J. R., WING, A. J. & COLEMAN, J. C. (1967). *Bacillus cereus* bacteraemia. A complication of intermittent haemodialysis. *Lancet*, **1**, 136.

CURTIS, J. R., WING, A. J., EASTWOOD, J. B., SMITH, E. K. M. & DE WARDENER, H. E. (1968). The control of metabolic bone disease by maintenance haemodialysis. *Proc. eur. Dial Transpl. Ass.*, **5**, 300.

DATHAN, J. R., THOMPSON, J. M. A. & WORTHINGTON, B. S. (1969). Angiographic studies of Quinton-Scribner arteriovenous cannulae. *Brit. med. J.*, **4**, 20.

DE PALMA, J. R., GOLDING, A. & MAZWELL, M. H. (1969). Shunt-angiography evaluation of A-V cannula malfunction in clotting. *Proc. eur. Dial. Transpl. Ass.*, **6**, 73.

DE VEBER, G. & MACDONALD, D. J. (1969). Psychological evaluation and management in haemodialysis and transplantation. *Proc. eur. Dial. Transpl. Ass.*, **6**, 140.

DITTRICH, P., GURLAND, H. J., KESSEL, M., MASSINI, M.-A. & WETZELS, E. (1969). *Hemodialyse und Peritonealdialyse*. Berlin: Springer-Verlag.

DRUKKER, W., SCHOUTEN, W. A. G. & ALBERTS, CHR. (1968). Report on regular dialysis treatment in Europe 4, 1968. *Proc. eur. Dial. Transpl. Ass.*, **5**, 3.

DRUKKER, W. (1968). The hard water syndrome. A potential hazard during regular dialysis treatment. *Proc. eur. Dial. Transpl. Ass.*, **5**, 284.

DRUKKER, W., HAAGSMA-SCHOUTEN, W. A. G., ALBERTS, CHR. & SPOEK, M. G. (1969). Report on regular dialysis treatment in Europe 5, 1969. *Proc. eur. Dial. Transpl. Ass.*, **6**, 99.

EASTWOOD, J. B., CURTIS, J. R., WING, A. J. & DE WARDENER, H. E. (1968). Hepatitis in a maintenance hemodialysis unit. *Ann. intern. Med.*, **69**, 59.

EDITORIAL (1969a). Hypertension in patients on regular dialysis. *Brit. med. J.*, **3**, 669.

EDITORIAL (1969b). Depletion on dialysis. *Brit. med. J.*, **2**, 778.

EDITORIAL (1969c). Hepatitis virus and renal dialysis. *Lancet*, **2**, 989.

EDITORIAL (1969d). Prophylaxis against infectious hepatitis. *Brit. med. J.*, **4**, 576.

EDITORIAL (1970). Australia antigen and hepatitis. *Brit. med. J.*, **1**, 247.

ELSTEIN, M., SMITH, E. K. M. & CURTIS, J. R. (1969). Reproductive potential of patients treated by maintenance haemodialysis. *Brit. med. J.*, **2**, 734.

ESCHBACH, J. W. JR. (1970). Anaemia and hemodialysis. *Proceedings of fourth International Congress of Nephrology*. In press.

FINE, R. N., DE PALMA, J. R., GORDON, A., MAXWELL, M. H., GRUSHKIN, C. M. & LIEBERMAN, E. (1969). Haemodialysis in children. *Proc. eur. Dial. Transpl. Ass.*, **6**, 149.

FLOYD, M., AYYAR, D. R., HUDGSON, P. & KERR, D. N. S. (1969). Myopathy in chronic renal failure. *Proc. eur. Dial. Transpl. Ass.*, 6, 203.

GAAN, D., MALLICK, N. P., BREWIS, R. A. L., SEEDAT, K. K. & MAHONEY, M. P. (1969). Cerebral damage from declotting Scribner shunts. *Lancet*, 2, 77.

GAZENFIELD, E. & ELIAHOU, H. E. (1969). Development of antibodies to endotoxins of dialysate-bacteria in patients on maintenance dialysis. *Abstracts of fourth International Congress of Nephrology*, 2, 118.

GENUTH, S. M., VERTES, V. & LEONARDS, J. R. (1969). Oral calcium absorption in patients with renal failure treated by chronic haemodialysis. *Metabolism*, 18, 124.

GLASHAN, R. W. & WALKER, F. (1968). A histological examination of veins used in artificial arteriovenous ("Quinton/Scribner") shunts. *Brit. J. Surg.*, 55, 198.

GLEADLE, R. I., BROWN, J. J., CURTIS, J. R., FRASER, R., LAWSON, D. H., LEVER, A. F., LINTON, A. L., MCVEIGH, S., ROBERTSON, J. I. S. & DE WARDENER, H. E. (1969). Plasma renin concentration and the control of blood pressure in patients with chronic renal failure: the effect of haemodialysis. *Proc. eur. Dial Transpl. Ass.*, 6, 131.

GOCKE, D. J. & KAVEY, N. B. (1969). Hepatitis antigen. Correlation with disease and infectivity of blood-donors. *Lancet*, 1, 1055.

GOODMAN, J. S., CREWS, H. D., GINN, H. E. & KOENIG, M. G. (1969). Bacterial endocarditis as a possible complication of chronic haemodialysis. *New Engl. J. Med.*, 280, 876.

GOVAN, J. R., POTER, C. A., COOK, J. G. H., DIXON, B. & TRAFFORD, J. A. P. (1968). Acute magnesium poisoning as a complication of chronic intermittent haemodialysis. *Brit. med. J.*, 2, 278.

HAMPERS, C. L. & SCHUPAK, E. (1967). *Long Term Hemodialysis*. London: Heinemann.

HARRISON, A. R. (Chairman). Round table on disturbances of calcium metabolism in transplanted patients and patients on maintenance haemodialysis. *Proc. eur. Dial. Transpl. Ass.*, 5, 404.

HOPEWELL, J. P., BLANDY, J. P., FESTENSTEIN, H. & MOORHEAD, J. F. (1969). Cooperation in transplantation services. *Brit. J. Hosp. Med.*, 2, 1194.

JOHNSON, W. J., WAGONER, R. D., HUNCT, J. C., MUELLER, G. J. & HALLENBECK, G. A. (1966). Long-term intermittent hemodialysis for chronic renal failure. *Proc. Mayo. Clin.*, 41, 73.

JOHNSON, J. W., WACHMAN, A., KATZ, A. I., HAMPERS, C. L., BERNSTEIN, D. S., WILSON, R. E. & MERRILL, J. P. (1969). Calcium metabolism after subtotal parathyroidectomy in chronic renal failure. *Trans. Amer. Soc. artif. intern. Organs*, 15, 333.

JENNEKENS, F. G. I., VAN DER MOST VAN SPIJK, D. & DORHOUT MEES, E. J. (1969). Nerve fibre degeneration in uraemic polyneuropathy. *Proc. eur. Dial. Transpl. Ass.*, 6, 191.

KALLITERAKIS, E., MARKETOS, S. G., TSEKOS, G. & PANDOS, A. P. (1968). Pericarditis urémique avec hémopéricarde et compression cardiaque. *Presse méd.*, 76, 265.

KAPLAN DE NOUR, A. & CZACZKES, J. W. (1968a). Psychological and psychiatric observations on patients in chronic haemodialysis. *Proc. eur. Dial. Transpl. Ass.*, 5, 67.

KAPLAN DE NOUR, A. & CZACZKES, J. W. (1968b). Emotional problems and reactions of the medical team in a chronic haemodialysis unit. *Lancet*, 2, 988.

KATZ, A. I., HAMPERS, C. L., WILSON, R. E., BERNSTEIN, D. S., WACHMAN, A., KAYE, M. & MERRILL, J. P. (1968). The place of subtotal parathyroidectomy in the management of patients with chronic renal failure. *Trans. Amer. Soc. artif. intern. Organs*, 14, 376.

KAYE, M. & COMTY, C. (1968). Nutritional repletion during dialysis. *Amer. J. clin. Nutr.*, 21, 583.

KAYE, M., COHEN, G. F., CHATTERJEE, G. & MANGEL, R. (1969). Regulation of the plasma ionised calcium and its therapeutic control in patients treated by regular haemodialysis. *Trans Amer. Soc. artif. intern. Organs*, 15, 341.

KENNEDY, A. C. & KERR, D. N. S. (1970). *Haemodialysis.* London: Arnold.

KERR, D. N. S. (1969). Testing new dialysers. *Proc. eur. Dial. Transpl. Ass.*, 6, 319.

KERR, D. N. S., WALLS, J., ELLIS, H., SIMPSON, W., ULDALL, P. R. & WARD, M. K. (1969). Bone disease in patients undergoing regular haemodialysis. *J. Bone Jt. Surg.*, 51, 578.

KIDD, E. E. (1964). Bacterial contamination of dialysing fluid of artificial kidney. *Brit. med. J.*, 1, 880.

KIM, D., BELL, N. H., BUNDESEN, W., PUTONG, P., SIMON, N. M., WALKER, C. & DEL GRECO, F. (1968). *Trans. Amer. Soc. artif. intern. Organs*, 14, 367.

KJELLSTRAND, C. M., LINDERGARD, R. & BOIJSEN, E. (1967). Treatment of clotted Quinton-Scribner arteriovenous shunts by streptokinase (Kanikinase^R). Results evaluated by angiographic and resistance studies. *Proc. eur. Dial. Transpl. Ass.*, 4, 61.

KOPPLE, J. D., SHINABERGER, J. H., COBURN, J. W., SORENSEN, M. & RUBINI, M. (1969). Optimal dietary protein treatment during chronic haemodialysis. *Trans. Amer. Soc. artif. intern. Organs*, 15, 302.

KULATILAKE, A. E., SAMPSON, D., PAPADIMITRIOU, M., VICKERS, J. & SHACKMAN R. (1969). A disposable parallel flow artificial kidney. *Proc. eur. Dial. Transpl. Ass.*, 6, 3.

LAWSON, D. H., WILL, G., BODDY, K. & LINTON, A. L. (1968). Iron metabolism in patients on regular dialysis treatment. *Proc. eur. Dial. Transpl. Ass.*, 5, 167.

LAZORTHES, F. (1969). Fistules arterio-veneuses chirurgicales et hémodialyse. *Imprimerie Fournie. Toulouse.*

LEONARD, C. D., WEIL, E. & SCRIBNER, B. H. (1969). Subdural haematomas in patients undergoing haemodialysis. *Lancet*, 2, 239.

LINDHOLM, D. D., PACE, R. L. & RUSSELL, H. H. JR. (1969). Anaemia of uremia responsive to increased dialysis treatment. *Trans. Amer. Soc. artif. intern. Organs*, 15, 360.

MACKENZIE, J. C., FORD, J. E., WATERS, A. H., HARDING, N. N., CATTELL, W. R. & ANDERSON, B. B. (1968). Erythropoiesis in patients undergoing regular dialysis treatment without transfusion. *Proc. eur. Dial. Transpl. Ass.*, 5, 172.

MAHER, J. H., FREEMAN, R. B., SCHMITT, G. & SCHREINER, G. E. (1965). Adherence of metals to cellophane membranes and removal by whole blood. A mechanism of solute transport during haemodialysis. *Trans. Amer. Soc. artif. intern. Organs*, 11, 104.

MARTIN, A. M., GLUNIE, G. J. A., TONKIN, R. W. & ROBSON, J. S. (1967). The aetiology and management of shunt infections in patients on intermittent haemodialysis. *Proc. eur. Dial. Transpl. Ass.*, 4, 67.

MATTER, B. J., PEDERSEN, J., PSIMENOS, G. & LINDEMAN, R. D. (1969). Lethal copper intoxication in hemodialysis. *Trans. Amer. Soc. artif. intern. Organs*, 15, 309.

McLeod, L. E., Mandin, H., Davidman, M., Ulan, R. & Lakey, W. H. (1966). Intermittent hemodialysis in terminal chronic renal failure. *Canad. med. Ass. J.*, **94**, 318.

Merikas, G., Marketos, S. & Konstantopoulos, E. (1966). Uremic pericardial tamponade. *Canad. med. Ass. J.*, **95**, 119.

Montgomerie, J. Z., Kalmanson, G. M. & Guze, L. B. (1968). Renal failure and infection. *Medicine*, **47**, 1.

Muth, R. G. & Wells, D. E. (1969). Four new coil hemodialysers. *Arch. intern. med.*, **124**, 179.

O'Riordan, J. L. H., Page, J., Kerr, D. N. S., Walls, J., Moorhead, J., Crockett, R. E., Franz, H. & Ritz, E. (1970). Hyperparathyroidism in chronic renal failure and dialysis oestodystrophy. *Quart. J. Med.* In press.

Nose, Y. (1970). Manual on Artificial Organs. *Vol. 1. The Artificial Kidney.*

Papadimitriou, M., Gingell, J. C. & Chisholm, G. D. (1968). Hypercalcaemia from calcium ion-exchange resin in patients on regular haemodialysis. *Lancet*, **2**, 948.

Papadimitriou, M., Carroll, R. N. P. & Kulatilake, A. E. (1969). Clotting problems with the Teflon-Silastic arteriovenous shunt in patients on regular haemodialysis. *Brit. med. J.*, **2**, 15.

Pendras, J. P. & Erickson, R. V. (1966). Hemodialysis: a successful therapy for chronic uremia. *Ann. intern. Med.*, **64**, 293.

PHLS (1968). Assessment of British gammaglobulin in preventing infectious hepatitis. A report to the director of the Public Health Laboratory Service. *Brit. med. J.*, **3**, 451.

PHLS (1969). Infection risks of hemodialysis—some preventive aspects: report to the Public Health Laboratory Service by working party on hemodialysis units. *Brit. med. J.*, **3**, 454.

Quinton, W. E., Dillard, D. H., Cole, J. J. & Scribner, B. H. (1962). Eight months' experience with Silastic-Teflon hypass cannulas. *Trans. Amer. Soc. artif. intern. Organs*, **8**, 236.

Quinton, W. E. & Baillod, R. (1970). Access to the blood stream for haemodialysis. In *Haemodialysis*. ed. A. C. Kennedy and D. N. S. Kerr. London: Arnold.

Rastogi, S. P., Frost, T., Anderson, J., Ashcroft, R. & Kerr, D. N. S. (1968). The significance of disequilibrium between body compartments in the treatment of chronic renal failure by haemodialysis. *Proc. eur. Dial. Transpl. Ass.*, **5**, 102.

Rastogi, S. P., Dewar, J., Frost, T. H. & Kerr, D. N. S. (1969). *In vivo* comparison of Kiil and Alwall-Gambro dialysers. *Proc. eur. Dial. Transpl. Ass.*, **6**, 363.

Reyman, T. A. (1968). Subacute constrictive uremic pericarditis. *Amer. J. Med.*, **46**, 972.

Ringertz, O., Nystrom, B. & Strom, J. (1969). Clinical aspects of an outbreak of hepatitis among personnel in hemodialysis units. *Scand. J. Infect. Dis.*, **1**, 51.

Roodvoets, A. P., Van Neerbos, B. R., Hooghwinkel, G. J. M., Hulsmans, H. A. M. & Beukers, H. (1967). Hyperlipidaemia in patients on regular dialysis treatment. *Proc. eur. Dial. Transpl. Ass.*, **4**, 257.

Shaldon, S. & McKay, S. (1968). Use of arteriovenous fistula in home haemodialysis. *Brit. med. J.*, **4**, 671.

Shaldon, S., Shaldon, J., McInnes, S., MacDonald, H. & Ogg, D. (1969). Long-term maintenance domestic haemodialysis in children. *Proc. eur. Dial. Transpl. Ass.*, **6**, 145.

SCHREINER, G. E., MAHER, J. F. & FREEMAN, R. B. (1967). Problems of haemodialysis. *Proceedings of Third International Congress of Nephrology*, **3**, 316. ed. E. L. Becker. Basel: Karger.

SCRIBNER, B. H. (1967). *Dialysis*. In *Renal Disease*. ed. D. A. K. Black, 2nd edition. London: Blackwell, p. 459.

SEEDAT, Y. K. (1969). Exchangeable potassium study in patients undergoing chronic haemodialysis. *Brit. med. J.*, **2**, 344.

SHEIL, A. G. R., STEWART, J. H., JOHNSON, J. R., MAYM, J., STOREY, B. G., ROGERS, J. H., CHARLESWORTH, J. A., WRIGHT, R., SHARP, A., JOHNSTON, J. M., SANDS, J. R. & LOEWENTHAL, J. (1969). Community treatment of end-stage renal failure by dialysis and renal transplantation from cadaver donors. *Lancet*, **2**, 917.

SHINABERGER, J. H. & GINN, H. E. (1968). A low protein, high essential amino acid diet for nitrogen equilibrium in chronic dialysis. In *Nutrition in Renal Disease*. ed. G. H. Berlyne. Edinburgh: Livingstone.

SPAUDLING, W. B. (1967). Subacute constrictive uremic pericarditis. *Arch. intern. Med.*, **119**, 644.

STEWART, W. K. & FLEMING, L. W. (1968). A diagnostic dilemma. A case of cholestasis due to anti-emetic treatment during regular dialysis treatment. *Proc. eur. Dial. Transpl. Ass.*, **5**, 324.

SYMONS, H. S. & WRONG, O. M. (1964). Uraemic pericarditis with cardiac tamponade, a report of four cases. *Brit. med. J.*, **1**, 605.

THOMSON, G. E., WATERHOUSE, K., McDONALD, H. P. JR. & FRIEDMAN, E. A. (1967). Haemodialysis for chronic renal failure. *Arch. intern. Med.*, **120**, 153.

TRAEGER, J., REVILLARD, J. P., TOURAINE, J. & BROCHIER, J. (1969). L'immunité cellulaire dans l'insuffisance rénale. *Proc. eur. Dial. Transpl. Ass.*, **6**, 165.

TRIGER, D. R. & JOEKES, A. M. (1969). Severe muscle cramp due to acute hypomagnesaemia in haemodialysis. *Brit. med. J.*, **2**, 804.

VERBERCKMOES, R. (1969). Calcium, magnesium and phosphate balance studies in patients under maintenance haemodialysis. *Proc. eur. Dial. Transpl. Ass.*, **6**, 269.

VERROUST, P. J., CURTIS, J. R., WING, A. J., EASTWOOD, J. B., STOREY, J., EDWARDS, M. S. & DE WARDENER, H. E. (1967). Maintenance haemodialysis without blood transfusion. *Proc. eur. Dial. Transpl. Ass.*, **4**, 12.

VERTES, V., CANGIANO, M. D., BERMAN, L. B. & GOULD, A. (1969). Hypertension in end-stage renal disease. *New Engl. J. Med.*, **280**, 978.

WALLS, J. & KOPP, H. (1968). Blood flow in arteriovenous shunts; observations and measurements. *Brit. med. J.*, **2**, 806.

WALSH, A. (1968). (Chairman). Round table discussion on the Cimino-Brescia fistula. *Proc. eur. Dial. Transpl. Ass.*, **5**, 391.

WATT, D. A. L., DUNN, B. P., LIVINGSTONE, W. R., MacDOUGALL, A. I., MacKAY, R. K. S., OBINECHE, E. N. & RENNIE, J. B. (1969). The use of urokinase in declotting of arteriovenous shunts. *Proc. eur. Dial. Transpl. Ass.*, **6**, 88.

WILKINSON, R., SCOTT, D. F., ULDALL, P. R., KERR, D. N. S. & SWINNEY, J. (1970). Plasma renin and exchangeable sodium in the hypertension of chronic renal failure. The effect of bilateral nephrectomy. *Quart. J. Med*. In press.

WING, A. J., CURTIS, J. R. & DE WARDENER, H. E. (1967). Reduction of clotting in Scribner shunts by long-term anticoagulation. *Brit. med. J.*, **3**, 143.

WING, A. J. (1968). Optimum calcium concentration of dialysis fluid for maintenance haemodialysis. *Brit. med. J.*, **3**, 150.

YPERSELE DE STRIHOU, C. VAN & STRAGIER, A. (1969). Effect of bilateral nephrectomy on transfusion requirements of patients undergoing chronic dialysis.
Lancet, **2**, 705.
ZUCKERMAN, A. J., TAYLOR, P. E. & ALMEDIA, J. D. (1970). Presence of particles
other than Australia-SH antigen in a case of chronic active hepatitis with
cirrhosis. *Brit. med. J.*, **1**, 262.

5 Haematology

MARTIN C. G. ISRAËLS

IRON-DEFICIENCY STATES. HAEMORRHAGIC DISEASES AND PLATELET FUNCTION. LEUKAEMIAS.

ANAEMIA DUE TO DISORDERS OF IRON METABOLISM

THE most common disorder of iron metabolism encountered in clinical medicine is iron deficiency and the anaemia it causes; other disorders are relatively rare but important when they occur, and they are sometimes confused with iron deficiency. Iron-deficiency anaemia is undoubtedly the commonest blood disorder seen in general practice, as several published surveys have shown. An average 70-kg man has about 3·5 g of elemental iron in his body; about two-thirds is in the form of haemoglobin in blood and bone marrow, about one-quarter is stored in the tissues in the form of haemosiderin or ferritin, and the remainder mostly in myoglobin and iron-containing enzymes; transport iron accounts for only 0·12 per cent of the total iron.

According to Harris (1963) three million red blood cells are produced and broken down *per second* in the normal human body; 6·3 g of haemoglobin containing 21 mg of iron are synthesized and degraded every 24 hours; so it is not surprising that continued iron deficiency soon produces clinically recognizable effects. However, to a certain extent the appearance of signs of iron deficiency is delayed by the fact that iron loss affects first the 25 per cent of body iron present in storage forms in the tissues; only when the store is exhausted does haemoglobin iron begin to be lost and only then do signs of iron deficiency appear in the blood and marrow cells.

The fact that there is a regular but small loss of iron from the body is now accepted, and normally there is a proper balance between loss and absorption. Many experiments have shown that in normal persons between 5 and 10 per cent of the iron in food is actually absorbed, but recent estimates by Jacobs and Greenman (1969) show how variable the availability of food iron can be and how many factors, including the method of cooking, can influence the proportion of food iron available for absorption in the alimentary tract.

G

Since the average western diet provides 10–15 mg of iron daily, the amount of iron normally absorbed is 1·0–1·5 mg. There are several sources of iron loss; the intestinal epithelium desquamates, and iron in the cells and iron in some red cells is lost this way; iron is also lost in leucocytes, skin cells, in sweat and a small amount in the urine. The total loss in the adult male or the non-menstruating female is about 1·0–1·5 mg daily, balancing the absorption. But in the menstruating female, and even more the pregnant female, and in the rapidly growing adolescent—male and female—more iron is needed; to a certain extent this need is met by increasing absorption, because in iron deficiency an increase of up to 40 per cent in the amount of iron absorbed from food can occur; even so, the balance is clearly precarious and consequently iron-deficiency anaemia frequently occurs in these groups of patients. Recently, some researches have been carried out on the detection of iron deficiency before anaemia appears, and this work is discussed below.

Growth, menstruation and pregnancy are almost physiological causes of iron deficiency and will respond to short-term treatment. The possible pathological causes of iron deficiency are very numerous; Beveridge and his co-workers (1965) at Oxford followed a group of 370 adult patients and found that the commonest cause of iron-deficiency anaemia was loss of blood from the alimentary tract; in this area, bleeding from peptic ulceration, from haemorrhoids, due to hiatus hernia, or produced by taking salicylates, particularly aspirin, were the most frequent causes. Like many others they found an increasing number of anaemic patients among those who had had a gastrectomy operation eight or more years before. Poor diet was an important cause, usually because the wrong types of foods were used, actual insufficiency being rare. Finally, they consider that menorrhagia is one of the most overlooked causes.

Iron deficiency nowadays is easily and effectively treatable in almost all patients, and current therapy will be described later; it is therefore very important to identify iron deficiency correctly and to ascertain the cause. With the facilities now available in the United Kingdom, the general practitioner should be able to sort out his iron-deficient patients into those with an easily definable cause and those in whom the cause is not clear, and he can thus decide which patients need further investigation.

Diagnosis of Iron Deficiency and its Cause

The first suggestion of iron-deficiency anaemia usually comes from the blood count carried out in a clinically anaemic patient. In these days of electronic counters it is reasonable to ask for a red-cell count, estimation of haemoglobin, colour index, packed cell volume and mean corpuscular haemoglobin concentration (MCHC); for a first blood count a white-cell count with differential count and a platelet count should be requested. The MCHC is the best indicator; if it is 30 per cent or less, iron deficiency is likely. In some patients the probable cause of the anaemia will be found at the initial clinical examination, but in the majority there is no such clue, and a decision has to be taken as to whether to ask for further laboratory investigation *before* any treatment is started. These further laboratory investigations are:

(1) estimation of serum iron level and total serum iron-binding capacity;
(2) examination of a marrow smear for presence of free iron and sideroblasts.

The serum iron level in adults is normally between 100 and 120 μg/ml, with a range of 75–175 μg/ml; in iron deficiency the figure is usually below 35 μg/ml. The total iron-binding capacity is normally 300–360 μg/ml and in anaemia it is usually raised to 350–460 μg/ml; normally the iron-binding capacity is 25 to 50 per cent saturated, but in iron deficiency the saturation is always less than 16 per cent.

In a normal marrow there will be some free iron, and sideroblasts are present, though often difficult to detect; the "ring" sideroblasts (see below) are always abnormal. In iron deficiency there is no free iron and no sideroblasts are present.

Since iron deficiency is relatively common, it is not practicable to carry out a full investigation in all patients. The best guide is age and sex. In menstruating females and in adolescent girls and boys it is reasonable to undertake a therapeutic test with an adequate course of an effective iron preparation (see below), remembering that a six-week period should be allowed for a response to appear. In all adult males and in women who are not menstruating, the serum iron and marrow investigations should be done; then if iron deficiency is present, investigations to determine the cause should be undertaken. The best order of investigation is first to look for a source of blood loss, and examination of the faeces for occult blood is the first step, since the alimentary tract is the most likely source. If there is no blood loss, malabsorption of iron is the next most likely cause, and finally a detailed enquiry about diet may produce the clue. The methods of investigating these possible causes of iron deficiency are well known, and are dealt with in standard textbooks. The use of radio-active chromium labelled red cells for the detection of the amount and source of alimentary tract bleeding has, however, been only recently developed. The principle of the method is that 10–20 ml of the patient's blood is withdrawn and the red cells are labelled with 50–200 microcuries of ^{51}Cr. The labelled cells are injected intravenously into the patient; if there is blood loss in the alimentary tract, radio-activity should appear in the faeces. All the faeces passed in the next seven to eight days must be collected; from their weight and from the estimate of radio-activity the daily blood loss can be calculated, but estimates of less than 2 ml daily are not significant. Then by finding out which specimen, in order, shows the highest radio-activity, an estimate can be given of the probable site of the bleeding; thus a peak in an early specimen suggests that the bleeding site is in the colon, whereas if the peak occurs in late specimens after six or seven days, the bleeding site is likely to be in the stomach or duodenum. Some overlap is inevitable, but it is significant that this method has proved most useful in detecting blood loss from the caecal area which is notoriously difficult to define by radiological methods. Even when barium studies have been negative, a second examination with refined techniques has often been successful in detecting a lesion when the radiologist knows that a particular area of the alimentary tract is thought to be the site of the blood loss.

If malabsorption of iron is suspected, much time can be saved by the use of a simple iron-absorption test. After an initial fasting-blood specimen for serum iron has been taken, a dose of 600 mg of ferrous sulphate is given orally; three hours later a further specimen is taken for serum iron. If absorption is normal the serum-iron level should have increased from the initial low level of less than 30 μg/ml to over 200 μg/ml. If the expected rise does not occur, the test should be repeated with the addition of 800–1000 mg of ascorbic acid, also orally; if this second test shows adequate absorption the patient is likely to respond to therapeutic doses of oral iron. If both tests give low results, parenteral treatment will be needed. A group of patients with iron deficiency who are appearing in increasing numbers are those who have had a gastrectomy eight or more years ago. These patients mostly give normal results with the iron-absorption test with ferrous sulphate, and the defect appears to be a failure to increase the absorption of food iron in the same way as the anaemic but otherwise normal patient is able to do. Their anaemia therefore usually responds well to oral iron therapy.

Iron Deficiency without Anaemia

Over 30 years ago, Jan Waldenström coined the name "sideropenia" for a condition in which clinical signs of iron deficiency such as koilonychia and glossitis with dysphagia occurred in the absence of anaemia, and he contended that the condition could be relieved by administering iron. The better techniques for investigating iron deficiency that have since been developed have supported his findings. The combination of a low serum iron, saturation of the total iron-binding capacity of serum below 16 per cent and the absence of free iron in a marrow specimen is currently accepted as evidence of iron deficiency. In 1960 Beutler and colleagues in America studied a group of 44 women with chronic fatigue who had haemoglobin levels in excess of 12 g/100 ml; they all showed evidence of iron deficiency judged by these criteria and those given iron treatment showed significantly more improvement than those given a placebo. Fielding and his colleagues (1965) working in London on their differential ferrioxamine test for estimating iron stores came across a group of women who were clinically well, and who had a haemoglobin level within normal range who had nevertheless no significant iron stores. This group formed no less than 35 per cent of the women tested, and Fielding reasonably pointed out that subject to menorrhagia or increased demand for iron in pregnancy such women would be liable to show iron-deficiency anaemia very soon. Two recent surveys have also drawn attention to the importance of sideropenia. Powell and his colleagues (1968) examined a group of elderly patients in a hospital in South Wales. If the serum iron was less than 50 μg/100 ml and the TIBC less than 16 per cent, they classed the patient as sideropenic, and found that out of their 333 patients 39 per cent of the men and 41 per cent of the women were sideropenic. The majority of these patients had some recognizable cause for their iron deficiency such as gastro-intestinal disease, but quite a few had conditions not usually associated with iron deficiency such as vascular disease; 55 per cent of patients with infections were also iron deficient. A group of 57 patients had haemoglobin levels in the normal range for their sex, but still had iron deficiency. McFarlane and others (1967) working in Glasgow examined a group of 500 women seen in general practices in Glasgow and estimated that 21 per cent had latent iron deficiency without overt anaemia and that, except in women over 80, latent iron deficiency was commoner than iron-deficiency anaemia; they gave the warning that some of these patients would develop anaemia within the next two years. Heinrich (1968) working in Germany has taken the matter even further and claims that there is a "pre-latent" stage of iron deficiency characterized by depleted iron stores and evidence of increased iron absorption while the serum iron and TIBC are still normal. It is not surprising that he claims that iron deficiency is in fact a very common condition, and he points out that in practical therapeutics we should allow for the fact that an oral dose of about 6 g of ferrous iron is needed simply to restore iron stores to normal.

These results suggest that the use of "iron tonics" for undue fatigue, especially in women, is not quite the old wives' tale that it is usually considered to be. Nowadays it is reasonable to ask the local pathological laboratory to estimate the serum iron and saturation of the iron-binding capacity of the serum. If these figures are low, a trial of oral iron therapy given for long enough is well worth while, always provided that proper clinical examination has not revealed any possible cause for iron deficiency that needs correction.

Sideroblastic Anaemias

"Sideroblasts" are normoblasts with cytoplasmic granules that contain iron, and therefore stain blue with the Prussian Blue reaction. Some sideroblasts are present in normal marrow smears, but the granules are scattered in the cytoplasm and are small and often difficult to see. Similarly scattered but more prominent granules are seen in conditions like haemolytic anaemias, megaloblastic anaemias and conditions in which the serum iron (transferrin) levels are increased, such as haemochromatosis. In the thalassaemias sideroblasts with prominent scattered cytoplasmic granules are common. But in the so-called sideroblastic anaemias the granules are found to be collected in a partial or complete ring round the normoblast's nucleus; the reason for this arrangement is unknown. These "ring sideroblasts" are found in marrow smears of some identified diseases such as erythroleukaemia, anaemia caused by drugs, particularly anti-tuberculous drugs, and haemolytic anaemias. But when these identifiable causes have been excluded there remains a group of "primary sideroblastic anaemias", some hereditary and some acquired. The cause of these anaemias is generally agreed to be a defect in haemoglobin synthesis, but how this is brought about has been much debated, and possible explanations have been well reviewed, for instance by Dacie and Mollin (1966).

These patients are usually referred to haematological clinics because they have been found to have an anaemia that does not respond to iron, vitamin B_{12} or folic acid. Physical signs other than those due to the anaemia are usually unimportant; sometimes the spleen may be just palpable. The hereditary and acquired groups present differences of incidence and laboratory findings. Hereditary sideroblastic anaemia is rare and almost entirely confined to the male sex; it is sometimes discovered in childhood and usually by early adult life. The anaemia is a hypochromic one which is chronic and will not respond to iron treatment; the MCHC is usually low, 28 per cent or less; sometimes the red cells appear dimorphic. Examination of the bone marrow shows the characteristic "ring sideroblasts". The serum iron level is raised and the iron-binding capacity often almost completely saturated, though the total may be normal. Haemoglobin analysis is normal, except perhaps for some reduction in haemoglobin A_2. The patients with a dimorphic blood may have reduced serum folate levels, but MacGibbon and Mollin point out that it is difficult to be sure that this means folic acid deficiency, since only some of these patients respond to treatment with folic acid. This anaemia is known to be related to an abnormality of pyridoxine metabolism. MacGibbon and Mollin (1965) have shown that about half the patients with sideroblastic anaemia of both hereditary and acquired forms excrete abnormal amounts of xanthurenic acid after a loading dose of 4 g of L-tryptophan given orally, and about one-third show improvement of the anaemia when treated with large doses of oral pyridoxine, such responses being more often seen in the hereditary group. The relation of sideroblastic anaemia to pyridoxine metabolism is not known at present. The inheritance in this disease follows a sex-linked, partially recessive pattern and several family trees have been published, e.g. by Bourne et al. (1965).

The primary acquired sideroblastic anaemia is less rare, and appears most often in middle-aged or elderly patients of either sex and there is no family history of similar cases. The anaemia is characteristically dimorphic with a variable proportion of hypochromic cells, and correspondingly the MCHC is rarely low, usually 30 to 34 per cent. By the time they are referred to a haematological clinic, many of these patients have received the full range of haematological treatment including parenteral iron, so that serum iron and serum folate estimations are useless. If no such treatment has been given the serum iron and the estimation of the saturation of a normal total iron-binding capacity is at the most only a little above normal. The bone marrow will provide the clue in the presence of "ring sideroblasts", and in untreated patients megaloblastic changes can often be found. About 50 per cent of these patients will show the abnormal response to a test dose of L-tryptophan mentioned above. In those that show megaloblasts, folic acid treatment will cause the marrow picture to revert to normoblastic, but this change is not often followed by much rise in the haemoglobin level. As in the hereditary group, about 30 per cent of patients will respond to doses of pyridoxine of the order of 150 mg daily orally when the treatment is maintained for some months. If the patient fails to respond to folic acid or pyridoxine, blood transfusion given at regular intervals becomes the only method so far available for relief. But repeated transfusion has to be used circumspectly in both groups of patients, since iron deposition in the tissues is very liable to occur and haemosiderosis soon becomes an undesirable complication. To a certain extent this effect can be mitigated by adding 1 g of desferrioxamine to the infusion when a blood transfusion is given.

Treatment of Iron-deficiency Anaemia

Two trends in iron therapy have become noticeable recently; one is the use of slow-release preparations for oral treatment, and the other is the increasing use of an intravenous infusion of the total dose of iron needed to make up the iron deficit in place of a series of small intravenous or intramuscular doses.

Israëls and Cook (1965) used the slow-release preparation "Ferrogradumet" in which the ferrous sulphate solution is soaked up by a plastic matrix of minute interstices which constitutes the "pill" which the patient takes *before* food in the morning. They showed that whereas a dose of 200 mg of Fe, whatever the iron salt used, had been known to give the optimum daily increase of haemoglobin in patients with iron-deficiency anaemia, when the slow-release preparation was used, a dose of only 105 mg of Fe produced the same daily rate of haemoglobin increase. The combination of a smaller daily dose and the slow release, mainly in the jejunum, reduced the incidence of unpleasant side-effects to a minimum. Another method of attaining the same result is the "Feospan" preparation in which the ferrous sulphate is incorporated into granules with coatings that ensure dissolution at different levels in the alimentary tract. The effectiveness of these preparations and the convenience of a single daily dose have led to the production of other slow-release iron preparations, some using other iron salts, and these are now being made available or are under trial. Such preparations are inevitably more expensive than the simple tablets of ferrous sulphate or ferrous gluconate. But if the patients will take these new preparations regularly, and if the incidence of side-effects is as low as with the original preparations, the extra expense may well be marginal as the desired effect will be obtained more quickly. It is now realized that, to prevent a quick relapse of iron deficiency, it is essential to fill the iron stores which have become depleted. In order to obtain this result, it is essential to continue iron therapy for some time after the haemoglobin concentration in the blood has become normal; it is likely that the period of continuing treatment should be about three months in women, and two months in men.

Parenteral iron treatment is recommended when the iron absorption test shows that absorption from the alimentary tract is defective, and in cases when it is essential to make sure that the iron is taken, where there is no time to risk failure of the patient to take the pills, as in late pregnancy. A less common indication is when it is necessary to build up iron stores in the face of continuing chronic blood loss, for example in patients with haemorrhagic telangiectasia. The standard parenteral technique is to calculate the dose of iron needed and administer it in a number of doses of convenient size; this may well mean that a patient will need ten or more doses of intramuscular iron. The discovery that the iron-dextran compound "Imferon" designed for intramuscular use can be safely given intravenously when well diluted has enabled the full dose to be given in one intravenous infusion.

The required dosage is calculated from the formula:

$$\text{Total iron required (mg)} = 0.3 \times WD,$$

where W = body weight in lb
D = haemoglobin deficit in percentage, taking 14.6 g/100 ml corresponding to 100 per cent.

Since 1 ml of Imferon contains 50 mg of iron, the total volume of Imferon to be administered can be calculated. This amount is diluted with 20 times the volume of normal saline and administered in a slowly running intravenous drip so that 500 ml of the iron-saline mixture takes at least three hours. A few patients have unpleasant reactions to this intravenous iron mixture; to avoid giving the full dose to such patients, the first 15 ml should be administered very slowly over 30 minutes or so. In such a patient, who really needed intravenous iron, the addition of chlorpheniramine ("Piriton") 4 mg to the drip and keeping her in bed for a few hours afterwards successfully prevented reactions. This technique is very useful in hospital practice and can be used when facilities are available for out-patient treatment as well as for in-patients, but at present it is less adaptable to the conditions of general practice.

REFERENCES

BEUTLER, E., LARSH, S. E. & GURNEY, C. W. (1960). Iron therapy in chronically fatigued non-anaemic women. A double blind study. *Ann. intern. Med.*, **52**, 389.

BEVERIDGE, B. R., BANNERMAN, R. M., EVANSON, J. M. & WITTS, L. J. (1965). Hypochromic anaemia: a retrospective study and follow-up of 378 in-patients. *Quart. J. Med.*, **34**, 145.

BOURNE, M. S., ELVES, M. W. & ISRAËLS, M. C. G. (1965). Familial pyridoxine-responsive anaemia. *Brit. J. Haemat.*, **11**, 1.

DACIE, J. V. & MOLLIN, D. L. (1966). Siderocytes, sideroblasts and sideroblastic anaemia. *Acta med. scand. Suppl.*, **445**, 237.

FIELDING, J., O'SHAUGHNESSY, M. C. & BRUNSTRÖM, G. M. (1965). Iron deficiency without anaemia. *Lancet*, **2**, 9.

HARRIS, J. W. (1963). Iron metabolism and iron-lack anaemia. In *The Red Cell*. Mass: Harvard University Press, chap 2.

HEINRICH, H. C. (1968). Iron deficiency without anaemia. *Lancet*, **2**, 460.

ISRAËLS, M. C. G. & COOK, T. A. (1965). New preparations for oral iron therapy. *Lancet*, **2**, 654.

JACOBS, A. & GREENMAN, D. A. (1969). Availability of food iron. *Brit. med. J.*, **1**, 673.

McFARLANE, D. B., PINKERTON, P. H., DAGG, J. H. & GOLDBERG, A. (1967). Incidence of iron deficiency, with and without anaemia, in women in general practice. *Brit. J. Haemat.*, **13**, 790.

MACGIBBON, B. H. & MOLLIN, D. L. (1965). Sideroblastic anaemia in man: observations on seventy cases. *Brit. J. Haemat.*, **11**, 59.

POWELL, D. E. B., THOMAS, J. H. & MILLS, P. (1968). Serum iron in elderly hospital patients. *Geront. Clin.*, **10**, 21.

HAEMORRHAGIC DISEASES

The clinical classification of haemorrhagic diseases at present divides the patients into those suffering from a clotting factor deficiency, such as haemophilia, and those suffering from a platelet deficiency. In addition there are those who have primarily a blood-vessel affection with normal blood; for example Henoch-Schönlein purpura. Most of the patients suffering from a clotting factor deficiency are in the haemophilia group, comprising classical haemophilia (Haemophilia A, Factor VIII deficiency) which accounts in this country for 85 per cent of the cases, and Christmas disease (Haemophilia B, Factor IX deficiency) which accounts for 15 per cent. It is pleasant to be able to record that since 1963, when the fibrin-stabilizing factor was recognized as Factor XIII, no new factor has been added to the list. Individual congenital deficiency of all the known factors in addition to Factors VIII and IX has been reported, their clinical presentation is well recognized and laboratory methods for detection of these deficiencies are well established.

Methods of managing haemophilic bleeding have been much improved lately by the introduction of new methods for concentrating the factors and of accessory drugs; these will be discussed in this section. Idiopathic thrombocytopenic purpura, the established type of platelet deficiency, is also well known, and most physicians are agreed about methods of confirming the diagnosis and planning the treatment. When these major groups have been dealt with, there remain an indefinite group of "bleeders", often with a history of family affection, that do not fit in; bleeding in this group may be just as troublesome as in haemophilia but how best to treat the patients is often uncertain. Investigation of this group has been much advanced by the newer techniques for the detection of abnormalities of platelet *function*, which may occur when platelet numbers remain within normal limits.

Abnormalities of Platelet Function

Until recent times, the only measure applicable to platelets was an estimate of their number in the blood, and the only measure of their function was the crude technique of estimating the bleeding time. It has been known for some time that in some haemorrhagic syndromes the bleeding time is definitely prolonged but the platelet count remains normal, the best example being von Willebrand's disease. This abnormality was originally attributed to inability of the capillary blood vessels to contract when traumatized, and this abnormality could be observed by studying the nail-bed capillaries under a suitable microscope; but this abnormality could, in practice, be found only in a minority of patients. Techniques have now been developed for studying some of the functions of platelets concerned with haemostasis in a quantitative manner, and in order to understand them it is necessary to consider briefly what happens when a small blood vessel is injured and allows blood to escape into the tissues.

When blood escapes through an aperture caused by injury, it comes into immediate contact with exposed collagen. Within seconds of this contact platelets *adhere* to the damaged area and this adhesion is followed by the release of adenosine diphosphate (ADP) from these adherent platelets and probably also from red blood cells in the area. This ADP causes more platelets to *aggregate* on top of those already adhering to the damaged surface, and in the process of aggregation the platelets release further ADP—the so-called "secondary release of ADP". Thus a chain reaction of aggregating platelets is set up resulting in the formation of a mass of platelets which will block the aperture in the vessel. Simultaneously with this platelet activity, the plasma coagulation processes will be in action; the intrinsic system is initiated by Factor XII and the extrinsic system through released tissue factor and Factor VII. The aggregating platelets themselves release a phospholipid, platelet factor 3, which acts by facilitating coagulation around the aggregating platelets. The coagulation soon proceeds to the release of thrombin which has two relevant actions in this situation: it causes viscous metamorphosis of the mass of aggregated platelets, a process whereby a loose mass of platelets still permeable to the blood stream is converted into an impermeable plug; thrombin catalyses the formation of fibrin which reinforces the platelet plug and produces a local firm clot. A further effect of the platelet aggregation is the release by the platelets of the vaso-constrictor substance, 5-hydroxytryptamine (serotonin). An excellent account of the interrelations between these different processes is given by Hardisty (1968).

The arrest of haemorrhage can be seen to be a complex process which begins with platelet adhesion and platelet aggregation. Methods for the quantitative estimation of these two platelet functions and of the availability of platelet factor 3 have now been developed and applied to the study of those disorders in which no deficiency of any of the 13 recognized clotting factors is known to occur. The distinction between platelet adhesiveness and aggregation is a convenient artificiality, and therefore it is essential to define these terms. Platelet *adhesiveness* (or stickiness) is the property of platelets to adhere to a foreign surface. Platelet *aggregation* is the property of platelets to adhere to each other. Platelet *agglutination* is the term reserved for the clumping of platelets caused by a known antigen-antibody reaction, e.g. in autoimmune conditions or caused by drug sensitivity. Platelet adhesiveness is measured by both *in vivo* and *in vitro* techniques; the latter are the more convenient and involve the exposure of platelets to a foreign surface, usually glass, under strictly controlled conditions, and the result is expressed as the percentage of platelets that are lost in passage over the surface. Platelet aggregation is usually estimated by a turbidometric technique introduced by O'Brien of Portsmouth. This is based on the observation that when ADP in a suitable concentration is added to a platelet-rich plasma, the platelets are aggregated and the plasma then becomes much clearer; if disaggregation occurs, as it does with lower concentrations of ADP, the optical density of the plasma increases again. Thus from observation of the records we can see whether the expected changes in aggregation are taking place, and a number of tests are now applied to the study of platelets in haemorrhagic conditions. These tests record the changes in platelet aggregation with different concentrations of ADP, in the presence of a standard connective tissue (collagen) extract, with thrombin and with adrenalin; the secondary release of ADP is recorded in the presence of connective tissue and also in the presence of kaolin. Platelet factor 3 is estimated by the ability of the platelets to restore the delayed recalcification time of a platelet-poor plasma. The details of these techniques would be inappropriate in this volume, and those interested should refer to the full discussion by Hellem and Stormorken (1969). The application of these methods to the group of patients with haemorrhagic diseases given such names as von Willebrand's disease, thrombasthenia and thrombopathia has already enabled us to sort out some more definable syndromes for which different methods of treatment are appropriate.

von Willebrand's disease

This hereditary bleeding disorder was originally described by von Willebrand in 1926. It is inherited as an autosomal dominant and affects both sexes equally, but the degree of disability suffered by affected individuals varies greatly, from trivial discomfort to life-threatening bleeding; fortunately really severely affected cases are rare. Spontaneous bleeding is usually confined to epistaxis; occasional patients have been recorded suffering from severe spontaneous gastro-intestinal haemorrhage or haematuria. Haemarthroses like those common in haemophilia do occur, but are rare. Several serious cases of menstrual bleeding are known, but again it is not common. The main trouble in this disease is the liability to severe haemorrhage after minor trauma, particularly after minor surgical procedures and after dental extraction. An odd and recognized clinical feature is that patients liable to prolonged bleeding after an extraction of a tooth may experience a major operation, such as appendicectomy, without undue loss of blood. Bleeding into subcutaneous and muscular tissue is very unusual spontaneously, but can be quite disproportionately severe after trauma.

Laboratory testing shows a prolonged bleeding time, normal clotting time, normal platelet count, and normal clot retraction. An unexpected feature has been the discovery that in many of the patients there is a deficiency of Factor VIII—the antihaemophilia factor. The reduction is usually mild, between 20 and 50 per cent of normal; a few severely affected patients have less than 20 per cent. Investigation of platelet function shows a constant reduction of platelet adhesiveness, but platelet aggregation is normal whether set off by ADP or any of the other "triggers" mentioned. Platelet factor 3 availability is normal. Prolonged observation of some of these patients has shown that both the clinical severity and the changes in the laboratory tests are variable, and patients known to be affected can sometimes give normal results with the usual tests.

The treatment of bleeding in von Willebrand's disease has been much influenced by the discovery of Factor VIII deficiency and by a further discovery that concentrates of Factor VIII will influence the prolonged bleeding time; in particular the snap-frozen plasma and cryoprecipitate preparations of Factor VIII will correct the bleeding time in von Willebrand patients who are not at the time short of Factor VIII, and is has been shown that this "von Willebrand factor" is present in haemophilic plasma, which has no

Factor VIII present. Therefore, if the patient is known to have a low Factor VIII level, or if an assay gives a low figure, treatment with snap-frozen plasma or cryoprecipitate should be given. Fortunately these patients respond very rapidly and quite a small dose suffices to raise the Factor VIII level above 30 per cent, so that a single day's treatment with two units of plasma or cryoprecipitate may be enough. The few patients who have an initial Factor VIII level below 20 per cent will, however, need to be treated in the same way as haemophilic patients with repeated doses until the bleeding stops. If the patient does not have a low Factor VIII level, the use of antihaemophilic preparations should be limited to severe haemorrhages such as gastro-intestinal bleeding or serious menorrhagia.

With most von Willebrand patients, superficial bleeding from cuts or grazes can be controlled by simple pressure for up to 30 minutes. *Epistaxis* is often persistent and troublesome; it can be checked by the application of topical thrombin powder on a gauze dressing; in serious cases the nose will have to be plugged, and it is important to use a non-adherent material. *Gastro-intestinal haemorrhage* is usually quite silent without any accompanying abdominal pain and, as in haemophilia, seems to be due to a "weeping" of an area of mucous membrane rather than a bleeding from a defined site. Treatment with antihaemophilic preparations should be given together with packed cells from stored blood if the haemoglobin level falls below 9 g/100 ml. *Menorrhagia* varies from troublesome to very serious; the use of one of the oral contraceptive preparations is advisable for a time. In serious cases antihaemophilic plasma will be needed as well. When *dental extraction* is required, the patient should be admitted to hospital and kept in bed for 24 hours afterwards, with the application of simple pressure dressings if needed. If the patient has low Factor VIII, 2 units of snap-frozen plasma should be given before the extraction; the few patients with really low Factor VIII need full haemophilic treatment and a splint should have been made beforehand. The anti-fibrinolytic agent, ε-aminocaproic acid (EACA), which has proved useful in the management of haemophilic bleeding, can also be used in von Willebrand's disease at the same dose of 0·1 mg/kg body weight four to six times daily, but in my own experience its use is not often needed.

Glanzmann's disease

This syndrome, also known as thrombasthenia, is much rarer than von Willebrand's disease. It appears to be inherited in a recessive manner and both sexes may be affected. The clinical picture resembles that of von Willebrand's disease in that spontaneous bleeding is unusual but bleeding after trauma and surgical operations can be serious. Laboratory tests show that the platelet count is normal, and the bleeding time is prolonged. But no Factor VIII deficiency has been found, clot retraction is defective, and the platelet function tests all give abnormal results. Platelet adhesiveness is diminished and platelet aggregation with ADP and other trigger materials hardly occurs at all; correspondingly platelet factor 3 availability is decreased.

Treatment of bleeding in Glanzmann's disease is difficult because the antihaemophilic preparations are of no value and blood transfusion simply makes up for blood loss. Transfusion of normal platelets has been tried but the results were disappointing. Local treatment of epistaxis with topical thrombin is effective.

Aspirin bleeding

O'Brien (1968) has shown that salicylates, particularly aspirin, can influence the results of platelet aggregation tests. The test most affected is the secondary release of ADP, with consequent secondary platelet aggregation which normally follows primary aggregation by collagen for example; the secondary release and platelet aggregation do not occur when the patient has been taking aspirin. It is therefore very important to enquire about drugs and household remedies before carrying out these tests. Other drugs are now known to influence platelet aggregation, for example "Arvin", the viper venom fraction being used as an anticoagulant.

The study of platelet functions is now being applied to many cases of haemorrhagic diathesis, and already some families have been reported which show defects in one or other of the tests available. This research is so far at the stage of collection of information and it may be some time before the syndromes other than those mentioned here are properly defined. The practical effect of this work at present is to warn clinicians that patients who say they are "bleeders" should be taken seriously and properly investigated, particularly before any surgical procedure is undertaken, however minor.

Management of Haemopia Syndromes

The clinical management of classical haemophilia and Christmas disease has been much improved by the advent of new methods of concentrating the haemophilia factor, and by the use of drugs to assist the action of the factor concentrates. Better methods of estimating the effect of treatment have also contributed to this improvement. It is essential to remember that in the haemophilia syndromes the bleeding tendency is due to the inherited lack of clotting factors, Factor VIII—antihaemophilic globulin (AHG)—in classical haemophilia and Factor IX in Christmas disease, or haemophilia B. To obtain control of haemorrhage, the missing factors must first be replaced; the drugs, like ε-aminocaproic acid (EACA), prolong the action of the factor replacement but will not themselves cause any rise in the plasma content of Factors VIII or IX.

Methods of assay of Factor VIII are now relatively simple and well established. Most workers use a one-stage technique, and if the assay method is being regularly used the results are consistent and can be employed for monitoring the effect of treatment. Assay of Factor IX, Christmas factor, is not so easy and a more elaborate two-stage technique still has to be employed to give sufficient accuracy for the control of treatment. Nevertheless, the regular use of these assays is mostly confined to the major haemophilia centres in this country, though any properly equipped pathological laboratory in a district general hospital can carry out the diagnostic tests with reasonable consistency. In classical haemophilia most of the patients have less than 1 per cent of normal AHG plasma level; a minority of "mild" patients have between 1 and 10 per cent of normal. In order to control spontaneous haemorrhage and bleeding into joints, it is sufficient to raise the plasma AHG to between 5 and 10 per cent of normal; but if there has been serious trauma or if major surgery has to be undertaken, for example any form of laparotomy, it is necessary to raise the level to 50 per cent of normal during the operative and immediately post-operative period and to keep the level at about 30 per cent thereafter until the wound is firmly healed. The difficulty in maintaining such levels is caused by two factors. The first is that the half-life of AHG is only 12 to 14 hours and consequently the dose must be repeated frequently, and the second is the sheer volume of fluid required to produce therapeutic levels; Rizza and Biggs (1969) who have discussed this problem in detail have calculated that a dose of 1500 ml of plasma given to a 70 kg man might raise the AHG level from zero to 23 per cent, but the final figure depends so much on the patient's reactions to fluid dilution that assays are essential to determine the real effect in an individual patient. The provision of effective concentrates has gone a long way to overcome this difficulty; at present concentrates are mostly available for the treatment of classical haemophilia (haemophilia A) and these will be first discussed.

There are at present two concentrates of human AHG available. The older, based on a method devised by Kekwick and Wolf of London, is used in Government-supported blood-products laboratories in this country and provides a lyophilized powder suitable for solution which yields a concentration of five to ten times. The supply of this AHG concentrate is limited, and has to be kept for the treatment of children, the management of major surgery, and the treatment of patients with cardiac failure; it is very effective. The newer method employs the concentrate prepared by the cryoprecipitate technique; this technique is simple enough to be employed by any laboratory which owns a refrigerated centrifuge capable of taking a plastic bag containing 450–500 ml of blood; the final product remaining in a plastic bag is a precipitated material which is redissolved in 5–10 ml of plasma. The cryoprecipitate preparation gives a concentration of up to 15 times, but the degree depends on losses during preparation and variation in the amount of AHG in the plasma of individual donors. The two important advantages of the cryoprecipitate preparation are its relatively simple preparation and storage, and the fact that the small volume can be administered by a syringe, so that it is not necessary to set up an intravenous drip apparatus. For haemorrhages needing only small amounts of AHG, such as the common haemarthroses in children, it is now feasible to give the equivalent of 1 pint (550 ml) of plasma in a single 10-ml injection which contains the concentrate from two cryoprecipitate units. Such an injection can be given in the out-patient clinic in a few minutes. It is not surprising therefore that the demand for cryoprecipitate preparation, especially by children's clinics, has grown and in this country the Regional Blood Transfusion Laboratories are mostly prepared to supply the concentrate on demand. However, experience has engendered some caution; the collection and transfer bags needed for each unit preparation are relatively expensive and difficulties with sterility, due to defects, have not been entirely overcome. Real care and expenditure of time are needed in the preparation if losses of AHG potency are not to become serious and if a preparation sufficiently free of red cells and suitably free of suspended particles is to be obtained. Thus, in Manchester, cryoprecipitate is restricted to the treatment of children, for the occasional major surgical operation when large amounts can be required, and in circumstances when fluid volumes must be restricted. It is sometimes very useful to be able to send cryoprecipitate units to another hospital so that the patient can be made fit for transfer to the haemophilia centre. In all other cases the standard fresh-frozen plasma preparation in the standard glass bottle continues to be used.

Recently, even more concentrated preparations of antihaemophilic globulin have been reported. When Brinkhous (1968) and his colleagues in North Carolina used the cryoprecipitate material as a starting-point, a large amount equivalent to that from 200 to 500 bottles of blood was needed. It was treated with glycine and a preparation representing a final concentration of AHG of 100 to 400 times that in the original plasma was obtained in the form of a lyophilized powder. A somewhat similar preparation utilizing polyethylene glycol as the purifying agent has been made by Johnson and workers at the American Red Cross; Rizza and Biggs (1969) report results with this material to be better than either cryoprecipitate or human AHG powder. Neither of these very concentrated materials is yet available either commercially or through the government blood-products laboratories, but they are likely to be prepared soon. The expense and the necessity of collecting the large amounts of blood required are limiting factors, and it is notable that one of Brinkhous' patients given a particularly large dose developed homologous serum hepatitis five months later.

Much less progress has been made in the treatment of Christmas disease (haemophilia B). The cryoprecipitate preparations are not suitable for the treatment of Christmas disease. Preparation of a concentrate from pooled human plasma by a method similar to that used for making the AHG concentrate has been moderately successful; at the Oxford Haemophilia Centre, a Factor IX concentrate has been made, using as a starting-point a residue rejected during the fractionation of plasma for the preparation of the standard AHG concentrate. This Oxford concentrate contains between 6 and 15 times the amount of Factor IX as normal plasma; but there seem to be difficulties in obtaining a sufficiently uniform product and the concentrate is not yet available for general distribution. Hoag and co-workers (1969) in San Francisco have described the preparation of a somewhat similar concentrate; one of the difficulties they experienced was that the activity actually obtained in the patient's plasma was less than 50 per cent of the activity expected from the assay of the concentrate. Nevertheless, this American concentrate has actually been advertised for commercial distribution. In the face of these difficulties the treatment of Christmas disease remains limited to the use of fresh-frozen plasma and this is, of course, satisfactorily effective.

Animal concentrates of AHG can be used in grave emergencies and to help to maintain AHG levels for the long periods needed when major surgery has to be undertaken. Porcine and bovine concentrates are commercially available in this country. Rizza and Biggs recommend an initial dose of 60–80 units per kg as an initial dose, and subsequent doses depend on the assay in the patient's blood which must be done daily; the rise of AHG titre is usually notably less than would be expected from the dose given and the reasons for this are not understood, so the daily assay is essential, and animal AHG should not be used unless facilities for this assay are assured. Such preparations usually provoke allergic reactions within seven to ten days, and even if these reactions are not prominent the response to the animal AHG becomes rapidly less; so the effective time for using these preparations is five to six days. Once an animal preparation has been given, a second course inevitably carries serious risks; Rizza and Biggs have in fact given six haemophiliacs second doses without serious effects and with a good rise in Factor VIII assay, but they recommend that the risk should be limited to emergencies when life is endangered. Fortunately there seems to be no cross antigenicity between porcine and bovine AHG. The animal concentrates have the considerable advantage that they are much more potent than human concentrates, and only small amounts of material in correspondingly small volumes of fluid are needed to maintain a proper level of plasma AHG.

Epsilon-amino-caproic acid (EACA)

This substance is an antifibrinolytic agent and the idea of using it in haemophilia was the possibility of protecting the often fragile blood clots that form from the normal processes. Experience in practice has shown that EACA is indeed a useful adjuvant, and that when it is employed the amount of plasma and other blood products used can be reduced. In Manchester we have found it most useful in the management of dental extraction and in the out-patient treatment of haemarthroses. It has been claimed that dental extraction can be carried out without undue bleeding by giving EACA alone, however, our experience has been that serious bleeding sometimes still occurs. We carried out a trial comparing patients managed on plasma alone, on EACA alone, and on a third regime, a combination of the two. The combined treatment was to give 2–4 units of plasma, according to the patient's weight, a short time before the dental extraction and on the first day after the extraction, and to give EACA in the usual dose of 0·1 mg/kg four to six times daily from the day of extraction for five to seven days according to the bleeding. In our experience this combined treatment was the most effective in reducing bleeding to a minimum. For the treatment of haemarthroses we give 2 units of cryoprecipitate to a child or 2 units of plasma to an older patient in the clinic, and then supply EACA at the same standard dose for five days. A definite contraindication to the use of EACA in haemophilia is haematuria; renal colic and even temporary loss of function of a kidney have been reported and we have met with these incidents. Consequently, haematuria is managed without EACA treatment. The only troublesome complication has been the tendency to vomiting and anorexia in some patients; in a few patients treatment has had to be stopped. A variant of EACA, "Cyclokapron", is now being given trial and may not have this undesirable effect. These drugs are of course effective in both types of the haemophilia syndrome.

Various other drugs, including steroids and oral contraceptives, have been suggested from time to time as adjuvants in the treatment of haemophilia but none have proved worth adopting for regular use.

REFERENCES

HARDISTY, R. M. (1968). Platelet function. In *Recent Advances in Clinical Pathology*, Series 5. London: J & A. Churchill, Chap. 11.

HELLEM, A. J. & STORMORKEN, H. (1969). Platelet adhesion-aggregation reaction and its clinical significance. In *Recent Advances in Blood Coagulation*. London: J. & A. Churchill, Chap. 5.

O'BRIEN, J. R. (1968). Effects of salicylates on human platelets. *Lancet*, 1, 779.

Management of haemophilia syndromes

BRINKHOUS, K. M., SHANBROM, E., ROBERTS, H. R., WEBSTER, W. P., FEKETE, L. & WAGNER, R. H. (1968). A new high-potency glycine-precipitated anti-hemophilic factor (AHF) concentrate. *J. Amer. med. Ass.*, 205, 613.

HOAG, M. S., JOHNSON, F. F., ROBINSON, J. A. & AGGELER, P. M. (1969). Treatment of Haemophilia B with a new clotting-factor concentrate. *New Engl. J. Med.*, 280, 581.

RIZZA, C. R. & BIGGS, R. (1969). The use of plasma fractions in the treatment of haemophilia and von Willebrand's disease. In *Progress in Hematology*, vol. VI. London: Heinemann Medical Books, p. 181.

THE LEUKAEMIAS

Our views on the possible causes of leukaemia are changing, but without affecting our methods of management to any degree. Three groups of theories are current: that leukaemia is a malignant neoplasm of the white-cell forming tissues like other malignant neoplasms, that it is set off by a virus infection, and that it is one of the group of immuno-proliferative disorders. The chromosome abnormalities that have been detected in acute leukaemias are regarded as secondary, and there is good evidence that the so-called "Philadelphia" chromosome characteristic of chronic myeloid leukaemia appears with the development of the disease, and is not a primary cause. Exposure to ionizing radiation is acknowledged to be a cause of leukaemia in cases of definite risk, such as occurs in the X-ray treatment of spondylitis or the use of ^{32}P in polycythaemia; but radiation is not now regarded as a general cause of leukaemia.

Leukaemia as a malignant neoplasm of white-cell tissue

This theory has been popular ever since leukaemia was first described. Superficially, the tissue changes of leukaemia suggest a neoplasm: the infiltration of organs with leukaemic cells to the detriment of their proper function, seen particularly in the bone marrow, and the occurrence in the later stages of acute leukaemias of apparently increased mitoses in the marrow and even in the blood. These suggest the "purposeless proliferation" that is a characteristic feature of neoplasms. This theory has influenced treatment predominantly: we use radiotherapy and cytotoxic drugs to destroy the abnormal proliferating cells in the hope that they will be replaced by normal cells. But although the malignant theory has been adopted as a working guide to management, research work, especially in the past five years, has produced results which do not fit in.

In chronic myeloid leukaemia there are several observations that fit in with the malignant hypothesis. For instance it has been found that in patients who were not yet treated and had an initial white cell count of less than 200,000 p.c.mm, the rate of increase of leucocytes in the blood follows an exponential curve, and if the leucocyte-doubling time is calculated for a group of patients, a definite correlation emerges between this time and the survival of the patients; the quicker the leucocytes increase, the shorter is the period of survival. Again in relapse after a period of successful control, the leucocyte-doubling time was found to have shortened, and this fits in with the clinical observation that each relapse is followed by deterioration and worsening of the prognosis. However, when the technique of thymidine-labelling is applied to bone marrow in chronic myeloid leukaemia, the rate of labelling turns out to be lower than in normal marrow, which suggests that there is in fact a slowing rather than a quickening of actual cell division.

Surprisingly this slowing of cell division noted in chronic myeloid leukaemia has also been found to occur in acute leukaemia. Experiments in which the DNA in cells is labelled with tritiated thymidine have shown that the blast cells in the blood in acute leukaemia are mostly non-dividing cells. In marrow, the range of labelling in acute leukaemia varies from 0·4 to 10 per cent, whereas in normal marrow 35 per cent of myelocytes and 61 per cent of basophil normoblasts show positive labelling. Such low labelling suggests that the blast cells have actually a prolonged life-span and the evidence available shows that there is a mixture of proliferating and non-proliferating blasts in acute leukaemic marrow. Even slow proliferation of cells will lead, under these circumstances, to a large accumulation of cells in the blood and tissues, such as is in fact found in clinical acute leukaemia. A supporting observation is that the rate of DNA labelling increases before a remission appears, and this fits in with the idea that normal maturation involves more, not less, rapid blast proliferation than in leukaemia.

Careful observation has shown that in leukaemic marrow it is the large blast cells which take the DNA label, whereas the small cells are only occasionally labelled. Furthermore, the large blast cells show decreasing grain counts, since at mitotic division the labelling material is shared between daughter cells. But the relatively few labelled small blast cells show no such change, and the experimenters suggest that they are derived from previously labelled large cells which have changed into a non-dividing phase. Examination of the marrow from patients with acute leukaemia shows that as a rule about 70 per cent of the cells remain unlabelled, and this suspected change from large proliferating to small non-dividing blasts has been further investigated and confirmed. It appears that the large blasts become smaller after one or two divisions and then cease to divide; if the large cells have been labelled with thymidine the label persists in the small cells, and such labelled small blasts can appear in the patient's blood, but the majority of the blast cells in the peripheral blood in acute leukaemia are of the non-dividing type. The reverse change from small non-divider to large dividing cell has not so far been reported.

The present view of acute leukaemia is therefore quite different from the classical idea of the replacement of normal marrow cells by a malignantly proliferating mass of blasts which overflow into the blood, and that the severe relapse stages occur when this proliferation becomes completely unrestrained in the manner of a spreading sarcoma. Instead we have the picture of a limited blast-cell proliferating population producing cells which fail to mature, become smaller and atypical in appearance and probably lose their capacity to divide; these non-dividing cells are preferentially released into the blood and accumulate in the tissues. Our present methods of treatment tend to kill off the mainly non-dividing cells and leave the stem-cells intact, so that relapse is almost bound to occur.

If, therefore, we are to continue to regard leukaemia as a variety of malignant disease, we have to qualify the statement by pointing out that it is very different from the accepted type of actively invasive and proliferative malignancy.

Leukaemia as a Virus Disease

The virus theory has always been attractive because it is well established that some fowl leukaemias are caused by a filtrable agent and leukaemia can be transmitted in mice from mother to foetus. Modern techniques of virus investigation have produced much new information about viruses in human leukaemia and two findings in particular are relevant. One is the demonstration of virus particles in the cells and blood of patients with acute leukaemias, and the second is the description of Burkitt's lymphoma, its apparent spread by an infective agent, and the discovery that several viruses occur in association with this tissue. Unfortunately, it now seems clear that these viruses are not aetiological agents and are probably no more than "passengers". Nevertheless, the search for a possible virus cause for leukaemia continues, because if this should be proved, effective prophylaxis and treatment would become possible. The virologists, however, agree that a different approach to the problem is needed. Bryan (1968) points out that the viruses of fowl and mouse leukaemia are RNA viruses which differ considerably in their properties from the viruses responsible for recognized infections, most of which are DNA viruses; the virus that induces warts in human patients is also a DNA virus. RNA viruses do not kill the infected cells, but stimulate growth and proliferation; in certain target cells they are known to cause temporary malignant transformation—temporary because after a number of divisions normal cells again appear under the conditions of tissue culture. The techniques used for detecting and assaying DNA viruses often fail when applied to RNA viruses. Bryan points out a particular difficulty caused by the fact that the amount of virus that can be recovered from infected tissue depends on the initiating dose of virus, whereas with most other types of virus the amount of virus increases as the infection progresses. Consequently, techniques for the detection of RNA viruses have to be able to respond to very small amounts; he concludes that new and more sensitive methods than we have at present will have to be developed if we are to be able to detect viruses that may cause leukaemia.

The present position is, therefore, that no practical measures designed to deal with virus infections can be adopted as yet in the management of leukaemias, but new methods may alter the picture in the future.

Leukaemia as an "Immuno-proliferative" Disorder

Dameshek is responsible for the idea of a group of disorders of abnormalities of growth, usually of a generalized character, involving cells of the immunocyte complex and associated with abnormalities of the immune mechanism. Lymphocyte, plasma cell and reticulum cell varieties of this group have been described, and chronic lymphatic leukaemia fits well into this group. Studies of mitotic cycles, and of RNA and DNA changes in lymphatic leukaemia have shown that, as in acute leukaemia, cell division is slower than normal; at the same time the life-span of the cells appears to be increased. Consequently there is good evidence for regarding chronic lymphatic leukaemia as an accumulative disease rather than as a proliferative disease; the infiltration of lymphocytes we find in so many organs may thus be due to an accumulation of cells which no longer go through the usual cycle. Abnormalities of immune reaction have indeed been demonstrated in the lymphocytes of chronic lymphatic leukaemia; they will not respond to antigens such as phytohaemagglutinin or other antigens to which the individual is known to be sensitive. Normal lymphocytes on the other hand, show the characteristic transformation to the so-called "PHA-blast" cells. Abnormalities of serum proteins affecting the immunoglobulins are known to occur in a proportion of patients.

Clinicians have long looked upon lymphatic leukaemia as different in prognosis from other leukaemias, and have recognized for some time that there is a group of patients who run a higher lymphocyte count than usual but that it remains constant for years in particular patients, and that there is no point in attempting to reduce it with treatment. In chronic lymphatic leukaemia too we are especially likely to meet the complication of an auto-immune haemolytic anaemia. It has also been suggested that the anaemia of chronic lymphatic leukaemia is due to inability of the erythroblasts to respond to the stimulus of anaemia in the same way as the lymphocytes in this disease fail to respond to normal stimuli, and in support of this there is the action of steroids in stimulating red-cell production.

There is thus a good case for classing chronic lymphatic leukaemia as an "immuno-proliferative disorder"; but there is little supporting evidence for including other leukaemias, including chronic myeloid leukaemia, in this group.

Diagnosis of Leukaemia

Nowadays, when it is standard practice to include bone marrow studies among the investigations of any patient with anaemia that is not quite straightforward, the diagnosis of leukaemia is rarely missed. The erythro-leukaemias sometimes present problems because the abnormal erythro-blasts resemble megaloblasts quite closely, and in the earlier stages of the disease may be more numerous than myeloblasts; this leads to a diagnosis of anaemia resistant to vitamin B_{12} or folic-acid therapy. The detection of erythroblasts with two or more nuclei of differing stages of development in the same cell is a useful pointer in favour of the leukaemic diagnosis.

In the past, considerable emphasis has been put on determining the type of acute leukaemia that is present; Hayhoe's monograph (1964) shows how far this can be done with the aid of current histochemical stains. The importance to the clinician is in the relation of leukaemic type to prognosis and management. Experience with modern therapy has shown that it is very important to distinguish the lymphatic leukaemias from the rest, since they are much more responsive to treatment and consequently have a considerably better prognosis, particularly in children.

Management of Leukaemia

Drug treatment is the accepted method at present. X-ray treatment is occasionally used in special circumstances—in chronic leukaemia, for example, to reduce a resistant mass of peripheral lymph glands in chronic lymphatic leukaemia. The drugs used are of three types: steroids, antinucleic acid substances like 6-mercaptopurine, and the truly cytotoxic drugs like mustine and its relations, busulphan and cyclophosphamide. The recent studies on the nature of the changes of cell kinetics in leukaemia, referred to at the beginning of this section, have shown that the destructive drugs act especially on the non-dividing or slowly-dividing cells, while leaving the potentially proliferative blast cells still able to go on producing cells that are liable to fail to mature and accumulate in the tissues. Practical experience has shown that these destructive drugs produce some valuable, if temporary, relief of symptoms, but we realize that by themselves they will not produce a remission of the leukaemia. The characteristic features of a true remission are that the normal cycle of cell maturation is resumed and that the normal distribution of cells between marrow and blood is restored. There is now firm evidence that steroids can induce this sort of remission, and there is suggestive evidence that mercaptopurine can do this and may not be a purely destructive type of drug; unfortunately, we have no idea as to how these drugs produce this effect. The clinical evidence from large series of cases like that collected by the Medical Research Council and the series seen at Manchester have shown quite clearly that steroids alone give just as good average results as other drugs and that without steroids, remission is unlikely. Remission is never impossible, because spontaneous remission in acute leukaemia is well known, though rare and temporary. At present, stimulated by American results, trials are being given to combinations of steroids, mercaptopurine and destructive drugs, and results with several such combinations have already been published. So far the results have not been spectacular, except in the acute lymphatic leukaemias of young children that are known to be particularly sensitive to treatment and in which almost any treatment will induce an initial remission in 80 per cent of patients; what these combined treatments aim at is prolonged remission and reduction of relapse, and it will clearly be some time before this sort of result can be properly assessed.

These schemes of combined treatment involve a great deal of trouble for the physician and considerable endurance for the patient. The Medical Research Council has initiated a trial of such a scheme with the assistance of haematologists all over the country. The scheme is aimed particularly at the acute lymphoblastic leukaemia of childhood, but adults and patients with myeloblastic leukaemia are also to be given a trial with the same plan. This scheme involves an initial period of 21 weeks chemotherapy; prednisone, vincristine given intravenously, and 6-mercaptopurine are given in defined combination for the first 15 weeks. This is followed by a course of six weeks' treatment with oral methotrexate and folinic acid, intravenous or intramuscular asparaginase and five doses of intrathecal methotrexate is given. This chemotherapy schedule is not continued if the patient fails to show remission by the sixth week. If all goes well, a trial of immunotherapy with BCG will be undertaken. The patient will, of course, have regular blood counts throughout the period and four marrow punctures during the chemotherapy phase, followed by a marrow puncture every eight weeks. Clinical experience with acute leukaemia suggests that only a minority of patients will fit in with the requirements of the full trial; patients taken off the trial will continue to be treated by more standard methods. It is clear that such an elaborate and taxing schedule will only be worth while if as a result a notable prolongation of life is obtained; so far such schemes have only succeeded in prolonging life by average periods measured in weeks.

There is some reason for taking the view that since none of our present drugs, alone or in combination, or methods involving bone-marrow destruction and replacement by transplants, have succeeded in eliminating the proliferating blast cells that seem to be the primary pathological abnormality in leukaemia, treatment is hardly worth while at all. But every clinic of any size numbers among its patients those who have shown really long remissions of many years, during which normal life and activity has been possible. Burchenal (1968) has lately gathered from world literature accounts of 159 patients who were still living five or more years after diagnosis. It is interesting to note that among 108 patients for whom full details of treatment are available, the largest single group was the 41 treated with steroids and mercaptopurine. It is this sort of record that makes it essential to offer at least one course of treatment to every patient with acute leukaemia who survives the first week after diagnosis. In acute leukaemia the treatment should be prednisolone 75 mg daily for adults and 50 mg daily for children combined with 6-mercaptopurine 150 mg daily (70 mg/sq. metre) for adults and corresponding dose for children; this combination should be given a trial of four to six weeks. If remission appears, the prednisolone can be reduced to 15 mg daily and finally stopped altogether; mercaptopurine can be reduced to 50 mg daily. There is some doubt about the necessity for continued drug treatment during a remission, but most physicians prefer to continue with a small dose of both drugs.

When a relapse occurs, steroids should be given again, but it is worth while giving a trial of vincristine therapy. Vincristine, one of the periwinkle alkaloids, is given intravenously at weekly intervals in a dose of 1·5 mg/M^2 for the first three weeks, reducing to 1·0 mg for a further three weeks. Vincristine is liable to produce peripheral nerve involvement, and then the dose must be reduced.

Blood transfusions are certain to be needed as supporting treatment, and occasionally folic acid deficiency appears and must be treated with oral folic acid, 5 mg daily.

Many new drugs have appeared and are still under trial, for example asparaginase, daunomycin and adriamycin. These are more toxic than present drugs, or have very limited activity and have not so far been regularly adopted.

In chronic leukaemias, busulphan remains the drug of choice for chronic myeloid leukaemia. But some odd side-effects which produce a syndrome resembling clinical Addison's adrenal insufficiency have appeared in some patients who have been on treatment for a period of years. The biochemical changes are not present, but the pigmentation and anorexia respond to a change of treatment to steroids sometimes combined with an oral mustard-type drug such as uromustine. The curious lung fibrosis reported in some patients taking busulphan is rare. In chronic lymphatic leukaemia it is important not to give treatment to the group who have a leukaemic blood picture, often found in the course of other investigations, but no clinical signs; it may be several years before signs like enlarged lymph glands appear. If clinical signs are present, the mustard group is best, beginning with chorambucil, but if there are prominent lymph-gland masses, expecially in the mediastinum, it is best to begin with the combination of steroids and intravenous mustine. Sooner or later these patients become anaemic, and then it is worth while to include steroids in a moderate dose of prednisolone 15–20 mg daily in the treatment.

REFERENCES

BRYAN, W. R. (1968). The viral study of leukemia and related neoplastic diseases: a problem apart. In *Perspectives in Leukemia*. New York: Grune and Stratton, p. 94.

BURCHENAL, J. H. (1968). Long-term survivors in acute leukemia. In *Proc. Internat. Conf. on Leukemia-Lymphoma*. ed. C. J. D. Zarafonetis. Philadelphia: Lea and Febiger, p. 469.

CRONKITE, E. P. (1968). Kinetics of leukemia cell proliferation. In *Perspectives in Leukemia*. New York: Grune and Stratton, p. 158.

HAYHOE, F. G. J., QUAGLINO, D. & DOLL, R. (1964). The cytology and cyto-chemistry of acute leukaemias. *Med. Res. Council Special Report Series no. 304.* London: H. M. Stationery Office.

ISRAËLS, M. C. G. (1968). Management of acute leukaemia. *Abstr. Wld. Med.,* **42,** 173.

6 Endocrine Disorders

R. I. S. BAYLISS

PATHOGENESIS OF GRAVES' DISEASE. PROPRANOLOL IN
THE TREATMENT OF GRAVES' DISEASE. ENDOCRINOPATHIES
ASSOCIATED WITH NON-ENDOCRINE TUMOURS

PATHOGENESIS OF GRAVES' DISEASE

UNDERSTANDING, admittedly still incomplete, of the mechanism by which
hypothyroidism develops in a patient with Hashimoto's thyroiditis has
opened a new vista in general medicine and in particular, endocrinology.
Here is a disease model in which the effects of autoantibodies can be followed
seriatim by study of the blood, by drill biopsies of the gland, and by repeated
assessment with radio-active iodine of the rate of thyroid hormone synthesis.
The resulting salient features of the goitre, a rising titre of antibodies to
thyroglobulin and thyroid cell microsomes, and lymphocytic and plasma
cell infiltration with eventual fibrosis and destruction of the gland, have given
to the clinician a clear concept of what may happen in an autoimmune
disease. Other organ-specific diseases, some proven and others still speculative, have been attributed to the development of autoantibodies. It has now
been shown that idiopathic Addison's disease of the adrenal glands, associated
in some instances with amenorrhoea, is linked with anti-adrenocortical
antibodies (Goudie *et al.*, 1966; Irvine *et al.*, 1967), and in patients with
amenorrhoea to the presence of antibodies against ovarian tissue (Irvine
et al., 1968).

It now seems likely that another disorder of the thyroid gland, Graves'
disease, may pave the way to a somewhat more surprising concept in autoimmune diseases. Hitherto, such processes have been equated with organ-
specific destruction, but there is increasing evidence that an autoantibody is
an important and probably the immediate cause of hyperthyroidism in
Graves' disease. If this proves to be the case, we shall be faced with what
at first sight may appear improbable and unexpected—an antibody stimulating rather than destroying a specific organ.

Role of Thyrotrophin in Graves' disease

The symptoms of Graves' disease were not ascribed to overactivity of the thyroid gland until the beginning of this century. The first rational explanation for the thyroid overactivity was advanced in the early 1930s when it was appreciated that the gland was under the control of a trophic hormone secreted by the anterior hypophysis. It was natural to suppose that Graves' disease was the consequence of increased secretion of thyroid stimulating hormone (TSH) by the pituitary gland. Was there not already good circumstantial evidence from the work of Harvey Cushing that adrenocortical hyperplasia and oversecretion resulted from increased pituitary production of adrenocorticotrophin? This analogy with Cushing's syndrome has proved incorrect, and has taken a long time to disprove because of the methodological difficulties in measuring the minute amounts TSH present in human plasma. Until recently, the bioassay procedures were demanding and imprecise. Failure to find increased amounts of plasma TSH in patients with Graves' disease was at first discounted as being due to the technical difficulties of the assay despite the fact that the same methods successfully showed high levels in patients with myxoedema due to primary thyroidal failure. More recently sensitive and specific radio-immune assay procedures have been developed for measuring TSH. Not only have these failed to show an increase in plasma TSH in Graves' disease, but they have gone further to emphasize that the plasma TSH level is actually reduced, indicating the depressed secretion of this trophic hormone by the pituitary (Lemarchand-Béraud et al., 1967; Odell et al., 1967). Of particular interest is the study by Adams and Kennedy (1965) of a hyperthyroid woman who before treatment had no detectable TSH (but a high LATS titre—vide infra) in her plasma; after she had been made myxoedematous with radio-iodine, the serum contained both TSH and LATS, but the TSH level fell when she was treated with thyroxine (T-4).

Response to thyroxine or tri-iodothyronine

More circumstantial evidence serves to exonerate excess TSH secretion as the cause of thyroid overactivity in Graves' disease. In Cushing's syndrome caused by excessive secretion of ACTH from the adenohypophysis adrenocortical function can be reduced substantially by administration of dexamethasone which depresses the output of corticotrophin from the pituitary, probably by inhibiting the release of corticotrophin release factor (CRF) from the hypothalamus. In Graves' disease no comparable suppression of thyroid hyperfunction can be induced by administration of thyroxine or of tri-iodothyronine (T-3). This observation, confirmed by many workers, strongly suggests that the thyroid gland is being stimulated by some substance other than TSH of pituitary origin.

Indeed this failure of T-4 or T-3 to depress thyroidal function, as measured by the uptake of radio-iodine, has proved a most useful confirmatory test in the diagnosis of hyperthyroidism, particularly when other findings and laboratory investigations are equivocal (Bayliss, 1967a and b). This non-suppressibility of radio-active iodine uptake in patients with Graves' disease is a characteristic feature, and is present in many, but not all, patients who exhibit unilateral exophthalmos before there is clinical or laboratory evidence of hyperthyroidism.

Findings in the pituitary

In patients with Cushing's syndrome associated with bilateral adrenal hyperplasia induced by excess ACTH production from a pituitary adenoma or ectopic source such as a bronchial carcinoma, characteristic hyalinization is found in the basophil cells of the adenohypophysis. Such histological changes are also found in patients given large doses of corticosteroids, and are now recognized as representing a resting phase in pituitary ACTH secretory activity. Similarly, in patients dying of a thyrotoxic crisis, the histological appearances of the pituitary are not those of hypersecretion but rather of a gland in a resting phase as a consequence of exposure to high circulating levels of T-4 (Radacot et al., 1965). Further evidence exonerating pituitary overactivity as the cause of Graves' disease are those rare instances in which hyperthyroidism has occurred in patients with well-documented panhypopituitarism (Fajans, 1968; Werner and Stewart, 1958; McKenzie, 1968), or has developed after hypophysectomy (Christensen and Binder, 1962; Wayne et al., 1964; Burke, 1967).

The Long-acting Thyroid Stimulator

That thyroid hyperfunction in Graves' disease might be induced by some substance other than TSH was first suggested by Adams and Purvis (1956, 1958) as an outcome of their endeavours to develop a new technique for bioassay of TSH. So much depends upon this method that some familiarity with the technique is important to the critical appreciation of the subsequent developments and ideas. In essence the procedure, as modified in certain important respects by McKenzie and Williamson (1966), is carried out in the mouse pre-treated with T-4 to suppress endogenous secretion of TSH. Radio-active ^{131}I is given intraperitoneally to label the iodine-containing compounds in the animal's gland. After injection of the serum under test (or the biologically calibrated standard), the increase of radio-iodine in serial blood samples is taken as a measure of the stimulus given to the thyroid gland (Munro et al., 1967). This technique suffers all the hazards and variables inherent in a bioassay procedure. Specificity cannot be guaranteed, nor is the response sensitive. Despite these limitations and differences between individuals in expressing their results, two different types of response are apparent. Serum from patients with myxoedema due to primary thyroid failure, which would be expected to have high TSH levels, and serum from euthyroid patients to which TSH has been added, induce a peak rise in plasma radio-activity two hours after injection, indicating the maximum release of ^{131}I-labelled compounds from the animal's gland at this time. In contrast, the sera from patients with Graves' disease usually if not always produce a response that differs significantly in its time relationship: the highest peak of plasma radio-activity does not occur until nine hours after the injection—hence the term *long-acting thyroid stimulator* (LATS). The basis of the distinction between LATS and TSH depends on this time-relationship, often not as clearly demarcated as one might wish. For example, with small doses of TSH and LATS there may be no statistical difference in the time at which the peak plasma radio-activity occurs, and the distinction is much clearer when large doses are used or the unknown serum contains high titres of TSH or LATS. The bioassay evidence that two distinct substances can stimulate the thyroid gland is further strengthened by demonstrating that antiserum to TSH will neutralize the TSH-type time response but not the delayed effect of LATS, whereas conversely anti-human IgG antiserum will nullify the more prolonged or delayed response so characteristic of LATS, but not the earlier response invoked by TSH (Dorrington and Munro, 1965). Much research has ensued to establish the differentiation between these two substances in terms of their chemical constitution and biological site of origin.

Nature of LATS. Not surprisingly, it has been proposed that LATS is a modified form of TSH consisting of the thyrotrophic hormone bound to a carrier protein which delays the onset of its biologically stimulating action (Major and Munro, 1962). That this is not the case depends on several pieces of evidence. Graves' disease has been observed in patients with Sheehan's syndrome who would not be expected to produce any TSH that could be bound to a carrier protein (Fajans, 1958; Irvine *et al.*, 1969). Furthermore, as was mentioned above, anti-TSH serum does not inhibit the activity of LATS in the mouse bioassay method, whereas anti-human IgG antiserum does inhibit the activity of LATS. Chemico-physical techniques indicate that LATS is a 7S gammaglobulin with all the characteristics of an IgG antibody irregularly distributed between the euglobulins and pseudoglobulins (Munro, 1967). It can be separated physically and enzymatically from TSH found in the 4S fraction. Some workers claim that LATS is a true immunoglobulin, and others that it is TSH bound to an IgG antibody (Meek *et al.*, 1964), but this view is difficult to sustain when Graves' disease can occur in a hypophysectomized patient. Munro *et al.* (1967) has found that enzymatic proteolysis of LATS yields small active fragments which induce a short-acting response similar to TSH in the mouse bioassay procedure. However, this shorter time-course of action and the diminished potency may be due to the abbreviated half-life of the protein in the circulation of the mouse.

Other enzymatic chromatographic and fractionation procedures suggest that LATS and TSH are distinct entities (Burke, 1968a), but the evidence cannot be accepted yet without some lingering reserve, because the ultimate distinction of the two substances depends on the imprecise bioassay technique in mice.

Site of origin of LATS

Further evidence that LATS and TSH are separate entities comes from studies to determine the site of origin of LATS. The long-acting stimulator has not been detected in extracts of the pituitary gland when even before hypophysectomy it was present in the patient's serum (McKenzie, 1962). The LATS levels in samples of jugular and mixed venous blood taken simultaneously are not significantly different (Major and Munro, 1962). LATS may also persist in the serum of patients with persisting Graves' disease who have undergone hypophysectomy (Becker and Furth, 1965; Burke, 1967). Thus it seems clear that LATS does not originate in the pituitary gland.

If LATS is an IgG antibody, one would expect its origin to lie in the lymphocytes and an antigen to be found to stimulate its production. Some progress has been made in both facets of the problem, particularly the first. McKenzie (1965) whose results have been confirmed by Miyai et al. (1967), has shown that LATS, or a substance very similar in its biological properties, is produced in vitro by the incubation of lymphocytes from patients with Graves' disease, and that the yield was enhanced by non-specific stimulation of the lymphocytes to produce antibodies by the addition of phytohaem-agglutinin. This effect, found in the lymphocytes of three out of five patients with Graves' disease who had high serum LATS titres, was not present in normal subjects.

Identification of the complementary antigen to LATS-IgG antibody is still uncertain even in terms of its very existence, but some evidence may be interpreted to suggest that it has its origin in the thyroid gland. Thus, after total ablation of the gland by surgery or radio-iodine in patients with Graves' disease the titre of thyroid antibodies, as measured by the agglutination of tanned red cells or the complement-fixation test, diminishes and in parallel there may be a reduction in the titre of LATS. It is possible that the microsomal fraction of the thyroid gland may have the required antigenic properties, because of all the fractions tested this is the most potent in inactivating the biological activity of LATS when various fractions from the human thyroid gland are incubated with LATS-containing serum and the supernatant subsequently assayed for long-acting stimulator activity (Beall and Solomon, 1966). However, in an attempt to induce a raised LATS titre in rabbits, whole human thyroid extract proved more potent than the microsomal fraction (Solomon and Beall, 1967).

Biological action of LATS

In mice LATS is a potent stimulator of thyroid activity as judged by several parameters. The uptake of radio-iodine by the gland is increased and the plasma levels of protein-bound ^{131}I, thyroxine and tri-iodothyronine are all raised. Histological support of increased glandular activity is reflected in a heightening of the acinar cells. These changes are found in hypophysec-tomized as well as intact animals; therefore, stimulation by LATS of the anterior hypophysis to enhance its secretion of TSH can be discounted.

Less direct experimental evidence of the biological effects of LATS in man is available because of the possible dangers attending the infusion of proteins or plasma extracts into normal controls. Serum known to have a high LATS titre by the mouse-bioassay method has, however, been infused into human volunteers: compared with the response obtained with serum from a myxoedematous subject which would contain a high TSH level, it produced a thyroid-stimulating response which had the characteristics expected of a long-acting thyroid stimulator (Arnaud et al., 1965).

The duration of the biological action of LATS can be assessed only from circumstantial evidence, but in the case of neonatal thyrotoxicosis there is a suggestion that the biological half-life is much longer than that of TSH. Neonatal hyperthyroidism may occur in infants born of thyrotoxic mothers, or of mothers formerly thyrotoxic but made euthyroid by thyroidectomy. The clinical syndrome of hyperthyroidism in the infant may last for up to two months, and the serum of both mother and infant have high LATS titres (McKenzie, 1964). One cannot be sure, however, that the high LATS titre in the infant is due to placental transfer of LATS from the mother. It is possible that the presumed antigen which promoted the high LATS levels in the mother has also the same effect in the infant, and that after birth the LATS level and the clinical features of hyperthyroidism in the infant gradually disappear due to the disappearance of the maternal antigen.

The fact that both TSH and LATS stimulate thyroid activity suggests that they may have certain chemical sequences in common and that they stimulate the same locus in the thyroid cells to promote the formation and secretion of thyroid hormones. Current cellular chemistry suggests that both may activate the adenyl-cyclase-cyclic-AMP enzyme system located in the membrane which separates the thyroidal cells from the plasma (McKenzie, 1968). This hypothesis is supported by in vivo studies showing that TSH given before LATS reduces the stimulating effect of the latter, whereas LATS given before TSH completely prevents any subsequent response to thyrotrophin (Burke, 1968b).

The fact less easy to comprehend is that an antibody, which LATS appears to be, can play a stimulatory role when because of the findings in Hashi-moto's thyroiditis most clinicians have come to look upon antibodies as destructive substances which suppress thyroidal activity. That an antibody can stimulate a biochemical process is at first sight surprising, but reflection on other antigen-antibody reactions may dispel this conventional view. The rejection of a renal transplant may be regarded as destructive—a negation—of the donor's kidney, but also as a very positive action, albeit a clinically unhelpful one, on the part of the recipient.

Clinical associations of LATS

If Graves' disease were the consequence of an increased LATS serum level, one might anticipate an increased titre in every patient with primary hyperthyroidism. The overall positive results from a number of different laboratories have ranged from as few as 6 per cent of cases to as many as 90 per cent. This variability is doubtless due to the imprecision of the bio-assay method. Using more up-to-date techniques, about 60 per cent of patients with Graves' disease have detectable LATS levels, and in 85 per cent positive results can be obtained by chemical concentration of the serum which may convert a negative to a positive response (Carneiro et al., 1966a). Furthermore, there is a positive correlation between the LATS level and the rate of radio-iodine turnover per unit weight of gland, which suggests that LATS is directly responsible for the increased thyroidal activity in these patients (Carneiro et al., 1966b). As would be expected, no increase in LATS or TSH titres has been found in hyperthyroidism induced by an autonomous toxic nodule.

Further indirect evidence to implicate LATS in the pathogenesis of Graves' disease is the relationship of the LATS titre to the clinical course of the disease in response to medical treatment. Patients with a high titre tend to relapse when antithyroid medication is stopped, and a permanent spontaneous remission may coincide with disappearance of the long-acting stimulator from the serum (McKenzie, 1961; McKenzie and Solomon, 1967). High LATS titres may persist in formerly hyperthyroid patients who have been rendered euthyroid with radio-iodine. The persistence of subclinical Graves' disease in these patients is evident from the failure of thyroxine to suppress thyroidal activity. Here McKenzie (1968) offers the logical and acceptable explanation that sufficient thyroid tissue remains to sustain euthyroidism but there is too little to be capable of further response to stimulation by the high LATS titre.

Relationship of LATS to non-hyperthyroid manifestations of Graves' disease

If the association between LATS and hyperthyroidism in Graves' disease is strong, the other features of the syndrome comprising the eye-signs and pre-tibial myxoedema are more dubiously attributable to the action of the long-acting stimulator. In general, there is a good correlation between the

H

presence of pre-tibial myxoedema and raised levels of LATS (Kriss *et al.*, 1964; Pimstone *et al.*, 1965; Der Kinderen, 1967), but conversely high LATS titres may be present without any skin change.

The data relating the LATS titre to the eye changes is conflicting. In some instances, high LATS levels have been associated with eye changes in 45 to 88 per cent of patients. Such an association may be fortuitous, because in 65 patients McKenzie and McCullagh (1968) found no correlation between the LATS titre and the degree of exophthalmopathy. Similarly high or very high LATS titres have been observed in some patients with active exophthalmos, though not in others with equally advanced eye changes (Der Kinderen, 1967). This Dutch worker suggests that both LATS and the proposed exophthalmos-producing-substance (EPS) are required before the eye-signs develop. By using a bioassay method, he has found the EPS level to be higher in those patients showing the most severe degree of exophthalmos and lower in those showing only minor changes. The origins and measurement of EPS are even more uncertain than those of LATS, and EPS has been found in the serum of patients with Graves' disease who showed no exophthalmos. The apparent relief of proptosis in one eye by hypophysectomy has been followed by the development of exophthalmos in the other, which suggests that the pituitary gland is not the site of formation of the exophthalmos-producing substance (Furth *et al.*, 1962).

Aetiology of Graves' Disease

If the hyperthyroidism of Graves' disease is due to the long-acting stimulator, the problem still unsolved is the nature of the primary aetiological factor. Does LATS arise because an antigen is liberated from the thyroid gland and hence the primary disorder is in the gland, or is LATS produced because of some primary dysfunction of the autoimmune system? It was originally suggested that in Hashimoto's thyroiditis the primary disturbance was the liberation of a thyroid antigen, presumed to be thyroglobulin because of the high titre of thyroglobulin antibodies found in the patients' serum. There is evidence, however, that thyroglobulin is constantly being released into the lymphatics draining the gland, and this suggests that the primary disorder is over-reactivity of the autoimmune system, which responds by the production of an abnormally high antibody titre. Genetic factors certainly play an important role in auto-immune diseases, and the evidence suggests that the hereditary disorder is more the consequence of an abnormal antibody response than the production of an enhanced antigenic stimulus. Graves' disease has a strong genetic component, the condition often occurring in several members of a family. Thus the formation of LATS may represent a primary disorder of the antibody-forming tissues. It is possible that those patients with Graves' disease who go into remission and remain euthyroid after treatment with antithyroid drugs for 18 to 24 months have only a transient disturbance of their autoimmune system, whereas in those with a high LATS titre, who repeatedly relapse when antithyroid drugs are stopped, the disturbance of antibody formation is permanent.

REFERENCES

ADAMS, D. D. (1958). The presence of an abnormal thyroid-stimulating hormone in the serum of some thyrotoxic patients. *J. clin. Endocr.*, **18**, 699.

ADAMS, D. D. & KENNEDY, T. H. (1965). Evidence of a normally functioning pituitary T.S.H. secretion mechanism in a patient with a high blood level of long-acting thyroid stimulator. *J. clin. Endocr.*, **25**, 571.

ADAMS, D. D. & PURVES, H. D. (1956). Abnormal responses in the assay of thyrotrophin. *Proc. Univ. Otago med. Sch.*, **34**, 11.

ARNAUD, C. D., KNEUBUALER, H. A., SEILING, V. L., WIGHTMAN, B. K. & ENGBRING, N. H. (1965). Responses of the normal human to infusions of plasma from patients with Graves' disease. *J. clin. Invest.*, **44**, 1287.

BAYLISS, R. I. S. (1967a). Stimulation and suppression tests of thyroid function. *Proc. roy. Soc. Med.*, **60**, 303.

BAYLISS, R. I. S. (1967b). Stimulation and suppression tests of thyroid function. In *Symposium on the thyroid gland. J. clin. Path.*, **20**, 360.

BEALL, G. N. & SOLOMON, D. H. (1966). Inhibition of long-acting thyroid stimulator by thyroid particulate fractions. *J. clin Invest.*, **45**, 552.

BECKER, D. V. & FURTH, E. D. (1965). Total surgical hypophysectomy in nine patients with Graves' disease: evidence for the extra-pituitary maintenance of this disorder. In *Current Topics in Thyroid Research. Proc. Int. Thyroid Conf., fifth, Rome.* ed. C. Cassano and M. Andreoli. New York: Academic Press, p. 596.

BURKE, G. (1967). Hyperthyroidism and demonstration of circulating long-acting thyroid stimulator following hypophysectomy for chromophobe adenoma. *J. clin. Endocr.*, **27**, 1161.

BURKE, G. (1968a). The long-acting thyroid stimulator of Graves' disease. *Amer. J. Med.*, **45**, 435.

BURKE, G. (1968b). On the competitive interaction of long-acting thyroid stimulator and thyrotropin *in vivo*. *J. clin. Endocr.*, **28**, 286.

CARNEIRO, L., DORRINGTON, K. J. & MUNRO, D. S. (1966a). Recovery of the long-acting thyroid stimulator from serum of patients with thyrotoxicosis by concentration of immunoglobulin G. *Clin. Sci.*, **31**, 215.

CARNEIRO, L., DORRINGTON, K. J. & MUNRO, D. S. (1966b). Relation between long-acting thyroid stimulator and thyroid function in thyrotoxicosis. *Lancet*, **2**, 878.

CHRISTENSEN, L. K. & BINDER, V. (1962). A case of hyperthyroidism developed in spite of previous hypophysectomy. *Acta med. Scand.*, **172**, 285.

DER KINDEREN, P. J. (1967). EPS, LATS and Exophthalmos. In *Thyrotoxicosis.* ed. W. J. Irvine. Edinburgh: Livingstone.

DORRINGTON, K. J. & MUNRO, D. S. (1965). Immunological studies on the long-acting thyroid stimulator. *Clin. Sci.*, **28**, 165.

FAJANS, S. S. (1958). Hyperthyroidism in a patient with postpartum necrosis of the pituitary. *J. clin. Endocr.*, **18**, 271.

FURTH, E. D., BECKER, D. V., RAY, B. S. & KANE, J. W. (1962). Appearance of unilateral exophthalmos of Graves' disease after the successful treatment of the same process in surgical hypophysectomy. *J. clin. Endocr.*, **22**, 518.

GOUDIE, R. B., ANDERSON, J. R., GRAY, K. K. & WHYTE, W. G. (1966). Auto-antibodies in Addison's disease. *Lancet*, **1**, 1173.

IRVINE, W. J., CHAN, M. M. W., SCARTH, L., COLB, F. O., BAYLISS, R. I. S. & DRURY, W. I. (1968). Immunological aspects of premature ovarian failure associated with idiopathic Addison's disease. *Lancet*, **2**, 883.

IRVINE, W. J., CULLEN, D. R., KIRKHAM, K. I. & EZRIN, C. (1969). Sheehan's syndrome associated with thyrotoxicosis and diabetes mellitus. *Proc. roy. Soc. Med.*, **62**, 40.

IRVINE, W. J., STEWART, A. G. & SCARTH, L. (1967). A clinical and immunological study of adrenocortical insufficiency (Addison's disease). *Clin. exp. Immunol.*, **2**, 31.

KRISS, J. P., PLESHAKOV, V. & CHIEN, J. R. (1964). Isolation and identification of long-acting thyroid stimulator and its relation to hyperthyroidism and circumscribed pretibial myxoedema. *J. clin. Endocr.*, **24**, 1005.

LEMARCHAND-BÉRAUD, T., VANOTTI, A. & SCAZZIGA, B. R. (1967). Plasma TSH levels in the different forms of thyrotoxicosis. In *Thyrotoxicosis*. ed. W. J. Irvine. Edinburgh: Livingstone.

MCKENZIE, J. M. (1960). Bio-assay of thyrotropin in man. *Physiol. Rev.*, **40**, 398.

MCKENZIE, J. M. (1961). Studies on the thyroid activator of hyperthyroidism. *J. clin Endocr.*, **21**, 635.

MCKENZIE, J. M. (1962). The pituitary and Graves' disease. *Proc. roy. Soc. Med.*, **55**, 539.

MCKENZIE, J. M. (1964). Neonatal Graves' disease. *J. clin Endocr.*, **24**, 660.

MCKENZIE, J. M. (1965). The origin of the long-acting thyroid stimulator and its role in Graves' disease. In *Proc. Pan-American Conf. Endocrinol., 6th, Mexico City*. ed. G. Gual. Amsterdam. *Excepta Med. Found.*, Int. Congr. Ser. No. 112, p. 375.

MCKENZIE, J. M. (1968). Humoral factors in the pathogenesis of Graves' disease. *Physiol. Rev.*, **48**, 252.

MCKENZIE, J. M. & McCULLAGH, E. P. (1968). Observations against a causal relationship between the long-acting thyroid stimulator and ophthalmopathy in Graves' disease. *J. clin. Endocr.*, **28**, 1177.

MCKENZIE, J. M. & SOLOMON, S. H. (1967). Neuro-endocrine factors in thyroid disease. In *An Introduction to Clinical Neuro-endocrinology*. ed. E. Bajusz. New York: Karger, p. 312.

MCKENZIE, J. M. & WILLIAMSON, A. (1966). Experience with the bio-assay of the long-acting thyroid stimulator. *J. clin. Endocr.*, **26**, 518.

MAJOR, P. W. & MUNRO, D. S. (1962). Observations on the stimulation of thyroid function in mice by the injection of serum from normal subjects and from patients with thyroid disorders. *Clin. Sci.*, **23**, 463.

MEEK, J. C., JONES, A. E., LEWIS, V. J. & VANDERLAAN, W. P. (1964). Characterization of the long-acting thyroid stimulator of Graves' disease. *Proc. Nat. Acad. Sci. U.S.*, **52**, 342.

MIYAI, K., FUKUCHI, M., KUMAHARA, Y. & ABE, H. (1967). LATS production by lymphocyte culture in patients with Graves' disease. *J. clin. Endocr.*, **27**, 855.

MUNRO, D. S., BROWN, J., DORRINGTON, K. J., SMITH, B. R. & ENSOR, J. (1967). Observations on the chemical structure of the long-acting thyroid stimulator and its influence on thyroid function in thyrotoxicosis. In *Thyrotoxicosis*. ed. W. J. Irvine. Edinburgh: Livingstone.

ODELL, W. D., UTIGER, R. D. & WILBER, J. (1967). Studies of thyrotropin physiology by means of immuno-assay. *Recent Progr. Hormone Res.*, **23**, 47.

PIMSTONE, B. L., HOFFENBERG, R. & BLACK, E. (1965). Parallel assays of thyrotropin, long-acting thyroid stimulator, and exophthalmos-producing substance in endocrine exophthalmos and pretibial myxoedema. *J. clin. Endocr.*, **24**, 976.

RADACOT, J., PEILLON, F., SABOUN, J. & DREYFUS, G. (1965). Regressive aspect of thyrotropin (TSH) pituitary cells in Graves' disease. In *Current Topics in Thyroid Research, Proc. Intern. Thyroid Conf., fifth, Rome*, ed. C. Cassono, and M. Andreoli. New York: Academic Press, p. 593.

SOLOMON, D. H. & BEALL, G. N. (1967). Production of LATS in rabbit by immunization. *Clin. Res.*, **15**, 127.

WAYNE, E. J., KONTRAS, D. A. & ALEXANDER, W. D. (1964). Clinical aspects of iodine metabolism. Oxford: Blackwell Scientific Publications.

WERNER, S. C. & STEWART, W. B. (1958). Hyperthyroidism in a patient with a pituitary chromophobe adenoma and a fragment of normal pituitary. *J. clin. Endocr.*, **18**, 266.

PROPRANOLOL IN THE TREATMENT
OF GRAVES' DISEASE

Although the fundamental control of patients with Graves' disease still resides in antithyroid drugs, radio-iodine or subtotal thyroidectomy, the advent of propranolol has contributed much to the amelioration of the symptoms and facilitated the management of patients with this condition. Propranolol has also helped to elucidate the genesis of some of the clinical manifestations of the hyperthyroidal state. It has long been suspected that the two thyroidal hormones, thyroxine and tri-iodothyronine, potentiated the action of catecholamines acting on the β-receptors. Thus patients with hyperthyroidism are abnormally responsive to adrenergic stimuli, and certain peripheral manifestations of Graves' disease such as the tremor, the excessive sweating, the warm hands consequent on vasodilatation, and the nervousness have been attributed to this rather than to the direct effect of excess thyroid hormones. Propranolol is a blocker of the β-adrenergic receptors. In a double-blind control trial (Shanks *et al.*, 1969) it was found that a high proportion of thyrotoxic patients experienced a reduction in palpitations, sweating, nervousness, tremor and peripheral vasodilation when propranolol was given in a dose of 40 mg four times daily. Propranolol also reduces the heart rate in the thyrotoxic patient whether sinus rhythm or atrial fibrillation is present (Howitt and Rowlands, 1966). In most cases this is associated with a reduction in cardiac output, and atrial fibrillation is better controlled than with digoxin alone. However, the tachycardia of hyperthyroidism is not solely attributable to adrenergic influences as the rate is not reduced to within the normal range until euthyroidism is achieved, and there is good evidence that thyroxine is in part responsible for the tachycardia by a direct action on the myocardium (McDevitt *et al.*, 1968).

The practical uses of propranolol in the treatment of the thyrotoxic patient are several. Slow intravenous injection of 5–15 mg has proved of value in patients with a thyrotoxic crisis, inducing a rapid reduction in pulse rate, tremor, hyperkinesia and mental disturbance (Parsons and Jewitt, 1967; McLean, 1967). Such treatment should be supplemented by tepid sponging to control hyperpyrexia, but in general, propranolol appears to achieve a degree of control only attainable before by using a number of different agents, namely pethidine, chlorpromazine and promethazine in combination. Propranolol is also of value in the alleviation of muscle weakness in thyrotoxic myopathy (Pimstone et al., 1968). The drug finds its chief use, however, in more common thyrotoxic situations. The time required for preparation of a patient for thyroidectomy can be shortened by giving propranolol 40 mg q.d.s. with carbimazole 10 mg eight-hourly for three to four weeks and adding potassium iodide 30 mg t.d.s. during the ten days before operation. The greatest value of propranolol may prove to be in the management of thyrotoxic patients treated with radio-iodine (Hadden et al., 1968). Since radio-iodine treatment does not induce its maximum effect for about three months, it has often been necessary in the past to control the patient's thyrotoxic symptoms with an antithyroid drug such as carbimazole after the dose of ^{131}I has been given. This practice makes it difficult to assess the patient's thyroid state three months later. First carbimazole has to be withdrawn; then three or four weeks later the clinical state of the patient and tests of thyroid function will show whether euthyroidism has been achieved, or whether a further dose of radio-iodine is required. The situation is further complicated by the knowledge that eventually hypothyroidism is likely to develop, with an incidence of about 40 per cent within five years. Two procedures have been advocated to avoid this eventual hypothyroidism. One is to give a small dose of ^{131}I initially and thereafter to control the thyroid hyperfunction with carbimazole; the other is to give a small dose of radio-iodine and control the hyperthyroid symptoms with propranolol. The second method has the advantage that tests of thyroid function are not influenced by propranolol. Using the present empiric dose of radio-iodine followed by propranolol it is possible after three months to assess by estimation of the free thyroxine index (Howorth and Maclagan, 1969) or the protein-bound iodine whether euthyroidism has been achieved. Satisfactory though this regime is, it does not preclude the development of hypothyroidism in the years to come. It has therefore been suggested that the ultimate development of hypothyroidism after ^{131}I treatment might be obviated by giving a smaller dose of radio-iodine (4 mc), and then controlling the patient's symptoms for as long as necessary with propranolol 40 mg q.d.s. (Hadden et al., 1968). Patients who respond to this smaller dose of radio-iodine show a fall in PBI, a significant gain in weight, and a fall in heart-rate within eight weeks, but as yet there is no proof that the high incidence of hypothyroidism will be eliminated. Patients who do not show such a satisfactory clinical or biochemical response require a further dose of ^{131}I and in them it can be inferred that the future incidence of hypothyroidism will be high.

Propranolol is also useful in the control of hyperthyroidism in the last four to six weeks of pregnancy. During this time it is advisable to stop anti-thyroid drugs for fear of rendering the baby hypothyroid at birth.

REFERENCES

HADDEN, D. R., MONTGOMERY, D. A. D., SHANKS, R. G. & WEAVER, J. A. (1968). Propranolol and iodine-131 in the management of thyrotoxicosis. *Lancet*, 2, 852.

HOWITT, G. & ROWLANDS, D. J. (1966). Beta-sympathetic blockade in hyper-thyroidism. *Lancet*, 1, 628.

HOWORTH, P. J. N. & MACLAGAN, N. F. (1969). Clinical application of serum-total-thyroxine estimation, resin uptake and free-thyroxine index. *Lancet*, 1, 224.

McDEVITT, D. G., SHANKS, R. G., HADDEN, D. R., MONTGOMERY, D. A. D. & WEAVER, J. A. (1968). The role of the thyroid in the control of heart-rate. *Lancet*, 1, 998.

McLEAN, A. G. (1967). Adrenergic beta blockade in the thyrotoxic crisis. *Med. J. Aust.*, 2, 229.

PARSONS, V. & JEWITT, D. (1967). Beta-adrenergic blockade in the management of acute thyrotoxic crisis, tachycardia and arrhythmias. *Postgrad. med. J.*, 43, 756.

PIMSTONE, N., MARINE, N. & PIMSTONE, B. (1968). Beta-adrenergic blockade in thyrotoxic myopathy. *Lancet*, 2, 1219.

SHANKS, R. G., HADDEN, D. R., LOWE, D. C., McDEVITT, D. G. & MONTGOMERY, D. A. D. (1969). Controlled trial of propranolol in thyrotoxicosis. *Lancet*, 1, 993.

ENDOCRINOPATHIES ASSOCIATED WITH NON-ENDOCRINE TUMOURS

In the last edition of this book, attention was paid to the various endocrine syndromes which sometimes develop in patients with carcinoma of the bronchus. It was clear at that time that the development of an endocrinopathy in a patient with cancer of the lung was seldom fortuitous, and evidence was accumulating as to the mechanism of this relationship. What was problematic in 1964 and 1965 is now well understood, and it is appreciated that many other tumours arising in non-endocrine tissues may induce endocrine disorders. It has been established that in those patients showing Cushingoid features, the primary tumour does not secrete adenocortical-like steroids, nor does it stimulate the hypothalamus or the adenohypophysis to produce increased amounts of ACTH. By biological and more precise immunoassay techniques, bronchial and other tumours of non-endocrine origin have been shown to secrete peptide compounds which are seemingly identical with those produced by the adenohypophysis or by other endocrine glands. Ultimate confirmation of the identity of these peptides must depend on determination of their exact amino-acid sequences, a tedious and complicated procedure. Such confirmation is most essential, because in many poly-peptide hormones biological activity resides in one portion of the molecule and species antigenic specificity in another.

The whole concept of endocrine disorders produced by tumours of non-endocrine organs has widened during recent years. Although lung cancers are statistically common and most frequently the promoters of endocrine disorders, a large number of other neoplasms may be responsible, particularly those arising in tissues or organs derived from the embryological foregut. These include the thymus, breast, thyroid, pancreas, kidney, trachea, ovary, uterus and mesenchymal tissue. Even such remote lesions as cerebellar haemangiomata may secrete a humoral substance that stimulates the bone marrow to produce an excess of red cells, and the tumours concerned may be benign, though more commonly malignant. It is not possible to associate one particular variety of endocrinopathy with one particular variety of tumour nor with its site of origin. Sometimes, admittedly, a particular hor-mone and endocrine disturbance is associated with a tumour arising in a particular organ, but such relationship is far from invariable. Indeed, some tumours, particularly those arising in the bronchus and of the oat-cell variety, may elaborate several hormones simultaneously and thereby pro-duce a "mixed" endocrine disturbance. By contrast, mesenchymal tumours are particularly associated with the production of hypoglycaemia, and renal tumours with a humoral substance that promotes increased red-cell pro-duction (Pennington, 1965).

The endocrine disorders induced by the secretion of hormones from organs not normally associated with endocrine function, and the secretion of humoral substances not usually produced by a particular endocrine gland, can give rise to considerable problems in differential diagnosis. It is not the purpose of this brief review to be comprehensive, but rather to point out these clinical difficulties and suggest how best the patient's symptoms can be ameliorated.

Adrenocorticotrophin

Of all the hormones elaborated by non-endocrine tumours, adrenocortico-trophin (ACTH) is the most common. The primary tumour is usually a bronchial carcinoma, but a wide variety of other neoplasms may be respons-ible. The subject has been very adequately reviewed by O'Riordan and his associates (1966). Very large amounts of an ACTH-like material may be secreted by these new growths, and induce intense hypersecretion of cortico-steroids from the adrenal glands. The clinical effects are extremely variable.

At one end of the spectrum, the findings are biochemical rather than clinical. The patient develops hypokalaemic alkalosis with associated vague weakness. The rate of progression of the primary tumour is such that no clinical features of Cushing's syndrome develop before the patient dies. Intermediate in the spectrum are Cushingoid features which may suggest an endocrine dysfunction of the pituitary gland causing bilateral adrenal hyperplasia or a primary tumour of the adrenal cortex. In these cases the clue to the ectopic secretion of ACTH by a non-endocrine tumour may lie in finding marked hypokalaemic alkalosis, though this is not an invariable concomitant (Friedman et al., 1966) and by an atypical clinical picture of Cushing's syndrome. At the other end of the spectrum is the classical picture of Cushing's syndrome, clinically and biochemically indistinguishable from that produced by primary pituitary or adrenocortical dysfunction. Such a situation may develop in patients with a benign bronchial adenoma, and the endocrinopathy may precede by months or years clinical or radiological evidence of the pulmonary tumour (Strott et al., 1968). Suspicion as to the "non-endocrine" origin of this type of Cushing's syndrome may be suggested by a disproportionately severe degree of diabetes mellitus and by the particularly high plasma and urinary levels of 11-hydroxycorticosteroids, often far greater than those found in Cushing's syndrome of primary endocrine origin. Confusion about the differentiation between Cushing's syndrome of endocrine origin and that induced by the ectopic secretion of ACTH from a tumour arising in non-endocrine tissue is made even worse by the unexpected finding that suppression of adrenocortical activity may be achieved with dexamethasone in the ectopic cases and that increased adrenocortical activity may be induced by exogenously administered ACTH, or by metyrapone (Strott et al., 1968; Jones et al., 1969). Thus to the physician the differential diagnosis of the aetiology of Cushing's syndrome in a particular patient has become harder rather than easier. In some instances, bilateral total adrenalectomy is rightly carried out, but several years later it is found that the cause of bilateral adrenal hyperplasia was ACTH produced by a non-endocrine tumour rather than by the pituitary gland. In every patient with Cushing's syndrome, it is important that the physician considers the possibility of a non-endocrine cause and excludes, as far as this is possible, a tumour of the bronchus, pancreas, ovary, thyroid, thymus, testis, oesophagus, colon, trachea, prostate or breast. Suspicion that the aetiology is of non-endocrine origin should be increased if there is marked alkalosis associated with hypokalaemia; also if the degree of Cushingoid features is less florid than would be expected in the presence of very high plasma or urinary corticosteroid levels.

From the point of view of treatment, it is important that a correct aetiological diagnosis of Cushing's syndrome is made. Hypophysectomy or the implantation of radio-active seeds into the adenohypophysis is clearly inappropriate when the primary cause is an ectopic source of ACTH or a primary adrenal tumour.

Control of hyperadrenocorticism in a patient with a non-endocrine tumour secreting ACTH should in the first instance be directed to the primary growth. If this is amenable to surgical extirpation or responsive to radiotherapy or cytotoxic drugs, the secretion of ACTH is reduced. When the primary non-endocrine tumour cannot be controlled by such means, or when its presence is suspected but cannot be located, bilateral adrenalectomy is indicated. In some instances the patient's clinical state is so precarious that such a major operation is not possible. In these circumstances the biosynthesis of adreno-cortical hormones may be inhibited by the administration of aminoglutetha-mide (Cash et al., 1967; Schteingart and Conn, 1967; Gordon et al., 1968) or the toxic compound o,p'-DDD (Southren et al., 1966).

Antidiuretic Hormone

The secretion of a humoral agent with immunological and biological properties identical with those of vasopressin may occur from a wide variety of tumours, particularly bronchial carcinomas but also such diverse new growths as cancer of the tongue and Hodgkin's disease (Spittle, 1966). In some instances the discovery of a low serum sodium concentration is a chance finding, and no symptoms derive from the hyponatraemia. In others there are clinical manifestations of water intoxication characterized by nausea, vomiting, irritability, mental confusion and psychotic behaviour. Such diverse symptoms may pose considerable problems in differential diagnosis involving physician, surgeon or psychiatrist.

The mechanisms responsible for the hyponatraemia were discussed in the last edition of this book. It is perhaps necessary to emphasize that the distinction between dilutional hyponatraemia due to ectopic inappropriate secretion of antidiuretic hormone and sodium depletion associated with adrenal insufficiency is easy to make. In the latter there is haemoconcentration with increased plasma levels of potassium, extrarenal azotaemia and a low blood pressure.

The clinical features produced by ectopic secretion of ADH may be relieved by treatment of the primary tumour by surgical resection, radio-therapy or cytotoxic drugs (Linton and Hutton, 1965). Restriction of water intake is a logical and effective form of treatment but often intolerable for the patient. For this reason Ross (1963) has advocated the use of fludrocortisone, a potent synthetic sodium-retaining compound, in doses as large as 4 mg daily. This amount, far greater than that required to control the Addisonian or totally adrenalectomized patient, who requires an amount of 0·1 mg daily, may relieve the patient's manifestations of water intoxication.

Parathormone

Hypercalcaemia, a low serum phosphate level and increased urinary excretion of calcium may occur without clinical, radiological or post-mortem evidence of skeletal metastases in a patient with a tumour of non-endocrine origin. Although the clinical picture may sometimes be dominated by the primary neoplasm, many such patients present with manifestations of hypercalcaemia characterized by thirst, polyuria, anorexia, nausea, vomiting, constipation, fever due to dehydration, or mental confusion. These symptoms might pose a considerable problem in differential diagnosis, and may even suggest cerebral metastases (Strickland *et al.*, 1967), unless the serum calcium level is estimated. This syndrome and true primary hyperparathyroidism are in practice more often diagnosed and subsequently confirmed by the chance discovery of hypercalcaemia than by any other means. The distinction between ectopic secretion of a parathormone-like substance (Tashjian *et al.*, 1964; Goldberg *et al.*, 1964) and primary hyperparathyroidism may be difficult unless the underlying malignancy is detected. In most instances the differentiation can be made by the application of the cortisol test advocated by Dent and Watson (1968). No reduction in hypercalcaemia occurs in patients with primary hyperparathyroidism but usually, but not invariably (Fry, 1962), cortisol induces a fall in the serum calcium level in patients with ectopic parathormone secretion from a malignant tumour, even though the achievement of normocalcaemia may be short-lived.

Relief of hypercalcaemic symptoms is best achieved by treatment of the underlying neoplasm, including the use of cytotoxic agents or mithramycin, an antibiotic with cytotoxic activity (Parsons *et al.*, 1967). Administration of phosphate or calcitonin may temporarily reduce the hypercalcaemia, and the corticosteroids may be helpful, although not effective for long.

Gonadotrophin Secretion

Excess gonadotrophin production has been observed in patients with tumours containing trophoblastic elements such as chorioncarcinoma and teratoma, and also in patients with primary tumours of the liver or bronchus. In the male the chief endocrine manifestation is gynaecomastia. Often, but not invariably, those with bronchial cancer also have pulmonary osteo-arthropathy, which is the probable consequence of ectopic secretion of growth hormone (*vide infra*). Fusco and his colleagues (1966) found very high levels of gonadotrophins in the urine by bioassay in four patients with lung cancer and gynaecomastia and confirmed that the origin of these hormones was from the neoplastic tissue by recovering large amounts from the primary tumour or from renal or lymph node metastases in contrast to low concentrations in the pituitary gland. Similar observations have been made in gynaecomastia associated with carcinomas of the adrenal cortex, stomach and kidneys (McFadzean, 1946; Chambers, 1949; Stokes, 1962).

More convincing confirmation of gonadotrophin production by a broncho-genic carcinoma has been obtained by Faiman *et al.* (1967) and Becker *et al.* (1968) using a radioimmunoassay technique that showed an arterio-venous gradient across the tumour bed for follicle-stimulating hormone. Removal of the tumour was associated with a reduction in the serum FSH level and a fall in the urinary excretion of oestradiol and oestrone. This particular patient also had pulmonary osteoarthropathy, but unfortunately growth hormone was not measured. Attention must be drawn to the seemingly unique case of a woman who developed recurrent clubbing of the fingers with successive pregnancies and more significantly osteoarthropathy (Cullen and Maskery, 1966); an observation suggesting that gonadotrophins or growth hormone or placental lactogen (which cannot yet be distinguished from growth hormone by radioimmunoassay) was responsible for the bone changes. In the case report by Faiman and his associates (1967) it seems more probable that in addition to gonadotrophin production, there was increased secretion of growth hormone from a tumour well recognized as having the capacity to secrete more than one peptide hormone.

Growth Hormone

The development of pulmonary osteoarthropathy with its marked increase in periosteal new bone formation is particularly associated with bronchial carcinoma. The pathogenesis of the painful bone changes remains uncertain. As long ago as 1943 Fried noted that patients with lung cancer who developed this syndrome and survived long enough sometimes exhibited clinical features suggestive of acromegaly, and subsequently others have commented on the clinical similarity between acromegaly and osteoarthropathy (Hammarsten and O'Leary, 1957; Vogl and Goldfischer, 1962). It is therefore of particular interest that Waldenström and his associates (Steiner *et al.*, 1968) have found high plasma levels of growth hormone in a patient with bronchial carcinoma and pulmonary osteoarthropathy. Resection of the tumour relieved bone pain and was accompanied by a fall in the plasma growth hormone level into the normal range. Similar findings have now been made by others (Bayliss, unpublished observation), with growth hormone levels as high as 98 ng/ml in one particularly severe case. In contrast, high plasma levels of the hormone have not been found in patients with finger clubbing unassociated with osteoarthropathy (Steiner *et al.*, 1968).

Excess growth hormone or related prolactin secretion may play a role in the pathogenesis of the gynaecomastia associated with neoplastic tumours, particularly in those patients who show no laboratory evidence of increased follicular stimulating or luteinizing hormones.

Relief of symptoms is achieved by resection of the primary tumour, indomethacin may also be effective in relieving bone pain.

Hypoglycaemia

The occurrence of hypoglycaemia, unrelated to an insulinoma of the pancreas, occurs most frequently in patients with large neoplasms of mesenchymal origin such as mesotheliomata or retroperitoneal fibrosarcomata (Fraser, 1965; Marks and Samols, 1966). Less common causes are carcinomas of lung, stomach, liver or adrenal glands. The mechanism responsible for the low blood glucose level is uncertain. In rare instances such as a primary bronchial carcinoma, insulin and glucagon have been extracted from the tumour but in most cases radioimmunoassay has failed to reveal high levels of plasma insulin. Such a finding makes it difficult to accept the proposition of Samaan et al. (1965) that a humoral agent promotes increased insulin production. It seems more likely that the low blood sugar level is the consequence of an unidentified compound that inhibits the release of glucose from the liver (Marks and Samols, 1966). As with other malignant tumours, the hypoglycaemia may be associated with additional endocrinopathies such as acromegaly, thyrotoxicosis, gynaecomastia and virilism (Marks and Rose, 1965).

The primary tumour responsible for the hypoglycaemia is easy to detect clinically, usually because of its size. Only rarely is the condition likely to be confused with an insulinoma. Under these circumstances the distinction can usually be made by the intravenous injection of 1 g tolbutamide. In patients with an insulinoma there is a striking increase in the plasma insulin level, whereas in patients with a non-pancreatic tumour the plasma insulin falls or remains unaltered; in both conditions there is a fall in the blood glucose level. Glucose tolerance tests and the responses to leucine or glucagon are less reliable in making this distinction.

Surgical removal of the tumour will relieve the symptoms of hypoglycaemia, but metastases are commonly a cause of further episodes of low blood glucose levels. Palliative radiotherapy or cytotoxic agents are relatively ineffective, but diazoxide may prove of value and possibly streptozotocin may be helpful, although this must be considered an experimental approach at the present time (Murray-Lyon et al., 1968).

Thyroid Stimulating Hormone

The production of hyperthyroidism by the secretion of a thyroid stimulating substance from a non-endocrine tumour is one of the least common endocrinopathies encountered. Even when hyperthyroidism is present in a patient with a carcinoma, proof of the aetiological relationship is difficult to obtain, partly because the two are common diseases and partly because of methodological difficulties in identifying thyroid stimulating hormone (TSH) by immunological and bioassay procedures. However, there does seem a particular relationship between chorioncarcinoma and excessive production of TSH, which may or may not be associated with clinical evidence of hyperthyroidism and increased levels of protein-bound iodine (Odell *et al.*, 1963; Steigbigel *et al.*, 1964). A substance antigenically related to TSH has been recovered from a chorioncarcinoma in a male (Hennen, 1966a) and also from another patient with a bronchial carcinoma (Hennen, 1966b).

Hydroxyindoles

Hyperperistalsis, diarrhoea and peripheral oedema may be produced by the secretion of 5-hydroxyindoles such as 5-hydroxytryptamine (5-HT or serotonin) and less commonly 5-hydroxytryptophan (5-HPT). Patients with such a syndrome may also exhibit episodic flushing which is probably attributable to the release of kinins (Oates *et al.*, 1964; Adamson *et al.*, 1969). The usual primary tumour responsible is an argentaffinoma of the gastro-intestinal tract and, less commonly, an adenoma of the bronchus. The tumour may rarely be an oat-cell carcinoma of the bronchus, a carcinoma of the stomach, pancreas, or ovary, or a carcinoma arising in the parafolli-cular cells of the thyroid gland (Brown and Lane, 1965; Kinloch *et al.*, 1965; Azzopardi and Bellau, 1965).

Difficulties in diagnosis arise when the presenting symptom is diarrhoea sometimes associated with colicky abdominal pain, and the primary tumour is clinically silent and radiologically undetectable. A correct diagnosis at this stage in the disease will be made only if the possibility of the carcinoid syndrome is borne in mind and the urine examined for 5-hydroxyindole-acetic acid, a metabolic degradation product of 5-HT and 5-HPT. Relief or partial control of the diarrhoea may be achieved with chlorpromazine or methysergide, a potent 5-HT antagonist (Peart and Robertson, 1961; Melmon *et al.*, 1965). Even more effective control of the diarrhoea may be achieved with para-chlorophenylalanine which inhibits the enzymatic conversion of tryptophan to 5-HT (Koe and Weissman, 1966; Engelman *et al.*, 1967).

Prostaglandins

Although they were discovered as long ago as 1934 by von Euler, prosta-glandins have only recently begun to achieve significance in clinical medicine. These compounds are long-chain fatty-acids with one or more unesterified –OH groups essential to their biological activity. At least six members of this group of compounds have been identified. Although their chemical structure is known, they are estimated and identified according to their chromatographic and biological properties because they are present in such small amounts. They can be detected in many tissues ranging from seminal fluid (in which they were first found) to pancreas, brain, kidney, heart, lung, liver, thymus and thyroid. Differing biological properties enable the prostaglandins to be separated into two, the E and F, groups. Both groups stimulate smooth muscle, but the E compounds are much more potent in reducing blood pressure by dilatation of small arterioles. This is not the appropriate place to review the increasing physiological literature on the action of prostaglandins in animals (*Lancet*, 1968). However, in the present context they are of possible importance as the cause of diarrhoea in patients with certain malignant tumours, since oral prostaglandins may cause hyperperistalsis, colicky abdominal pain, diarrhoea and a rapid transit time through the intestine in normal subjects (Misiewicz *et al.*, 1969).

Diarrhoea may be a prominent feature in patients with medullary carcinoma of the thyroid gland (Clinicopathological Conference, 1967; Williams, 1966). This diarrhoea has been attributed in the past to the production of 5-hydroxyindoles by the malignant parafollicular cells which may also produce calcitonin and kinins. In four out of seven such cases appreciable amounts of prostaglandins have been found in the tumour tissue, and in two of the patients who had diarrhoea raised prostaglandin levels were present in the blood, with an amount considerably higher in the blood stream draining the tumour than in the peripheral venous blood (Williams *et al.*, 1968). Proof that prostaglandins were responsible for the diarrhoea is difficult to obtain, but there was no evidence of increased amounts of 5-HT, histamine, acetylcholine or catecholamines in extracts of the tumours. Similarly, high prostaglandin levels have been detected (Sandler *et al.*, 1968) in three patients with diarrhoea associated with a bronchial carcinoid tumour, an alpha-cell islet tumour of the pancreas and a ganglioneuroma. The aetiological role of prostaglandins as the cause of the diarrhoea is hard to prove, because these tumours may secrete other humoral substances and there is evidence that prostaglandins may act synergistically with 5-HT, histamine and kinins.

Mechanism of Ectopic Hormone Production

To the clinician it is perhaps sufficient that he should know that a variety of malignant tumours may produce hormones, and that in practice he distinguishes an endocrinopathy due to a primary endocrine disorder from that associated with a neoplasm of non-endocrine tissue because the treatment and prognosis are so different. It is also important to enquire why malignant cells are capable of secreting such a variety of hormones. This fundamental question will doubtless be answered by the cellular biologiss. It seems improbable that a malignant cell should synthesize the 84-amino-acids by chance and arrange them in the correct sequence to produce parathormone. Even if the biological activity of parathormone resides in only 20 of its 84 amino-acids it would be a remarkable turn of the wheel of fate for such a compound to be synthesized, and even less probable that one particular type of malignant tissue should produce two or more peptide hormones with widely differing biological actions.

All undifferentiated cells, except the sex cells, are endowed with an identical genetic code and are therefore totipotential and have an inherent capacity to produce any peptide normally found in the body. As cells become more specialized and confine their activity in the body to a particular function, the genetic information for the reproduction of proteins is suppressed. Present evidence suggests that this repression of DNA coded information is achieved by RNA or histones. Thus the secretion of peptide hormones by malignant tissue may be due to the de-repression of DNA, with the resultant synthesis of one or more peptide hormones (*Lancet*, 1967).

REFERENCES

ADAMS, D. D., KENNEDY, T. H. & PURVES, H. D. (1969). Comparison of the thyroid stimulating hormone content of serum from thyrotoxic and euthyroid people. *J. clin. Endocr.*, **29**, 900.

ADAMSON, A. R., GRAHAME-SMITH, D. G., PEART, W. S. & STARR, M. (1969). Pharmacological blockade of carcinoid flushing provoked by catecholamines and alcohol. *Lancet*, **2**, 293.

AZZOPARDI, J. G. & BELLAU, A. R. (1965). Carcinoid syndrome and oat-cell carcinoma of the bronchus. *Thorax*, **20**, 393.

BECKER, K. L., COTTRELL, J., MOORE, C. F., WINNACKER, J. L., MATTHEWS, M. J. & KATZ, S. (1968). Endocrine studies in a patient with a gonadotrophin-secreting bronchogenic carcinoma. *J. clin. Endocr.*, **28**, 809.

BROWN, H. & LANE, M. (1965). Cushing's and malignant carcinoid syndromes from ovarian neoplasm. *Arch. intern. Med.*, **115**, 490.

CASH, R., BROUGH, A. J., COHEN, M. N. P. & SATOH, P. S. (1967). Aminoglutethimide (Elipten-Ciba) as an inhibitor of adrenal steroidogenesis: mechanism of action and therapeutic trial. *J. clin Endocr.*, **27**, 1239.

CHAMBERS, W. L. (1949). Adrenal cortical carcinoma in male with excess gonadotrophin in urine. *J. clin. Endocr.*, **9**, 451.

CLINICOPATHOLOGICAL CONFERENCE (1967). A case of diarrhoea and goitre. *Brit. med. J.*, **2**, 293.

CULLEN, D. R. & MASKERY, P. J. K. (1966). Clubbing of fingers and hypertrophic osteoarthropathy in pregnancy. *Lancet*, **2**, 473.

DENT, C. E. & WATSON, L. (1968). The hydrocortisone test in primary and tertiary hyperparathyroidism. *Lancet*, **2**, 662.

ENGELMAN, K., LOVENBERG, W. & SJOERDSMA, A. (1967). Inhibition of serotonin synthesis by para-chlorophenylalanine in patients with the carcinoid syndrome. *New Engl. J. Med.*, **277**, 1103.

FAIMAN, C., COLWELL, J. A., RYAN, R. J., HERSHMAN, J. M. & SHIELDS, T. W. (1967). Gonadotropin secretion from a bronchogenic carcinoma: demonstration by radioimmunoassay. *New Engl. J. Med.*, **277**, 1395.

FRASER, R. T. (1965). Hypercalcaemia and hypoglycaemia associated with tumours. *Proc. roy. Soc. Med.*, **58**, 483.

FRIED, B. M. (1943). Chronic pulmonary osteoarthropathy; dispituitarism as a probable cause. *Arch. intern. Med.*, **72**, 565.

FRIEDMAN, M., MARSHALL-JONES, P. & ROSS, E. J. (1966). Cushing's syndrome: adrenocortical hyperactivity secondary to neoplasms arising outside the pituitary-adrenal system. *Quart. J. Med.*, **35**, 193.

FRIEDMAN, M., MIKHAIL, J. R. & BHOOLA, K. D. (1965). Cushing's syndrome associated with carcinoma of the bronchus in a patient with normal plasma electrolytes. *Brit. med. J.*, **1**, 27.

FRY, L. (1962). Pseudohyperparathyroidism with carcinoma of bronchus. *Brit. med. J.*, **1**, 301.

FUSCO, F. D. & ROSEN, S. W. (1966). Gonadotrophin-producing anaplastic large-cell carcinomas of the lung. *New Engl. J. Med.*, **275**, 507.

GOLDBERG, M. F., TASHJIAN, A. H., ORDER, S. E. & DAMMIN, G. J. (1964). Renal adenocarcinoma containing a parathyroid hormone-like substance and associated with marked hypercalcemia. *Amer. J. Med.*, **36**, 805.

GORDON, P., BECKER, C. E., LEVEY, G. S. & ROTH, J. (1968). Efficacy of amino-glutethimide in the ectopic ACTH syndrome. *J. clin. Endocr.*, **28**, 921.

HAMMARSTEN, J. F. & O'LEARY, J. (1957). Features and significance of hypertrophic osteoarthropathy. *Arch. intern. Med.*, **99**, 431.

HENNEN, G. (1966a). Detection of a thyroid-stimulating factor in a choriocarcinoma occurring in a male. *Arch. intern. physiol. Biochim.*, **74**, 303.

HENNEN, G. (1966b). Thyrotropin-like factor in a non-endocrine cancer tissue. *Arch. intern. physiol. Biochim.*, **74**, 701.

JONES, J. E., SHANE, S. R., GILBERT, E. & FLINK, E. B. (1969). Cushing's syndrome induced by the ectopic production of ACTH by a bronchial carcinoid. *J. clin. Endocr.*, **29**, 1.

KINLOCK, J. D., WEBB, J. N., ECCLESTON, D. & ZEITLIN, J. (1965). Carcinoid syndrome associated with oat-cell carcinoma of bronchus. *Brit. med. J.*, **1**, 1533.

KOE, B. K. & WEISSMAN, A. (1966). *p*-chlorophenylalanine: a specific depletor of brain serotonin. (1966). *J. Pharmacol. exp. Ther.*, **154**, 499.

LANCET EDITORIAL (1967). Hormones and histones? **1**, 86.

LANCET EDITORIAL (1968). Prostaglandins, **1**, 30.

LINTON, A. L. & HUTTON, I. (1965). Hyponatraemia and bronchial carcinoma: therapy with nitrogen mustard. *Brit. med. J.*, **2**, 277.

MCFADZEAN, A. J. S. (1946). Feminisation associated with carcinoma of adrenal cortex. *Lancet*, **2**, 940.

MARKS, V. & SAMOLS, E. (1966). Hypoglycaemia of non-endocrine origin. *Proc. roy. Soc. Med.*, **59**, 338.

MARKS, V. & ROSE, F. C. (1965). *Hypoglycaemia*. Oxford: Blackwell Ltd.

MELMON, K. L., SJOERDSMA, A., OATES, J. A. & LASTER, L. (1965). Treatment of malabsorption and diarrhoea of the carcinoid syndrome with methysergide. *Gastroenterology*, **48**, 18.

MISIEWICZ, J. J., WALLER, S. L., KILEY, N. & HORTON, E. W. (1969). Effect of oral prostaglandin E_1 on intestinal transit in man. *Lancet*, **2**, 648.

MURRAY-LYON, I. M., EDDLESTON, A. L. W. F., WILLIAMS, R., BROWN M., HOGBIN, B. M., BENNETT, A., EDWARDS, J. C. & TAYLOR, K. W. (1968). Treatment of multiple-hormone-producing malignant islet-cell tumour with streptozotocin. *Lancet*, **2**, 895.

OATES, J. A., MELMON, K., SJOERDSMA, A., GILLESPIE, L. & MASON, D. T. (1964). Release of a kinin peptide in the carcinoid tumour. *Lancet*, **1**, 514.

ODELL, W. D., BATES, R. W., RIVLIN, S., LIPSETT, M. B. & HERTZ, R. (1963). Increased thyroid function without clinical hyperthyroidism in patients with choriocarcinoma. *J. clin. Endocr.*, **23**, 658.

O'RIORDIAN, J. L. H., BLANSHARD, G. P., MAXHAM, A. & NABARRO, J. D. N. (1966). Corticotrophin-secreting carcinomas. *Quart. J. Med.*, **35**, 137.

PARSONS, V., BAUM, M. & SELF, M. (1967). Effect of mithramycin on calcium and hydroxyproline metabolism in patients with malignant disease. *Brit. med. J.*, 1, 474.

PEART, W. S. & ROBERTSON, J. I. S. (1961). Effect of serotonin antagonist (UML 491) in carcinoid disease. *Lancet*, 2, 1172.

PENNINGTON, D. G. (1965). Polycythaemia in neoplastic diseases. *Proc. roy. Soc. Med.*, 58, 488.

ROSS, E. J. (1963). Hyponatraemic syndromes associated with carcinoma of the bronchus. *Quart. J. Med.*, 32, 297.

ROSS, E. J. (1966). Endocrine syndromes of non-endocrine origin. *Proc. roy. Soc. Med.*, 59, 335.

SAMAAN, H., LAL, F., FRASER, R. T. & WELBOURNE, R. B. (1965). Insulin assay in two cases of spontaneous hypoglycaemia due to retroperitoneal mesothelioma. *Brit. med. J.*, 2, 195.

SANDLER, M., KARIM, S. M. M. & WILLIAMS, E. D. (1968). Prostaglandins in amine-peptide-secreting tumours. *Lancet*, 2, 1053.

SCHTEINGART, D. E. & CONN, J. W. (1967). Effects of aminoglutethimide upon adrenal function and cortisol metabolism in Cushing's syndrome. *J. clin. Endocrinol. Metab.*, 27, 1657.

SOUTHREN, A. L., TOCHIMOTO, S., STROM, L., RATUSCHNI, A., ROSS, H. & GORDON, G. (1966). Remission in Cushing's syndrome with o,p'-DDD. *J. clin. Endocr.*, 26, 268.

SPITTLE, M. F. (1966). Inappropriate anti-diuretic hormone secretion in Hodgkin's disease. *Postgrad. med. J.*, 42, 523.

STEIGBIGEL, N. H., OPPENHEIM, J. J., FISHMAN, L. M. & CARBONE, P. P. (1964). Metastatic embryonal carcinoma of the testis associated with elevated plasma TSH-like activity and hyperthyroidism. *New Engl. J. Med.*, 27, 345.

STEINER, H., DAHLBÄCK, O. & WALDENSTRÖM, J. (1968). Ectopic growth-hormone production and osteoarthropathy in carcinoma of the bronchus. *Lancet*, 1, 783.

STOKES, J. F. (1962). Unexpected gynaecomastia. *Lancet*, 2, 911.

STRICKLAND, N. J., BOLD, A. M. & MEDD, W. E. (1967). Bronchial carcinoma with hypercalcaemia simulating cerebral metastases. *Brit. med. J.*, 2, 590.

STROTT, C. A., NUGENT, C. A. & TYLER, F. H. (1968). Cushing's syndrome caused by bronchial adenomas. *Amer. J. Med.*, 44, 97.

TASHJIAN, A. H., LEVINE, L. & MUNSON, P. L. (1964). Immunochemical identification of parathyroid hormone in non-parathyroid neoplasms associated with hypercalcemia. *J. exp. Med.*, 119, 467.

VOGL, A. & GOLDFISCHER, S. (1962). Pachydermoperiostosis: primary or idiopathic hypertrophic osteoarthropathy. *Amer. J. Med.*, 33, 166.

WILLIAMS, E. D. (1966). Diarrhoea and thyroid carcinoma. *Proc. roy. Soc. Med.*, 59, 602.

WILLIAMS, E. D., KARIM, S. M. M. & SANDLER, M. (1968). Prostaglandin secretion by medullary carcinoma of the thyroid. *Lancet*, 1, 22.

7 Cardiology

RAYMOND DALEY

TRANSPLANTATION. CORONARY HEART DISEASE. INTENSIVE
CORONARY CARE UNITS. THROMBOEMBOLISM. CARDIO-
MYOPATHY. MITRAL REGURGITATION. ARRHYTHMIAS.
REPLACEMENT OF HEART VALVES

PROGRESS in cardiology has been continuous. The major advances have
been in the fields of cardiac surgery and cardiac physiology. They have been
concerned with cardiac transplantation, valve replacement, the surgery of
coronary artery disease, thromboembolism and the arrhythmias. Future
developments are difficult to predict.

CARDIAC TRANSPLANTATION

In mid-1969, over 100 heart transplants were performed. There is virtually
only one technique, which was originated by Shumway (1966). This procedure retains the atria and is not a difficult operation. Following transplantation, it is of great interest that the heart can speed up on effort, and
this is presumably due to intrinsic sympathetic synapses. The catecholamine
supply must be conjectural but is worthy of study.

The main practical problem in transplantation is, of course, immunosuppressive treatment. The techniques of this are rapidly improving and the
aim is to manage with minimal dosage of steroids and immunosuppressives.

It is believed that the first heart transplant in man was performed in
Mississippi on 23rd January 1964, after laboratory experimentation beginning
in 1956. The recipient was a 68-year-old white man in a preterminal state
from atherosclerotic coronary artery disease. The prospective human donor
could not be used because of his survival in a respirator and accordingly, a
chimpanzee heart was used. This is described by Hardy and Chavez (1968).
They state that the cardiac output of the primate donor was 3·6 l/min. The
transplanted heart was easily defibrillated, but they thought that because of

the advanced metabolic deterioration of the recipient and the size of the donor heart, the fatal outcome two hours after defibrillation was almost inevitable. However, the initial feasibility of heart transplantation was established.

In a compilation of cases of heart transplantation in man between 1st January 1964 and 23rd October 1968, the total number was 66. In eight, the donors were older than the recipients of the transplant. The youngest recipient was a five-year-old girl, and there were four recipients over the age of 60: none of these survived. The oldest survivors are aged 59 and 58. There is a striking improvement in results in the later transplants. However, including Hardy's first case mentioned above, and Barnard's first case in March 1967, the survival record on 23rd October 1968 is 32 out of 65 patients, with 33 dead.

Messmer et al. (1969) analysed 15 patients who underwent cardiac transplantation for "end-stage heart-disease". They compared their survival time with those 42 potential recipients who did not receive allografts. The mean survival time of the potential recipients was 74 days; the average for the transplant patients was 111 days (including 22 days waiting time before operation). They say that the difference does not justify the wide application of cardiac transplants, but they think that it is an indication for its use in suitable cases in which it may prolong life and relieve symptoms.

The main criticism of this argument is the length of time that recipients have to wait before a suitable donor is available. Nevertheless, the figures are not very impressive. The causes of death at operation have been critically analysed by all the transplant teams, and the operation is rarely at fault. Ross (1968) in considering his patients, believes that insufficient removal of the recipient atria may have led to death by multiple pulmonary emboli. He intends in future to remove as much of the recipient atria as possible; there may be many more such anatomical surgical difficulties, but these are probably insignificant in comparison to the immunological problems.

The immunological obstacles are considerable, and there have been no significant advances in combating them. The processes involved are mediated by lymphocytes involving and invading fibrous tissue, thrombosis, oedema and perivascular thrombosis obliterating the smaller arteries. The transplant may then be destroyed by necrosis. Immunosuppressive treatment consists of azothioprine, corticosteroids and antilymphocytic globulin. These are in part effective, but they are somewhat empirical and may not only suppress signs of rejection, but they may also make the control of infection difficult. It is assumed that lymphocytic activity is the greatest menace to rejection, but safe and potent antisera have yet to be developed.

Barnard (1968) discusses the diagnosis of rejection and concludes that "no single parameter permits an unequivocal diagnosis". He found that decrease in exercise tolerance, cardiac failure and dilatation were important findings. A fall in gamma M levels may help in predicting rejection.

The functional activity of a transplanted heart must depend upon haemodynamic, nervous and chemical considerations. There is no reason why Starling's Law should not apply, and such hearts increase in rate on effort, but there is little knowledge about the availability of increased force of contraction and consequent cardiac output. It is known that a denervated heart is unduly sensitive to medullary catecholamines. This "drive" is mainly lost when adrenal-medullary catecholamines are deficient. This is an interesting contrast to *in situ* denervated hearts in which this does not obtain. It will be very interesting to know how these factors affect cardiac failure, irregularities and even chest pain on effort—the last still being so poorly understood that heart transplantation may help in its explanation.

The ethics of cardiac transplantation evoke perpetual controversy. The British Medical Association Planning Unit have expressed their views strongly, and probably reasonably, that there will never be sufficient heart transplant donors in this country, and support the proposition that "even if heterografts from animals were ever utilized, and if double the number of cardiac teams did nothing else, the demand would not be met" (1968). The comparison is made between renal and heart transplants. In paired organs, the difference is obvious and the success of renal transplantation is now established. However, the argument that one form of transplantation is established and that the other is not, should surely not be the deciding factor against heart transplantation, otherwise progress will never be made.

The final count on organ transplantation must concern the liver and the lung. Efforts to increase the "take" of liver transplants by Calne (see Chapter 12) have been described.

Lung transplantation has hardly begun and the indications for recipients are not clear. It has been described from Edinburgh in a case of Paraquat poisoning, which "would seem to be a good indication, provided sufficient time can be allowed to elapse for the complete elimination of the drug; otherwise, the graft may be destroyed".

Thus, grafting is in its infancy. The heterograft, homograft or zenograft will probably play a greater part in our next edition.

REFERENCES

BARNARD, C. N. (1968). Human tissue transplantation. *Amer. J. Cardiol.*, **22**, 811.

BMA PLANNING UNIT (1968). *Brit. med. J.*, 1969, **1**, 106.

HARDY, J. D. & CHAVEZ, C. M. (1968). The first heart transplant in man. *Amer. J. Cardiol.*, **22**, 772.

MESSMER, B. J., NORA, J. J., LEACHMAN, R. D. *et al.* (1969). Survival-times after cardiac allografts. *Lancet*, **1**, 954.

ROSS, D. (1968). Report of a heart transplant operation. *Amer. J. Cardiol.* **22**, 838.

SHUMWAY, N. E. (1966). The present status of cardiac transplantation. *Angiology*, **17**, 289.

CORONARY HEART DISEASE

There is no improvement in the total mortality figures for coronary artery disease. McDonald (1968) has reviewed the risk factors in coronary heart disease and makes the following points concerning the subjects of undue risk.

The first unfavourable omen is first-degree relatives affected by the disease, especially if there is impairment of lipoprotein lipase. Men and women after the menopause, or women who have had bilateral oophorectomy are also susceptible, as are those affected by abnormalities of metabolism such as hyperglyceridaemia and abnormal carbohydrate metabolism. Twenty per cent of those suffering from cardiac infarction have a raised level of serum uric acid; the disease is also more prevalent in localities where the water is hard. The study of daily variations of uric acid, creatinine and blood-urea levels, and renal clearances supports the hypothesis that the hyperuricaemia is the result of the variable interactions of the two mechanisms; impaired renal disposal and overproduction of uric acid (Rizzon *et al.*, 1968).

There is a higher incidence in subjects of systemic hypertension. Other factors include unusual platelet behaviour, obesity (excessive animal fat and sugar intake) and excessive cigarette smoking.

Occupational hazards of population groups are interesting, even if difficult to evaluate (Morris, 1962). The highest risk group is radio and telegraph operators, and the lowest rag, bone and bottle sorters. Roman Catholic priests, doctors, brokers and managers all appear high on the list.

McDonald further discusses the frequency of thrombus formation in coronary artery occlusion and stresses the difficulty of distinguishing between occlusion thrombi, recanalizing thrombi and arterial plaques. He believes that most cases of cardiac infarction depend on thrombosis and that "the flowing of blood may be of prime importance in ischaemic heart disease, and more so than the changes in the arterial blood".

The coronary arterial flow is unique in that it occurs mainly in diastole, which may enhance the possibility of thrombosis because of turbulence.

Intravascular thrombosis is associated with abnormal platelet behaviour, such as turnover, aggregation and possibly adhesiveness. These changes in platelets may indicate other abnormalities in the blood such as those involving catecholamines, free fatty acids and red blood cells.

INTENSIVE CORONARY CARE UNITS

Eighty per cent of acute coronary artery occlusions are complicated by some form of disordered rhythm. Whether or not this is discovered by patient monitoring in a ward or in an intensive care unit is probably not very important. Oliver (1968) discusses four levels of coronary care units. The first is a simple monitoring system with a bedside oscilloscope for electrocardiographic display and a defibrillator. Oliver believes that such simple units may have considerable dangers.

The second consists of grouping a few beds in an open ward with electrocardiograms linked to a central oscilloscope. The objection to this is the approximation of patients studying the behaviour of their neighbours, which must be set against the estimated value and necessity of resuscitative procedures.

The third level is represented by a unit of individual rooms with bedside and exteriorized monitoring systems. This may include means of inserting cardiac pacemaking catheters and apparatus for measuring haemodynamic and biochemical events.

The fourth is the incorporation of a coronary unit into the framework of a general intensive care unit, and this may well be the most satisfactory and economic arrangement.

Since many ventricular arrhythmias occur within the first two hours of cardiac infarction, it has been thought that appropriately equipped flying-squad teams should be available. One of the pioneer studies was carried out in Belfast by Pantridge and Geddes (1967), and they have shown that resuscitation can be as effective in the home as in intensive care units. While home treatment of this type with specially equipped ambulances may help to reduce mortality, there are difficulties in getting such care to the patient's home rapidly after the infarction. One of the worst problems is the understandable difficulty that neither the patient nor the doctor may realize the seriousness of the symptoms. In analysing these delays Oliver (1968) finds that the "patient delay" is usually about one hour and that other delays are concerned with the call to and the arrival of the doctor, the ambulance, and finally, "hospital admission delays". In the Edinburgh Royal Infirmary Coronary Care Unit, 57 per cent of all patients are admitted within four hours of the onset of symptoms, but others have suggested that if mortality is to be significantly affected even this period is too long.

It is doubtful whether there is any important recent contribution in treatment, apart from the effective management of dysrhythmias, and Julian (1968) has reviewed this subject. Sinus bradycardia may complicate inferior myocardial infarction. It may be part of the ill-understood vasovagal reactions, or may occur as an isolated event. The danger lies in the warning of ventricular ectopic activity. If ventricular ectopic beats associated with hypotension are present, 1 mg of atropine should be given intravenously.

Interesting observations of early bradyarrhythmia complicating acute myocardial infarction have been made by many authors. Posterior infarction complicated by bradyarrhythmias has been found in 60 per cent of patients who come under intensive care within one hour of the arrival of a mobile coronary care unit. It has been suggested that excessive vagal discharge manifested by this rhythm may be an important precursor of ventricular fibrillation. It is postulated that as vagal neuroceptors have been described in the region of the coronary sinus, severe vagotonia may complicate posterior infarction and block of the right coronary artery. Such infarcts may be quite small, and if vagotonia of this kind can be relieved by atropin, repeated aliquots of atropin can make the ultimate outlook very good.

REFERENCES

JULIAN, D. G. (1968). The management of dysrhythmias in cardiac infarction. *J. roy. Coll. Physicians (Lond.)*, **3**, 54.

LASSERS, B. W. & JULIAN, D. G. (1968). Artificial pacing in management of complete heart block, complicating acute myocardial infarction. *Brit. med. J.*, **2**, 142.

McDONALD, L. (1968). Thrombosis in coronary heart disease. *Brit. med. J.*, **30**, 151.

MORRIS, J. M. (1962). Coronary disease in England. *Cardiol. prat. (Firenze)*, **13**, 85.

OLIVER, M. F. (1968). The place of a coronary care unit. *J. roy. Coll. Physicians (Lond.)*, **3**, 47.

PANTRIDGE, J. F. & GEDDES, J. S. (1967). A mobile intensive care unit in the management of myocardial infarctions. *Lancet*, **2**, 271.

RIZZON, P., HUMAN, G. P. & SNYMAN, H. W. (1968). Incidence, pattern and mechanism of transient hyperuricemia in patients with acute myocardial infarction. *Mal. cardiovasc.*, **9**, 423.

SUTTON, R., CHATTERJEE, K. & LEATHAM, A. (1968). Heart block following acute myocardial infarction. *Lancet*, **2**, 645.

WEINBLATT, E., SHAPIRO, S. & SAGER, R. V. (1968). Prognosis of men after first myocardial infarction; mortality and first recurrence, in relation to selected parameters. *Amer. J. publ. Hlth.*, **58**, 1329.

THROMBOEMBOLISM

Thromboembolism has been the subject of much attention and a more aggressive attack during the past few years. There has been considerable discussion about the various values of vein ligation, anticoagulants and fibrinolytic agents in the treatment of thrombosis of the leg and pelvic veins. The embolic risk in *thrombophlebitis* is small, since the thrombus is usually firmly adherent to the venous wall. In fact an embolic episode occurs in only 15 per cent of patients, and this is associated with suppurative liquification of the clot.

In *phlebothrombosis*, the story is quite different. Clots form in the deep veins of the sole and calf, and embolism is frequent. Deep-vein thrombosis classically occurs about the tenth day after operation, especially if there has been immobility. It has been said that thrombosis is promoted by altered blood such as alteration in the fibrinogen content and increased platelet adhesiveness, but doubt has recently been cast upon the latter. The abnormal physical signs comprise the "chart" sign, in which the temperature and pulse rate are increased. When there is accompanying pulmonary embolism there will also be an increase in the respiration rate. The appearance of a leg in which there is a phlebothrombosis is dusky with dilated superficial veins, with or without oedema. The most important physical sign however is tenderness of the sole. The importance of calf tenderness is that it should be bi-directional; that is, tenderness is elicited by squeezing a calf not only from the front to the back, but from side to side. Homan's sign is late, and is not entirely reliable. The prophylaxis of "rest" phlebothrombosis is the encouragement of frequent dorsi-flexion of the feet, which has been shown by radio-sodium tracer studies to be the most effective method of increasing the velocity of calf blood flow. Obviously, anything which leads to venous occlusion must be discouraged. In a recent survey in a London Hospital it was found that 15 per cent of patients in medical wards who had no relevant symptoms had phlebothrombosis. The detection of deep sole and calf vein thrombosis has therefore become very important and there are now new techniques which are complementary to each other and very promising.

The first is phlebography. This is a surprisingly benign procedure but puts the patient to some inconvenience, and if an urgent diagnosis is required the technique is cumbersome. Browse *et al.* (1969) studied 50 patients by bilateral phlebography following their first, or sometimes recurrent, pulmonary embolus. Nineteen were found to have fresh loose peripheral thrombus, and in eight of them the thrombus appeared big enough to cause a major pulmonary artery obstruction and death. They treated these 19 patients by vein ligation in addition to anticoagulants. They suggest that anticoagulants will not prevent all recurrent pulmonary emboli, and that phlebography, and if necessary surgery, might well become part of the routine investigations and treatment of all patients after their first pulmonary embolus.

Secondly, radio-active fibrinogen can be introduced into the foot or ankle veins and its course "tracked" up the venous pathway by counters.

Thirdly, ultrasonic methods of assessing venous blood flow will detect recent thrombi rapidly and with minimal distress to the patients (Evans and

Cockett, 1969). These authors describe a technique of examining the venous system from the calf to the inferior vena cava, and they report that their results compare favourably with those from phlebography. This ultrasonic Doppler principle clearly has considerable promise, and in a survey of general medical wards it has been surprising how many previously un-suspected deep-vein thromboses have been found.

If a pulmonary embolus occurs in a previously normal pulmonary circu-lation it will be lethal only if at least one-third of the lung vasculature is obliterated. The symptom of pulmonary embolism is dyspnoea. Pulmonary infarction will only occur when there has been pre-existing pulmonary venous hypertension, and the symptoms of infarction are dyspnoea, chest pain and haemoptysis.

There is very little evidence that there is any reflex pulmonary vaso-constriction consequent upon embolism, and the seriousness of the effects depend on mechanical blockage. Dyspnoea is vagally mediated and so is the "call for the bed pan". In animals, both phenomena can be abolished if vagotomy is done prior to experimental pulmonary embolism.

Repeated pulmonary emboli, packed together, may lead to progressive pulmonary hypertension and it is possible that primary pulmonary hyper-tension is caused in this way. This suggestion leads at once to the conclusion that more attention should be paid to looking for an embolic source in such patients.

The micro-embolic forms of pulmonary emboli are altogether different. Experimentally, foreign materials such as spores are often trapped deeply in the lung circulation if they are more than $5\,\mu$ in diameter, depending on their adhesiveness. Glass spheres will traverse the lungs with greater facility than lycopodium spores. In pulmonary arteries up to 1 mm in diameter, thrombi have been found which could well be microscopic emboli containing fibrin, platelets and leucocytes. They have been found especially in elderly people immobilized after injuries and with venous stasis. Smaller micro-emboli are usually less than $100\,\mu$ in diameter. They are found in the terminal arterioles or capillaries of patients who have had major surgery, especially vascular operations, and who go through a stage of post-haemorrhagic hypercoagulability.

In a recent survey by Vessey and Doll (1969), 84 patients were found to have deep-vein thrombosis or pulmonary embolism, 50 per cent of whom had used oral contraceptives during the month preceding the onset of their illness, while only 14 per cent of the 168 "controls" had done so. Of 17 patients with coronary thrombosis two had been using oral contraceptives, compared with an expected figure of 2·1. The patients with coronary thrombosis smoked more than the control patients, and were on the average 8·3 lbs heavier than "control" women of the same age and height. They conclude that "the new evidence strengthens the belief that oral contraceptives are a cause of venous thromboembolism and cerebral thrombosis, but does not indicate that they are a cause of coronary thrombosis".

In man, pulmonary embolism may cause right ventricular failure, so-called "shock" being accompanied by peripheral vasoconstriction, hypotension and a climbing jugular venous pulse. Right ventricular angina produces the same symptoms as those arising in the left heart and the differential diagnosis from myocardial infarction is very difficult. The presence of a right ventricular heave and a right ventricular fourth heart sound may be helpful. Atrial fibrillation complicates either event with equal frequency, and pulmonary embolism must always be considered in the aetiology of atrial fibrillation of acute onset. The electrocardiogram will be helpful only when the central venous pressure is raised, and the most important electrical sign is right bundle branch block. The radiology of pulmonary embolism is disappointing, the most likely early sign being a raised diaphragm. The shadows cast by pulmonary infarction are of any shape and are vague. With repeated pulmonary embolism, the main pulmonary artery enlarges and the periphery of the lungs becomes increasingly translucent and avascular.

Of all patients with acute pulmonary embolism, with or without infarction, two-thirds will die and probably about half the deaths will occur in the first year. Active treatment is, therefore, imperative. If time allows and there has not been an episode of cardiac arrest, it is highly desirable for an accurate diagnosis of the site of the block to be made. This can be done either by pulmonary angiography, which of necessity implies right heart catheterization, or by ultra-sound. The injection of radio-active tagged albumin aggregates followed by lung scanning will demonstrate any area of non-perfused lung, but this last test is vitiated by lung disease.

There are still newer methods of detecting pulmonary arterial block, such as drilling through the main pulmonary artery. The management of acute pulmonary embolism depends on the clinical state of the patient. If shock is not severe and the patient's condition is improving, the immediate problem resolves itself into thrombolytic therapy, defibrination or conventional anticoagulants.

One course of treatment is repeated injection of streptokinase; an initial loading dose of 0·6 mega units in 30 minutes is followed by 0·1 mega units per hour for two or three days.

Hirsch et al. (1968) describe their treatment of 18 patients. Twelve out of sixteen cases investigated showed angio-cardiographic improvement after 24 to 48 hours' treatment. They think that this treatment is most effective in aiding resolution after a single embolic episode.

The difficulties of treatment are that streptokinase has to be given through a pulmonary artery catheter and patient monitoring is very important with reference to arrhythmias, while repeated measurement of fibrinolytic activity must be made. If there is no evidence of embolic resolution after 24 hours, embolectomy should be considered. Defibrination by Arvin is a similar approach to treatment; this intriguing drug is the venom of the Malayan viper and has been described by Bell *et al.* (1968). Fibrinogen concentrations were measured and dosage was slowly increased taking about three weeks to reach pre-treatment fibrinogen level. These results were initially encouraging. There were no haemorrhagic episodes and two patients had normal menstrual periods while on Arvin treatment. In seven patients, there was rapid resolution of venous thrombosis. A point of interest is that there was improvement in venous thrombosis in patients who had previously received conventional anticoagulants. However, in early 1968, Petney and his colleagues reported two patients who underwent a second course of treatment with Arvin and were found to be refractory to it. Plasma from these patients neutralized the clotting effect of Arvin added *in vitro*. It appears, therefore, to be weakly antigenic and this precludes long-term treatment.

The use of anticoagulants of the coumarin variety is satisfactory in patients who have had a single venous thrombosis, and such an episode is usually safely treated in this way. However, in patients with a continuing predisposition to embolism, such as those with heart failure and atrial fibrillation, there is slight evidence that embolic resolution does occur, or is incomplete.

The use of heparin is a different matter, especially if given in high dosage. This is because the bronchoconstriction which accompanies pulmonary embolism is related to amine production resulting from thrombin-platelet interactions. Heparin blocks this, but only in much higher doses than are required to alter the thrombin-fibrinogen interation. If heparin is used it should be continued for about a week. Oral anticoagulants can be started on the second day of heparin treatment and continued for about a month, until all evidence of the thrombotic source has gone.

However, the ultimate decision must be made as to where the emboli have arisen, by methods mentioned above, and measures such as venous ligation undertaken in order to stop repetition. When pulmonary arteries are occluded with emboli, blood begins to flow past in minutes. The degree of perfusion will decide whether the patient dies or improves or whether his condition remains unstable. If the condition is deteriorating, or if shock or cardiac arrest have occurred, embolectomy has to be done. A decision must be made within the first two hours and the site of the embolus must be located if at all possible. The patient will probably already have been receiving heparin. If embolectomy is decided upon, the next step is to provide circulatory assistance with veno-arterial by-pass, and surprisingly low flows can be very helpful. The pulmonary artery is approached through a medium sternotomy. When the chest is opened the emboli are removed from central and peripheral arteries. The operative mortality is about 50 per cent. Embolectomy performed in hospital, without by-pass facilities, can at the best only be done by occluding the cavae (for a maximum of three minutes) and help the circulatory load by partial embolic removal. However, such operations can be completely life-saving, leaving no residual morbidity.

Dexter (1969) believes that in a 320-bed hospital only one or two patients a year will require embolectomy. This may be an under-estimate. However, the important fact is that definitive treatment is now available.

REFERENCES

BELL, W. R., PITNEY, W. R., OAKLEY, C. M. & GOODWIN, J. F. (1968). Therapeutic defibrination in the treatment of thrombotic disease. *Lancet*, **1**, 490.

BLOOMFIELD, D. K. & RUBINSTEIN, L. I. (1969). Mitral-valve prosthesis, warfarin anticoagulation and pregnancy. *Lancet*, **2**, 290.

BROWSE, N. L., LEA THOMAS, M., SOLAN, M. J. & YOUNG, A. E. (1969). Prevention of recurrent pulmonary embolism. *Brit. med. J.*, **3**, 382.

DEXTER, L. (1969). The management of pulmonary embolism. *J. roy. Coll. of Physicians (Lond.)*, **3**, 162.

EVANS, D. S. & COCKETT, F. B. (1969). Diagnosis of deep-vein thrombosis with an ultrasonic Doppler technique. *Brit. med. J.*, **2**, 802.

HIRSCH, J., HALL, G. S., McDONALD, I. G., McCARTHY, R. A. & PITT, A. (1968). Streptokinaise therapy in acute major pulmonary embolism; effectiveness and problems. *Brit. med. J.*, **4**, 729.

IONESCU, M. I. & ROSS, D. N. (1969). Heart-valve replacement with autologous fascia lata. *Lancet*, **2**, 335.

VESSEY, M. P. & DOLL, R. (1969). Investigation of relation between use of oral contraceptives and thromboembolic disease. *Brit. med. J.*, **2**, 651.

CARDIOMYOPATHY

Goodwin and his colleagues (1964) and Harris *et al.* (1968) have grouped cardiomyopathies into a practical classification of *congestive*, *restrictive*, and *obstructive* types. The term "cardiomyopathy" has probably had its use over-stretched because it is now used to describe not only abnormal cardiac muscle, but also metabolic and infective lesions of the myocardium.

Harris *et al.* (1968) have classified cardiomyopathies in children as *idiopathic* and *non-obstructive*. In their series there was no suggestion of an obstructive aetiology, but they have not suggested any alternative causation. They think that the pattern of the disease that they are describing is most consistent with the South African type of endomyocardial fibrosis, with frequent embolic episodes. They point out that the condition differs from the dense endomyocardial fibrotic inflow tract obstruction with destruction of the endocardium described by Davies (1948) in Uganda, but they quote only one case of ventricular restriction in their series in which compliance was reduced due to ventricular hypertrophy. In the remainder, there was patchy endocardial thickening containing both fibrous and elastic tissue, affecting the outflow more than the inflow tract and associated with cardiomegaly. Systemic embolism was common. There was sometimes cardiac enlargement, pulsus alternans and tall "a" waves in the jugular venous pulse, an atrial fourth heart sound, and electrocardiographic bi-ventricular enlargement.

Goodwin (1967) discusses *primary* cardiomyopathy in which the heart muscle is affected primarily, rather than secondarily to other diseases in the heart or elsewhere in the body, and *secondary* cardiomyopathy in which the heart lesion is just part of a generalized disease.

Primary cardiomyopathy

This may be due to viruses, endomyocardial fibrosis, endocardial fibro-elastosis, alcohol, pregnancy and the puerperium, or the aetiology may be unknown as in hypertrophic obstructive cardiomyopathy.

Endomyocardial fibrosis occurs in the humid districts of Africa. It has been attributed to various dietary deficiencies, infection, or even an African variant of acute rheumatism. However, it may occur in Europeans many years after they have left an endemic area. Despite lack of knowledge of its aetiology, there is considerable knowledge of the pathology, and it is constant. There is thick fibrous tissue covering the walls of the ventricles and invading the myocardium. When the right heart is involved the cusps of the tricuspid valves may be distorted, and gross right atrial enlargement and tricuspid incompetence ensue. The right ventricular cavity becomes increasingly obliterated. In the left ventricle a similar process occurs, leading to mitral incompetence and pulmonary venous hypertension. There may be a pericardial effusion and atrial fibrillation is common. Similar remarks apply to endocardial fibroelastosis except that the disease is not climatically determined, occurs usually during the first year of life, and mainly involves the left ventricle. The endocardium is covered with thick fibrous tissue which does not invade the endocardium. Mitral incompetence is common.

The virus about which most is known is the Coxsackie-B. Not only may this produce myocarditis, but also pericarditis, with or without effusion. There is now increased knowledge about the effect of Q fever on the myocardium. This disease is associated with myocarditis, usually valve regurgitation, fever, a normal white count, a low sedimentation rate, negative blood cultures, and suggestive blood titres.

Puerperal cardiomyopathy has evoked much discussion. It may not be a separate entity, but merely another form of cardiomyopathy brought to light by the altered hormonal environment of pregnancy. There is generalized "T" wave inversion in the electrocardiogram, which may persist for months or even years. The disease does not respond to any form of treatment, but a further pregnancy occurring in the presence of continuing electrocardiographic abnormalities may be lethal. Walsh *et al.* (1955) describe a number of undernourished negro women with this condition, but it also occurs in normally nourished European women.

Alcoholic cardiomyopathy is now regarded as a true entity. Unlike beri-beri, it is associated with a low cardiac output. Atrial fibrillation is common, and as in other forms of myocardial intoxication there is often a left ventricular third heart sound.

There is a further syndrome of cryptogenic primary cardiomyopathy, which begins with a series of febrile episodes and has a progressive and fatal course. The myocardium is fibrotic and infiltrated with round cells.

Obstructive cardiomyopathy most commonly involves the outflow tract of the left ventricle and there is asymmetrical hypertrophy of the myofibrils. The number of myofibrils in man is constant and each fibril is supplied by a single capillary. In the rat, partial occlusion of the aorta leads to left ventricular hypertrophy only if the pituitary is intact. Whether or not myofibrils are replaced is a matter of conjecture and interest. In obstructive cardiomyopathy the signs are those of subvalvular aortic stenosis, and the recognition of the condition is important, since it is amenable to surgical treatment.

When the right ventricle is involved, there is impairment of diastolic filling, and the signs are similar to those of constrictive pericarditis. Radiologically, there may or may not be cardiac enlargement and there is no calcification. Cardiac catheterization reveals a raised end-diastolic right ventricular pressure, and consequently the pressure may be raised in both atria.

Secondary cardiomyopathy

This condition may be due to a wide variety of diseases, amongst which are amyloidosis, scleroderma, leukaemia and polyarteritis nodosa. In cardiac amyloidosis, the electrocardiogram shows steep inversion of the anterior "T" waves, which is probably an indication of the duration of the disease. There is also macroglossia in this form of amyloidosis. In polyarteritis nodosa, there is not only arteritis of the smaller arteries and arterioles, but there may be aneurysm formation in the larger coronary arteries. In disseminated lupus erythematosus, there is often myocardial disease as well as nodules on the atrioventricular valves (Libman-Sack's disease). Myeloid leukaemia betrays itself by the blood count, splenomegaly and leukaemic retinal deposits. Retinal haemorrhages reflect the degree of anaemia rather than the total white cell count.

With the exception of surgery for an obstructed outflow there is no specific treatment in the majority of these conditions and treatment is therefore empirical, including that of the heart failure, with or without the use of steroids. Bacterial endocarditis is a hazard only recently recognized; it occurs at the atrioventricular valves and is presumably due to turbulence of flow because of distorted valves.

REFERENCES

GOODWIN, J. F. (1967). The cardiomyopathies. *Hosp. Med.*, **2**, 1008.

GOODWIN, J. F., GORDON, H., HOLLMAN, A. & BISHOP, M. B. (1964). Clinical aspects of cardiomyopathy. *Brit. med. J.*, **26**, 16.

HARRIS, L. C., RODIN, A. E. & NGHIEM, Q. X. (1968). Idiopathic non-obstructive cardiomyopathy in children. *Amer. J. Cardiol.*, **2**, 153.

WALSH, J. J., BURCH, G. E., BLACK, N. C., FERRANS, V. J. & HIBBS, R. G. (1965). Idiopathic myocardiopathy of the puerperium (post-partum heart disease). *Circulation*, **32**, 19.

MITRAL REGURGITATION

Regurgitation of blood through the mitral valve may be congenital (as in the cleft mitral cusp associated with a septum primum defect); or due to abnormal cusp tissue or chordae as in Marfan's syndrome; or it may arise from rheumatic or other acquired causes. Goodwin (1968) has given a very full account of the last. He points out that whereas deformity and perforation of mitral cusps often occur in bacterial endocarditis, many patients who develop regurgitation have a disordered sub-valvular apparatus, i.e. the papillary muscles and the chordae tendinae. He lists the following causes:

1. papillary muscle failure due to infarction, infection or infiltration;
2. rupture of one or more chordae tendinae, which may be spontaneous, the result of infection, or occasionally trauma;
3. papillary muscle function may be disordered in the cardiomyopathies, particularly in congestive cardiomyopathy, endomyocardial fibrosis, and hypertrophic obstructive cardiomyopathy.

The haemodynamic effects of papillary muscle failure and ruptured chordae tendinae are the same. If the patient suddenly develops pulmonary oedema following infarction (especially inferior infarction) it may well be due to papillary muscle failure, and there are the associated physical signs of mitral regurgitation, an apical "diamond" shaped murmur being associated with a third heart sound.

It has been suggested that failure of a posterior papillary muscle may lead to radiation of the murmur to the base of the heart, but not so with anterior papillary failure. Catastrophic pulmonary oedema is probably due to the presence of a previously normal left atrium with normal compliance. If death does not occur quickly, chronic pulmonary oedema may follow for weeks, or months. In a few instances it slowly improves due to hypertrophy of other papillary muscles and adaptation of the valve structure. In most instances surgery offers the only hope of relief, and repair of papillary muscles can produce dramatic improvement.

Rupture of a single chorda is not disastrous. It is probable that several chordae have to be ruptured before there is pulmonary oedema. It has been suggested that where there is spontaneous rupture of the chordae the mitral valve has been previously abnormal and unable to accept excessive strain.

In both these situations, atrial fibrillation is rare. In congestive cardiomyopathy, there is dilatation of the valve ring and it is associated with the physical signs found in rheumatic incompetence; i.e. low cardiac output, an apical presystolic murmur and a third heart sound at the apex.

In hypertrophic obstructive cardiomyopathy, mitral regurgitation is due to papillary muscle failure, with or without hypertrophy, unco-ordinated contraction and reduction in size of the left ventricular cavity. The regurgitant murmur is usually not pan-systolic.

"Sub-valvular" regurgitation can result from papillary muscle infiltration by such diseases as sarcoidosis (Raftery et al., 1966) or dermatomyositis.

In all these conditions, if the cardiac symptoms and signs are not associated with generalized disease, direct repair of papillary muscles should be attempted or the valve should be replaced. The terminology of cardiomyopathy is rather confused because it now incorporates myocarditis, which should really be an infective lesion. The aetiology of such infection is obscure, and may be associated with any systemic disease.

Brock (1958) described the first patient with obstruction of the left ventricular outflow tract and the subsequent descriptions of Teare show that there was asymmetrical hypertrophy of the myofibrils in this area.

There have now been many operations described in which there has been extraction of the excessive outflow load. This disease occurs not only in the left heart, but also in the right. It is probably unrelated to the other form of cardiomyopathy, which is so-called "congestive" and, therefore, it must be clear that one or two of these separate diseases must be defined. Surgery is clearly available to one, and not to the other. Infective cardiomyopathy, apart from such diseases as amyloidosis, is probably at the moment unstable. The aetiology of other cardiomyopathies is not adequately understood.

REFERENCES

BROCK, R. (1958). Principles in the surgical treatment of aortic stenosis. *Actachir. belg.*, **57**, 759.

GOODWIN, J. F. (1968). Acquired non-rheumatic mitral disease. *J. roy. Coll. Physicians (Lond.)*, **3**, 61.

RAFTERY, E. B., OAKLEY, C. M. & GOODWIN, J. F. (1966). Acute subvalvular mitral incompetence. *Lancet*, **2**, 360.

CARDIAC ARRHYTHMIAS

It has been calculated that the optimum pulse rate in a normal heart is 140 per minute: at this rate the heart is behaving most efficiently. It is probable

I

that in a normal heart, excessive rate of whatever duration will not lead to heart failure. Sinus tachycardia can be provoked by fever, emotion, hyperthyroidism, anaemia, etc. A low heart rate of 50 or 60 per minute is comparatively common in athletes with large hearts and an increased stroke volume.

Sinus bradycardia has been discussed under "Coronary Artery Disease". It is probably worth treating after a myocardial infarction if the electrocardiogram shows the "P on T pattern", because this may be a prelude to ventricular fibrillation. It is appropriately treated by 0·3 to 0·6 mg of atropine intravenously. Sinus tachycardia, without any underlying detectable pathological basis, should either be ignored or treated only by sedation.

Digitalis preparations

The main effect of any form of digitalis, whether it be the leaf or an alkaloid, is to increase cardiac efficiency. It is probably not important that it reduces ventricular rate, which it presumably does by increased vagal activity. Except for atrial flutter digitalis probably has little effect on the control of arrhythmias. In paroxysmal atrial fibrillation it will probably reduce the ventricular rate during an attack, but will have no influence in prevention of attacks. Digoxin is the most favoured alkaloid but it sometimes causes vomiting. Digitoxin is equally effective in improving myocardial efficiency and does not usually lead to nausea or vomiting. This may disguise the other toxic effects of the drug. It is always difficult to know whether a patient is adequately digitalized or not, and probably the most satisfactory means of doing this is to give an intravenous injection of acetyl-strophanthidin while the patient is under electrocardiographic control, because if this does not lead to further depression of the "junction J" of the "ST" segment, the patient is probably under-digitalized. Over-digitalization can lead to the dangerous situation of paroxysmal atrial tachycardia with block (PAT). The distinction between this and atrial flutter can be extremely difficult, and further digitalization may not only aggravate but also prolong the situation. Therefore, if there is doubt in this connection, the appropriate course of action is electrical cardioversion.

Electrical cardioversion as described by Lown *et al.* (1963) has altered the entire situation of arrhythmias. His major contribution was the placing of the "shock" in watt-seconds just after the nadir of the "R" wave. If the shock is put in later, ventricular fibrillation may ensue.

Electrical cardioversion is, therefore, the treatment of choice for any ventricular or supra-ventricular arrhythmias.

Other therapy

Quinidine depresses excitability, conduction velocity and contractility of the heart. Using quinidine sulphate, the blood level is not adequately maintained throughout the night hours. It is now more common practice to use

Kinidin (quinidine bisulphate) because the blood level is more likely to be sustained. Idiosyncrasy to any form of quinidine may cause nausea, vomiting, diarrhoea, tinnitus, erythematous or purpuric rashes and disturbed vision. The last is by far the most important, although it is very rare, because it may lead to optic atrophy. The suggestions that quinidine therapy may lead to embolic episodes is not substantiated. It is probable that patients requiring quinidine therapy are already prone to emboli, and the relation is probably coincidental rather than causal.

Patients who require cardioversion should be taken off digitalis and given quinidine at least a day prior to the procedure. The long-term effect of any form of quinidine in maintaining normal rhythm is very doubtful.

Procainamide has rather similar properties to quinidine; it has no value in supraventricular tachycardias, but is very valuable in ventricular arrhythmias. It is given in doses of 250–500 mg every six hours and has few complications, hypotension not being a disadvantage. The "PR", "QRS", and "QT" intervals are prolonged. The main value of this drug, therefore, is probably in repetitive ventricular tachycardia, which cannot be controlled by simpler means.

Lignocaine is a local anaesthetic and the most effective drug which can be used to prevent ventricular arrhythmias. There is therefore a case for its wide use immediately after myocardial infarction. The dose is 1–2 mg/kg of body weight, followed by 1–2 mg per minute. The initial dose can be given as 2 per cent solution intravenously. There are very few side-effects, but the drug has been implicated in thromboembolism; it is therefore wise to give heparin concurrently. Lignocaine should therefore be the first drug given to a patient with a cardiac infarction, accompanied of course by an analgesic.

In the case of other drugs, too little is known of their pharmacology. Propranalol decreases cardiac contractility which is a negative inotropic effect. It slows the heart rate which again is a negative chronotropic effect and it may have actions similar to quinidine, and also an anti-catecholamine effect. Propanalol reduces heart rate, stroke volume, cardiac output and systemic blood pressure. It has been used for a variety of arrhythmias but it arouses progressively less enthusiasm. It should not be given in the face of cardiac failure, because of reduction of "cardiac drive".

Diphenylhydantoin has long been used as an anti-epileptic agent, and it has more recently been used with success in ventricular arrhythmias. The dose is 3·5 mg/kg of body weight. Given in larger doses, it has been known to cause cardiac arrest.

Digitalis should be given in atrial arrhythmias not only with the idea of preventing left ventricular failure, but also to control the ventricular rate in atrial infarction, or events secondary to ventricular infarction.

Prolonged ventricular arrhythmias are often preceded by ventricular ectopic beats, especially if the ectopic beat is so close to the previous normal beat that the so-called "R on T pattern" is produced. Lignocaine intravenously is the drug of choice; it has fewer side-effects than quinidine or procainamide, but either of these drugs should be continued orally for about a month following an infarction. The initial dose of lignocaine is 100 mg intravenously, followed by an infusion of 2 g in 500 ml of laevulose at the rate of 2 mg a minute over 24 hours, and this is continued for about 48 hours. The same procedure is employed for ventricular tachycardia, but if it is unsuccessful, direct current shock is used. Therefore, a warning of a serious ventricular arrhythmia may be preceded by suggestive electrocardiographic changes and it is certain that these patients should be monitored.

Julian (1968) found that 17 of his 20 patients with ventricular fibrillation left hospital and were alive six months to two years later. His experience in patients with cardiac failure or shock were not nearly so good.

If complete heart block occurs it is usually within a few hours after myocardial infarction, and it may be preceded by bundle branch block or atrio-ventricular defects. It can be treated either by an infusion of 2–5 g of Isoprenaline in 500 ml of laevulose, or by a pacemaker inserted when the block occurred and therefore available for immediate use (Lassers and Julian, 1969).

Sutton *et al.* (1968) (p. 236) found a mortality of 45·5 per cent in 55 patients treated with artificial pacing for atrioventricular conduction defects. There was no statistical difference between the use of fixed-rate or demand pacemakers and the latter did not remove the risk of ventricular fibrillation. Adverse features associated with a high mortality were myocardial failure, anterior infarction and syncopal attacks.

Finally, a disorder known as "accelerated idioventricular rhythm" is fairly common. There are chains of complexes resembling a bundle branch block pattern at a slow rate, and either sinus bradycardia or atrioventricular interference dissociation; it requires no treatment.

Balcon *et al.* (1966) investigated the use of propanalol in acute myocardial infarction and found that its prophylactic or therapeutic value was negligible. In a controlled trial of 114 patients with a confirmed diagnosis, the mortality at 28 days was 23·3 per cent in the treated group, and 24·1 per cent in the control group.

Cardiac arrest leads rapidly to acidosis and many attempts have been made to combat it. In a multicentre controlled clinical trial by the Medical Research Council, the value of potassium, glucose and insulin was assessed. In the treated group, the mortality was 23·9 per cent and in the control groups, 25·3 per cent. Hence, there was no significant advantage in this type of therapy, nor was there any decrease in arrhythmias. This emphasizes how little is known about cell membrane equilibrium.

The prognosis for patients after their first myocardial infarction has been studied by Weinblatt *et al.* (1968) (p. 236). They present their findings of 881 men with a first myocardial infarction diagnosed over a four-year period in the Health Plan of Greater New York. Within one month of the attack, 36 per cent of the men experiencing their first myocardial infarction were dead. "For the 564 men who survive the first month after their initial myocardial infarction, the overall probability of surviving to 4·5 years after the event is 81 per cent. Survival over this period varies inversely with age—from 88 per cent of the men under 45 to 79 per cent of those aged 55 to 64, at the time of the myocardial infarction."

There is a higher mortality rate when angina has been present for two or more months prior to infarction. Pre-existence of hypertension is probably not important in increasing mortality rates except in the older age-groups. Once survived, the so-called severity of the attack has little bearing on the future. If this is judged by the severity of the pain, there is probably an inverse relationship between it and survival. Small areas of ischaemic muscle can be very painful, whereas large necrotic areas are often painless. A better guide to the future is probably the presence or absence of "Q" waves. Their presence means a transmural infarction which carries with it the inherent dangers of cardiac arrest, ventricular aneurysm, or even cardiac wall rupture.

In the New York series, the probability of surviving four to five years after the initial attack in males is 52 per cent. The correct value to put on the many parameters possibly concerned with prognosis have been ably attacked by Wolff *et al.* (1968), who conclude that "analysis of this data does not permit useful interpretation or, even worse, provides misleading statements that become embalmed in the literature of the field".

The obliteration of heart pain is a very interesting and rather confused matter. The cardiac afferent sympathetic fibres run alongside the coronary arteries. They can be interrupted by insertion of some foreign substance into the myocardium, such as omentum, talc or parts of the lung. It is probable that the result is the same in all these instances.

Another method of achieving the same end is to divide the first to fourth dorsal posterior roots. This operation can be done from a supra-clavicular approach. It is often argued that patients can take more exercise without pain after operation; this may be because of adequate denervation, or because the heart rate does not speed up to the same extent on effort. There are other approaches to persistent angina; one is the introduction of artificial myxoedema. This is an unsatisfactory procedure if one is dealing with people of high intellectual calibre. The serum cholesterol rises in two to three years after they have been treated, indicating that idiopathic myxoedema must usually be a disease of long standing. In the present context it also seems that the cholesterol level is not important.

The other approach to myocardial ischaemia is the Veinberg operation, which involves implantation of one or both of the internal mammary arteries into the heart. It is pointless to implant an internal mammary artery into fibrous tissue, and before the operation is contemplated the site of the arterial block should be known by coronary angiography, and it ought also to be known whether the ventricle is viable—that is expanding. If such a situation has been proven, the insertion of an internal mammary artery can be helpful, probably not through direct anastomoses, but through arterio-taxis. This process will take two to three months to develop and can be very effective, with the reservation that the operation involves opening the pericardium and hence the probable interruption of afferent sympathetic fibres.

REFERENCES

BALCON, R., JEWITT, D. E., DAVIES, J. P. H. & OSRAM, S. (1966). A controlled trial of propanolol in acute myocardial infarction. *Lancet*, **2**, 917.

JULIAN, D. G. (1968). The management of dysrhythmias in cardiac infarction. *J. roy. coll. Physicians (Lond.)*, **3**, 54.

JULIAN, D. G., LASSERS, B. W. & GODMAN, M. J. (1969). Pacing for heart block in acute myocardial infarction. *Ann. N.Y. Acad. Sci.*, **167**, 911.

LASSERS, B. W. & JULIAN, D. G. (1968). Artificial pacing in management of complete heart block complicating acute myocardial infarction. *Brit. Med. J.*, **2**, 142.

LOWN, B., PERLROTH, M. G., KAIDLREY, S., ABE, T. & HARKEN, D. E. (1963). "Cardioversion" of atrial fibrillation. A report on the treatment of 65 episodes in 50 patients. *New Eng. J. Med.*, **269**, 325.

WOLFF, G. A., VEITH, F. & LOWN, B. (1968). A vulnerable period for ventricular tachycardia following myocardial infarction. *Cardiovascular Res*, **2**, 111.

REPLACEMENT OF HEART VALVES

Over 15,000 Starr-Edwards silicone rubber-ball type of prosthetic valves have been manufactured. In an analysis of the late complications, Roberts and Morrow (1968) have encountered thrombosis of the prosthesis, diffuse secondary left ventricular fibroelastosisis after mitral valve replacement, aortic intimal proliferation with narrowing of the coronary ostia after aortic valve replacement, bleeding secondary to Warfarin-induced hypopro-thrombinaemia, aneurysm formation at the site of the excision of left ventricular papillary muscles, and degeneration of the silicone rubber aortic ball (ball variance). In each of the 12 necropsies carried out four months or more after aortic valve replacement, the rubber ball had degener-ated, and in all but one of these subjects ball variance was the cause of death. In this series, five out of six patients showed evidence of intravascular haemo-lysis. The incidence of ball variance is very much less in mitral prosthesis, presumably because of the difference in work done in relationship to velocity of blood flow.

The incidence of aortic ball variance is very difficult to assess, but it may complicate a third of operations carried out two years previously. The catastrophic suddenness of ball variance has naturally emphasized the importance of prediction. Probably the best available means is phono-cardiography, which should be carried out at frequent intervals. If the aortic opening click disappears or becomes muffled, a very good case can be made for replacement of the ball or the whole prosthesis. In view of the number of patients involved in this situation, diagnostic evidence of possible variance is very important.

In the future, stainless steel or cloth-covered balls may solve some of these problems and valve replacement is bound to continue.

When to replace heart valves

Braimbridge (1969) states that "the indications for any cardiac operation are the presence of symptoms preventing the patient from leading a reason-ably normal life, or the prognosis of the patient's disease being worse than the risks of surgery". He goes on to say that the average patient is referred for valve replacement because he is too breathless to lead a normal life. The mortality for prosthetic valve replacement is 10 per cent for a single valve and about 20 per cent for multiple valve replacement.

The problem of the moribund patient is emphasized by Emanuel (1968). He described four moribund patients who were restored to normal life by valve replacement. This outlines the point that cardiac failure is no longer a bar to cardiac surgery, and indeed at times, operation is life-saving.

With regard to the aortic valve, an isolated lesion of this can be treated either by a prosthetic valve, or by a "homograft". The advantage of the homograft is that long-term anticoagulants are unnecessary. Recently Ross (1968) has used the pulmonary valve cusps as an aortic graft with considerable success. Heterographic aortic valves avoid two disadvantages of homografts, the supply and size problems. The heterograft valve has been obtained usually from the pig and is sewn to a dacron-covered metal ring with struts for holding up the commissures. The "upside-down" valve has been shown to function well for at least two years, but long-term survival is uncertain, and some centres have already abandoned its use.

Grafted valves have the disadvantage of early calcification. How many valves to replace is a matter of great difficulty, and it has now been shown that many tricuspid valves thought to be competent are in fact found not to be so at operation.

Ionescu and Ross (1969) report a search for a better substitute for diseased heart-valves, and describe a technique using autologous fascia-lata grafts mounted on a supportive frame. They state that these grafts have been inserted into seven patients since April 1969 in the mitral, aortic, or tricuspid area, with good immediate results. No systemic emboli have occurred, and this is the more remarkable because anticoagulants were not used.

Bacterial endocarditis and prosthetic valves

This problem mainly involves the aortic valve. Continued malaise and fever following valve replacement are highly suspicious. These findings should lead to repetitive blood cultures, especially if aortic valve regurgitation develops. Secondly, when aortic valves become infected, it is either impossible or increasingly difficult to control the infection, and the only possible course of action may be valve replacement with or without previous catheterization and angiography. The same remarks apply to infected prosthetic seatings. When there has been multiple valve replacement it is obvious that a correct diagnosis presents insuperable difficulties. An interesting complication of these disorders is valve disease due to "Q" fever, and it would appear that such patients, once infected, do not respond to medical treatment: they must have their valves excavated and replaced.

Pregnancy and valve replacement

There are many young women who have had valve replacement who subsequently become pregnant. A report by Oakley (1968) discusses the dangers of anticoagulants and valve replacement during pregnancy. Other authors have pointed out that while coumarin derivatives pass the placental barrier, heparin does not, and it is therefore reasonable to allow such women to continue with coumarin until about the 36th week, and then replace it with heparin. This routine has proved to be effective.

Bloomfield and Rubinstein (1969) describe an uncomplicated pregnancy in a 27-year-old patient with rheumatic heart disease who had had a Starr-Edwards mitral valve prosthesis. During pregnancy, the patient took Warfarin sodium for 36 weeks and switched to heparin 18 days before delivery. A normal girl was born with a prothrombin-time that was only slightly prolonged. They believe that successful pregnancy and delivery in patients with mitral valve prosthesis is possible when careful control of anticoagulants is maintained.

REFERENCES

BENNETT, G. G. & OAKLEY, C. M. (1968). Pregnancy in a patient with a mitral-valve prosthesis. *Lancet*, **1**, 616.

BLOOMFIELD, D. K. & RUBINSTEIN, L. T. (1969). Mitral valve prosthesis, warfarin anticoagulation and pregnancy. *Lancet*, **2**, 290.

BRAIMBRIDGE, M. V. (1969). When to replace heart valve. *Med. News*, **1**, 5.

EMMANUEL, R. (1968). Too ill for cardiac surgery? *Brit. med. J.*, **2**, 400.

IONESCUE, M. I. & ROSS, D. N. (1969). Heart-valve replacement with autologous fascia lata. *Lancet*, **1**, 335.

ROBERTS, W. C. & MORROW, A. G. (1968). Fatal degeneration of the silicone rubber ball of the Starr-Edwards prosthetic aortic valve. *Amer. J. Cardiol.*, **22**, 614.

ROSS, D. (1968). Homograft replacement of the aortic valve. *Surgery*, **63**, 382.

8 The Medical Treatment of Malignant Disease

G. HAMILTON FAIRLEY

ACUTE LEUKAEMIA. CHRONIC MYELOID LEUKAEMIA. POLYCYTH-
AEMIA VERA. CHRONIC LYMPHOCYTIC LEUKAEMIA. HODGKIN'S
DISEASE. RETICULUM CELL SARCOMA. GIANT FOLLICULAR
LYMPHOMA. MYELOMATOSIS. MACROGLOBULINAEMIA. OTHER
MALIGNANT DISEASES.

IT is now nearly 100 years since Billroth (1871) first recommended arsenic for the treatment of Hodgkin's disease, but it is only in the last 25 years that significant advances have been made in the chemotherapy of malignant disease. Surgery and radiotherapy still remain the treatment of choice for localized tumours, but once spread has occurred beyond the point at which these two methods can be applied, one has to turn to medical treatment. Initially, this simply took the form of some drug that would attack all dividing cells, but additional methods are now available which include the use of hormones, enzymes and possibly in the future, immunotherapy.

It would not be possible, nor is this the place, to list all the various cancer chemotherapeutic agents with their modes of action, or to deal with every form of malignant disease. Instead, it is proposed to give a general outline of the commonly available forms of treatment, and to show how both the aims and the approach of chemotherapy have changed, with particular reference to the reticuloses (leukaemias and lymphomas) because it is in these diseases that the greatest advances have been made in the past decade.

Cytotoxic drugs

Most of the chemotherapeutic drugs used in malignant disease today interfere by one mechanism or another with the synthesis of DNA, RNA, or protein, and act against both malignant and normal cells. Figure 8.1 shows in a diagrammatic and very simplified form some of the points at which the more commonly used drugs act (modified from Connors, 1969).

Many cytotoxic drugs act as alkylating agents, and the first to be introduced was nitrogen mustard, at the end of the 1939–45 war. This was first used by Gilman and Philips (1946) and Wilkinson and Fletcher (1947). It is given in the form of mustine hydrochloride, by injection into a fast-running intravenous infusion to prevent burning of the tissues, and acts rapidly. Clearly it had disadvantages and many further compounds have been introduced

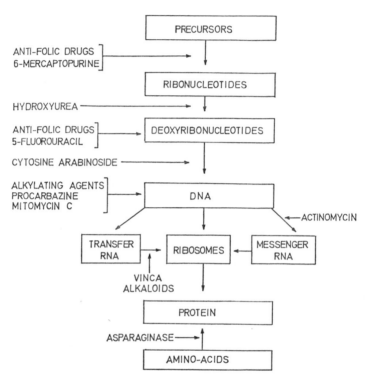

FIG. 8.1 Simplified diagram of the site of action of the agents most commonly used in the treatment of malignant disease.

which carry the nitrogen mustard warhead. The ones in common use at the present time are chlorambucil, melphalan, and cyclophosphamide. Other alkylating agents include busulphan (used in chronic granulocytic leukaemia) and a nitrosourea BCNU (used in acute leukaemia).

Another group of cytotoxic drugs are the antimetabolites. These compounds owe their action to the fact that they obstruct the working of an enzyme system because chemically they are very similar to but not identical with an enzyme substrate, and once combined with the enzyme prevent further reaction. The first to be used in man were the folic acid antagonists, by Farber et al. (1948) in acute leukaemia, the one in common use now being amethopterin (methotrexate). This was followed by the introduction of the purine antagonists, 6-Mercaptopurine, and more recently azathioprine (Hitchings and Elion, 1967); there are many more including cytosine arabinoside, hydroxyurea and 5-Fluorouracil.

Another group of cytotoxic agents come from bacteria and plants. The antibiotics—actinomycin, mitomycin, daunorubicin and adriamycin, and the vinca alkaloids—vinblastine and vincristine (from the plant Vinca rosea) have marked anti-tumour effects both in man and animals.

Hormones

Some tumours grow especially well in an environment where androgens predominate over oestrogens (e.g. carcinoma of the prostate) and the reversal of this balance by giving a synthetic oestrogen may lead to tumour regression and control of the disease for several years (see reviews by Hall, 1967; Fergusson, 1969). Similarly, treatment with androgens may be successful in controlling some cases of carcinoma of the breast for many years. In breast carcinoma also, changing the hormonal state by adrenalectomy, pituitary ablation, and the administration of synthetic adrenocortical hormones may also have a beneficial effect on the tumour (Hayward, 1968). More recently, progestational hormones have been used in malignant disease, particularly in carcinoma of the body of the uterus, ovaries and breast, and in hypernephroma (Briggs et al., 1967).

Adrenocortical steroids such as prednisone and prednisolone are widely used in the management of leukaemia. They have a direct effect on the malignant cells in acute lymphoplastic and chronic lymphatic leukaemia as well as in lymphosarcoma, and have additional advantageous actions in lessening the degree of haemolysis in a variety of malignant diseases. This decreases the tendency to haemorrhage in thrombocytopenia, and possibly protects the marrow to some extent against the toxic effects of other forms of chemotherapy and radiotherapy.

Enzymes

The observation by Kidd (1953) that guinea-pig serum would lead to the regression of some transplanted lymphomas led to the discovery by Broome (1961) that it was the presence of the enzyme L-asparaginase which was responsible for this effect. Broome showed that some malignant cells, particularly in leukaemia, were unable to synthesize asparagine and would die unless asparagine was present in the medium, or if the asparagine was destroyed by the enzyme asparaginase. From the theoretical viewpoint this is one of the most exciting developments in the treatment of malignant disease, for at last we have a metabolic defect in the malignant cell which is not present in a normal cell, and an enzyme which will therefore act specifically against the malignant cell, leaving the normal cells unaffected.

Unfortunately, although this enzyme is effective in killing some malignant cells in man, particularly in acute lymphoblastic leukaemia, (Hill *et al.*, 1967; Oettgen *et al.*, 1967; Beard *et al.*, 1970) resistance to L-asparaginase invariably develops, which limits its usefulness.

Immunotherapy

The value of immunotherapy has yet to be proved. There is no doubt that in experimental animals various immunological procedures can both prevent the induction of malignant disease, and cause some regression of existing tumours (Alexander and Fairley, 1964). However, all the evidence suggests that a powerful immune response is required to kill even a small number of malignant cells, and this form of treatment can be expected to be of value only in patients with minimal amounts of malignant disease (Fairley, 1969).

These agents may be used in a variety of ways:

1. As adjuvants to radiotherapy and surgery.
2. Singly:
    (*a*) continuous treatment
    (*b*) cyclical treatment
    (*c*) intermittent (pulse) treatment.
3. In combinations.

The problems of which method to use and the integration of medical with surgical treatment and radiotherapy are well illustrated by a consideration of the changes in the treatment of the reticuloses. These will therefore be considered in some detail and the problem of other forms of malignant disease briefly discussed in the light of these results.

ACUTE LEUKAEMIA

The change in the treatment of acute leukaemia reflects the altered attitude towards the treatment of malignant disease in general. At first, single agents were used in a continuous manner, and only when there was obvious resistance to a compound was another drug used. Fortunately resistance to one group of drugs is not necessarily accompanied by resistance to a different drug, and Table 8.1 shows that as more agents became available the prognosis of acute leukaemia in children improved.

One of the obvious facts about continuous chemotherapy is that the malignant cells eventually become resistant to the agent employed and the treatment has to be changed. Based on this fact the idea has developed that to give the known effective agents in a deliberate cyclical manner, changing from one drug to another at specific time-intervals, might lessen the chances of resistant populations of malignant cells emerging. This has been used most successfully in the maintenance treatment of acute lymphoblastic leukaemia of childhood by Zuelzer (1964), although a study undertaken by the Australian Cancer Society (1968) failed to reveal any difference between the cyclic and non-cyclic use of vincristine, 6-Mercaptopurine, methotrexate and cyclophosphamide in maintaining remissions in this disease.

TABLE 8.1

Median survival in children with Acute Lymphoblastic Leukaemia as more treatments have become available, based on the patients treated at the Memorial Hospital, New York

	Median Survival
No specific treatment	5 months
Folic-acid antagonists and corticosteroids	9 months
Purine antagonists	12 months
Vincristine and cyclophosphamide	14 months
Intensive combination chemotherapy	> 3 years

Originally, in acute leukaemia, single drugs were administered every day, but the work of Skipper (1968) has shown that with some agents, particularly methotrexate, intermittent administration is more effective both in animal leukaemia and in man. The probable reason for this is that the old concept that malignant cells are dividing rapidly is untrue (Cronkite, 1968). Indeed, in some malignant diseases the "cell-doubling time" may be much longer than with normal cells. The use of methotrexate in an intermittent manner enables the normal cells to recover more rapidly than the malignant cells between the doses of the drug, and when used in this way it can be given in larger doses and is much more effective in prolonging remissions in acute leukaemia in man (Djerassi, 1967; Frei, 1967) (Fig. 8.2) and in curing the L1210 leukaemia in mice. It is interesting that this concept does not apply to all drugs, e.g. 6-Mercaptopurine is no more effective when given intermittently than continuously.

Another concept which has proved to be of great value is the use of drugs in combination, and Figure 8.3 shows how the use of combinations of drugs is superior to the use of single agents in acute lymphoblastic leukaemia (Holland, 1968), the best combination being vincristine and prednisone.

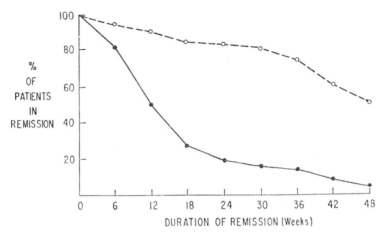

FIG. 8.2. Graph taken from an article by Frei (1967) showing the comparative effects of two dose schedules of methotrexate in maintaining remission in acute leukaemia in children
● 3 mg/m²/ day orally)
○ 30 mg/m² twice weekly by injection)
(Reproduced from an article by Frei in *Cancer Chemotherapy*, ed. I. Brodsky and S. B. Kahn, 1967. New York and London: Grune & Stratton.

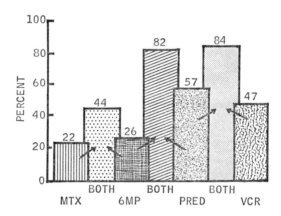

FIG. 8.3. Effect of single drugs and of combinations (shown in adjacent pairs) in inducing remissions in acute lymphoblastic leukaemia in children. (Reproduced from an article by Holland, J. F. in *Perspectives in Leukaemia*, ed. W. Dameshek and R. M. Dutcher, 1968. New York and London: Grune & Stratton.

There have been many in the past who have been critical of subjecting patients to intensive chemotherapy with all its accompanying toxicity in what is regarded as an inevitably fatal disease. However, an aggressive approach to the treatment of acute leukaemia is justified by the results of Burchenal

(1967), who has collected from the entire world 157 cases of proven acute leukaemia of all types, of whom 103 are alive and free from disease between five and seventeen years later (Table 8.2).

It is against this background that one must consider the present treatment of acute leukaemia.

TABLE 8.2

Long-term Survival in Acute Leukaemia
(Burchenal 1967)

	Number alive at 5+ years	Number free from disease at 5–17 years
Adults	30	16
Children	127	87
Total	157	103

The treatment of acute lymphoblastic leukaemia

It is now clearly established that failure to obtain a complete remission in this disease carries grave prognostic significance. Figure 8.4, which is taken from a paper by Frei (1967), shows the survival of patients in whom a remission was obtained on the first occasion, and those in whom it was not.

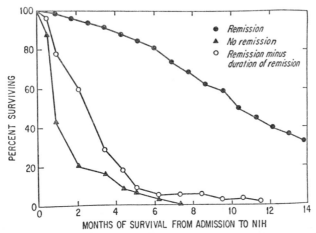

FIG. 8.4. The effect of obtaining a remission on the survival of children with acute lymphoblastic leukaemia admitted to the National Institutes of Health, Bethesda. (Reproduced from an article by Frei in *Cancer Chemotherapy*, ed. I. Brodsky and S. B. Kahn, 1967. New York and London: Grune & Stratton.)

The treatment most commonly used to achieve this is prednisolone or prednisone* 40 mg/m² (40 mg/per square metre of body surface) daily by mouth, together with vincristine 1·4 mg/m² weekly by intravenous injection.

Between 85 and 95 per cent of the patients will gain a complete remission with this combination. Some workers still use more intensive chemotherapy from the start, as given in the VAMP, POMP and BIKE regimes (see Table 8.3).

TABLE 8.3

Intensive Treatment Schedules for Acute Lymphoblastic Leukaemia carried out at the National Cancer Institute, Bethesda

1. *Vamp*
    5 courses each lasting 10 days were given during remission consisting of:
       Vincristine 2 mg/m²/week (2 injections per course)
       Methotrexate 20 mg/m² every four days I.V.
       6-mercaptopurine 60 mg/m²/day by mouth
       Prednisone 40 mg/m²/day by mouth

2. *Pomp*
    5 courses each consisting of:
       Vincristine 2 mg/m²/week I.V. (2 injections per course)
       Methotrexate 7·5 mg/m²/day I.V. for 5 days
       6-mercaptopurine 600 mg/m²/day I.V. for five days
       Prednisolone 1000 mg/m²/day I.V. for five days
          After five courses have been given courses are repeated monthly for twelve months

3. *Bike*
    First course (remission induction):
       Prednisone 40 mg/m²/day by mouth
       Vincristine 2 mg/m²/week I.V.
    Second course:
       Methotrexate 15 mg/m²/day I.V. for 5 days
    Third course:
       6-mercaptopurine 1000 mg/m²/day I.V. for 5 days
    Fourth course:
       Cyclophosphamide 1000 mg/m²/ I.V.—single dose
       Courses 2 and 4 were then repeated

A complete remission may be defined as the absence of any abnormal physical signs, such as lymphadenopathy and hepatosplenomegaly, a return to normal of the blood and bone marrow, and no evidence of leukaemia involving the nervous system or other organs. Once this has been achieved,

* In adults in Britain the dose of prednisone is often 40 mg per individual patient, but higher doses are used, particularly in the U.S.A.

further treatment is necessary, for without it the patients relapse quite rapidly—usually within a few months. This phase of treatment is termed consolidation or cyto-reduction, and it appears that some drugs are more efficacious in this phase than others. For example, when used alone to prolong remissions 6-Mercaptopurine is more effective than vincristine (Holland, 1968), and some authorities prefer to reserve some drugs for the induction of remissions, and others for maintenance (Fig. 8.5), although the distinction is

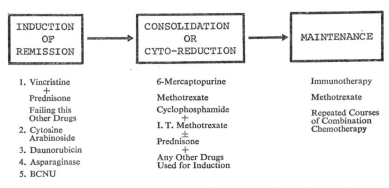

FIG. 8.5. Scheme for the treatment of acute lymphoblastic leukaemia.

not clear-cut. For example, it is still not clear in which phase of the disease it is best to use the enzyme L-asparaginase. It is, however, established that used alone, either in relapse or at the onset of the disease, remissions are obtained in over 30 per cent of the patients (Hill *et al.*, 1967; Oettgen *et al.*, 1967; Beard *et al.*, 1970). Unfortunately, resistance to this drug occurs quite easily, and it should now almost certainly be used in combination with other drugs and not as a single agent. Whether it is best used in remission or in the presence of detectable disease has yet to be established.

A further complication in the management of leukaemia in remission is that disease may exist undetected in organs which appear to be inaccessible to conventional treatment (Mathé *et al.*, 1965). For this reason it is necessary to give prophylactic intra-thecal methotrexate in the period of consolidation, and radiotherapy may be required for isolated masses arising in the bone, testis, ovaries, etc. It is interesting that these lesions often arise at a time when the blood and bone marrow are normal.

It is immediately apparent that the possible permutations and combinations are very considerable, and this creates one of the major problems in determining treatment at the present time. Many centres use different treatments, in an uncontrolled manner, and in insufficient numbers of patients to make analysis of the results possible. For this reason, in many countries large-scale trials are organized (in Britain by the Medical Research Council) to compare different regimes, and it is essential that as many centres as possible should collaborate in such trials, which have already proved to be of great value. For example, Holland (1969) reporting on the work of the Acute Leukaemia Group B in the U.S.A. has shown that after induction of re-mission, followed by various regimes of consolidation, a very effective form of maintenance is methotrexate given twice weekly by mouth. Mathé (1969) has also achieved long-maintained remissions using immunotherapy follow-ing intensive chemotherapy, with non-specific stimulation with BCG and/or specific immunization with irradiated leukaemic cells.

There is another reason why the treatment of acute lymphoblastic leuk-aemia should be based on centres with special knowledge and facilities. This is that the complications of the disease, particularly the occurrence of a haemorrhagic state due to thrombocytopenia and infections due to neutro-penia, have been accentuated due to the use of intensive chemotherapy. Indeed it is highly undesirable that such chemotherapy should be given unless facilities for platelet transfusions and nursing in a sterile environment are available. This does not mean that patients have to be treated in such centres all the time, but their treatment should be planned by such a centre and the facilities used for those periods during the disease when they are required (James et al., 1967; Fairley, 1969).

If a remission is not obtained with the combination of vincristine and pred-nisolone, the other drugs listed in Figure 8.5 should be used, and if these fail the compounds normally reserved for the consolidation period should be tried. When a patient in remission relapses, vincristine and prednisolone should be used again, and often another remission is obtained. Failing this, the other drugs should be used.

Quite deliberately, no attempt has been made to give a specific regime for the treatment of acute lymphoblastic leukaemia, because the detail changes so rapidly. However, the principles are unlikely to alter greatly in the immediate future, and are worth reiterating.

First, the treatment should be planned in collaboration with a special centre whose facilities may be required at a time when intensive chemo-therapy is used.

Secondly, the essential initial aim is to produce a remission. This should be followed by further intensive chemotherapy to reduce the number of malig-nant cells as far as possible. Finally, some form of maintenance treatment should follow this, as shown in Figure 8.5. The Medical Research Council in this country has a controlled trial for the treatment of acute lympho-blastic leukaemia, and the more cases admitted to this study the more quickly we will be able to determine the best forms of treatment.

Acute myeloblastic leukaemia

Until very recently, treatment for this form of leukaemia has been most disappointing, and there has even been a controversy between Crosby

(1968) and Boggs *et al.* (1969) as to whether myeloblastic leukaemia should be treated at all. However, the introduction of the newer drugs such as cytosine arabinoside and daunorubicin have changed the attitude to treatment, although the prognosis is still much worse than in acute lymphoblastic leukaemia.

It is clearly logical to apply the same principles to the treatment of myeloblastic leukaemia as those already discussed for lymphoblastic leukaemia, though the individual drugs used may differ. For example, vincristine and prednisone, which are so effective in acute lymphoblastic leukaemia, are less effective than daunorubicin and cytosine arabinoside in acute myeloblastic leukaemia. As with lymphoblastic leukaemia, if a remission is not obtained other drugs must be used.

The position in acute myeloblastic leukaemia is not as clear as in acute lymphoblastic leukaemia, and further studies are required to determine which combinations are likely to be most effective. For example, the place of asparaginase is uncertain. It readily clears blast cells from the blood without materially affecting the marrow, so it may have a role if used in combination with other agents (Beard *et al.*, 1970). A suitable scheme is shown in Figure 8.6, and trials are being arranged to assess the effect of different combinations of drugs in this disease, one of which is now under way, organized by the Medical Research Council.

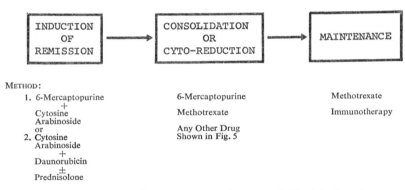

METHOD:

1. 6-Mercaptopurine + Cytosine Arabinoside or 2. Cytosine Arabinoside + Daunorubicin ± Prednisolone	6-Mercaptopurine Methotrexate Any Other Drug Shown in Fig. 5	Methotrexate Immunotherapy

FIG. 8.6. Scheme for the treatment of acute myeloblastic leukaemia.

CHRONIC MYELOID OR GRANULOCYTIC LEUKAEMIA

This disease belongs to the group of diseases termed "chronic myeloproliferative disorders" by Dameshek and Gunz (1964). This group is characterized by chronic proliferation of the cells in the bone marrow, and although clear syndromes may be recognized by the cell line chiefly involved, there is usually proliferation of the other elements as well.

For this reason the treatment of these syndromes, which include poly-cythaemia vera, essential thrombocythaemia and myelofibrosis as well as chronic granulocytic leukaemia, is very similar and involves either radio-therapy in the form of ^{32}P, or chemotherapy, usually in the form of busulphan.

The aims of treatment in chronic granulocytic leukaemia differ from those in acute leukaemia. As acute leukaemia is fatal unless treated, and relapse occurs rapidly unless intensive chemotherapy is given, the aim of treatment is to attempt to kill all the malignant cells with the goal, rarely achieved, of curing the disease. This has not been done in the chronic stage of chronic granulocytic leukaemia for two main reasons: first, intensive chemotherapy inevitably carries a mortality, particularly if special isolation facilities and platelet infusions are not readily available; since it is now established that conventional chemotherapy can keep patients in good health for several years without any real risk, such a procedure would be unjustified. Secondly, since the hallmark of chronic granulocytic leukaemia (the Philadelphia chromosome) has been found not only in the cells of the granulocyte series, but also in the normoblasts, it is suggested that to cure the basic defect one would have to destroy all the cells in the bone marrow, a hazardous under-taking (Clein and Flemans, 1966; Rastrick et al., 1968; Rastrick, 1969). Most authorities would now agree that the best treatment at the present time is to control the disease during the chronic phase, and to use intensive chemo-therapy only during the terminal blastic phase of the disease.

There are two main forms of treatment for controlling the chronic phase of this disease: ^{32}P (Osgood et al., 1956) and busulphan (Galton, 1969). Until busulphan was introduced by Haddow and Timmis (1953) and Galton (1953), radiotherapy in the form of external irradiation of the spleen or ^{32}P was probably the best way of controlling the disease. However, busulphan has been shown to be superior to ^{32}P in a Medical Research Council trial reported in 1968. Both the survival and the control of the disease were better in those treated with busulphan than with radiotherapy. It is interesting to note that although the quality of life has been improved by controlling the size of the spleen, correcting the anaemia and keeping the white blood count in the region of 10,000–15,000/cu.mm by treatment with busulphan, the time-interval between the diagnosis and the onset of the blastic phase of the disease has not been significantly prolonged. Indeed, the entire life-span may not have been greatly lengthened since treatment for the blastic phase is rarely successful. The mean survival is between three and four years from diagnosis (Scott, 1957).

Busulphan is given initially in a dose of 4 mg daily by mouth, and the subsequent dose is titrated against the clinical response, particularly the blood count. There are two major disadvantages in the use of busulphan; first, if too much is given bone marrow aplasia occurs, which is usually irreversible and may prove fatal; secondly, long-term treatment for several years produces the complications of pulmonary fibrosis (Oliner *et al.*, 1961), pigmentation, anorexia, and weight loss in a syndrome resembling Addison's disease (Kyle *et al.*, 1959; Harrold, 1966). For this reason, busulphan treatment may have to be stopped and then either dibromomannitol (Eckhardt *et al.*, 1963) or hydroxyurea (Fishbein *et al.*, 1964; Kennedy and Yarbro, 1966; Malpas, 1967; Weil and Tanzer, 1967) should be used.

Once the blastic phase of the disease occurs, busulphan ceases to be effective, and the various forms of treatment used for acute myeloblastic leukaemia can be tried, but usually without any marked success.

POLYCYTHAEMIA VERA

The problem of the management of polycythaemia vera has recently aroused great interest. Before embarking on treatment for any disease, it is important to know whether it is really necessary; i.e. what happens to patients who are treated, compared with those who are not.

The most impressive evidence that polycythaemia vera must be treated comes from Denmark. Videbaek (1950) reviewed 125 patients diagnosed between 1920 and 1945. Many of these patients were inadequately treated by modern standards, and the median survival time (i.e. the time when 50 per cent of the patients were dead) was only four and a half years for men and eight and a half years for women. As with many diseases, the prognosis was better in women than in men. Chievitz and Thiede (1962) analysed 250 cases of polycythaemia vera who died between 1933 and 1961 and found that 50 per cent of the patients who received no treatment were dead in eighteen months. Of those treated with venesection alone 50 per cent were dead in three and a half years, and of those treated with radiotherapy 50 per cent were dead in 12 years (Fig. 8.7). This showed first that polycythaemia vera must be treated, and secondly that venesection alone is not enough, although it may form an essential part of the treatment. Additional treatment in the form of chemotherapy or radiotherapy must be given.

By venesection it is possible to lower the PCV rapidly, whereas both radiotherapy and chemotherapy may take many weeks to produce their effect. The reason that venesection alone is inadequate is that it fails to influence the white cell and platelet counts, and hence does not control the vascular complications, which account for most of the early deaths in this disease.

As with chronic granulocytic leukaemia, the two ways of controlling this disease are by chemotherapy or radiotherapy. The most commonly used drug is busulphan (Myleran), which was introduced by Galton (1953) and Haddow and Timmis (1953) for the treatment of chronic myeloid leukaemia. It was therefore logical to use it in other myeloproliferative disorders. There is no doubt that some patients can be successfully controlled using this drug

(Perkins *et al.*, 1964) although Killman and Cronkite (1961) found that the dose was limited by thrombocytopenia, and venesection was needed to control the PCV. In addition, continuous treatment with busulphan needs very careful supervision, and the patients must be seen at frequent intervals since bone marrow suppression may be irreversible and pigmentation and interstitial pulmonary fibrosis may occur (Galton, 1953; Leake *et al.*, 1963; Harrold, 1966).

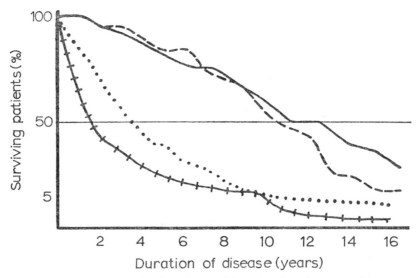

Fig. 8.7. Survival of patients with polycythaemia vera with different forms of treatment. (Reproduced from an article by Chievitz, E. and Thiede, T. in *Acta med. Scand.* (1962), **172**, 513).
+++++ Untreated
.... Venesection alone
————— X-ray therapy alone
- - - - - - - Various combinations with X-ray therapy.

The other drug, pyrimethamine (Daraprim), which is a folic acid antagonist, was first used by Isaacs in 1954 in the treatment of polycythaemia vera. It may also cause a pancytopenia, but this is rapidly reversible with folic acid. As with busulphan, the patients have to be seen at frequent intervals since folic-acid deficiency may precipitate a sudden fall in the white cell and platelet counts, and even cause a marked anaemia unless the dose is carefully controlled. Other side-effects include nausea and vomiting, buccal ulceration and exfoliative dermatitis (Perkins *et al.*, 1964).

The other major treatment for polycythaemia vera is radiotherapy. Initially, it was given as total irradiation (spray treatment) but this was replaced by ^{32}P which was first used by Lawrence in California (Lawrence, 1940). The advantages of ^{32}P are considerable: it is easily given by intravenous injection, the exact dose each patient has received is known, which is not always the case with oral chemotherapeutic agents, and there are no side-effects. The only disadvantage of ^{32}P is that it may cause acute leukaemia.

There has been much confusion in the past about leukaemia in poly-cythaemia. There is no doubt that whether polycythaemic patients are treated with ^{32}P or chemotherapy, or not treated at all, a blood picture closely resembling chronic myeloid leukaemia may occur. This is not surprising, since polycythaemia is a myeloproliferative disorder and the white cell count is frequently raised at some point in the disease: nor is it surprising that thrombocythaemia occurs, or that the proliferation of cellular elements may give way to proliferation of fibrous tissue, causing myelofibrosis. These changes occur as a natural part of the disease.

However, the occurrence of acute leukaemia, which is infiltration of the marrow with blast cells, is quite different. There is no doubt that acute leukaemia, when it occurs in polycythaemia, is much commoner in patients treated with ^{32}P. The incidence of acute leukaemia in four published series of patients treated without any form of irradiation was one out of 233 deaths (0·4 per cent) (Tinney et al., 1945; Chievitz and Thiede, 1962; Perkins et al., 1964; Modan and Lilienfeld, 1965). In patients treated with ^{32}P, acute leukaemia was responsible for between 8 and 30 per cent of the deaths in the series described by Stroebel et al. (1951); Wiseman et al. (1951); Wasserman (1954); Lawrence (1955); Ledlie (1960); Modan and Lilienfeld (1965); and Watkins et al. (1967). From this there can be no doubt that the incidence of acute leukaemia is greatly increased if the patients receive ^{32}P, which is hardly surprising in view of the reports of leukaemia following nuclear explosions (Moloney and Kastenbaum, 1955), and therapeutic irradiation of the marrow in ankylosing spondylitis and other diseases (Moloney, 1959; Court Brown and Doll, 1965).

This situation can be resolved only by comparing the results in patients treated with and without irradiation. In patients who have not been treated or who have received inadequate treatment, over 50 per cent die of thrombosis or haemorrhage (Videbaek, 1950; Chievitz and Thiede, 1962) compared with 25 to 40 per cent of patients treated with ^{32}P (Wasserman, 1954; Stroebel et al., 1951; Lawrence, 1955; Ledlie, 1966). In the series of 127 patients managed without radiation therapy reported by Perkins et al. (1964) 46 per cent died of haemorrhage, thrombosis or ischaemic heart disease.

Apart from the cause of death, the survival of patients treated with and without ^{32}P appears to be the same. The median survival of patients treated with ^{32}P was found to be 13·3 years by Massouredis and Lawrence (1957) and 13·6 years in patients managed without radiotherapy (Perkins et al., 1964). It is interesting that another group of workers in Manchester

(Halnan and Russell, 1965) have treated 107 patients with ^{32}P and compared their results with those of Perkins *et al.* (1964), finding no significant difference in survival. Our results at St Bartholomew's Hospital, where we have used ^{32}P extensively, support this conclusion (Watkins *et al.*, 1967).

Hume *et al.* (1966) found that, by measuring the red cell volume, using ^{51}Cr, and relating this to lean body mass, the dose of ^{32}P required to reduce the red cell volume to normal could be predicted, and was in fact less than the dosage customarily used. This is of considerable importance in avoiding over-treatment and unnecessary irradiation.

It would seem, therefore, that there is no statistically significant difference between the survival of patients treated with chemotherapy and those treated with radiotherapy, and yet the matter cannot be allowed to rest with this conclusion; for Osgood (1964), using the same data as Modan and Lilienfeld (1965) concluded that although ^{32}P increased the risk of acute leukaemia, it prolonged life in polycythaemia more effectively than any other treatment.

One has to weigh the advantages of ^{32}P (the ease of administration, the lack of side-effects, the accurate control of the dosage, and the fact that it is always given by experts) against the disadvantage of causing acute leukaemia. Similarly, with chemotherapy the advantage of a low incidence of acute leukaemia must be weighed against the presence of side-effects, the difficulty of controlling dosage, and the possibility of irreversible and fatal damage to the marrow. If Osgood (1964) is right in saying that ^{32}P is the most effective treatment for polycythaemia, it would be a great pity to abandon it in favour of chemotherapy without good reason.

It is, therefore, our policy at the present time to control the red cell count by means of venesection and to give ^{32}P for the control of the platelet count. We try to give as small a dose of ^{32}P as possible, and reserve chemotherapy in the form of busulphan for the later stages of the disease, particularly if a chronic myeloid leukaemic blood count develops.

CHRONIC LYMPHOCYTIC OR LYMPHATIC LEUKAEMIA

This lymphoproliferative disorder differs greatly from either acute leukaemia or chronic granulocytic leukaemia. First, the age distribution is the same as for carcinomas, becoming more frequent with advancing years; secondly, it very rarely becomes transformed into a terminal "blastic" phase, but the behaviour can change to that of an invasive lymphosarcoma; thirdly, immunological abnormalities arise with impairment of antibody formation and sometimes auto-immune haemolytic anaemia, both of which may require treatment; fourthly, in the absence of symptoms, excessive glandular enlargement, anaemia, or thrombocytopenia, the disease may remain stationary for many years without treatment, unlike the other forms of leukaemia where deterioration inevitably occurs in untreated cases.

There are three main forms of treatment for chronic lymphocytic leukaemia: radiotherapy, cytotoxic drugs, and corticosteroids, each of which may be used under different circumstances. First, it must be emphasized that it may be quite unnecessary to give any treatment at all, and there is certainly no indication simply to reduce the number of lymphocytes in the peripheral blood if this is the only abnormality.

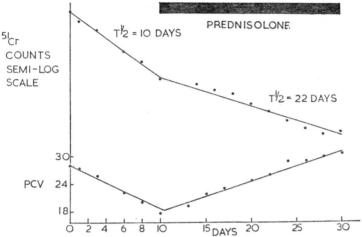

FIG. 8.8. The changes in the packed cell volume and survival of 51Cr-labelled red cells in a patient with chronic lymphocytic leukaemia and a negative Coombs test, before and during treatment with prednisolone.

The best group of drugs for the treatment of this disease is the nitrogen mustard group, and the one most commonly used is chlorambucil (Galton et al., 1961) although cyclophosphamide is equally effective (Fairley, 1964). As with chronic myeloid leukaemia, the aim is to control the disease, not to attempt a radical cure, and most people use conventional doses of these drugs, the starting dose for chlorambucil being 0·2 mg/kg, and the dose is slowly reduced as the disease is controlled. Some authorities now recommend the use of larger doses intermittently rather than conventional doses given continuously. In addition to reducing the number of lymphocytes in the blood and marrow, these drugs usually cause a reduction in the size of the enlarged lymph nodes, liver and spleen as well, but have less effect on anaemia and thrombocytopenia.

If anaemia and thrombocytopenia are present corticosteroids should be used (Galton et al., 1961; Dameshek and Gunz, 1964) and may be rapidly effective. Autoimmune haemolytic anaemia may occur in this disease, but even in the absence of a positive Coombs test there may be a marked haemolytic component in the anaemia. For example, Figure 8.8 shows the effect of treatment with prednisolone on both the packed cell volume and the rate of destruction of the red blood cells in a patient with chronic lymphocytic leukaemia in whom the Coombs test was negative. Before receiving prednisolone (40 mg daily), the PCV was falling and the $T\frac{1}{2}$ (half-life) of ^{51}Cr-labelled red cells was ten days. Immediately prednisolone was given the PCV started to rise, and the $T\frac{1}{2}$ of the labelled red cells was lengthened to 22 days. A similar effect may occur with thrombocytopenia, and in the presence of anaemia, thrombocytopenia, marked lymphocytosis and enlarged glands it is often desirable to treat the patient with prednisolone first, and to add chlorambucil later.

Radiotherapy has been used in the past in the form of ^{32}P to control the disease, but it is now reserved for the local treatment of large glandular masses which may respond more rapidly to irradiation than to chemotherapy. The tumours also tend to be very radio-sensitive, responding to much smaller doses than are required for reticulum cell sarcoma and Hodgkin's disease.

Finally, a further complication in the management of this disease is liability to infection, due both to granulocytopenia and to an inability to form circulating antibody. Hypogammaglobulinaemia is a constant feature which becomes more pronounced as the disease progresses. Infections may be prevented by regular injections of gammaglobulin (Shaw et al., 1960; Fairley and Scott, 1961), but these are expensive and have only a slight advantage over the use of antibiotics.

HODGKIN'S DISEASE

Considerable advances have recently been made in the treatment of Hodgkin's disease. There is now no doubt that patients with localized disease (Stages I and II—Table 8.4) should be treated with intensive wide-field radiotherapy, with the result that as many as 80 per cent will be permanently cured (Peters and Middlemiss, 1958; Easson and Russell, 1963; Kaplan, 1966). This dramatic improvement is due to improved radiotherapeutic techniques, so that large doses of irradiation can be given not only to the involved area but to the adjacent lymph node areas as well. Another factor may be that with improved methods of investigation, particularly the introduction of lymphangiography to demonstrate the iliac and para-aortic glands, the exact anatomical extent of the disease can be assessed more accurately and correct staging carried out.

Because radiotherapy is the treatment of choice for patients with localized disease, chemotherapy is reserved for those patients who have disseminated disease at the time of presentation, or who have recurrence in previously irradiated areas making further radiotherapy impossible.

Until recently, the effective drugs such as the nitrogen mustards (mustine hydrochloride, chlorambucil, cyclophosphamide) vinblastine, and procarbazine, were used as single agents. We found that definite objective improvement occurred in about 70 per cent of the patients (Fairley *et al.*, 1966). However, Lacher and Durrant (1965), using a combination of vinblastine and chlorambucil, obtained complete remissions in 63 per cent, and partial remissions in a further 18 per cent in disseminated Hodgkin's disease. At the National Cancer Institute, Bethesda, Carbone and his colleagues (Carbone, 1967; DeVita *et al.*, 1969) using four agents simultaneously—prednisone, vincristine, nitrogen mustard and procarbazine—obtained 80 per cent complete remissions, and 90 per cent complete + partial remissions in patients with Hodgkin's disease who had previously received no treatment. Similar results have been obtained by Bernard and his colleagues in Paris (Bernard *et al.*, 1967; Goguel *et al.*, 1969).

TABLE 8.4

Rye Method of Staging Hodgkin's Disease
(Peters *et al.*, 1966)

Stage 1	Disease limited to one anatomical region
Stage II	Disease confined to one side of the diaphragm
Stage III	Disease on both sides of the diaphragm but limited to involvement of lymph nodes and spleen
Stage IV	Involvement of bone marrow, lung, pleura, liver, bone, skin, kidneys, gastrointestinal tract or any tissue other than lymph nodes and spleen

If the systemic symptoms of fever, sweating, pruritus and weight loss are absent the patients are classified as "A", and if they are present as "B".

As these results are so much better than those obtained using single agents, we have also been using combination chemotherapy for the past two years. Our regime has changed slightly in detail, but not in principle from that used at N.I.H. (Carbone, 1967) and by Bernard *et al.* (1967). First, we have used a smaller dose of prednisone but have given it with every course. Secondly, we have used vinblastine rather than vincristine because vinblastine is known to be very effective as a single agent in Hodgkin's disease, and is less neurotoxic than vincristine. Thirdly, we have lengthened the time interval between courses from two to four weeks. Our regime is as follows:

Prednisolone 40 mg. (for an adult patient) by mouth days 0–14 inclusive.
Procarbazine 100 mg/m^2 daily by mouth days 0–14 inclusive.
Vinblastine 10 mg (for an adult patient) on days 0, 7, and 14 intravenously.
Mustine hydrochloride 6 mg/m^2 on days 0 and 7.

Prednisone, or prednisolone, was included in this regime for two reasons. First, to protect in some degree against the toxic effects on the bone marrow, and secondly, because steroids have a limited but useful role in the treatment of Hodgkin's disease, even when used alone, by reducing fever, lessening haemolysis, and in some instances causing gland regression.

Our results (Nicholson *et al.*, 1970) are very similar to those obtained by both the French and American groups (DeVita *et al.*, 1969; Goguel *et al.*, 1969) and are summarized in Table 8.5. As one would expect, the best

TABLE 8.5

Initial Response to Combination Chemotherapy in Hodgkin's Disease

Group	Total	Complete Remission	Partial Remission	Failure
No previous treatment	5	4	1	0
Only radiotherapy in the past	10	10	0	0
Chemotherapy ± radiotherapy in the past	18	4	10	4
Total	33	18	11	4

patients were those who had been treated with radiotherapy only in the past, i.e. they had initially presented with localized disease which had been successfully treated but had developed recurrence. Patients who had had no previous treatment, i.e. those who had presented initially with generalized disease, responded reasonably well, but those who had received both chemotherapy and radiotherapy in the past, i.e. the most advanced cases, did not respond so well.

There is no doubt that combination chemotherapy produces a higher proportion of both complete and partial remissions than the use of single agents in Hodgkin's disease. Furthermore, the response to treatment is more rapid than with single agents, and the time interval between each course probably gives the normal tissues, particularly the bone marrow, an opportunity to recover, enabling a larger total amount of chemotherapy to be given. We still do not know whether remissions obtained in this way will last longer than those obtained by using single agents, but the results of DeVita *et al.* (1969) suggest that they may.

Our results suggest that the bone marrow toxicity of combination chemotherapy is much greater in patients who have previously received continuous treatment with single cytotoxic agents, and such treatment should be given with caution to these patients, probably with modified doses. With patients who have had no previous chemotherapy it has been gratifying that the leucopenia and thrombocytopenia have always recovered.

These results raise another and very important problem in the treatment of Hodgkin's disease, which is the indication for using chemotherapy as opposed to radiotherapy. Using the Rye classification shown in Table 8.4, everyone is now agreed that Stage I and II disease, i.e. disease confined to lymph nodes situated on one or other side of the diaphragm, must be treated with high dosage wide-field irradiation, and that Stage IV disease, i.e. disease which is disseminated to involve organs other than lymph nodes or spleen, should be treated with chemotherapy. The problem centres around the treatment of patients with Stage III disease, i.e. disease confined to lymph nodes but present on both sides of the diaphragm. Smithers (1969) recommends treating patients with Stage IIIA disease with radiotherapy, and Kaplan (1968) includes IIIB as well. Others are still treating Stage III disease with chemotherapy. Certainly the initial response to combination chemotherapy in those patients in whom chemotherapy is being used for the first time compares very favourably with Kaplan's patients treated with radiotherapy. It remains to be seen which group has the better ultimate prognosis. A controlled trial of the two forms of treatment in Stage III is highly desirable.

RETICULUM CELL SARCOMA

The same principles apply to the treatment of this disease as in Hodgkin's disease. Radiotherapy is undoubtedly the treatment of choice for localized disease, although as yet there has been no large series of patients treated with wide-field radiotherapy including the adjacent non-involved lymph node areas. There are two main reasons for this: first, reticulum sarcoma is not as common as Hodgkin's disease, and secondly, although on many occasions Hodgkin's disease recurs in adjacent lymph node areas, this is not so in reticulum cell sarcoma (Smithers, 1967).

Similarly, with chemotherapy, single agents were used until recently on a continuous basis for generalized disease. Now, following the success of combination chemotherapy in Hodgkin's disease and acute leukaemia, this form of treatment is being used in reticulum cell sarcoma. We have used the same combination as in the National Institutes of Health programme (Carbone, 1967) using vincristine, prednisolone, procarbazine (Natulan) and mustine hydrochloride, as already stated in the section on Hodgkin's disease. It is too early to assess the long-term effect of this form of treatment, but some of the initial results have been most encouraging. Hoogstraten et al. (1969) compared the use of cyclophosphamide alone with a combination of cyclophosphamide, vincristine, and prednisone, and found the latter to be superior.

However, both radiotherapy and chemotherapy are less effective in reticulum cell sarcoma than in Hodgkin's disease, and the prognosis is usually poor, although occasional long-term survivors exist.

GIANT FOLLICULAR LYMPHOMA AND LYMPHOSARCOMA

Once again, the principles of treatment are identical with those for Hodgkin's disease and reticulum cell sarcoma, with radiotherapy for local lesions and chemotherapy for generalized disease. Giant follicular lymphoma (Brill-Symmers disease) frequently presents as localized disease, and if it is treated at this stage there may be an interval of many years before any evidence of recurrence occurs. Indeed, with isolated involvement of the spleen, splenectomy has led to long survival or even "cures" in some cases. The drugs used in this group of diseases may be given either as single agents or in combination. The best single agent is some form of nitrogen mustard, e.g. chlorambucil or cyclophosphamide, but more centres are now turning to combination chemotherapy using either the National Institutes of Health scheme (Carbone, 1967) or a combination of cyclophosphamide, vincristine and prednisone (Hoogstraten et al., 1969).

There is one special form of lymphosarcoma occurring chiefly in Africa described first by Mr. Denis Burkitt, and known as Burkitt's lymphoma. This frequently presents as a jaw tumour, and one injection of a chemotherapeutic agent such as cyclophosphamide, vincristine or methotrexate may lead to remarkable regression, and in some cases may cure the disease completely (Burkitt, 1967). It is inconceivable that one injection could kill all the malignant cells, and other host factors—particularly some form of immunity—may play a part, but these have yet to be clarified.

MYELOMATOSIS

In myelomatosis the malignant proliferation of plasma cells within the bone marrow and the excessive production of immunoglobulin in the form of IgG, IgA, IgD or as light chains (Bence-Jones protein) gives rise to five major manifestations which require treatment. First, there may be *anaemia* due to marrow infiltration, which is sometimes accompanied by leucopenia and thrombocytopenia, or sometimes presents a leucoerythroblastic picture. Secondly, the *osteolytic lesions* in the bones may cause considerable pain, particularly if pathological fractures occur. Thirdly, there may be *renal failure*, particularly if there is Bence-Jones protein in the urine. Fourthly, *hypercalcaemia*, presumably due to excessive resorption from bone, may be found. Finally, a *haemorrhagic state* may occur due to the presence of large amounts of immunoglobulins in the plasma.

There is no doubt that the best treatment for the relief of bone pain is radiotherapy. The effect is much faster than that of chemotherapy, but of course there is no effect on the disease in other parts of the body and it must therefore be regarded as purely palliative.

Chemotherapy for myelomatosis has proved disappointing in the past, although both cyclophosphamide and melphalan have produced a definite increase in survival (Waldenström, 1964; Korst *et al.*, 1964; Speed *et al.*, 1964). A comparison between melphalan and cyclophosphamide used on a continuous basis was made in a Medical Research Council trial and demonstrated no difference between these two drugs (Galton and Peto, 1968). By contrast, urethane, which has been used extensively in the past, is not effective (Holland *et al.*, 1966). Corticosteroids have also been used and are of particular value in the presence of anaemia and uraemia, and have a dramatic effect in lowering the serum calcium, particularly if a low calcium diet is also given.

The best results so far recorded have been obtained by Alexanian *et al.* (1969), using intermittent melphalan and prednisone. They observed objective improvement in 19 per cent of patients on daily melphalan, 35 per cent on intermittent melphalan, and 70 per cent on intermittent melphalan and prednisone. The median survival was six months longer in the intermittent melphalan plus prednisone group than in the continuous melphalan group.

Melphalan is, however, especially dangerous in myelomatosis if uraemia is also present, and under these circumstances the dose of the drug should be reduced (Galton and Peto, 1968).

A controlled Medical Research Council trial is now in progress comparing the effect of cyclophosphamide with intermittent melphalan and prednisone in this disease.

MACROGLOBULINAEMIA

Macroglobulinaemia may arise in a number of diseases such as chronic lymphatic leukaemia, lymphosarcoma, and even Hodgkin's disease, which themselves require treatment. However, the presence of the macroglobulin in the plasma may cause symptoms; for example, a haemorrhagic diathesis with epistaxis, haemoptysis, and bleeding gums; a retinopathy and heart failure probably due to a mixture of increased viscosity of the blood; and anaemia. Treatment may therefore be directed either against the proliferating cells forming the macroglobulin, that is cells of the lymphocyte-plasma cell series, or a direct attack may be made against the protein itself, or the macroglobulin may be removed from the serum by plasmapheresis.

Treatment directed against the cells forming macroglobulin

The two groups of drugs most commonly used are the nitrogen mustards and corticosteroids; they have often been given together, so that it is sometimes difficult to assess which of the two has been responsible for any improvement. However, in some cases they have been used alone, and each may be of value. Chlorambucil has also proved effective, but it must be given for a period of many months and usually leads to symptomatic improvement and to reduction, but not disappearance of the abnormal protein (Bayrd, 1961; Kok, 1962). Similar results may be obtained with cyclophosphamide. Symptomatic improvement and a reduction in the amount of circulating macroglobulin has also been reported following treatment with prednisone (Glenchur et al., 1958; Pitney et al., 1958). Probably the best treatment is the continuous use of chlorambucil, with or without corticosteroids.

Treatment designed to cause dissociation of the macroglobulin

Macroglobulins are aggregates of smaller globulin fractions joined by sulphydryl linkages, and are therefore capable of being split into these smaller components by sulphydryl-reducing agents (Deutsch and Morton, 1957). This can readily be accomplished in the laboratory by a variety of such compounds, including penicillamine, and this has been used in man. Some workers have reported a reduction in the concentration of circulating macroglobulin (Block et al., 1960; Ritzmann et al., 1960), but many have been unsuccessful (Dacie, 1962; Fairley, 1969). Thus it seems certain that although macroglobulins can always be dissociated in vitro by sulphydryl-reducing compounds, the results in vivo are variable and usually disappointing, probably because a sufficient concentration of penicillamine in the plasma cannot be attained.

Removal of macroglobulin by plasmapheresis

Removal of macroglobulin from the body can be achieved by plasmapheresis, although the protein will accumulate again, and therefore to obtain any long-term benefit it has to be repeated at weekly intervals. Plasmapheresis is certainly useful in an emergency when there is severe cardiac failure or retinopathy, both of which may resolve completely after the concentration of macroglobulin in the serum is reduced (Schwab and Fahey, 1960; Schwab et al., 1960; Conway and Walker, 1962). Conway and Walker (1962) adopted the simple technique of taking blood from the patient into citrate, and then inverting the bottle. The very high ESR produced virtually complete separation of the cells from the plasma within one hour, enabling the red cell layer to be transfused back into the patient without the plasma.

More recently, the IBM Continuous Blood Cell Separator has been used for plasmapheresis in both myelomatosis and macroglobulinaemia (Powles and Hamilton Fairley, 1970), but this will remain a research procedure until more machines are available.

OTHER MALIGNANT DISEASES

Chorioncarcinoma

Until recently, once this tumour had metastasized it invariably proved fatal, but intensive combination chemotherapy using methotrexate and 6-Mercaptopurine has produced some remarkable results with complete remissions obtained in 50 to 75 per cent of the patients, many of whom remain free from disease for many years and are presumably cured (Bagshawe, 1967; Hertz, 1967). One of the factors responsible for this may be that in this disease there is a very sensitive index of the presence of cancer cells in the excretion of human chorionic gonadotrophin hormone (HCG) in the urine. This means that it is possible to detect recurrence long before it is clinically apparent. Also, the excretion of HCG is a guide by which to judge how long to continue treatment after clinical remission has occurred. One of the most difficult decisions in chemotherapy is to know when to stop successful treatment, but in this disease there is a scientific basis both for stopping the drugs and for starting treatment again. This is illustrated in Figure 8.9, taken from Bagshawe (1968) showing the effect of methotrexate and 6-Mercaptopurine on the urinary excretion of the hormone.

Hormonal Dependent Tumours

Carcinoma of the prostate

This grows best in an androgenic environment and reversing this either by bilateral orchidectomy or by treatment with oestrogens may produce remarkable control of disseminated disease for many years. There has been some question in the past as to whether orchidectomy is necessary in addition to the administration of oestrogens, but it has been claimed that there is a better prognosis in cases with established metastases if both forms of treatment are given (Nesbit and Baum, 1950). Stilboestrol is still the most commonly used oestrogen, starting with a dose of 50 mg daily by mouth. This carries the hazard of salt and water retention, and may precipitate heart failure.

Once the tumour has escaped from control by oestrogens, other forms of endocrine treatment may be beneficial. Bilateral adrenalectomy has produced some transient benefit, but destruction of the pituitary gland by irradiation with ^{90}yttrium introduced into the gland via a fine catheter has produced a good response, with abolition of pain in 31 out of 74 patients, and partial responses in a further 20 patients reported by Fergusson (1969). Relapse at

K

this point may be treated with cytotoxic drugs such as cyclophosphamide used alone or in combination, but the results are disappointing.

Carcinoma of the breast

This, unlike carcinoma of the prostate, arises in different endocrine contexts, and the treatment varies depending on whether the patient is pre-menopausal or post-menopausal.

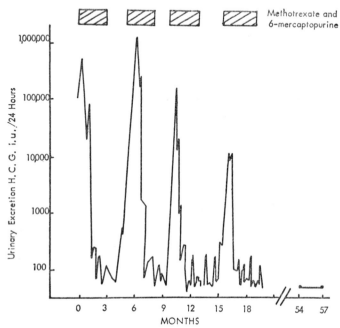

FIG. 8.9. Graph taken from an article by Bagshawe (1968) showing the urinary excretion of human chorionic gonadotrophin (HCG) by a patient with chorioncarcinoma. There was a relapse following each of the first three courses of methotrexate and 6-Mercaptopurine, but following a longer fourth course complete remission was obtained and the patient is free from disease over three years later.

Ⴁ Once the disease has become generalized in pre-menopausal women, the best initial treatment is bilateral oophorectomy, which is much more effective than an irradiation menopause as this sometimes fails to prevent all oestrogen activity. If a remission is not obtained following this or if the patient relapses, androgens are used and most clinicians now prefer to use Nandrolone phenylpropionate (Durabolin) 25–50 mg weekly by intramuscular injection as it produces the same remission rate with less side-effects than testosterone. This may control the situation for a variable time ranging from months to several years, but when the disease again escapes other forms of endocrine treatment are given. These include bilateral adrenalectomy, pituitary ablation with ⁹⁰yttrium and the use of prednisolone. Hayward(1968)considers that prednisolone is not as effective as pituitary ablation, but may be used if the latter is not possible for some reason, or following it when relapse occurs. Another kind of endocrine treatment may then be given in the form of progestational hormones, which produced a remission in 25 per cent of 634 patients reviewed by Briggs *et al.* (1967). Finally, chemotherapy in the form of methotrexate or an alkylating agent such as cyclophosphamide may produce prolonged remissions in some patients (Krakoff, 1967).

In post-menopausal women, the initial treatment is different. First, it is essential to be sure that all oestrogen activity has in fact ceased, and this is done by examining a vaginal smear. Providing there is no oestrogen activity, oestrogens should be given as in carcinoma of the prostate. About half the patients will respond, but when relapse occurs the principles of treatment are the same as in the pre-menopausal state.

Suitable schemes for the treatment of patients with recurrent or inoperable breast cancer are shown in Figures 8.10 and 8.11, taken from Krakoff's paper (1967).

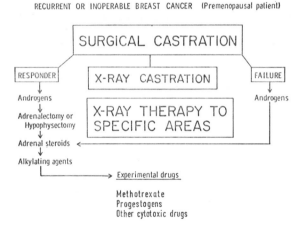

FIG. 8.10. Scheme for the treatment of inoperable breast cancer (pre-menopausal patient).

Various progestational hormones

These may have an effect on disseminated carcinomas of the endometrium in 31 per cent, cervix 27 per cent, ovary and breast 25 per cent, and possibly in renal carcinomas as well (see review by Briggs *et al.*, 1967).

Other Tumours

It would be impossible to list all the various tumours and the different forms of treatment which have been used. Most other carcinomas, such as those of bronchus, stomach, colon and pancreas, as well as malignant melanoma, are unresponsive to chemotherapy, but occasionally a surprising but gratifying regression may be obtained by using one of the alkylating agents, or the newer anti-metabolites such as 5-Fluorouracil, particularly when they are used in combination. It is therefore worth while giving at least one course of treatment, and of the newer regimes Costanzi *et al.* (1969) have reported some beneficial responses in various carcinomas, including malignant melanoma and adenocarcinoma of the pancreas, using a mixture of cyclophosphamide, vincristine, methotrexate and 5-Fluorouracil. Similarly, with the sarcomas, combinations of drugs may produce remarkable results in some patients.

RECURRENT OR INOPERABLE BREAST CANCER (Late postmenopausal patient)

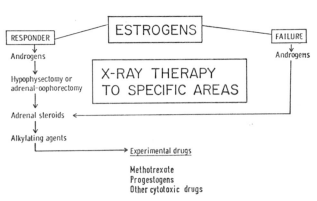

FIG. 8.11. Scheme for the treatment of inoperable breast cancer (late post-menopausal patient).

CONCLUSION

Much of this chapter has deliberately been devoted to the treatment of the reticuloses, for it is here that the drugs are most effective and where the best methods of administration can be studied. Applying what has been learned in these diseases to the treatment of other malignant diseases will improve our management of many forms of malignant disease. The present position of cancer treatment may be summarized in the following way:

1. The best treatment for malignant disease is surgery or radiotherapy, and chemotherapy should only be given to diseases which are disseminated beyond the points at which these can be used.
2. The advent of many more cytotoxic drugs, and the discovery of an enzyme active only against malignant cells and not normal cells has

greatly improved the value of chemotherapy in the control of malignant disease.

3. The use of drugs in combination and the techniques of giving them in a cyclical manner or by "pulse" therapy rather than by using them singly and continuously has further improved the results to the point at which in some patients with certain diseases the malignant process may be permanently arrested. It can no longer be said that chemotherapy has never cured anyone.

REFERENCES

ALEXANDER, P. & FAIRLEY, G. H. (1964). *Clinical Aspects of Immunology*, 2nd edn. ed. P. G. H. Gell and R. R. A. Coombs. Oxford: Blackwell.

ALEXANIAN, R., HAUT, A., KHAN, A. U., LANE, M., McKELVEY, E. M., MIGLIORE, P. J., STUCKEY, W. J. JR. & WILSON, H. E. (1969). Treatment for multiple myeloma. *J. Amer. med. Ass.*, 208, No. 9, 1680.

AUCHINCLOSS, J. H. & DUGGAN, J. J. (1957). Effects of venesection on pulmonary and cardiac function in patients with chronic pulmonary emphysema and secondary polycythemia. *Amer. J. Med.*, 22, 74.

AUSTRALIAN CANCER SOCIETY: Report by Childhood leukaemia Study Group (1968). Cyclic drug regimen for acute childhood leukaemia. *Lancet*, 1, 313.

BAGSHAWE, K. D. (1967). Choriocarcinoma: Transactions of a conference of the International Union against Cancer. eds. J. F. Holland and M. M. Hreshchyshyn. Berlin: Springer-Verlag.

BAGSHAWE, K. D. (1968). Tumour growth and anti-mitotic action. *Brit. J. Cancer*, 22, 698.

BAYRD, E. D. (1961). Continuous chlorambucil therapy in primary macroglobulinaemia of Waldenström. Report of four cases. *Proc. Staff Meet. Mayo Clinic, New York*, 36, 135.

BEARD, M. E. J., CROWTHER, D., GALTON, D. A. G., GUYER, R. J., HAMILTON FAIRLEY, G., KAY, H. E. M., KNAPTON, P. J., MALPAS, J. S. & BODLEY SCOTT, R. (1970). L-asparaginase in the treatment of acute leukaemia and lymphosarcoma. *Brit. med. J.*, 1, 191.

BERNARD, J., BOIRON, M., GOGUEL, A., JACQUILLAT, CL., TANZER, J. & WEIL, M. (1967). Traitement de la maladie de Hodgkin par une polychimiothérapie associant moutarde à l'azote, vincristine, méthylhydrazine et prednisone. *Presse Méd.*, 75, No. 52, 2647.

BLOCH, H. S., PRASAD, A., ANASTASI, A. & BRIGGS, D. R. (1960). Serum protein changes in Waldenström's macroglobulinaemia during administration of a low molecular weight thiol (penicillamine). *J. Lab. clin. Med.*, 56, 212.

BOGGS, D. R., WINTROBE, M. M. & CARTWRIGHT, G. E. (1969). To treat or not to treat acute granulocytic leukaemia. II. *Arch. intern. Med.*, 123, 568.

BRIGGS, M. H., CALDWELL, A. D. S. & PITCHFORD, A. G. (1967). The treatment of cancer by progestogens. *Hosp. Med.*, October, 63.

BRODSKY, I. (1964). The use of ferrokinetics in the evaluation of busulphan therapy in polycythaemia vera. *Brit. J. Haemat.*, 10, 291.

BROOME, J. D. (1961). Evidence that the L-asparaginase activity of guinea-pig serum is responsible for its antilymphoma effects. *Nature*, **191**, 1114.

BURCHENAL, J. H. (1967). Long-term survival in Burkitt's tumor and in acute leukemia. *Cancer Res.*, **27**, Part I, 2616.

BURKITT, D. (1967). *The Treatment of Burkitt's Lymphoma*. ed. J. H. Burchenal and D. P. Burkitt. U.I.C.C. Monograph Series 8. Berlin: Springer.

CARBONE, P. P. (1967). Hodgkin's disease: combined clinical staff conference at the National Institutes of Health. *Ann. intern. Med.*, **67**, No. 2, 424.

CHIEVITZ, E. & THIEDE, T. (1962). Complications and causes of death in polycythaemia vera. *Acta med. scand.*, **172**, 513.

CLEIN, G. P. & FLEMANS, R. J. (1966). Involvement of the erythroid series in blastic crisis of chronic myeloid leukemia. Further evidence for presence of Philadelphia chromosome in erythroblasts. *Brit. J. Haemat.*, **12**, 754.

CONNORS, T. A. (1969). *Scientific Basis of Cancer Chemotherapy*. ed. G. Mathé. p. 1.

CONWAY, N. & WALKER, J. M. (1962). Treatment of macroglobulinaemia. *Brit. med. J.*, **2**, 1296.

COSTANZI, J. J. & COLTMAN, C. A. (1969). Combination chemotherapy using cyclophosphamide, vincristine, methotrexate and 5-fluorouracil in solid tumours. *Cancer*, **23**, 589.

COURT BROWN, W. M. & DOLL, R. (1965). Mortality from cancer and other causes after radiotherapy for ankylosing spondylitis. *Brit. med. J.*, **2**, 1327.

CRONKITE, E. P. (1968). *Perspectives in Leukaemia*. ed. W. Dameshek and R. M. Dutcher. London and New York: Grune & Stratton, p. 158.

CROSBY, W. H. (1968). To treat or not to treat acute granulocytic leukemia. *Arch. intern. Med.*, **122**, 79.

DACIE, J. V. (1962). *The Haemolytic Anaemias*. 2nd edn. Part II. London: Churchill.

DAMESHEK, W. & GUNZ, F. (1964). *Leukaemia*. 2nd edn. London and New York: Grune & Stratton.

DEUTSCH, H. F. & MORTON, J. I. (1957). Dissociation of human serum macroglobulins. *Science*, **125**, 600.

DEVITA, V. T., SERPICK, A. & CARBONE, P. P. (1969). Combination chemotherapy of advanced Hodgkin's disease: the NCI program. *Proc. Amer. Ass. Cancer Res.*, **10**, 18.

DJERASSI, I. (1967). Methotrexate infusions and intensive supportive care in the management of children with acute lymphocytic leukemia: follow-up report. *Cancer Res.*, **27**, 2561.

EASSON, E. C. & RUSSELL, M. H. (1963). The cure of Hodgkin's disease. *Brit. med. J.*, **1**, 1704.

ECKHARDT, S., SELLEI, C., HORVATH, I. P & ISTITORIS, L. (1963). Effect of 1,6-dibromo-1, 6-dideoxy-D-mannitol on chronic granulocytic leukemia. *Cancer Chemotherapy Reports*, **33**, 57.

FAIRLEY, G. H. (1964). *Cyclophosphamide*. eds. G. H. Fairley and J. M. Simister. Bristol: Wright.

FAIRLEY, G. H. (1969). Immunity to malignant disease in man. *Brit. med. J.*, **2**, 467.

FAIRLEY, G. H. (1969b). Unpublished observation.

FAIRLEY, G. H., PATTERSON, M. J. L. & SCOTT, R. B. (1966). Chemotherapy of Hodgkin's disease with cyclophosphamide, vinblastine and procarbazine. *Brit. med. J.*, **2**, 75.

FAIRLEY, G. H. & SCOTT, R. B. (1961). Hypogammablobulinaemia in chronic lymphatic leukaemia. *Brit. med. J.*, **2**, 920.

FARBER, S., DIAMOND, L. K., MERCER, R. D., SYLVESTER, R. F. & WOLFF, J. A. (1948). Temporary remissions in acute leukemia in children produced by folic-acid antagonist 4-aminopteroylglutamic acid, aminopterin. *New Engl. J. Med.*, **238**, 787.

FERGUSSON, J. D. (1969). The management of prostatic cancer. *Brit. J. Hosp. Med.*, **2**, 585.

FISHBEIN, W. N., CARBONE, P. P., FREIREICH, E. J., MISRA, D. & FREI, E. IIIrd (1964). Clinical trials of hydroxyurea in patients with cancer and leukemia. *Clin. Pharmacol. Ther.*, **5**, 574.

FREI, E. (1967). Chemotherapy of acute leukemia. In *Cancer Chemotherapy*. eds. I. Brodsky and S. B. Kahn. London and New York: Grune & Stratton.

GALTON, D. A. G. (1953). Myleran in chronic myeloid leukaemia. *Lancet*, **1**, 208.

GALTON, D. A. G. (1969). Chemotherapy of chronic myelocytic leukaemia. In *Seminars in Haematology*, Vol. 6, No. 4, October, p. 323.

GALTON, D. A. G. & PETO, R. (1968). A progress report on the Medical Research Council's therapeutic trial in myelomatosis. *Brit. J. Haemat.*, **15**, 319.

GALTON, D. A. G., WILTSHAW, E., SZUR, L. & DACIE, J. V. (1961). The use of chlorambucil and steroids in the treatment of chronic lymphocytic leukaemia. *Brit. J. Haemat.*, **7**, 73.

GARDNER, F. H. & PRINGLE, J. C. (1961). Androgens and erythropoiesis. *New Engl. J. Med.*, **264**, 103.

GILMAN, A. & PHILIPS, F. S. (1946). The biological actions and therapeutic applications of the β-chloroethyl amines and sulfides. *Science*, **103**, 409.

GLENCHUR, H., ZINNEMAN, H. H. & BRIGGS, D. R. (1958). Macroglobulinaemia—report of two cases. *Ann. intern. Med.*, **48**, 1055.

GOGUEL, A., WEIL, M., JACQUILLAT, CL. & BOIRON, M. (1969). Polychimiothérapie de la maladie de Hodgkin. In *Actualités Hématologique*, Series 3. ed. J. Bernard, p. 124.

HADDOW, A. & TIMMIS, G. M. (1953). Myleran in chronic myeloid leukaemia. Chemical constitution and biological action. *Lancet*, **1**, 207.

HALL, THOMAS, C. (1967). The present status of chemotherapy for genitourinary malignancies. In *Cancer Chemotherapy*. eds. I. Brodsky and S. B. Khan. London and New York: Grune & Stratton.

HALNAN, K. E. & RUSSELL, M. H. (1965). Polycythaemia vera. *Lancet*, **2**, 760.

HARROLD, B. P. (1966). Syndrome resembling Addison's disease following prolonged treatment with busulphan. *Brit. med. J.*, **1**, 463.

HAYWARD, J. L. (1968). Breast cancer—treatment of the advanced case. *Hospital Medicine*, **2**, 408.

HERTZ, T. (1967). *Choriocarcinoma*. Transactions of a conference of the International Union against Cancer. eds. J. F. Holland and M. M. Hreshchyshyn, Berlin: Springer-Verlag.

HILL, J. M., ROBERTS, J., LOEB, E., KHAN, A., MacLELLAN, A. & HILL, R. W. (1967). L-asparaginase therapy for leukemia and other malignant neoplasms—remission in human leukemia. *J. Amer. med. Ass.*, **202**, 882.

HITCHINGS, G. H. & ELION, G. B. (1967). Mechanisms of action of purine and pyrimidine analogs. In *Cancer Chemotherapy*. eds. I Brodsky and S. B. Kahn. London and New York: Grune & Stratton.

HOLLAND, J. F. (1968). Progress in the treatment of acute leukaemia, 1966. In *Perspectives in Leukemia*. eds. W. Dameshek and R. M. Dutcher. London and New York: Grune & Stratton, p. 217.

HOLLAND, J. F. (1969). Proceedings of the meeting of the O.E.R.T.C. held in Paris, July, 1969. To be published.

HOLLAND, J. F., HOSLEY, H., SCHARLAU, C., CARBONE, P. P., FREI, E., IIIrd, BRINDLEY, C. O., HALL, T. C., SHNIDER, B. I., GOLD, G. L., LASAGNE, L., OWENS, A. H. (JR.) & MILLER, S. P. (1966). A controlled trial of urethane treatment in multiple myeloma. *Blood*, **27**, 328.

HOOGSTRATEN, B., OWENS, A. H., LENHARD, R. E., GLIDEWELL, O. J., LEONE, L. A., OLSON, K. B., HARLEY, J. B., TOWNSEND, S. R., MILLER, S. P. & SPURR, C. L. (1969). Combination chemotherapy in L.S.A. and R.C.S. *Blood*, XXXIII No. 2, Part II, 370.

HOWARTH, S., MCMICHAEL, J. & SHARPEY-SCHAFER, E. P. (1948). Effects of oxygen, venesection and digitalis in chronic heart failure from diseases of the lungs. *Clin. Sci.*, **6**, 187.

HUME, R., COWELL, M. A. & GOLDBERG, A. (1966). Prediction of the dose of radio-active phosphorus in the treatment of polycythaemia vera. *Clin. Radiol.*, **17**, 295.

JAMES, K. W., JAMESON, B., KAY, H. E. M., LYNCH, J. & NGAN, H. (1967). Some practical aspects of intensive cytotoxic therapy. *Lancet*, **1**, 1045.

ISAACS, R. (1954). Treatment of polycythaemia vera with daraprim. *J. Amer. med. Ass.*, **156**, 1491.

KAPLAN, H. S. (1966). Role of intensive radiotherapy in the management of Hodgkin's disease. *Cancer*, **19**, 356.

KAPLAN, H. S. (1968). Clinical evaluation and radiotherapeutic management of Hodgkin's disease and the malignant lymphomas. *New Engl. J. Med.*, **278**, 892.

KENNEDY, B. J. & YARBRO, J. W. (1966). Metabolic and therapeutic effects of hydroxyurea in chronic myeloid leukaemia. *J. Amer. med. Ass.*, **195**, 1038.

KIDD, J. G. (1953). Regression of transplanted lymphomas induced *in vivo* by means of normal guinea-pig serum. *J. exp. Med.*, **98**, 565.

KILLMAN, S. A. & CRONKITE, E. P. (1961). Treatment of polycythaemia vera with myleran. *Amer. J. med. Sci.*, **241**, 218.

KOK, D'A. (1961). Response to chlorambucil therapy in two cases of Walden-ström's macroglobulinaemia. *Proc. 8th Congress, European Soc. of Haematology*, Vienna.

KORST, D. R., CLIFFORD, G. O., FOWLER, W. M., LOUIS, J., WILL, J. & WILSON, H. E. (1964). Multiple myeloma. Analysis of cyclophosphamide therapy in 165 patients. *J. Amer. med. Ass.*, **189**, 758.

KRAKOFF, I. H. (1967). Chemotherapy and hormonal therapy in carcinoma of the breast. In *Cancer Chemotherapy*. eds. I. Brodsky and S. B. Khan. London and New York: Grune & Stratton, p. 77.

KYLE, R. A., SCHWARTZ, R. S., OLINER, H. L. & DAMESHEK, W. (1959). A syndrome resembling adrenal cortical insufficiency associated with long-term busulphan (myleran) therapy. *Blood*, **18**, 497.

LACHER, M. J. & DURRANT, J. R. (1965). Combined vinblastine and chlorambucil therapy in Hodgkin's disease. *Ann. intern. med.*, **62**, 468.

LAWRENCE, J. H. (1940). Nuclear physics and therapy: preliminary report on a new method for the treatment of leukaemia and polycythaemia. *Radiology*, **35**, 51.

LAWRENCE, J. H. (1955). Polycythemia; physiology, diagnosis and treatment. In *Modern Medical Monograph*. New York & London: Grune & Stratton.

LEAKE, E., SMITH, W. G. & WOODLIFF, H. J. (1963). Diffuse interstitial pulmonary fibrosis after busulphan therapy. *Lancet*, **2**, 432.

LEDLIE, E. M. (1960). The incidence of leukaemia in patients with polycythaemia vera treated by 32P. *J. Fac. Radiol. (Lond.)*, **11**, 130.

LEDLIE, E. M. (1966). Treatment of polycythaemia vera by 32P. *Proc. roy. Soc. Med.*, **59**, 1095.

MALPAS, J. S. (1967). Assessment of hydroxyurea in leukaemia. *Clinical Trials Journal*, November, p. 873.

MASSOUREDIS, S. P. & LAWRENCE, J. H. (1957). The problem of leukemia in polycythemia vera. *Amer. J. med. Sci.*, **233**, 268.

MATHÉ, G. (1969). Approaches to the immunological treatment of cancer in man. *Brit. med. J.*, **4**, 7.

MATHÉ, G., SCHLUMBERGER, J. R., SCHNEIDER, M., CATTAN, A., AMIEL, J. L., SCHWARZENBERG, L. & MERY, A. M. (1965). Étude histologique et cytologique approfondie de la remission dite complète des leucemies aiguès. Abstracts of 10th Congress of the European Society of Haematology, Strasbourg. p. 178.

MEDICAL RESEARCH COUNCIL (1968). Working party for therapeutic trials in leukaemia. Chronic granulocytic leukaemia: comparison of radiotherapy and busulphan therapy. *Brit. med. J.*, **1**, 201.

MODAN, B. & LILIENFELD, A. M. (1965). Polycythemia vera and leukemia—the role of radiation treatment. A study of 1222 patients. *Medicine (Baltimore)*, **44**, 305.

MOLONEY, W. C. (1959). Leukaemia and exposure of X-ray: a report of six cases. *Blood*, **14**, 1137.

MOLONEY, W. C. & KASTENBAUM, M. A. (1955). Leukaemogenic effects of ionising radiation on atomic bomb survivors in Hiroshima city. *Science*, **121**, 308.

NESBIT, R. M. & BAUM, W. C. (1950). Endocrine control of prostatic carcinoma: clinical and statistical survey of 1818 cases. *J. Amer. med. Ass.*, **143**, 1317.

NICHOLSON, W. M., BEARD, M. E. J., CROWTHER, D., STANSFIELD, A. G., MALPAS, J. S., FAIRLEY, G. H. & SCOTT, R. B. (1970). Combination chemotherapy in disseminated Hodgkin's disease. *Brit. med. J.*, **3**, 1970.

OETTGEN, H. F., OLD, L. J., BOYSE, E. A., CAMPBELL, H. A., PHILIPS, F. S., CLARKSON, B. D., TALLAL, L., LEEPER, R. D., SCHWARTZ, M. K. & KIM, J. H. (1967). Inhibition of leukemias in man by L-asparaginase. *Cancer Research, Part I*, **27**, 2619.

OLINER, H., SCHWARTZ, R., RUBIO, F. & DAMESHEK, W. (1961). Interstitial pulmonary fibrosis following busulphan therapy. *Amer. J. Med.*, **31**, 134.

OSGOOD, E. E. (1964). Leukaemogenic effect of ionising-irradiation treatment in polycythaemia. *Lancet*, **2**, 967.

OSGOOD, E. E., SEAMAN, A. J. & KOLER, R. D. (1956). Results of the 15-year program of treatment of chronic leukemias with titrated regularly spaced total body irradiation with phosphorus 32 or X-ray. Congress for the International Society of Haematology, Boston, published 1958. p. 44.

PERKINS, J., ISRAËLS, M. C. G. & WILKINSON, J. F. (1964). Polycythaemia vera: clinical studies on a series of 127 patients managed without radiation therapy. *Quart. J. Med.*, **33**, 499.

PETERS, M. V. & MIDDLEMISS, K. C. H. (1958). A study of Hodgkin's disease treated with irradiation. *Amer. J. Roentgenol.*, **79**, 114.

PITNEY, W. R., O'SULLIVAN, W. J. & OWEN, J. A. (1958). Effect of prednisolone on anaemia associated with macroglobulinaemia. *Brit. med. J.*, **2**, 1508.

POWLES, R. L. & HAMILTON FAIRLEY, G. (1970). (In press.)

RASTRICK, J. M. (1969). A method for the positive identification of erythropoietic cells in chromosomal preparations of bone marrow. *Brit. J. Haemat.*, 16, 185.

RASTRICK, J. M., FITZGERALD, P. H. & GUNZ, F. W. (1968). Direct evidence for the presence of the Ph. chromosome in erythroid cells. *Brit. med. J.*, 1, 96.

RITZMANN, S. E., COLEMAN, S. L. & LEVIN, W. C. (1960). The effect of some mercaptanes upon a macro-cryoglobulin; modification induced by cysteamine, penicillamine and penicillin. *J. clin. Invest.*, 39, 1320.

SCHWAB, P. J. & FAHEY, J. L. (1960). Treatment of Waldenström's macroglobulinaemia by plasmapheresis. *New Engl. J. Med.*, 263, 574.

SCHWAB, P. J., OKUN, E. & FAHEY, J. L. (1960). Reversal of retinopathy in Waldenström's macroglobulinaemia by plasmapheresis. *Arch. Ophthal.*, Chicago, 64, 515.

SCOTT, R. B. (1957). Leukaemia. *Lancet*, 1, 1099.

SHAW, R. K., SZWED, C., BOGGS, D. R., FAHEY, J. L., FREI, E., MORRISON, E. & UTZ, J. P. (1960). Infection and immunity in chronic lymphocytic leukaemia. *Arch. intern. Med.*, 106, 467.

SKIPPER, H. E. (1968). Cellular kinetics associated with "curability" of experimental leukemia. In *Perspectives in Leukemia*. eds. W. Dameshek and R. M. Dutcher. London and New York: Grune & Stratton, p. 187.

SMITHERS, D. W. (1967). Hodgkin's disease. *Brit. med. J.*, 2, 337.

SMITHERS, D. W. (1969). Clinical research in Hodgkin's disease. *The Scientific Basis of Medicine Annual Review*, 1969. p. 95.

SPEED, D. E., GALTON, D. A. G. & SWAN, A. (1964). Melphalan in the treatment of myelomatosis. *Brit. med. J.*, 1, 1664.

STROEBEL, C. F., HALL, B. E. & PEASE, G. L. (1951). Evaluation of radiophosphorus therapy in primary polycythemia. *J. Amer. med. Ass.*, 146, 1301.

TINNEY, W. S., HALL, B. E. & GIFFIN, H. Z. (1945). The prognosis of polycythemia vera. *Proc. Mayo Clin.*, 20, 306.

VIDEBAEK, A. (1950). Polycythaemia vera: cause and prognosis. *Acta. med. scand.*, 138, 179.

WALDENSTRÖM, J. (1964). Melphalan therapy in myelomatosis. *Brit. med. J.*, 1, 859.

WASSERMAN, L. R. (1954). Polycythemia vera—its cause and treatment in relation to myeloid metaplasia and leukemia. *Bull. N.Y. Acad. Med.*, 30, 343.

WATKINS, P. J., HAMILTON FAIRLEY, G. & BODLEY SCOTT, R. (1967). Treatment of polycythaemia vera. *Brit. med. J.*, 2, 664.

WEIL, M. & TANZER, J. (1967). The effect of hydroxyurea on chronic myeloid leukaemia. *Clinical Trials Journal* (November), p. 895.

WETHERLEY-MEIN, G., JONES, N. F. & PULLAN, J. M. (1961). Effects of splenectomy on red-cell production in myelofibrosis. *Brit. med. J.*, 1, 84.

WILKINSON, J. F. & FLETCHER, F. (1947). Effect of β-chlorethylamine hydrochlorides in leukaemia, Hodgkin's disease, and polycythaemia vera. *Lancet*, 2, 540.

WISEMAN, B. K., ROHN, R. J., BOURONCLE, B. A. & MYERS, W. G. (1951). The treatment of polycythaemia vera with radioactive phosphorus. *Ann. intern. Med.*, 64, 311.

ZUELZER, W. W. (1964). Implications of long-term survival in acute stem-cell leukaemia of childhood treated with composite cyclic therapy. *Blood*, 24, 477.

9 Metabolic and Endocrine Diseases

REGINALD HALL

VARIETIES OF HYPERPARATHYROIDISM. CALCITONIN.
ADDISON'S DISEASE. MAGNESIUM METABOLISM. AMYLOIDOSIS

VARIETIES OF HYPERPARATHYROIDISM

Primary hyperparathyroidism

PRIMARY hyperparathyroidism is not a rare disease, and may be recognized more often when radioimmunoassays of parathyroid hormone become readily available. Several recent surveys suggest that hyperparathyroidism, usually identified by asymptomatic hypercalcaemia, may be present in 0·1 per cent of the general population. The condition should always be considered in any patient with obscure bone or renal disease, particularly if renal calculi or nephrocalcinosis can be demonstrated. The condition usually results from a single adenoma, but may less frequently be due to multiple adenomas, diffuse hyperplasia of all four glands or parathyroid carcinoma. Multiple adenomas, often familial, of the pituitary, adrenal, pancreas or thyroid may be associated with primary hyperparathyroidism due to one or more tumours or to diffuse hyperplasia of the parathyroids.

An analysis of Dent's patients by Lloyd (1968) produced evidence of two main types of parathyroid tumour: one fast-growing, highly active, causing overt bone disease; the other slow-growing, of low activity, causing renal stones. It was originally suggested by Dent (1962) that these two types of parathyroid disease could result from secretion of different parathyroid hormones, but recent studies by Potts et al. (1966) have provided no evidence as to the existence of two biologically distinct hormones. Primary hyperparathyroidism in all its forms must therefore be accepted as due to excessive secretion of one parathyroid hormone, though it is conceded that modifying factors such as an increased absorption of dietary calcium may prevent the development of overt bone disease in some patients with renal calculi, despite high circulating levels of parathyroid hormone (Hodgkinson, 1963).

Clinical manifestations of hyperparathyroidism may be divided into three main categories depending on the presence of:

1. skeletal involvement;
2. renal and urinary tract involvement;
3. hypercalcaemia.

Parathyroid adenomas are rarely palpable, and most lumps in the necks of patients with hypercalcaemia turn out to be thyroid adenomas.

(1) **Skeletal manifestations** are variable, ranging from bone pain to pathological fractures usually through bone cysts, dorsal kyphosis and loss of height. An epulis of the jaw or osteoclastomas at other sites may be the presenting feature of the condition. Joint pain, sometimes occurring in acute episodes termed "pseudo-gout" and associated with chondrocalcinosis, is another rare manifestation of hyperparathyroidism (Bywaters *et al.*, 1963). Clubbing of the fingers due to fracture and compression of the tips is rarely present.

(2) **Renal and urinary tract involvement** is a frequent cause of symptoms, the earliest of which are polyuria and polydipsia sometimes mimicking diabetes insipidus. A serum calcium estimation is mandatory in any patient with polyuria not due to diabetes mellitus or overt urinary infection. Later, small calculi (described as sand or gravel) or definite stones, usually composed of calcium phosphate or oxalate, may be passed. Renal impairment may be due to nephrocalcinosis, secondary infection, or obstruction.

(3) **Hypercalcaemia** should be considered as a cause of unexplained anorexia, nausea, vomiting, constipation, thirst or lethargy. Depression, stupor or psychosis may also occur. The nails may be unusually strong and thick and there may be hypermotility of the joints. Calcium may be deposited in the eyes (band keratopathy). Neonatal hypoparathyroidism should always alert the clinician to the possibility of maternal hyperparathyroidism.

Laboratory diagnosis of hyperparathyroidism is still based on the finding of an elevated serum calcium level, blood being taken from the fasting patient without venous occlusion. Following demonstration of an elevated serum calcium, other possible causes of hypercalcaemia must be excluded, though this can be difficult since more than one cause can be present in the same patient (sarcoidosis, metastatic carcinoma of bone, tumours without bone metastases (producing a parathyroid hormone-like material), myelomatosis, milk-alkali syndrome, vitamin D intoxication (often iatrogenic), thyrotoxicosis, idiopathic hypercalcaemia of childhood, and extensive Paget's disease with immobilization).

In an attempt to rule out the other causes of hypercalcaemia mentioned above, Dent (1956) and Dent and Watson (1968) have devised a hydrocortisone suppression test. The test is unnecessary if the clinical evidence is strongly in favour of hyperparathyroidism and when there is no other obvious cause of hypercalcaemia. In most cases of hypercalcaemia not due to hyperparathyroidism, hydrocortisone leads to a rapid fall in serum calcium, whereas in hyperparathyroidism the serum calcium remains elevated (in 45/46 of the patients studied by Dent and Watson, 1968). In the test, hydrocortisone 40 mg is given eight-hourly for ten days and blood samples are taken in the fasting state at nine a.m. immediately before and five, eight and ten days after commencement of the therapy. The accuracy of the test can be improved by correcting the calcium levels for variations in total plasma protein, adding or subtracting 0·25 mg for each unit change down or up in the third decimal place of the plasma specific gravity as determined by the copper sulphate method, taking 1·027 as normal. If electrophoresis shows the protein distribution to be abnormal, the correction is inaccurate and should not be applied. Estimation of the serum ionized calcium may be of value in such cases.

Elevation of the urinary calcium and a lowered serum phosphate level may also be of value in diagnosis. In 1964, Wills and McGowan reported that the plasma chloride was raised in hyperparathyroidism, usually to levels greater than 102 mEq per litre, and this finding has been confirmed by Pyrah *et al.* (1966). Urinary hydroxyproline excretion is generally increased in patients with a raised alkaline phosphatase or radiological evidence of bone disease.

Elevated levels of circulating parathyroid hormone can now be detected in the majority of patients with primary hyperparathyroidism by radio-immunoassay. In general, this technique depends on the ability of radio-iodine-labelled hormone to compete with unlabelled hormone, which is being measured, for combination with a specific antibody. Hormone bound to antibody (B) is separated from unbound or free hormone (F), and the ratio between them is determined. In the presence of increasing known amounts of hormone there is a progressive displacement of labelled hormone from combination with antibody and a lowering of the B/F ratio so that a standard curve can be drawn. The amount of hormone in any unknown plasma can then be calculated by comparing its B/F value with that of the standard curve. As yet, standard human parathyroid hormone is not available, and results are expressed in terms of a bovine preparation (Buckle, 1968).

Treatment. Once the diagnosis of primary hyperparathyroidism has been established, the neck is explored and the parathyroid adenoma removed. However, the surgeon must be aware that multiple tumours may be present, and an attempt should be made to identify all four parathyroids (sometimes up to six glands may exist). The tumour may be in an ectopic site, e.g. in the mediastinum, and the clinical diagnosis should be so firm that it indicates to the surgeon the necessity of exploring the mediastinum if no tumour is found in the neck. Hyperplasia of all four glands should be treated by removal of three glands and subtotal resection of the fourth. Post-operative tetany is common and requires treatment with vitamin D and calcium, and sometimes magnesium.

If the serum calcium level fails to fall after operation, whether or not one or more adenomas have been removed, additional autonomous parathyroid tissue is obviously present. So long as the serum calcium level is not dangerously elevated it is best to wait a few months before further attempts are made to localize the tumour. Arteriography, filling the inferior thyroid artery by way of the brachial artery, may allow demonstration of the tumour by displacement of the inferior thyroid artery. Venous catheterization with removal of serial blood samples for parathyroid hormone estimation at different levels of the neck has recently proved useful. Parathormone can be released from a tumour by massage of the relevant side of the neck, and the increased level of the hormone detected by radioimmunoassay of serial blood samples. Scanning the neck after administration of 75Se-Selenomethionine along with thyroid suppression by triiodothyronine allows the demonstration of some large tumours, although these are not usually difficult to find by exploration.

If severe, hypercalcaemia (serum calcium greater than 15 mg/100 ml), may require emergency treatment because of the danger of cardiac arrest. As mentioned previously, the hypercalcaemia of hyperparathyroidism is resistant to corticosteroid therapy. Three kinds of treatment have been advocated: calcitonin and the sodium salts of phosphate and sulphate. Calcitonin is sometimes able to lower the calcium levels in hypercalcaemia, but supplies of the hormone are not readily available. Phosphate is very effective though the mechanism of its action is not well understood. Tetany and metastatic calcification may result from phosphate administration, and the initial dose of phosphate should not exceed 50 millimoles (Goldsmith and Ingbar, 1966). Intravenous sodium sulphate infusions are well tolerated; usually 3 litres of isotonic sodium sulphate solution are given intravenously over a nine-hour period causing a fall in serum calcium as well as a rise in urinary calcium excretion (Chakmakjian and Bethune, 1966). Phosphate infusions may be preferable in patients with heart failure because a smaller volume of the solution is required.

Secondary hyperparathyroidism

This is a well-recognized entity defined by Albright and Reifenstein (1948) as "a condition when more parathyroid hormone is manufactured than is normal but where this hormone is needed for some compensatory purpose". It can develop in response to any long-maintained hypocalcaemic stimulus such as malabsorption or chronic renal failure. All four parathyroids are usually hyperplastic, and serum calcium levels are low or normal (but never raised) depending on the extent to which the parathyroids are able to compensate for the hypocalcaemia. The bones show evidence of the previous hypocalcaemia—rickets or osteomalacia—as well as *osteitis fibrosa cystica*. Treatment with vitamin D corrects the hypocalcaemia, removes the stimulus to the parathyroids and allows the bone disease to heal.

Tertiary hyperparathyroidism

This term was first suggested by Walter St Goar (1963) to describe patients who develop parathyroid adenomas causing hypercalcaemia on the basis of reactive or secondary parathyroid hyperplasia. Davies *et al.* (1968) have recently established a firm foundation for this syndrome. Amongst their first 200 cases of primary hyperparathyroidism they found 12 patients with parathyroid adenomas, which probably developed as a result of long-standing hyperplasia due to malabsorption or chronic renal glomerular failure.

Both primary and tertiary hyperparathyroidism were found more frequently in women than in men. The ages of the patients ranged from 28 to 72 years. More cases were associated with malabsorption syndromes than with chronic renal failure: gluten-induced enteropathy (six cases), post-gastrectomy osteomalacia (three cases) and adult-presenting "vitamin-D-resistant" osteomalacia, polycystic kidneys and prolonged renal glomerular failure of unknown cause (one case each). Tertiary hyperparathyroidism should be suspected in any patient with long-standing malabsorption or renal failure who develops hypercalcaemia. In some cases the hypercalcaemia is observed during treatment with vitamin D, but persists after this is withdrawn. When total plasma calcium levels are only marginally raised, estimation of the ionized calcium or the hydrocortisone suppression test may be of value. In three-quarters of the patients bone X-rays or biopsies showed signs of osteomalacia, and in a similar number there was evidence of increased parathyroid action on bone—*osteitis fibrosa cystica*. Thus it appears that tertiary hyperparathyroidism, like the primary variety, can occur with or without *osteitis fibrosa cystica*. It is possible that some patients with tertiary hyperparathyroidism were suffering from the primary form which had been missed initially, though the evolution of the syndrome was observed in four of the patients described by Davies *et al.* (1968). These patients had typical secondary hyperplasia when first seen, and during the period of observation hypercalcaemia developed and was cured by removal of a parathyroid adenoma.* As in other disorders of calcium metabolism the role of calcitonin needs to be defined. Treatment is to remove the adenoma unless renal failure is too advanced to allow operation, when haemodialysis can sometimes be helpful. After removal of the adenoma, long-term treatment with vitamin D may be needed to prevent hypocalcaemia.

* Keynes and Caird (1970) suggest that in some patients with autonomous hyperparathyroidism associated with steatorrhoea and osteomalacia the manifestations of primary parathyroid disease are masked by vitamin-D deficiency, a state in which the action of parathyroid hormone may be blocked.

Tertiary hyperparathyroidism provides an opportunity to study the process of tumour formation in man, because the prolonged hypocalcaemic stimulus leads to hyperplasia, adenoma and possibly carcinoma. The situation is analogous to that occurring in other endocrine glands in which prolonged physiological stimuli eventually culminate in the formation of benign or malignant tumours.

REFERENCES

ALBRIGHT, F. & REIFENSTEIN, E. C. (1948). *The Parathyroid Glands and Metabolic Bone Disease*. London: Baillière, Tindall and Cox.

BUCKLE, R. M. (1968). Radioimmunoassay of parathyroid hormone in primary hyperparathyroidism. *J. roy. Coll. Phycns.*, 3, 77.

BYWATERS, E. G. L., ST J. DIXON, A. & SCOTT, J. T. (1963). Joint lesions of hyperparathyroidism. *Ann. rheum. Dis.*, 22, 171.

CHAKMAKJIAN, Z. H. & BETHUNE, J. E. (1966). Sodium sulfate treatment of hypercalcemia. *New Engl. J. Med.*, 275, 862.

DAVIES, D. R., DENT, C. E. & WATSON, L. (1968). Tertiary hyperparathyroidism. *Brit. med. J.*, 3, 395.

DENT, C. E. (1956). Cortisone test for hyperparathyroidism. *Brit. med. J.*, 1, 230.

DENT, C. E. (1962). Some problems of hyperparathyroidism. *Brit. med. J.*, 2, 1495.

DENT, C. E. & WATSON, L. (1968). The hydrocortisome test in primary and tertiary hyperparathyroidism. *Lancet*, 2, 662.

GOLDSMITH, R. S. & INGBAR, S. H. (1966). Inorganic phosphate treatment of hypercalcemia of diverse etiologies. *New Engl. J. Med.*, 274, 1.

HODGKINSON, A. (1963). Biochemical aspects of primary hyperparathyroidism: An analysis of 50 cases. *Clin Sci.*, 25, 231.

LLOYD, H. M. (1968). Primary hyperparathyroidism: an analysis of the role of the parathyroid tumour. *Medicine (Baltimore)*, 47, 53.

POTTS, J. T. JR., AURBACH, G. D. & SHERWOOD, L. M. (1966). Parathyroid hormone: chemical properties and structural requirements for biological and immunological activity. *Recent Progr. Hormone Res.*, 22, 101.

PYRAH, L. N., HODGKINSON, A. & ANDERSON, C. K. (1966). Primary hyperparathyroidism. *Brit. J. Surg.*, 53, 245.

ST GOAR, W. (1963). In Case records of Massachusetts General Hospital. *New Engl. J. Med.*, 268, 943.

WILLS, M. R. & MCGOWAN, G. K. (1964). Plasma chloride levels in hyperparathyroidism and other hypercalcaemic states. *Brit. med. J.*, 1, 1153.

CALCITONIN

Copp was the first to observe that dogs from whom the thyroids and parathyroids had been removed were unusually sensitive to an acute calcium load. Subsequently, he carried out a series of experiments which demonstrated the presence of a circulating hypocalcaemic factor which he named calcitonin. He originally considered that this new hormone derived from the parathyroid glands, but later research work revealed that in many species, including man, calcitonin was produced mainly in the thyroid gland. Foster *et al.* (1964) suggested that calcitonin was formed in the parafollicular or "C" cells of the thyroid. These parafollicular cells arise independently of the follicular cells of the thyroid, from the ultimobranchial body originating from the last branchial pouch. In fish, reptiles and birds the ultimobranchial body remains separate from the thyroid, which does not contain any calcitonin. However, it has only recently been possible to demonstrate "C" cells in the human thyroid. These cells, which are either less numerous than in many other species or more difficult to identify by standard "C" cell stains, are mainly localized in the postero-medial portions of the lateral lobes. Despite the demonstration of a hypocalcaemic factor in the human parathyroid and thymus (Galante *et al.*, 1968), no histological confirmation of "C" cells in these sites has as yet been obtained.

Structure of calcitonin

MacIntyre and his colleagues, and Neher and his associates, have recently isolated the human hormone in pure form, and the full amino-acid sequence of the molecule has been deduced and confirmed by total synthesis. The structure of human calcitonin is shown in Figure 9.1. It is a single-chain

STRUCTURE OF HUMAN CALCITONIN (3419 M.Wt.)

```
     ┌─────────────────────────────────────────┐
H  -  Cys - Gly - Asn - Leu - Ser - Thr - Cys - Met - Leu - Gly -
      1     2     3     4     5     6     7     8     9     10

   - Thr - Tyr - Thr - Gln - Asp - Phe - Asn - Lys - Phe - His - Thr -
     11    12    13    14    15    16    17    18    19    20    21

   - Phe - Pro - Gln - Thr - Ala - Ile - Gly - Val - Gly - Ala - Pro* - NH₂
     22    23    24    25    26    27    28    29    30    31    32
```

$$H - Cys - Gly - Asn - Leu - Ser - Thr - Cys - Met - Leu - Gly -$$

* (Prolinamide)

FIG. 9.1

32 amino-acid polypeptide which differs extensively in structure from porcine calcitonin, 18 of the 32 amino-acids being different. Such a marked dissimilarity is unique among peptide hormones from related species. Bovine calcitonin differs from porcine calcitonin by only three amino-acid residues. Isolation of human calcitonin was aided by the fact that medullary carcinomas of the thyroid are exceedingly rich in the hormone. Both calcitonin monomer and calcitonin dimer have been isolated from human tissue, and it is uncertain which of these is the active form of the hormone. Because of the dissimilarities between human and animal calcitonin it is obvious that results of immunoassays based on antibodies to animal calcitonin should be inter-

preted with caution when applied to man, and it is probably preferable to use human calcitonin rather than porcine material in clinical trials.

Salmon calcitonin, extracted from the ultimobranchial glands, appears to be much more active than porcine calcitonin, possibly due to the slower degradation. Results of its use in man, however, are not yet available.

Actions of calcitonin

Calcitonin has its major action on bone, inhibiting bone resorption by reducing osteoclastic osteolysis. The hormone is effective in parathyroidectomized animals, indicating that its effect is independent of parathyroid hormone, though it inhibits the action of parathyroid hormone on bone. The precise interrelationship of the effects of the two hormones is still poorly understood. MacIntyre has postulated that calcitonin minimizes the action of parathyroid hormone on bone, but does not oppose its effects on the kidney and gut. Under conditions of calcium deprivation, calcitonin levels fall and parathyroid hormone is able to mobilize bone calcium.

Calcitonin reduces serum calcium, urinary calcium and hydroxyproline in patients with high osteoclastic resorption irrespective of the initial calcium levels, but in patients with normal resorption the serum calcium remains unchanged although urinary calcium may be increased.

To conclude: calcitonin is not a calcium lowering factor but a bone resorption or bone metabolism lowering agent.

Control of calcitonin secretion. Calcitonin secretion can occur at normal serum calcium levels, but the major stimulus for calcitonin release from the "C" cells is an increase in the serum calcium level. An abnormally high magnesium level can also cause secretion of calcitonin.

Assay of calcitonin. Calcitonin can be assayed by its hypocalcaemic action in rats, the sensitivity of the assay being increased by phosphate administration to the assay animal. A radioimmunoassay of calcitonin is now available and the technique, which involves the use of antibodies to porcine calcitonin, is far more sensitive than that employing antibodies to human calcitonin. Normal levels of calcitonin are less than 5 ng/ml, which is the lower limit of sensitivity in the human system.

Calcitonin in disease

A striking elevation of serum calcitonin levels is found in patients with medullary carcinoma of the thyroid (*vide infra*). Raised serum levels are also found in some patients with hyperparathyroidism, presumably due to the hypercalcaemic stimulus. Decreased serum levels have been observed in some cases of hypoparathyroidism and in osteopetrosis. In some patients with pseudohypoparathyroidism the calcitonin content of the thyroid is increased. However, calcium infusion studies suggest that neither pseudohypoparathyroidism nor osteopetrosis is due to increased secretion of calcitonin.

After total thyroidectomy, patients maintained on 1-thyroxine usually have normal fasting serum calcium levels unless the parathyroid glands are damaged. However, these patients show impaired ability to restore the calcium level to normal after a calcium infusion (Williams *et al.*, 1966). This is unlikely to be due to calcitonin deficiency because calcitonin levels in the circulation are normal, and alternative sites of calcitonin production in the thymus and parathyroids have been demonstrated. So far there is no convincing evidence in man of any disease caused by over- or under-secretion of calcitonin.

Calcitonin therapy

Calcitonin has been used in three clinical situations: Paget's disease, osteoporosis and hypercalcaemia. In Paget's disease, calcitonin tends to lower the serum calcium if the rate of bone turnover is raised and there is an increased renal clearance of phosphate. Marked symptomatic improvement has been reported after calcitonin administration in patients with this disease. The effects of calcitonin on patients with osteoporosis are more variable, probably due to the heterogeneity of this clinical syndrome. Calcium balances tend to become positive, bone resorption is inhibited and some workers have reported an increase in bone mineralization. Definite clinical improvement has not yet been proved, and prolonged treatment with human or salmon calcitonin is necessary in order to clarify the situation. Calcitonin is usually effective in lowering the serum calcium in hypercalcaemic states, particularly in those associated with increased bone turnover.

Medullary carcinoma of the thyroid—a calcitonin-producing tumour

The medullary carcinoma is a distinct variety of thyroid cancer. It is a solid tumour composed of islands of regular cells with abundant granular cytoplasm and a variable amount of amyloid in the stroma. Despite the lack of cellular differentiation, the prognosis of patients with this type of tumour is usually quite good.

It was first suggested by Williams (1966) that the tumour arises from the parafollicular or "C" cells, now known to be the source of calcitonin. Milhaud *et al.* (1968) described two cases of medullary carcinoma with high levels of a hypocalcaemic factor in the tumour, and in one of them a hypocalcaemic agent was also present in the circulation. Cunliffe *et al.* (1968) described a patient who had mucosal neuromas, a known association of medullary carcinoma of the thyroid. Calcitonin was demonstrated in the circulation of this patient, the thyroid origin was proved by the finding of a very high thyroid vein content of the hormone, and the excised medullary carcinoma had a calcitonin content 5000 times greater than normal. After total thyroidectomy, calcitonin disappeared from the circulation with a half-life of about 15 minutes. It is of interest that pre-operative calcium infusions in this patient caused an elevation of the plasma calcitonin level, demonstrating that the tumour was still responsive to stimuli which normally raise calcitonin output.

In most patients with medullary carcinoma the serum calcium level is normal despite the hypercalcitoninaemia. If bone resorption does not normally play a significant part in the maintenance of the serum calcium, it would be expected that its inhibition by calcitonin would not cause hypocalcaemia. It may be possible to diagnose medullary carcinoma pre-operatively by measuring the calcitonin levels, and by the same method a recurrence can also be detected at an early stage.

REFERENCES

CALCITONIN (1968). *Proceedings of the Symposium on Thyrocalcitonin and the "C" Cells, July* 1967. London: Heinemann Medical Books Ltd.

COPP, D. H. (1969). Review: Endocrine control of calcium homeostasis. *J. Endocr.*, 43, 137.

CUNLIFFE, W. C., BLACK, M. M., HALL, R., JOHNSTON, I. D. A., HUDGSON, P., SHUSTER, S., GUDMUNDSSON, T. V., JOPLIN, G. F., WILLIAMS, E. D., WOODHOUSE, N. J. Y., GALANTE, L. & MACINTYRE, I. (1968). A calcitonin-secreting thyroid carcinoma. *Lancet*, 2, 63.

FOSTER, G. V., MACINTYRE, I. & PEARSE, A. G. E. (1964). Calcitonin production and the mitochondrion-rich cells of the dog thyroid. *Nature (Lond.)*, 203, 1029.

GALANTE, L., GUDMUNDSSON, T. V., MATTHEWS, E. W., TSE, A., WILLIAMS, E. D., WOODHOUSE, N. J. Y. & MACINTYRE, I. (1968). Thymic and parathyroid origin of calcitonin in man. *Lancet*, 2, 537.

MILHAUD, G., TUBIANA, M., PARMENTIER, C. & COUTRIS, G. (1968). Epithélioma de la thyroïd sécrétant de la thyrocalcitonine. *C.R. Acad. Sci. (Paris)*, Sér. D., 266, 608.

ILLIAMS, E. D. (1966). Histogenesis of medullary carcinoma of the thyroid. *J. clin. Path.*, 19, 114.

WILLIAMS, G. A., HARGIS, G. K., GALLOWAY, W. B. & HENDERSON, W. J. (1966). Evidence of thyrocalcitonin in man. *Proc. Soc. exp. Biol. (N.Y.)*, 122, 1273.

ADDISON'S DISEASE

Immunological aspects

Addison's disease can be divided into two main aetiological categories: idiopathic and tuberculous. The idiopathic form has now been shown to belong to a group of diseases characterized clinically by a predominantly female incidence, a familial tendency and the presence of organ-specific antibodies in the serum, and histologically by lymphocytic infiltration and atrophy. Pernicious anaemia (autoimmune gastritis), Hashimoto's disease and myxoedema (autoimmune thyroiditis) as well as some forms of hypo-parathyroidism also belong to this group. The diseases tend to be associated with vitiligo and diabetes mellitus.

Serological evidence of adrenalitis is rare in patients with thyroid disease or pernicious anaemia, but thyroiditis and gastritis are common in patients with adrenalitis (Irvine *et al.*, 1967). It has been suggested that if the term autoimmune adrenalitis is to be preferred to that of idiopathic Addison's disease, it should be on the understanding that while autoimmune mechanisms may be of major importance in the pathogenesis of this variety of adrenal disease, it still remains to be proved.

Irvine *et al.* (1967) have studied the clinical and serological details of 51 patients with adrenocortical insufficiency. Idiopathic and probable idiopathic adrenal insufficiency had a predominantly female sex ratio (2·5 to 1) with a mean age of onset of 33 years. Antibodies to adrenal cortex could be detected by immunofluorescence or complement-fixation techniques in the serum of 80 per cent of the women but in only 10 per cent of the men and the titre was usually low. No adrenal antibodies were found in the circulation of patients with tuberculous Addison's disease.

Blizzard *et al.* (1967) also found adrenal antibodies in approximately 50 per cent of their patients with idiopathic Addison's disease. In 51 of their 118 patients one or more associated diseases had been diagnosed—hypoparathyroidism (18), pernicious anaemia (7), moniliasis (7), diabetes mellitus (10), hepatic cirrhosis (2), alopecia areata (3), thyroid disease (30). A further 24 patients had antibodies to gastric, thyroid or parathyroid tissue. It can be concluded from these studies that patients with idiopathic Addison's disease run the risk of developing a variety of other disorders.

Premature gonadal failure in Addison's disease

Turkington and Lebovitz (1967) were the first to report abnormalities of gonadal function in patients with idiopathic Addison's disease. Amongst 32 patients with this condition they found seven with primary gonadal failure, three with atrophic testes, three with premature menopause and one with cystic ovaries. Premature ovarian failure usually preceded the development of clinical Addison's disease by several years. Studies by Irvine and his associates (1968) provide a possible explanation for gonadal failure associated with idiopathic Addison's disease. They demonstrated antibodies reactive with the theca interna of the ovary, the interstitial cells of the testis and the adrenal cortex in 5/77 patients with this variety of Addison's disease. Negative results were obtained in tuberculous Addison's disease and in normal controls. All five of the women with antibodies had either complete failure of menstruation or an early menopause. The finding of antibodies reacting with more than one steroid-producing tissue probably reflects the presence of common antigens, presumably enzymes involved in steroid biosynthesis. Primary gonadal failure may therefore be added to the variety of endocrinopathies associated with idiopathic Addison's disease, but further studies are required before the immunological aetiology of the condition can be accepted.

Epidemiology of Addison's disease

Mason and his colleagues (1968) have studied the epidemiology of Addison's disease. On 1st January 1960, they carried out a prevalence count in the North-east Metropolitan Hospital region and identified 82 patients with Addison's disease in a population of 3,200,000 of all ages. In the age-range 25 to 69 years the disease affected 39 per million, 12 with tuberculous and 27 with non-tuberculous hypoadrenalism. It was found that tuberculous disease was commoner in men and non-tuberculous disease in women. During a five year follow-up period of 74 of these 82 patients only one died of Addison's disease, but 11 other deaths from the disease occurred in the region during this period, all in patients who first presented after the prevalence count had been completed. In the four Metropolitan Hospital Board areas the annual death rate from Addison's disease in the age-group mentioned above appeared to be 1·4 per million. Of a total of 56 deaths in the four areas, 28 were due to tuberculous and 28 to non-tuberculous disease.

The value of this community study lies in the finding of a different clinical picture from that presenting in hospital practice. Two major clinical courses were found: the chronic and the acute.

The chronic course usually associated with non-tuberculous disease occurred more frequently in women than men. The prognosis was good and the fatality rate low, probably because the patients were under regular medical care.

The acute course of Addison's disease tended to be due to tuberculous disease and atrophy of the glands with equal frequency, and no difference in incidence between the sexes could be established. The onset was sudden, the course rapid, the outlook poor and the death rate high. The patients often had difficult social and psychiatric problems. In many cases a firm diagnosis was not possible until autopsy.

It is concluded that the Registrar-General's mortality figures showing nearly four deaths from non-tuberculous to one from tuberculous Addison's disease substantially underestimate the tuberculous form because of inaccurate recording of death certificates. Further epidemiological studies of other endocrine diseases are required to correct the bias in the clinical picture which has emerged from hospital-based studies.

Diagnosis of Addison's disease

Addison's disease is suspected in many patients who present with lethargy, nausea and vomiting, hypotension and weight loss, particularly if there is an increase in pigmentation of the skin. Most of these patients do not suffer from Addison's disease but from psychiatric disorders, malnutrition, malignant disease or chronic renal disorders. The demonstration of a low 17-oxosteroid and 17-hydroxycorticosteroid excretion in the urine may appear to support a diagnosis of hypoadrenalism in many of these patients, but this finding is not specific and can be made in any patient affected by a chronic wasting disease. Moreover it is often forgotten that urinary steroid excretion is lowered in the elderly. The apparent improvement by cortico-steroid administration may be due to the non-specific stimulation of appetite and well-being which is a transient effect of cortisol.

The diagnosis of hypoadrenalism is based firstly on the demonstration of adrenal hypofunction by the estimation of cortisol, aldosterone and androgen output and secondly on tests determining the pathogenesis of the disease. Cortisol deficiency can be diagnosed clinically, the patient complaining of weakness, nausea and vomiting, headaches, muscle and joint pains and faintness when standing. Indirect tests of cortisol deficiency do not require any special apparatus and are easily carried out. Patients with hypoadren-alism may or may not have electrolyte disturbances (hyponatraemia, hyperkalaemia) and elevation of the blood urea. Failure to excrete a water load is due to many causes, but correction of the defect by the adminis-tration of cortisol indicates hypoadrenalism. Ahmed and his colleagues (1967) have provided an explanation for this hitherto puzzling phenomenon. They have demonstrated that plasma levels of antidiuretic hormone (arginine vasopressin) are elevated in patients with untreated adrenocortical insufficiency. They suggest that hypersecretion of antidiuretic hormone (or impaired degradation) may play an important role in the abnormal water metabolism of hypoadrenalism, and that glucocorticoids promote normal water diuresis by inhibiting the over-secretion of arginine vasopressin by the neurohypophysis.

Electrocardiographic abnormalities can also provide indirect evidence of cortisol deficiency. Hartog and Joplin (1968) analysed the ECG pattern of 16 patients with proven hypoadrenalism. Thirteen showed flattening or inversion of the T waves in the standard and unipolar limb leads, six showed prolongation of the $Q-T_c$ interval and three showed a fall in voltage of the QRS complex. In the majority of these patients a striking regression of the changes occurred after cortisol repletion. There appears to be no correlation between these abnormalities and changes in the serum electrolytes, but alterations in the intracellular electrolytes may be responsible.

Although disease of an endocrine gland may not be reflected in the basal output of hormones, it always results in an impairment of the hormonal reserve. Modern endocrine function tests are therefore based on the change in hormone output induced by some agent known to stimulate the gland which is being tested. The synthetic corticotrophin (ACTH) preparation

Synacthen is β^{1-24} corticotrophin which contains the first 24 amino-acids of the ACTH chain in which biological activity resides. Any patient suspected of hypoadrenalism can be quickly, safely and accurately assessed by the 30-minute Synacthen-test which does not require hospitalization. It is based on the increase in plasma cortisol, usually measured as 11-hydroxy-corticosteroids, 30 minutes after a single intramuscular injection of 0·25 mg of Synacthen. The criteria for a normal test should be as follows:

1. The initial plasma cortisol should be greater than $5\mu g/100$ ml.
2. The plasma cortisol increment 30 minutes after Synacthen injection should be more than 7 $\mu g/100$ ml.
3. The plasma cortisol level at 30 minutes should be greater than $18\mu g/100$ ml whatever the initial level.

All three criteria should be satisfied for a normal response.

If the response to Synacthen is normal, significant adrenocortical disease can be excluded. If it is subnormal, more prolonged stimulation may be required before truly impaired adrenal function can be established, which is particularly important when distinguishing primary hypoadrenalism from that secondary to pituitary insufficiency. An intravenous infusion of 0·5 mg of Synacthen over five hours has been used, but the development of Synacthen Depot where the hormone is adsorbed on to a zinc-phosphate complex has prolonged the period of action and allowed a single intramuscular injection to be used. After administration of 1 mg of Synacthen Depot intramuscularly the plasma cortisol levels from nine normal patients were (mean $\pm$ SEM in $\mu g/100$ ml): $\frac{1}{2}$ hour $31\cdot4\pm4\cdot7$, 1 hour $36\cdot3\pm2\cdot7$, 2 hours $43\cdot3\pm3\cdot5$, 3 hours $45\cdot3\pm3\cdot3$, 4 hours $48\cdot7\pm3\cdot6$ and 5 hours $52\cdot4\pm5\cdot6$. These results do not differ from those obtained by the intravenous infusion of 0·5 mg of Synacthen (Nuki et al., 1969). An impaired response is again an indication for at least three days' treatment with ACTH after which the test should be repeated, any abnormality being then conclusive proof of primary adrenocortical disease.

Tests which help to determine the underlying cause of hypoadrenalism include serological tests for adrenal and other antibodies, flat X-ray of the abdomen to demonstrate the calcification of tuberculous adrenals, and the more recent 2-deoxy-D-glucose (2-DG) test. Infusions of 2-DG cause a consistent and marked increase in adrenaline output in normal subjects and in patients with idiopathic Addison's disease, but not in those with tuber-culous disease of the adrenals (Wegienka et al., 1966). The substance 2-DG, a glucose analogue, blocks the intracellular utilization of glucose, inducing a relative glucose deficiency, particularly in the nervous system, which leads to adrenaline output from the intact adrenal medulla. In idiopathic Addison's disease the presumed autoimmune process is confined to the adrenal cortex leaving the medulla intact, whereas tuberculous disease causes a pan-adrenalitis with destruction of both cortex and medulla, and therefore loss of the capacity to secrete adrenaline.

REFERENCES

AHMED, A. B., GEORGE, B. C., GONZALEZ-AUVERT, C. & DINGMAN, J. F. (1967). Increased plasma arginine vasopressin in clinical adrenocortical insufficiency and its inhibition by glucosteroids. *J. clin. Invest.*, **46**, 111.

BLIZZARD, R. M., CHEE, D. & DAVIS, W. (1967). The incidence of adrenal and other antibodies in the sera of patients with idiopathic adrenal insufficiency (Addison's disease). *Clin. exp. Immunol.*, **2**, 19.

HARTOG, M. & JOPLIN, G. F. (1968). Effects of cortisol deficiency on the electrocardiogram. *Brit. med. J.*, **2**, 275.

IRVINE, W. J., CHAN, M. M. W., SCARTH, L., KOLB, F. O., HARTOG, M., BAYLISS, R. I. S. & DRURY, M. I. (1968). Immunological aspects of premature ovarian failure associated with idiopathic Addison's disease. *Lancet*, **2**, 883.

IRVINE, W. J., STEWART, A. G. & SCARTH, L. (1967). A clinical and immunological study of adrenocortical insufficiency (Addison's disease). *Clin. exp. Immunol.*, **2**, 31.

MASON, A. S., MEADE, T. W., LEE, J. A. H. & MORRIS, J. N. (1968). Epidemiological and clinical picture of Addison's disease. *Lancet*, **2**, 744.

NUKI, G., SHEPHERD, J., DOWNIE, W. W., DICK, W. C. & HAINSWORTH, I. R. (1969). Adrenocorticotrophic responses to a single injection of Tetracosactrin Depot and to a standard Tetracosactrin infusion. *Lancet*, **1**, 188.

TURKINGTON, R. W. & LEBOVITZ, H. E. (1967). Extra-adrenal endocrine deficiencies in Addison's disease. *Amer. J. Med.*, **43**, 499.

WEGIENKA, L. C., GRASSO, S. G. & FORSHAM, P. H. (1966). Estimation of adrenomedullary reserve by infusion of 2-deoxy-D-glucose. *J. clin. Endocr.*, **26**, 37.

MAGNESIUM METABOLISM

Magnesium is the second most plentiful intracellular cation, the body content of magnesium being about 2000 mEq. Approximately half of the body's magnesium is in bone and the rest is equally distributed between muscle and other soft tissues, liver and striated muscle having high concentrations (15–20 mEq/kg). Measurements of serum magnesium by atomic absorption techniques indicate values ranging from 1·6 to 2·1 mEq/litre. In adults, the average daily magnesium intake is of the order of 25 mEq, mostly derived from green vegetables. Absorption is normally from the small intestine, though colonic absorption can also take place. Calcium appears to influence magnesium absorption, possibly by competition in a common absorptive process. Usually about one-third of the magnesium intake is excreted in the urine, though under conditions of deprivation renal excretion is markedly reduced (to less than 1 mEq/day).

Magnesium is a co-factor in many key enzyme systems, especially those which hydrolyze and transfer phosphate groups, including the phosphatases and those involved in the reactions of adenosine triphosphate. It is essential for the stabilization of DNA, RNA and ribosomes and in the binding of messenger RNA to ribosomes.

Magnesium or calcium depletion causes increased neuronal excitability and neuromuscular transmission, whereas magnesium excess has a curare-like action on the neuromuscular junction and may cause general anaesthesia.

Magnesium Deficiency

It has not been possible to induce symptomatic magnesium depletion by dietary restrictions alone, probably because marked renal conservation of magnesium occurs. To produce clinical effects, it is necessary for an inadequate intake to be aggravated by loss of gastro-intestinal fluids or malabsorption.

Magnesium depletion can exist without reduction in serum magnesium levels; conversely hypomagnesaemia may be present when the cellular magnesium content is normal. However, a lowered serum level is usually indicative of magnesium depletion in the appropriate clinical context. Estimation of erythrocyte magnesium or urinary excretion is also useful in detecting depletion of the element.

Magnesium deficiency causes neuromuscular dysfunction indicated by hyperexcitability and sometimes behaviour disorders. Tetany, major or minor epilepsy, ataxia, vertigo, tremor, muscle weakness, depression, irritability and psychosis may be associated with magnesium deficiency and are reversed by repletion. There is no clinical difference between the tetany of calcium and that of magnesium depletion. The electrocardiogram can be helpful in distinguishing hypocalcaemia from magnesium deficiency. In the former there is prolongation of the QT interval, whereas in the latter there is depression of ST segments and inversion of T waves in the precordial leads. Manifestations of magnesium deficience rarely occur unless the serum magnesium level is less than 1 mEq/litre.

The main causes of symptomatic hypomagnesaemia are indicated in Table 9.1.

Gastro-intestinal disorders

Magnesium deficiency can complicate a wide range of gastro-intestinal disorders, depletion occurring by a variety of mechanisms. Steatorrhoea from any cause results in magnesium depletion, probably due to excretion of large quantities of magnesium soaps. Vigorous oral calcium therapy may aggravate magnesium depletion because of competition for a common transport process of the two ions. Nasogastric suction removes about 1 mEq of magnesium per litre fluid and if this procedure is prolonged and intravenous infusions without magnesium are given this may lead to magnesium depletion. Alcoholic cirrhosis is a potent cause of magnesium deficiency which has been implicated, probably erroneously, in the pathogenesis of delirium tremens. Many factors may be involved including poor dietary intake, steatorrhoea from liver and pancreatic malfunction, and secondary aldosteronism if there is ascites. It should be stressed again that poor dietary intake alone does not cause symptomatic hypomagnesaemia in man.

TABLE 9.1

Causes of Symptomatic Hypomagnesaemia
(from Wacker and Parisi, 1968 by
permission of the editor of the *New Engl. J. Med.*)

Gastro-intestinal disorders
  Malabsorption syndromes, including non-tropical sprue
  Malabsorption due to extensive bowel resection
  Bowel and biliary fistulas
  Prolonged nasogastric suction with administration of
    magnesium-free parenteral fluids
  Prolonged diarrhoea
  Protein-calorie malnutrition
  Alcoholic cirrhosis
  Pancreatitis

Endocrine disorders
  Hyperparathyroidism and hypoparathyroidism
  Hyperaldosteronism
  Diabetic coma

Renal diseases
  Glomerulonephritis, pyelonephritis, hydronephrosis,
    nephrosclerosis and renal tubular acidosis (acute
    renal failure and chronic renal failure can cause
    hypermagnesaemia)

Alcoholism

Diuretic therapy
  Mercurials, ammonium chloride and thiazides

Malignant osteolytic disease

*Porphyria with inappropriate secretion of antidiuretic
hormone*

Excessive lactation

"Idiopathic"

Endocrine disorders

Magnesium depletion may complicate *hyperparathyroidism*, sometimes in the presence of a normal serum magnesium. Hypomagnesaemia may become manifest only after removal of the parathyroid adenoma, and the resulting tetany may require treatment with magnesium.

Aldosterone causes increased urinary and faecal magnesium excretion, and hypomagnesaemia may be responsible for symptoms in patients with *primary or secondary aldosteronism.*

Hypoadrenalism is a cause of *increased* serum magnesium which is however symptomless.

Diabetic ketosis may be associated with hypermagnesaemia but, as in the case of potassium, low serum levels of magnesium may rapidly follow the institution of effective therapy. It has been suggested that 5 mEq/litre of magnesium should be added to the intravenous therapy in diabetic ketosis, preferably an hour or two after commencement of the treatment.

Hyperthyroidism is a cause of asymptomatic hypomagnesaemia and conversely hypothyroidism results in hypermagnesaemia.

Diuretics

Many diuretics increase the renal excretion of magnesium. It is mandatory to estimate the serum magnesium in any patient on diuretic therapy who has evidence of neuromuscular irritability. Magnesium depletion, like potassium deficiency, may sensitize the myocardium to digitalis and predispose to arrhythmias.

Magnesium Excess

Magnesium excess occurs most frequently in acute or severe chronic renal failure and it is dangerous to give magnesium salts to such patients. Cardiac conduction defects develop at serum levels of 5–10 mEq/litre, with an increase in the PR interval and QRS duration and an increased amplitude of the T wave. Tendon reflexes are reduced as the concentration reaches 10 mEq/litre, and respiratory paralysis and general anaesthesia occur at about 15 mEq/litre. Still higher concentrations cause cardiac arrest in diastole.

Magnesium therapy

Magnesium therapy is indicated when the clinical features of magnesium depletion are present and when this is confirmed by low serum, erythrocyte, urinary or tissue magnesium levels. The sulphate salt is available in solutions of 10, 25 and 50 per cent concentrations; the rate of intravenous infusion should not exceed 1·5 ml of a 10 per cent solution per minute. Magnesium sulphate has also been used as a sedative in the treatment of pre-eclampsia and eclampsia. Oral magnesium supplements are preferable to intravenous injections when there is no urgency, and up to 10 mEq of magnesium hydroxide can be given daily by mouth without causing any alteration of bowel habit in many instances.

REFERENCES

HANNA, S., MacINTYRE, I., HARRISON, M. & FRASER, R. (1960). The syndrome of magnesium deficiency in man. *Lancet*, **2**, 172.

WALKER, W. E. C. & PARISI, A. F. (1968). Medical progress: magnesium metabolism. *New Engl. J. Med.*, **278**, 658, 712, 772.

AMYLOIDOSIS

Amyloidosis is the term applied to a group of conditions with the common characteristic of a deposition of a metachromatically staining protein (amyloid) in various tissues. Amyloid itself does not cause any tissue reaction and it is only when the deposits occur in strategic positions such as the bundle of His, or in massive amounts, that clinical sequelae result.

Amyloidosis can arise either as a complication of a number of different diseases (Table 9.2) and is then called secondary, or without any obvious cause when it is referred to as primary or idiopathic. Both sporadic and genetically determined varieties of primary amyloidosis can occur.

TABLE 9.2

Diseases Associated with Secondary Amyloidosis

1. Tuberculosis, leprosy

2. Chronic suppuration, e.g. osteomyelitis, bronchiectasis, decubitus ulcers following paraplegia

3. Rheumatic diseases and the "collagenoses"
   - (a) Rheumatoid arthritis and Still's disease
   - (b) Sjögren's syndrome
   - (c) Psoriatic arthropathy
   - (d) Ankylosing spondylitis
   - (e) Systemic lupus erythematosus

4. Ulcerative colitis

5. Regional ileitis

6. Sarcoidosis

7. Reticuloses

8. Malignant tumours, especially of the kidneys

In both types of the disease amyloid tissue is deposited in connective tissue, but the distribution differs to a certain extent in the two forms. In primary amyloidosis the deposits are usually found in cardiac, smooth and skeletal muscle, the tongue, skin and nerves, whereas in the secondary type the lesions are present in the liver, spleen, kidneys, intestine and adrenals. It has, however, become increasingly recognized that this classification is unsatisfactory since a direct relationship between the distribution and the two different forms of the disease does not always exist.

Missmahl (1959, 1969) has suggested a new classification based on the relationship between the amyloid deposits and particular connective tissue fibres. Perireticular amyloid (deposition along reticulin fibres) is said to be a generalized vascular disease, with amyloid deposition starting in the basement-membrane area and spreading to the tunica media. Included in this variety of amyloidosis are the hereditary nephropathic amyloidoses (e.g. familial Mediterranean fever) and the secondary amyloidoses associated with diseases listed in Table 9.2. The pericollagen type (deposition initially along collagen fibres) is described as involving connective tissue starting with the tunica adventitia of the blood vessel and spreading into the media. This variety includes the hereditary amyloidoses of neuropathic and cardiopathic types, acquired amyloidosis of multiple myeloma and idiopathic amyloidosis of the primary or localized varieties. Table 9.3 shows a comprehensive classification of the amyloidoses after Muckle (1969).

It should, however, be stressed that the distribution of these fibril types can be ascertained in early deposits only by meticulous technique, and as the deposition progresses the distribution becomes less obvious. Cohen (1967) emphasizes the uniformity of the amyloid fibrils themselves in all types of amyloidosis, and prefers to retain the old clinical classification such as the presence or absence of other disease and genetic associations, and relegates the tissue distribution of the amyloid fibrils to the background.

Incidence

While amyloidosis rarely causes death, it is more prevalent than is generally realized. Significant amyloid deposits are found in 0·5 to 1·0 per cent of routine hospital autopsies. In certain ethnic groups the disease is not uncommon e.g. the dominantly-inherited, atypical neuropathic form seen in a part of Portugal and the recessively-inherited, typical nephropathic type associated with fever affecting certain Mediterranean races (familial Mediterranean fever). The major form of sporadic primary amyloid disease occurs in the fifth and sixth decades, whereas secondary amyloidosis can appear at any age.

Clinical Manifestations

The clinical manifestations of secondary amyloidosis may be masked by the underlying disease process and depend on the organs affected by the deposits. *Renal* involvement leads characteristically to a nephrotic syndrome and later to chronic renal failure. When the rate of deposition of amyloid is slower and less extensive, blood vessels tend to be involved causing nephrosclerosis and hypertension, and protein loss may be less marked. Renal vein thrombosis can complicate amyloidosis affecting the kidneys and may lead to a rapid exacerbation of the nephrotic syndrome.

TABLE 9.3

Classification of the Amyloidoses
(after Muckle, 1969)

Distribution	Fibre Association	Hereditary	Sporadic
Generalized	Pericollagen	1. Neuropathy, legs (Portugal) 2. Neuropathy, arms (N. America) 3. Neuropathy+carpal tunnel syndrome (N. America) 4. Cardiomyopathy (Denmark)	Secondary: with myelomatosis Idiopathic: classical "primary"
Generalized	Perireticulin	1. Nephropathic (familial Mediterranean fever, Israel) 2. Nephropathic (similar syndrome, Derbyshire in United Kingdom)	Secondary: 1. chronic infection 2. malignancy Idiopathic: nephropathic
Localized	Pericollagen	—	Dermal
Localized	Mostly pericollagen, others not known	1. Senile cerebral 2. Dermal 3. Corneal	1. Senile (cerebral, pancreatic pulmonary, cardiac, seminal) 2. Diabetic (pancreatic islets) 3. Tracheo-bronchial diffuse 4. Focal, nodular (pulmonary, ureteric) 5. In or with neoplasms (carcinoma of skin, medullary carcinoma of thyroid)
Humoral	Mostly pericollagen others not known	—	Hepatic, dermal, pulmonary

Hepatomegaly

This is common, but evidence of liver failure such as jaundice and hepatic coma rare. A specific deficiency of plasma coagulation factor X has been described in some cases of severe hepatic amyloidosis. *Splenomegaly* is seldom more than moderate. *Gastro-intestinal* involvement leads to chronic diarrhoea and a malabsorption syndrome. In secondary amyloidosis extensive deposition in the *adrenals* may cause adrenocortical failure. Amyloid *neuropathy* may be the result of vascular lesions or compression atrophy. *Myopathy* principally affects the tongue and heart. In *cardiomyopathy* lesions are frequent in the bundle of His, and heart failure is accompanied by a low

ECG voltage, arrhythmias and digitalis sensitivity. *Skin* involvement is manifested by purpura or by flat brownish papules, and the elements of the triple response may be impaired.

Diagnosis

Amyloidosis may be suspected clinically, but as in sarcoidosis the diagnosis depends on the histological appearance of biopsy material. The Congo red test is unreliable and not without risk; it should not be used. There is a high incidence of rectal infiltration in most varieties of amyloidosis and rectal biopsy is now the diagnostic procedure of choice. It is essential that the biopsy includes a substantial portion of submucosa with its vasculature, and it is usually possible to distinguish between perireticulin and pericollagen deposits. Renal biopsy is also a valuable method of diagnosis, though because of the risks involved and because the kidney may be little affected in primary amyloidosis, this procedure should be used only for patients with evidence of renal involvement, e.g. albuminuria, hypertension, haematuria or uraemia. Due to the risk of haemorrhage, liver biopsy is not often indicated. Moreover, since hepatic deposits are frequently uneven the procedure is unreliable. Gum biopsy is painful and may give negative results even in advanced disease.

Nature and pathogenesis of amyloid

Amyloid is a form of connective tissue which can be shown by electron-microscopy to consist of fibrils measuring 80–100 Å in diameter and several thousand Å in length. The fibrils are coated with small amounts of most of the connective tissue acid mucopolysaccharides (particularly heparin sulphate) and plasma proteins. One of these proteins which is invariably present in human amyloid substance is a glycoprotein designated amyloid "P" protein. This has not been detected in normal tissues, but traces of it exist in adult plasma.

It is now generally agreed that amyloid fibrils are produced within the cytoplasm of reticuloendothelial cells, either those which normally form reticulin or those which synthesize collagen. These fibrils are subsequently extruded from the cells. The exact nature of the stimulus which causes these cells to produce amyloid is unknown, but in secondary amyloidosis the major factor appears to be over-exposure to antigens or toxins.

REFERENCES

BRITISH MEDICAL JOURNAL (1968). Tests for amyloidosis. 4, 564.
COHEN, A. S. (1967). Amyloidosis. *New Engl. J. Med.*, 277, 522, 574.

MISSMAHL, H. P. (1959). What is the relation between the various forms of amyloidosis and the connective tissue fibres? *Verh. dtsch. Ges. inn. Med.*, **65**, 439.

MISSMAHL, H. P. (1969). Amyloidosis. In *Textbook of Immunopathology*, Vol. 2. ed. P. Miescher. London: Grune & Stratton, p. 421.

MUCKLE, T. J. (1969). Association of clinical pathologists, trainee pathologists teaching tape. A short account of human amyloidosis.

10 Diseases of the Nervous System

PETER HUDGSON AND HENRY MILLER

GENERAL CONSIDERATIONS. CONGENITAL CERVICO-MEDULLARY ABNORMALITIES. HYDROCEPHALUS. PARA-NEOPLASTIC NEUROLOGICAL SYNDROMES IN MALIGNANT DISEASE. VIRAL INFECTIONS OF THE CENTRAL NERVOUS SYSTEM. THE PERIPHERAL NEUROPATHIES. THE NEUROLOGICAL COMPLICATIONS OF CHRONIC RENAL FAILURE. THE NEUROLOGICAL COMPLICATIONS OF LIVER DISEASE. LUMBAR CANAL STENOSIS. RECENT ADVANCES IN THE STUDY OF MUSCLE DISEASE

GENERAL CONSIDERATIONS

In a review of this kind it is clearly impossible to include all the major clinical problems confronting neurologists. Cerebral vascular disease and its management were discussed at length in the fourth (1961) and fifth (1966) editions of this book, and the treatment of Parkinson's disease was reviewed in the fifth edition. Because of this these subjects will not be discussed in detail. However, there have been several important advances in our knowledge of these diseases with respect to their natural history, investigation and treatment since the fifth edition. These will be discussed briefly hereunder.

Cerebral Vascular Disease

As far as the natural history of cerebral vascular disease is concerned, the most important recent advance has been the recognition of increasing numbers of cerebrovascular accidents of various kinds in young women taking oral contraceptives (the high-dose oestrogen-progestogen combination). The magnitude of the risk is still uncertain, principally because of the difficulty in obtaining data susceptible to statistical evaluation. However, the clinical study of Bickerstaff and Holmes (1967) and the recent statistical survey of Vessey and Doll (1969) leave little doubt that the risk exists, although it is certainly less than the risk of thrombo-embolism during pregnancy or in the puerperium. It can probably be ignored with safety in perfectly healthy young women, but "the pill" should not be prescribed for women with bad varicose veins or with a previous history of thrombo-embolic episodes of any kind.

The principles underlying investigation and treatment of patients with cerebral vascular disease have not altered materially since the last edition, and have recently been reviewed by Miller and Hudgson (1970). Since then, a variety of isotopic tracer techniques for measuring regional cerebral blood flow have become available. It has yet to be shown that they will be applicable to the clinical study of cerebral vascular disease in general, but they may be of considerable value in certain situations.

Regional cerebral perfusion rates can be estimated by pursuing the clearance of a freely diffusable tracer from the brain following its introduction either by internal carotid artery injection or by inhalation. The most commonly used tracer is ^{133}Xenon whose gamma emissions can be recorded through the intact skull. After saturation of the brain the rate of clearance is recorded, and this is proportional to the blood flow. A multi-exponential curve is produced which can be analysed into two principal components which are related to perfusion in the cortex (fast component) and white matter (slow component). The principles underlying these methods have been reviewed by Harper (1967).

Cerebral blood flow measurement has been shown to be of value in assessing patients for carotid artery surgery (O'Brien et al., 1967), since the washout methods of blood flow measurement reflect the perfusion rate at cellular level and hence blood flow in the smallest vessels. Blood-flow measurements have also been used to predict the occurrence of cerebral ischaemia following elective carotid occlusion, usually carried out for aneurysm. Jennett (1967) has shown that if the blood flow is reduced to below 25 per cent following clipping of the carotid artery then the patient is likely to develop ischaemic complications. Finally, when a large number of counters are used simultaneously, cerebral blood flow measurement in small areas may be a useful adjunct to scanning and angiography in the assessment of patients with cerebral vascular disease, vascular malformations and tumours.

The Treatment of Parkinson's Disease

It is now clear that the recent introduction of L-dopa in the treatment of Parkinsonism heralds a new era in the medical treatment of the disease. It originated in the neurochemical observation that in Parkinsonian syndromes, whether "idiopathic", post-encephalitic or secondary to manganese poisoning there is a selective and striking reduction in the normally concentrated dopamine content of the *substantia nigra*. The administration of dopamine itself is without benefit in Parkinsonism, and initial trials with small doses of its precursor L-dopa (Barbeau, 1962) were suggestive rather than impressive. It was not until 1967 that Cotzias et al. increased the dose to 8 g daily, with excellent therapeutic results that have now been widely confirmed, initially in North America and now in this country (Calne *et al.*, 1969; Godwin-Austen *et al.*, 1969).

About two-thirds of all patients are significantly improved and even in some severe cases the physical signs of the disease may virtually disappear. However, rigidity and akinesia are much more conspicuously relieved than tremor, and where the latter is the most troublesome symptom, stereotactic thalamotomy seems likely to retain its place as the treatment of choice.

Side-effects are troublesome and only partly due to initial difficulties in the purification of the drug. Dosage must be very slowly built up from 1 g daily in divided doses if nausea, vomiting and orthostatic hypotension are to be avoided. However, the most important side-effect is involuntary movements which may reach dystonic proportions. The avoidance of this complication is chiefly a matter of dosage, which in any case can often be progressively reduced after a few months. One of the patients reported by Godwin-Austen *et al.* (1969) became hypomanic on a dose of 8 g daily, but this disappeared when the dose was reduced to 5 g daily. This did not alter the beneficial effect on his Parkinsonism in any way.

The drug is expensive and in short supply chiefly because of the need to provide a purely laevo-rotatory form, but technical difficulties can no doubt be overcome: it may also be possible to reduce effective dosage materially by the concurrent administration of a decarboxylase inhibitor.

With increased availability and clinical experience it seems likely that L-dopa will become a routine treatment for Parkinsonism. The Medical Research Council has just initiated a multi-centre trial of L-dopa in Parkinson's disease in the United Kingdom and it is hoped that this will confirm its beneficial effects in a short time. Since, at present prices, free use of the drug could impose an extra cost of £15m. annually on the National Health Service, cheaper manufacture and measures to reduce dosage deserve urgent attention.

REFERENCES

BARBEAU, A. (1962). The pathogenesis of Parkinson's disease: a new hypothesis. *Canad. med. Ass. J.*, **87**, 802

BICKERSTAFF, E. R. & HOLMES, J. McD. (1967). Cerebral arterial insufficiency and oral contraceptives. *Brit. med. J.*, **1**, 726.

CALNE, D. B., STERN, G. M., LAWRENCE, D. R., SHARKEY, J. & ARMITAGE, P. (1969). L-dopa in postencephalitic Parkinsonism. *Lancet*, **1**, 744.

COTZIAS, G. C., VAN WOERT, M. H. & SCHIFFER, L. M. (1967). Aromatic aminoacids and the modification of Parkinsonism. *New Engl. J. Med.*, **276**, 374.

GODWIN-AUSTEN, R. B., TOMLINSON, E. B., FREARS, C. C. & KOK, H. W. L. (1969). Effects of L-dopa in Parkinson's disease. *Lancet*, **2**, 165.

HARPER, A. M. (1967). Measurement of cerebral blood flow in man. *Scot. med. J.*, **12**, 349.

JENNETT, W. B. (1967). The diagnostic use of radioisotopes in brain disorders. *Hosp. Med.*, **1**, 1037.

MILLER, H. & HUDGSON, P. (1970). Neurological emergencies. In *Compendium of Emergencies*, 3rd edition, ed. H. Gardiner-Hill. London: Butterworth.

O'BRIEN, M. D., VEALL, N. J., LUCK, R. J. & IRVINE, W. T. (1967). Cerebral cortex perfusion rates in extracranial cerebral vascular disease and the effects of operation. *Lancet*, **2**, 392.

VESSEY, M. P. & DOLL, R. (1969). Investigation of relation between use of oral contraceptives and thromboembolic disease. A further report. *Brit. med. J.*, **2**, 651.

CONGENITAL CERVICO-MEDULLARY ABNORMALITIES

It was pointed out in the previous edition (Stern, 1966) that lesions of various kinds in the upper cervical canal and the foramen magnum may simulate "untreatable" degenerative conditions, particularly syringomyelia. Gardner (1965) had previously suggested that many cases of so-called syringomyelia may in fact be due to chronic hydromyelia (congenital dilatation of the central canal) associated with one or other of the Chiari anomalies at the cervico-medullary junction. He further suggested that surgical decompression of these anomalies might arrest the progress of neurological deficit in affected persons. In a personal series of 74 cases he reported arrest of deterioration or even improvement in 68 surgically treated cases. Interest in Gardner's views has been re-awakened by the work of Appleby *et al.* (1968) and Foster *et al.* (1969), who reported 20 patients with syringomyelia or syringomyelia-like syndromes who were found to have a variety of congenital cervico-medullary abnormalities. In three of these the anomalies were studied in detail at autopsy (Foster *et al.*, 1969). The clinical features of these patients corresponded to the five types of presentation of foramen magnum lesions described by Symonds and Meadows (1937), viz. syringomyelia or atypical syringomyelia; spastic tetraparesis; profound loss of joint-position sense in the upper limbs and, to a lesser extent, the lower limbs; hydrocephalus; and brain-stem and cerebellar manifestations. With respect to the latter, we have noted that many of our own patients have experienced oscillopsia and have had striking postural nystagmus. The frequency of this finding has also been emphasized by Gordon (1969) who found vocal cord paralyses in a number of patients, presumably due to damage to the central connections of the vagus. In spite of the fact that the underlying anomalies must have been present since birth, none of the patients had a history of neurological illness in early life. Age at the time of presentation varied from 17 to 56 years and the majority presented in early adult life. The sex incidence was unremarkable.

The diagnosis of "symptomatic" syringomyelia is essentially radiological. The association of syringomyelia with a variety of skeletal abnormalities in the upper cervical spine and the base of the skull has been recognized for many years (Spillane *et al.*, 1957). The presence of anomalies such as simple fusion of vertebral bodies or spinous processes, the Klippel-Feil anomaly, or basilar impression should alert the observer to the possible existence of an underlying congenital abnormality of the neuraxis. However, the presence of bony anomalies is by no means a *sine qua non* for the diagnosis of congenital anomalies of the cervico-medullary junction, gross abnormalities sometimes being found in patients with completely normal cervical spines and skull bases (Appleby *et al.*, 1968). The definitive diagnosis of these conditions rests on myelography of the upper cervical cord and the foramen magnum regions in the supine position (Appleby *et al.*, 1968). This examination demonstrates descent of hind-brain structures, particularly the cerebellar tonsils, into the cervical canal behind the cord, whereas in routine examinations in the prone position the contrast medium passes straight through the foramen magnum into the pre-pontine cistern. Use of this technique on a wide scale has led to identification of increasing numbers of these anomalies (Appleby, 1969; Gordon, 1969; Newton, 1969; Smith and Ridley, 1969) and their presence has been confirmed at surgical exploration in many instances (Appleby *et al.*, 1968; Gordon, 1969; Hankinson, 1970). Gardner (1965) has consistently advocated surgical decompression of the upper cervical canal as the only rational method of treatment for "syringomyelia". Encouraging results of surgical treatment have also been reported by Appleby *et al.* (1968), Gordon (1969) and Hankinson (1970), although follow-up has been too short as yet to permit confidence about the long-term outcome. Indeed, Appleby *et al.* (1969) have separated seven cases from a group of over 50 because of deterioration in their neurological deficits after decompression of the foramen and upper cervical canal. In two instances deterioration was rapid, culminating in central respiratory failure and necessitating urgent ventricular drainage. At operation these patients were shown to have dense arachnoidal adhesions around the exit foramina of the fourth ventricle and in the upper canal, but no congenital anomalies were found. Review of their myelograms showed that the changes were consistently different from those in the patients with congenital anomalies, most of whom had improved post-operatively. Because of this, Appleby and his colleagues suggested that only those patients in whom congenital anomalies could be demonstrated with confidence by myelography should be submitted to decompression of the canal and foramen. They further suggested that patients with obvious adhesive arachnoiditis on myelography might best be treated by elective insertion of some form of ventriculo-atrial shunt.

The clinical and radiological studies have rekindled controversy about the pathogenesis of "syringomyelia" and syringobulbia. In spite of its known association with congenital anomalies of the axial skeleton, it has traditionally been regarded as a primary degenerative condition of the spinal cord. Gardner (1965) challenged this view, suggesting that most cases were in fact due to chronic *hydromyelia* produced by partial or complete obstruction to the egress of cerebrospinal fluid (CSF) from the foramina of Magendie and Luschka. He postulated that the pulsatile CSF, unable to leave the ventricular system, gradually distends the central canal of the cord which is normally in communication with the fourth ventricle until late in foetal life. His views have been supported by Appleby *et al.* (1968) and by Hankinson (1970) who has found persistent communications between the "syrinx" and the fourth ventricle in a number of personal cases. Williams (1969) has recently summarized the various hypotheses for the pathogenesis of syringomyelia and has presented his own view that distension of the central canal may be due to venous pressure swings rather than arterial pulse waves transmitted through the CSF. It should be emphasized however that the communication between the central canal and the ventricular system that is central to all theories of pathogenesis deriving from Gardner's work is not always found at operation, so a healthy scepticism should be preserved about the above speculation until final proof is forthcoming. In this context it is of interest that Wadia (1967) has described a late-onset myelopathy in Indians with congenital atlanto-occipital dislocations. The dislocations were often accompanied by other congenital anomalies of the cervical skeleton, e.g. the Klippel-Feil syndrome, but no evidence of the Chiari malformations was found radiologically or at operation. Clinically the patients presented with attacks of weakness and sensory loss in all four limbs, spastic tetraparesis and loss of proprioception, but not with syringomyelic syndromes.

REFERENCES

APPLEBY, A. (1969). Craniovertebral anomalies. *Proc. roy. Soc. Med.*, **62**, 729.

APPLEBY, A., BRADLEY, W. G., FOSTER, J. B., HANKINSON, J. & HUDGSON, P. (1969). Syringomyelia due to arachnoiditis at the foramen magnum. *J. neurol. Sci.*, **8**, 451.

APPLEBY, A., FOSTER, J. B., HANKINSON, J. & HUDGSON, P. (1968). The diagnosis and management of the Chiari anomalies in adult life. *Brain*, **91**, 131.

FOSTER, J. B., HUDGSON, P. & PEARCE, G. W. (1969). The association of syringomyelia and congenital cervico-medullary anomalies: Pathological evidence. *Brain*, **92**, 25.

GARDNER, W. J. (1965). Hydrodynamic mechanism of syringomyelia; its relationship to myelocele. *J. Neurol. Neurosurg. Psychiat.*, **28**, 247.

GORDON, D. S. (1969). Neurological syndromes associated with craniovertebral anomalies. *Proc. roy. Soc. Med.*, **62**, 725.

HANKINSON, J. (1970). Syringomyelia and the surgeon. In *Modern Trends in Neurology*, *5th* Series, ed. D. Williams. London: Butterworth.

NEWTON, E. J. (1969). Syringomyelia as a manifestation of defective fourth ventricular drainage. *Ann. roy. Coll. Surg. Engl.*, **44**, 194.

SMITH, J. & RIDLEY, A. (1969). Cerebellar ectopia presenting in adult life. *Brit. med. J.*, **1**, 353.

SPILLANE, J. D., PALLIS, C. & JONES, A. M. (1957). Developmental abnormalities in the region of the foramen magnum. *Brain*, **80**, 11.

STERN, G. M. (1966). Diseases of the nervous system. In *Progress in Clinical Medicine*, 5th edition, ed. R. Daley and H. Miller. London: Churchill.

SYMONDS, C. P. & MEADOWS, S. P. (1937). Compression of the spinal cord in the region of the foramen magnum. *Brain*, **60**, 52.

WADIA, N. H. (1967). Myelopathy complicating congenital atlanto-axial dislocation. *Brain*, **90**, 449.

WILLIAMS, B. (1969). The distending force in the production of communicating syringomyelia. *Lancet*, **2**, 189.

HYDROCEPHALUS

Hydrocephalus, communicating or obstructive, has long been recognized as a potentially treatable cause of progressive dementia in adults. Interest in this problem has been re-awakened by the recent introduction of a new pathophysiological concept to explain some cases of hydrocephalus and by the use of a new technique for the diagnosis of communicating hydrocephalus. In 1965, Hakim and Adams, and Adams *et al.*, described a group of individuals who presented with progressive dementia and ataxia, some of whom had previously sustained head injury, meningitis or subarachnoid haemorrhage. All had normal or slightly raised spinal fluid pressure, and they improved for short periods after lumbar puncture. Air encephalography revealed hydrocephalus of varying severity, *with no passage of air over the surfaces of the hemispheres*. All the patients studied had ventriculo-atrial shunts inserted and were said to have improved significantly. These workers proposed the name "normal pressure" hydrocephalus for this syndrome and Adams (1966) suggested a mechanism for the development of this kind of hydrocephalus similar to that invoked by Gardner (1965) to explain syringomyelia and outlined above. The validity of this concept must remain in doubt for the time being, and the writers can only say that their personal experience lends little support to the hypothesis to date.

However, it is generally agreed that ventricular drainage produces improvement or at least arrest of progress in dementia due to communicating hydrocephalus with *high* spinal fluid pressure. One of the difficulties associated with the management of such cases is the deterioration which often follows confirmation of the diagnosis by air encephalography. The application of isotope cisternography, a scanning technique introduced by Di Chiro (1964a and b), may avoid such complications, and there are now a number of reports of its successful use in this situation, e.g. Bannister *et al.* (1967). In this test, radio-iodinated serum albumin (RISA) containing a small dose (100 μC) of ^{131}I is injected into the lumbar theca, and its passage through the spinal fluid pathways is scanned at two, six, 24 and 48 hours. Under normal circumstances no tracer enters the ventricular system, but in communicating hydrocephalus the isotope can be detected in the ventricles by 24 hours. According to Bannister *et al.* (1967) the total radiation dose to the central nervous system was only one rad and to the body one millirad, although Sear and Cohen (1968) suggested that it may have been much higher. Brocklehurst (1968), Bull (1968) and Di Chiro (1968) have subsequently confirmed that the radiation dose is in fact small. Ommaya *et al.* (1968) have emphasized the value of isotope cisternography with RISA in locating the fistulae in cases of non-traumatic spinal fluid rhinorrhoea. Di Chiro *et al.* (1968) modified the technique, substituting isotopic Technetium (^{99m}Tc) attached to serum albumin for RISA, and found this to be particularly useful for the investigation of spontaneous spinal fluid rhinorrhoea.

REFERENCES

ADAMS, R. D. (1966). Further observations on normal pressure hydrocephalus. *Proc. roy. Soc. Med.*, **59**, 1135.

ADAMS, R. D., FISHER, C. M., HAKIM, S., OJEMANN, R. G. & SWEET, W. H. (1965). Symptomatic occult hydrocephalus with "normal" cerebrospinal fluid pressure. *N. Engl. J. Med.*, **273**, 117.

BANNISTER, R., GILFORD, E. & KOCEN, R. (1967). Isotope encephalography in the diagnosis of dementia due to communicating hydrocephalus. *Lancet*, **2**, 1014.

BROCKLEHURST, G. (1968). Radiation dose in isotope encephalography. *Lancet*, **1**, 358.

BULL, J. W. D. (1968). Radiation dose in isotope encephalography. *Lancet*, **1**, 357.

DI CHIRO, G. (1964a). New radiographic and isotopic procedures in neurologic diagnosis. *J. Amer. med. Ass.*, **188**, 524.

DI CHIRO, G. (1964b). Movement of the cerebrospinal fluid in human beings. *Nature (Lond.)*, **204**, 290.

DI CHIRO, G. (1968). Radiation dose in isotope encephalography. *Lancet*, **1**, 526.

DI CHIRO, G., ASHBURN, W. L. & BRINER, W. H. (1968). Technetium Tc99m serum albumin. *Arch. Neurol.*, **19**, 218.

GARDNER, W. J. (1965). Hydrodynamic mechanism of Syringomyelia: its relationship to myelocele. *J. Neurol. Neurosurg. Psychiat.*, **28**, 247.

HAKIM, S. & ADAMS, R. D. (1965). The special clinical problem of symptomatic hydrocephalus with normal cerebrospinal fluid pressure. *J. Neurol. Sci.*, **2**, 307.

OMMAYA, A. K., DI CHIRO, G., BALDWIN, M. & PENNYBACKER, J. B. (1968). Non-traumatic cerebrospinal fluid rhinorrhoea. *J. Neurol. Neurosurg. Psychiat.*, **31**, 214.

SEAR, R. & COHEN, M. (1968). Radiation dose in isotope encephalography. *Lancet*, **1**, 249.

PARANEOPLASTIC NEUROLOGICAL SYNDROMES IN MALIGNANT DISEASE

A variety of what have been called "neuromyopathic" disorders may occur in association with malignant neoplasms of one kind or another. The development of such disorders, which is not due to the physical presence of the primary tumour or its metastases, is presumed to be a manifestation of metabolic disturbance engendered by the tumour. Such an association was first reported by Brouwer (1919) and it was Brouwer and Biemond (1938) who suggested that the neoplasm may have been responsible for the neurological lesion. Current interest in this group of disorders was stimulated by Denny-Brown's (1948) description of a pure sensory neuropathy in association with a bronchogenic carcinoma, and the accounts of subacute cerebellar degeneration in association with carcinoma, in papers by Brain, Daniel and Greenfield (1951) and Henson, Russell and Wilkinson (1954). The incidence of these disorders has been the subject of recent controversy. It is likely that the figures quoted in the past by the London Hospital workers have been too high, although it is now generally accepted that their overall incidence (including non-symptomatic cases) is approximately 6 per cent in epithelial tumours (Brain, 1965) and 2 per cent in the reticuloses (Currie et al., 1970). This figure rises steeply in bronchogenic carcinoma and ovarian carcinoma, where incidences of 16 per cent and 11 per cent respectively have been reported (Croft and Wilkinson, 1965). Wilner and Brody (1968) recently claimed that the incidence of the neuromyopathies was equally high in patients with chronic non-cancerous lung disease. These patients were controls in a comparative study with bronchogenic carcinoma and were all inmates of Veterans Administration hospitals in the U.S.A. Many of them drank large quantities of alcohol, which can produce similar neurological conditions, e.g. dementia, cerebellar degeneration, peripheral neuropathy, myopathy. For this reason, together with the small number of patients studied, their claim must be regarded with some reservation.

The various para-neoplastic syndromes reported in association with visceral neoplasms are as follows:

1. Subacute cerebellar degeneration
2. Sensory neuropathy
3. Mixed sensorimotor neuropathy
4. Myopathy
5. Myasthenic-myopathic syndrome (the Eaton-Lambert syndrome)
6. Motor neurone disease
7. Encephalomyelitis
8. Neurological disturbances produced by para-neoplastic metabolic syndromes, e.g. hypercalcaemia or inappropriate antidiuretic hormone (ADH) secretion.

It should be noted that more than one of these disturbances may occur in association with a single neoplasm. The writers have recently seen a case of subacute cerebellar degeneration which presented in the first instance with dementia and epileptic seizures due to inappropriate ADH secretion and water retention. It is also important to remember that in some of these patients pathological evidence of degeneration elsewhere in the central nervous system, e.g. in the corticospinal tracts or the extrapyramidal pathways, may be found at autopsy although clinical evidence of its existence had been absent or minimal.

Carcinoma of the lung is the commonest neoplasm producing these syndromes, 85 cases of bronchogenic carcinoma occurring in a recent series of 162 (Croft and Wilkinson, 1965). The oat-cell carcinoma of the bronchus was the commonest histological type represented in this group. In the same study Croft and Wilkinson (1965) found that breast, stomach and ovary were other relatively common primary sites.

These conditions have about the same incidence in the lymphomas and the myeloproliferative disorders (Currie et al., 1970). Cerebellar degeneration, the peripheral neuropathies and polymyositis have been reported in Hodgkin's disease and other lymphomas, but the incidence of the other disorders seems to be less than in epithelial neoplasms. A number of other "para-neoplastic" conditions occur in association with the lymphomas, e.g. myelopathies, progressive multifocal leucoencephalopathy. Their relationship with the underlying neoplasm is likely to be different from the conditions listed above and they will be discussed separately (see viral infections of the central nervous system).

Subacute cerebellar degeneration

The principal pathological changes in this syndrome include loss of Purkinje cells, degeneration of the direct spinocerebellar tracts, and meningeal and perivascular lymphocytic infiltration, often accompanied by patchy minor changes elsewhere in the central nervous system. The condition usually progresses steadily over a period of weeks or a few months at the most, and may antedate clinical evidence of the underlying neoplasm. The longest recorded delay between the onset of cerebellar degeneration and the appearance of the cancer is eight years, in a case described by Brain and Wilkinson (1965). This naturally raises the question of the genuineness of the relationship in such instances. The patients usually have ataxia of the limbs and of the trunk, sometimes so severe that they cannot sit up in bed, with dysarthria and sometimes nystagmus. The latter has been claimed in the past to be uncommon, but affected half the patients in the recent London Hospital survey (Brain and Wilkinson, 1965). The progress of the condition is sometimes apparently arrested by successful resection of the underlying neoplasm, but gradual deterioration continues in most cases (Brain and Wilkinson, 1965).

Sensory neuropathy

Pathologically, this condition is characterized by gross degenerative changes in the neurones of the dorsal root ganglia, with sparse lymphocytic infiltration of the ganglia and demyelination in the dorsal columns and the sensory fibres of peripheral nerves. The patients present clinically with loss of all modalities of sensation and pain in the extremities, the lower being more severely affected than the upper limbs. Pain is often severe and persistent, variously described as "tearing", "dragging", or "burning", and sometimes accompanied by nausea. The deep tendon reflexes are usually lost but weakness of the limb muscles is absent or minimal. Motor nerve conduction velocities are usually normal but sensory nerve action potentials cannot be recorded. The sera and spinal fluid of some of these patients contain complement-fixing antibodies to neural tissue (Wilkinson, 1964), and some cases are steroid-responsive, suggesting that the neuropathy may have an immunological basis. Once again the clinical onset of neuropathy may precede that of the underlying malignancy. In practice, malignancy should be excluded in all cases of peripheral neuropathy presenting in middle or late adult life. The index of suspicion will clearly be higher if the symptoms are predominantly sensory and severely painful.

Mixed sensorimotor neuropathy

This is more often encountered than the sensory form described above. Its symptomatology is essentially the same as in any other mixed peripheral neuropathy and in general it is a less dramatic and more slowly progressive illness than the purely sensory form. However, occasional cases of rapidly progressive mainly motor neuropathy resembling the Guillain-Barré syndrome have been described in association with bronchogenic carcinoma and Hodgkin's disease (Currie *et al.*, 1970). Some of these cases also are steroid-responsive. The clinical approach to the individual case is the same as in sensory neuropathy.

Myopathy

It has been claimed that a non-specific proximal myopathy may occur in patients with cancer, especially in males (Henson, 1969). It is probable, however, that the only myopathic conditions associated with malignant disease are polymyositis, dermatomyositis (Walton, 1969) and the so-called myasthenic-myopathic syndrome described below. The overall incidence of malignant neoplasms in polymyositis or dermatomyositis is about 20 per cent, the figure rising to over 50 per cent in males over 40 years (Arundell *et al.*, 1960) and to 71 per cent in males over 50 years (Shy, 1962). In females over 50 years, the incidence is stated to be 24 per cent (Shy, 1962). The clinical presentation of polymyositis associated with malignancy is the same as that in any other form of the disease. The patients present with proximal muscular weakness and wasting, which may be rapidly or gradually progressive and is often accompanied by muscle pains. There may be no involvement of the skin or this may vary from Raynaud's phenomenon to the florid eruption of dermatomyositis. There may also be general malaise, anorexia, weight loss and feverishness suggesting an associated systemic disturbance. The diagnosis can be confirmed by electromyography and by finding a raised serum creatine kinase level, while in some cases focal necrosis, regeneration and inflammatory changes can be found on muscle biopsy. However, the latter investigation is notoriously unreliable in polymyositis, and, because of the patchy pathological changes, a normal biopsy does not exclude the diagnosis. Many patients with polymyositis associated with malignancy improve with steroid therapy, though Pearson (1969) claims that the response is less impressive than in other forms of the disease. The comments made previously about the investigation of peripheral neuropathy in middle or late life are germane in this context. A patient in this age-group presenting with proximal myopathy should be thoroughly screened to exclude an occult and possibly surgically treatable neoplasm.

Myasthenic-myopathic syndrome (the Eaton-Lambert syndrome)

The association of fatiguable muscle weakness with bronchogenic carcinoma was first described by Anderson *et al.* (1953), and further cases were reported by Henson *et al.* (1954), and by Heathfield and Williams (1954) who considered that their symptoms were not due to typical myasthenia gravis. Subsequently Lambert, Eaton and Rooke (1956) described an unusual defect of neuromuscular transmission in a similar group of patients. This has subsequently been shown to be characteristic of the condition, which has a number of important clinical, physiological and pharmacological differences from classical myasthenia gravis. The extraocular muscles are only rarely involved, the deep tendon reflexes are diminished or absent, and the response to the anticholinesterases including edrophonium (Tensilon) is unimpressive. Electromyographic studies show an incremental response of the compound muscle action potentials evoked by supramaximal stimulation of the appropriate motor nerve at tetanic rates. In sharp contrast to classical myasthenia, these patients are extremely sensitive to ganglion-blocking agents though still relatively sensitive to curare. The fatiguability and electrophysiological abnormality are usually improved by treatment with guanidine hydrochloride given orally in doses ranging from 15 to 30 mg/kg body weight per day. Detailed accounts of the myasthenic syndrome and the nature of the neuromuscular transmission defect are given by Lambert and Rooke (1965), McQuillen and Johns (1967), and Kennedy and Jimenez-Pabon (1968). A similar defect can be produced by the administration of certain antibiotics, notably neomycin, streptomycin and kanamycin (McQuillen *et al.*, 1958).

Motor neurone disease

Brain, Croft and Wilkinson (1965) reported a number of patients with syndromes apparently indistinguishable from motor neurone disease who also had carcinomas of the lung, breast stomach or small bowel. They claimed that the particular kind of motor neurone disease in this group of patients differed from the classical variety in that its progression tended to be very much slower. They suggested that when the diagnosis of motor neurone disease is made and the progression of symptoms appears to be unusually slow, an intensive search should be made for an occult carcinoma, because of the relatively good prognosis of the neurological disturbance. However, they conceded that a minority of cases of classical motor neurone disease survive for many years and the validity of this association must remain in doubt for the time being.

Encephalomyelitis

Henson *et al.* (1954) described two patients with oat-cell carcinomas of the bronchus and clinical disturbances pointing to lesions in the brain stem and spinal cord. Autopsy revealed what they described as a chronic progressive poliomyelitis. Henson and his colleagues (1965) have recently reported another five cases of a similar nature and noted an association with sensory neuropathy in four of these. They suggest that this condition is inflammatory, possibly due to activation of latent viral infection, producing lesions in the limbic system, the motor nuclei of the brain stem, and the anterior horn cells of the cord. In this context it is interesting that Walton *et al.* (1969) reported what they called subacute poliomyelitis in a patient with Hodgkin's disease who died with a bizarre neurological illness. Limbic encephalitis in isolation may be the substrate for the organic psychiatric breakdown that sometimes occurs in malignant disease. Most cases of this nature are associated with oat-cell carcinoma of the bronchus.

Neurological disturbances in hypercalcaemia and inappropriate ADH secretion

Oat-cell carcinomas of the bronchus especially may secrete polypeptide hormones closing resembling parathormone and vasopressin. These hormones produce hypercalcaemia and water retention respectively, and these in turn may be accompanied by a variety of neurological disturbances. Hypercalcaemia may be accompanied by lethargy, irritability and muscle hypotonia. Water retention can produce psychiatric syndromes of various kinds, a confusional state, stupor leading to coma, and epileptic seizures. Focal neurological signs such as hemiparesis may be found during any of these phases. Inappropriate ADH secretion should be suspected if a patient has consistently low serum sodium levels (usually 120 milliequivalents per litre or less) and can be confirmed by finding low plasma osmolality. The treatment of this condition is water restriction.

REFERENCES

ANDERSON, H. J., CHURCHILL-DAVIDSON, H. C. & RICHARDSON, A. T. (1953). Bronchial neoplasm with myasthenia. *Lancet*, 2, 1291.

ARUNDELL, F. D., WILKINSON, R. D. & HASERICK, J. R. (1960). Dermatomyositis and malignant neoplasms in adults. *Arch. Derm. Syph. (Chic).*, 82, 772.

BRAIN, LORD (1965). In *The Remote Effects of Cancer on the Nervous System*, ed. Lord Brain and F. H. Norris Jr. New York and London: Grune & Stratton.

BRAIN, LORD, CROFT, P. B. & WILKINSON, M. (1965). Motor neurone disease as a manifestation of neoplasm. *Brain*, 88, 479.

BRAIN, W. R., DANIEL, P. B. & GREENFIELD, J. G. (1951). Subacute cerebellar degeneration and its relation to carcinoma. *J. Neurol. Neurosurg. Psychiat.*, 14, 59.

BRAIN, LORD & WILKINSON, M. (1965). Subacute cerebellar degeneration associated with neoplasms. *Brain*, 88, 465.

BROUWER, B. (1919). Beitrag zur Kenntnis der chronischen diffusen Kleinhirner-krankungen. *Neurol. Zbl.*, 38, 674.

BROUWER, B. & BIEMOND, A. (1938). Les affections parenchymateuses du cervelet et le signification due point de vue de l'anatomie et de la physiologie de cet organe. *J. Belg. Neurol.*, 38, 691.

CROFT, P. B. & WILKINSON, M. (1965). The incidence of carcinomatous neuro-myopathy in patients with various types of carcinoma. *Brain*, 88, 427.

CURRIE, S., HENSON, R. A., MORGAN, H. G. & POOLE, H. J. (1970). The incidence of the non-metastatic neurological syndromes of obscure origin in the reticu-loses. *Brain*, 93, 629.

DENNY-BROWN, D. (1948). Primary sensory neuropathy with muscular changes associated with carcinoma. *J. Neurol. Neurosurg. Psychiat.*, 11, 73.

HEATHFIELD, K. W. G. & WILLIAMS, J. R. B. (1954). Peripheral neuropathy and myopathy associated with bronchogenic carcinoma. *Brain*, 77, 122.

HENSON, R. A. (1969). Neuromuscular disorders associated with malignant disease. In *Disorders of Voluntary Muscle*, 2nd edition, ed. J. N. Walton. London: Churchill.

HENSON, R. A., HOFFMAN, H. L. & URICH, H. (1965). Encephalomyelitis with carcinoma. *Brain*, 88, 449.

HENSON, R. A., RUSSELL, D. S. & WILKINSON, M. (1954). Carcinomatous neuropathy and myopathy, a clinical and pathological study. *Brain*, 77, 82.

KENNEDY, W. R. & JIMENEZ-PABON, E. (1968). The myasthenic syndrome associated with small-cell carcinoma of the lung (Eaton-Lambert syndrome). *Neurology (Minneap.)*, 18, 757.

LAMBERT, E. H., EATON, L. M. & ROOKE, E. D. (1956). Defect of neuromuscular conduction associated with malignant neoplasms. *Amer. J. Physiol.*, 187, 612.

LAMBERT, E. H. & ROOKE, E. D. (1965). Myasthenic state and lung cancer. In *The Remote Effects of Cancer on the Nervous System*, ed. Lord Brain and F. H. Norris Jr. New York and London: Grune & Stratton.

McQUILLEN, M. P., CANTOR, H. E. & O'ROURKE, J. R. (1958). Myasthenic syn-drome associated with antibiotics. *Arch. Neurol.*, 18, 402.

McQUILLEN, M. P. & JOHNS, R. J. (1967). The nature of the defect in the Eaton-Lambert syndrome. *Neurology (Minneap.)*, 17, 527.

PEARSON, C. M. (1969). Polymyositis and related disorders. In *Disorders of Volun-tary Muscle*, 2nd edition, ed. J. N. Walton. London: Churchill.

SHY, G. M. (1962). The late onset myopathy. *Wld. Neurol.*, 3, 149.

WALTON, J. N. Personal communication.
WALTON, J. N. (1969). (Ed.) *Disorders of Voluntary Muscle*, 2nd edition. London: Churchill.
WILKINSON, P. C. (1964). Serological findings in carcinomatous neuromyopathy. *Lancet*, 1, 1301.
WILNER, E. C. & BRODY, J. A. (1968). An evaluation of the remote effects of cancer on the nervous system. *Neurology (Minneap.)*, 18, 1120.

VIRAL INFECTIONS OF THE CENTRAL NERVOUS SYSTEM

Acute viral infections of the central nervous system were discussed in the third (1956) and fourth (1961) editions of this book. As a result of effective vaccination programmes in Europe, North America and Australasia, poliomyelitis no longer constitutes a public health problem. Nevertheless, an appreciation of its clinical features and behaviour remains important for a generation of physicians who know it only as a difficult and rarely encountered diagnostic exercise. Viral encephalitis of the St Louis B and Murray Valley types is uncommon in north-western Europe, but interest in infective encephalitis has been maintained for several reasons. An increasing number of cases of subacute sclerosing panencephalitis and of acute necrotizing encephalitis due to the herpes simplex virus is being recognized. A large body of evidence that the former is a late complication of measles virus infection has accumulated, together with the emergence of some new concepts in the fields of slow and latent virus infection. To date, only one slow virus infection, kuru, has been positively identified in man, although the speculative incrimination of slow virus infection in other and more common neurological conditions such as multiple sclerosis and motor neurone disease is intriguing. Subacute sclerosing panencephalitis and herpes simplex encephalitis will be discussed in detail, and our present knowledge of slow virus infections reviewed.

Subacute sclerosing panencephalitis (SSPE)

This condition is a nosologically distinct entity with a variety of morbid anatomical abnormalities which have essentially the same clinical expression. The spectrum of SSPE includes the subacute inclusion body encephalitis of Dawson (1933) in which the cerebral cortex is principally involved and numerous inclusion bodies are found, subacute sclerosing leucoencephalitis (Van Bogaert and De Busscher, 1939; Van Bogaert, 1945) which is characterized by patchy demyelination, and all possible combinations of these two.

The disease has a subacute evolution over a period of weeks or months. It usually affects adolescents or young adults, and presents initially with disturbances of behaviour and affect followed by epileptic seizures, myoclonic jerks which can be violent, progressive dementia and a variety of focal neurological signs. The disease process is nearly always fatal, treatment with steroids and antiviral drugs such as the thiosemicarbazones apparently failing materially to effect its course. However, three cases have been reported in which spontaneous recovery occurred (Pearce and Barwick, 1964; Cobb and Morgan-Hughes, 1968), whilst arrest of the progress of the disease has been described by Legg (1967). In the fully-developed syndrome the EEG abnormality is virtually diagnostic: the record is marked by runs of electrical silence punctuated at regular intervals by symmetrical complexes of high-voltage slow wave activity. The total protein and gammaglobulin levels in the spinal fluid are usually elevated, but final confirmation of the diagnosis rests on either brain biopsy or autopsy. The pathological changes include chronic perivascular inflammation, neuronal fall-out, gliosis, and patchy demyelination. However, the characteristic abnormality is the presence of both intranuclear and cytoplasmic inclusion bodies, the former being of the Cowdry type A variety.

The presence of Cowdry type A inclusions suggested the possibility of viral infection, and this thesis was strengthened by the demonstration of particles resembling measles virus in ultrastructural studies of biopsy and autopsy material (Tellez-Nagel and Harter, 1966; Dayan et al., 1967). More direct virological evidence in favour of a relationship between measles virus infection and SSPE has been provided by the studies of Connolly et al. (1967) and Legg (1967), who found antibodies to the virus in high titre in blood from affected subjects. In one of the cases described by Connolly and colleagues the titre of measles virus antibody rose during the course of the illness. These workers (Connolly et al., 1968) have also demonstrated the presence of measles virus antigen in the brains of patients with SSPE by fluorescent antibody staining.

In short, there is sound reason for associating measles virus infection of the central nervous system, presumably contracted during childhood, with the subsequent development of SSPE. The implications for the individual patient are uncertain, although more effective antiviral chemotherapy may help in the future. The risk of this "latent" infection may also be a further argument for vaccination against measles in the unaffected child.

Herpes simplex encephalitis

Infection of the human central nervous system with the *Herpesvirus hominis* was first reported in 1941 (Smith et al.), but the frequency with which it can cause a fulminating meningoencephalitis has only recently been appreciated. An increasing number of reports of herpes simplex encephalitis has appeared in the literature in the last five years, and the diagnosis must now be seriously considered in any rapidly evolving encephalitic or meningitic illness of uncertain nature. Indeed it seems likely that many cases previously labelled as acute haemorrhagic leuco-encephalopathy may have been due to *Herpesvirus* infection.

In herpes simplex encephalitis, the expected pathological changes of a viral infection are found in destruction of neurones, perivenous inflammatory cell accumulation (primarily lymphocytic) and gliosis. In addition there is gross vascular congestion and cerebral oedema, often followed by massive haemorrhagic infarction. In many cases both intranuclear and intracytoplasmic inclusions are seen in the neurones and glia, and the latter change seen in brain biopsy material in the acute illness is virtually diagnostic of herpes simplex infection. These changes may be seen anywhere in the brain but have a curious predilection for one or other temporal lobe, and this may lead to a mistaken diagnosis of a focal lesion such as tumour or infarction in these situations.

The condition may affect individuals of any age and of either sex. Murray et al. (1966) felt on the basis of autopsy experience in southern Australia that the condition was more likely to occur in the summer, but Olson et al. (1967) were unable to find a particular seasonal incidence in their much larger American series. Herpes simplex encephalitis does not appear to follow any characteristic antecedent illness nor have any other particular precipitants.

Olson et al. (1967) have recently analysed the clinical features of 49 patients with *Herpesvirus* infections of the nervous system seen in the Walter Reed Army Institute of Research, Washington, D.C. All these cases presented as acute non-bacterial neurological infections which were subsequently shown to be due to *Herpesvirus hominis*. Thirty-six patients presented with or developed encephalitis, and in this group the mortality rate was very high (25/36). Two-thirds of these patients developed epilepsy at some stage in their illness and many presented with major seizures, often with a focal onset. In such cases the disease usually pursues an unremittingly severe course to deep coma, though lateralizing signs of some kind are often demonstrable. In a minority of cases, progress may be more gradual with a variety of focal neurological disturbances such as aphasia, sensory disturbances, or hemiparesis. Most patients run a high fever and some show signs of meningeal irritation, particularly in the early stages of their illness. Until recently the outcome of the disease was fatal in almost every case, but early treatment now offers some prospect of recovery. The clinical pattern emerging from the group of patients analysed by Olson et al. (1967) is in keeping with that in other recent case reports (Adams and Jennett, 1967; Breeden et al., 1966; Marshall, 1967) and with personal experience.

The diagnosis should be suspected in any patient presenting with an encephalitic illness of explosive onset, particularly with an epileptic seizure of some kind. Suspicion should be heightened if unconsciousness rapidly supervenes, especially with signs of an apparently focal lesion in one or other hemisphere, particularly in the temporal lobes. Other indirect evidence in favour of herpes simplex encephalitis includes a slow wave EEG focus in one or other temporal lobe,* demonstration of a temporal lobe "mass" radiologically, and bloody spinal or ventricular fluid. Definitive diagnosis during life depends on demonstration of intranuclear and intracytoplasmic inclusion bodies in nuerones or glia in brain biopsy material. Confirmation of a tentative diagnosis of herpes simplex encephalitis by these means was first reported by MacCallum *et al.* (1964), and this is now a standard investigation in suspected cases. More recently the morphological diagnosis of herpes simplex encephalitis has been taken a step further by the electron-microscopic identification of *Herpesvirus* particles in biopsy and autopsy material from seven cases (Harland *et al.*, 1967). The diagnosis can also be confirmed by finding a rising titre of complement-fixing antibodies to the virus in sera from affected persons. The serological diagnosis of herpes simplex infection in the nervous system has been discussed in detail by Johnson *et al.* (1968) and at a recent Clinico-pathological Conference (*Brit. med. J.*, 1969). In many cases surgical decompression of the grossly swollen brain will have been carried out as a life-saving measure before the diagnosis has been confirmed. In any case, where this has proved necessary and no obvious cause is found such as a tumour or haematoma, a cortical biopsy should be routinely taken. The patient should also be given steroids, preferably Dexamethasone in high dosage (up to 5 mg six-hourly), to reduce cerebral oedema, though Bøe *et al.* (1965) claimed that the prognosis in herpes simplex encephalitis was worse if the patient was treated with steroids alone. The most significant single advance in the treatment of this condition has been the introduction of the substituted pyrimidine base, 5-iodo, 2'-deoxyuridine (idoxuridine, IDU) which has an apparently specific inhibiting effect on *Herpesvirus hominis*.

The successful use of this antiviral agent has been reported in a number of patients (Breeden *et al.*, 1966; Marshall, 1967), and it should now be regarded as routine treatment. The drug is administered intravenously in a total dose of 0·5 g per kg body weight over a period of five days. A number of toxic side-effects have been reported, bone marrow depression being the most common (Calabresi, 1963; Breeden *et al.*, 1966), though gastro-intestinal irritation and impaired renal function have also been personally encountered.

In conclusion, it should be emphasized that the possibility of herpes simplex infection should be considered in any fulminating encephalitic illness. The treatment of the condition includes urgent surgical decompression and steroids to reduce cerebral oedema. The only specific measure available at present is exhibition of idoxuridine after confirmation of the diagnosis by brain biopsy.

* Upton and Gumpert (1970), *Lancet*, 1, 650, have recently described what may be a characteristic EEG abnormality in herpes simplex encephalitis. They described six patients who rapidly developed periodic complexes against a background of diffuse slow wave activity between the 2nd and 15th days of their illnesses. These complexes then disappeared without any clinical improvement.

Kuru

The concept of "slow" virus infection was introduced by the Icelandic virologist Sigurdsson (1954). The term implies that the virus produces a gradually progressive degenerative illness after an unusually prolonged incubation period. The general problem of slow virus infections of the nervous system has recently been reviewed by Gajdusek (1967). It was believed at first that slow virus infections affected only animals, but at least one human disease, kuru, is now considered to be due to such an agent. Kuru is a progressive degenerative neurological condition with an inevitably fatal outcome, which occurs only in the Fore linguistic group in the Eastern Highlands of New Guinea. The condition was first described by Gajdusek and Zigas in 1957, and a considerable literature has accumulated on the subject. There has been some uncertainty about its clinical features, but the recent detailed study of Hornabrook (1968) leaves little doubt that its predominant manifestations are subacute cerebellar degeneration and dementia. The possibility that this condition was due to a transmissible agent was strongly suggested by Gajdusek (1967) who succeeded in producing a syndrome indistinguishable from kuru in champanzees inoculated with brain from fatal human cases. The disease is characterized pathologically by loss of neurones, gliosis, spongioform degeneration and especially by the development of strongly PAS-positive kuru "plaques". These changes can be found throughout the nervous system (Fowler and Robertson, 1959; Klatzo et al., 1959) but are most severe in the cerebellum and the limbic system (Kakulas et al., 1967). The resemblance of these abnormalities to those seen in scrapie, mink encephalomyelitis and subacute spongioform encephalopathy has been noted by various workers including Beck and Daniel (1965), Beck et al. (1966), and Field (1967).

There is no neurological disorder exactly comparable with kuru in European or North American experience though Jakob-Creutzfeld disease may provide the closest analogy. It is of considerable interest that successful transmission of this condition to chimpanzees has recently been claimed (Gibbs et al., 1968). The importance of kuru lies in the fact that it is the first chronic progressive "degenerative" disease of the nervous system for which an infective cause had been demonstrated. The possible implications of this finding in relation to commoner diseases, particularly multiple sclerosis and motor neurone disease, are evident.

Progressive multifocal leucoencephalopathy

This obscure condition, a demyelinating process which complicates the course of lymphomas, particularly Hodgkin's disease, was first recognized by Aström et al. (1958). It presents with fits, dementia and a variety of focal disturbances of neurological function. Rapid progression to a fatal conclusion is usual, though a histologically confirmed case which survived for five years has recently been described (Hedley-Whyte *et al.*, 1966). Pathologically disseminated foci of softening are found in both the white and grey matter. In these foci surviving axons denuded of their myelin sheaths and attendant oligodendroglia may be seen, though these also disappear in the larger foci. Characteristic histopathological abnormalities are found in oligodendrocytes and astrocytes. The nuclei of the former are greatly enlarged, and those of the latter are enlarged and polyploid and often contain abnormal mitotic figures. Aström *et al.* (1958) and Cavanagh *et al.* (1959) both pointed out the similarity between these changes and those seen in the nervous system after exposure to ionizing radiations. Eosinophilic intranuclear inclusions have been found in some material, particularly in the nuclei of the oligodendroglia. This finding prompted the suggestion that the condition may have been associated with viral infection. The possibility of such an association was greatly strengthened by the electron-microscopic demonstration of particles closely resembling polyoma virus in the nuclei of oligodendrocytes from affected subjects (Zu Rhein and Chou, 1965). While it is clearly dangerous to infer a direct cause-and-effect relationship, it seems to be reasonable to assume that the glia in progressive multifocal leucoencephalopathy are parasitized by a papova virus of some kind. If this is true, it may well be that the virus is directly responsible for the nuclear abnormalities and indirectly for demyelination by eventually destroying the host cells (*Lancet*, 1966). In this context it is of interest that Walton *et al.* (1969) found inflammatory changes in the spinal cord of a patient with Hodgkin's disease who died with an obscure neurological illness. They likened these changes to "subacute poliomyelitis" and suggested they may have been due to latent viral infection.

REFERENCES

ADAMS, J. H. & JENNETT, W. B. (1967). Acute necrotizing encephalitis: a problem in diagnosis. *J. Neurol. Neurosurg. Psychiat.*, **30**, 248.

ASTRÖM, K. E., MANCALL, E. L. & RICHARDSON, E. P. JR. (1958). Progressive multifocal leukoencephalopathy: Hitherto undescribed complication of chronic lymphatic leukemia and Hodgkin's disease. *Brain*, **81**, 93.

BECK, E. & DANIEL, P. M. (1965). Kuru and scrapie compared: Are they examples of system degeneration? In *Slow, Latent and Temperate Virus Infections*, NINDB Monograph No. 2, ed. D. C. Gajdusek, C. J. Gibbs, Jr. and M. Alpers. Washington, D.C.: U.S. Department of Health, Education and Welfare.

BECK, E., DANIEL, P. M., ALPERS, M., GAJDUSEK, D. C. & GIBBS, C. J. JR. (1966). Experimental "kuru" in chimpanzees. *Lancet*, **2**, 1056.

BØE, J., SOLBERT, C. O. & SAETER, T. (1965). Corticosteroid treatment for acute meningo-encephalitis: A retrospective study of 346 cases. *Brit. med. J.*, **1**, 1094.

BREEDEN, C. J., HALL, T. C. & TYLER, H. R. (1966). Herpes simplex encephalitis treated with systemic 5-iodo-2'-deoxyuridine. *Ann. int. Med.*, **65**, 1050.

Brit. med. J. (1969), **2**, 33. A short fatal illness for discussion (Clinicopathological Conference).

CALABRESI, P. (1963). Current status of clinical investigations with 6-azauridine, 5-iodo-2'-deoxyuridine and related derivatives. *Cancer Res.*, **23**, 1260.

CAVANAGH, J. B., GREENBAUM, D., MARSHALL, A. H. E. & RUBINSTEIN, L. J. (1959). Cerebral demyelination associated with disorders of the reticulo-endothelial system. *Lancet*, **2**, 524.

COBB, W. A. & MORGAN-HUGHES, J. A. (1968). Non-fatal subacute sclerosing leucoencephalitis. *J. Neurol. Neurosurg. Psychiat.*, **31**, 115.

CONNOLLY, J. H., ALLEN, I. V., HURWITZ, L. J. & MILLAR, J. H. D. (1967). Measles virus antibody and antigen in subacute sclerosing panencephalitis. *Lancet*, **1**, 542.

CONNOLLY, J. H., ALLEN, I. V., HURWITZ, L. J. & MILLAR, J. H. D. (1968). Subacute sclerosing panencephalitis. Clinical, pathological epidemiological and virological findings. *Quart. J. Med.*, **37**, 625.

DAWSON, J. R., JR. (1933). Cellular inclusions in cerebral lesions of lethargic encephalitis. *Amer. J. Path.*, **9**, 7.

DAYAN, A. D., GOSTLING, J. V. T., GREIVES, J. L., STEVENS, D. W. & WOODHOUSE, M. A. (1967). Evidence of a pseudomyxovirus in the brain in subacute sclerosing leucoencephalitis. *Lancet*, **1**, 980.

FIELD, E. J. (1967). The significance of astroglial hypertrophy in scrapie, kuru, multiple sclerosis and old age together with a note on the possible nature of the scrapie agent. *Deutsch. Z. Nervenheilk*, **192**, 265.

FOWLER, M. & ROBERTSON, E. G. (1959). Observations on kuru. Part III. Pathological features in five cases. *Aust. Ann. Med.*, **8**, 16.

GAJDUSEK, D. C. (1967). Slow virus infections of the nervous system. *N. Engl. J. Med.*, **276**, 392.

GAJDUSEK, D. C. & ZIGAS, V. (1957). Degenerative disease of the central nervous system in New Guinea. The endemic occurrence of "kuru" in the native population. *N. Engl. J. Med.*, **257**, 974.

GIBBS, C. J. JR., GAJDUSEK, D. C., ASHER, D. M., ALPERS, M. P., BECK, E., DANIEL, P. B. & MATTHEWS, W. B. (1968). Creutzfeldt-Jakob disease (spongiform encephalopathy): Transmission to the chimpanzee. *Science*, **161**, 388.

HARLAND, W. A., ADAMS, J. H. & McSEVENEY, D. (1967). Herpes simplex particles in acute necrotising encephalitis. *Lancet*, **2**, 581.

HEDLEY-WHYTE, E. T., SMITH, B. P., TYLER, H. R. & PETERSON, W. P. (1966). Multifocal leukoencephalopathy with remission and five year survival. *J. Neuropath. exp. Neurol.*, **25**, 107.

HORNABROOK, R. W. (1968). Kuru—a subacute cerebellar degeneration. The natural history and clinical features. *Brain*, **91**, 53.

JOHNSON, R. T., OLSON, L. C. & BEUSCHER, E. L. (1968). Herpes simplex infections of the central nervous system. Problems in laboratory diagnosis. *Arch. Neurol.*, **18**, 260.

KAKULAS, B. A., LECOURS, A-R. & GAJDUSEK, D. C. (1967). Further observations on the pathology of kuru. *J. Neuropath. exp. Neurol.*, **26**, 85.

KLATZO, I., GAJDUSEK, D. C. & ZIGAS, V. (1959). Pathology of kuru disease. *J. Neuropath. exp. Neurol.*, **18**, 335.

Lancet (1966) **1**, 353. Polyoma virus and leucoencephalopathy (Leading article).

LEGG, N. J. (1967). Viral antibodies in subacute sclerosing penencephalitis: a study of 22 patients. *Brit. med. J.*, **3**, 350.

MACCALLUM, F. O., POTTER, J. M. & EDWARDS, D. H. (1964). Early diagnosis of herpes simplex encephalitis by brain biopsy. *Lancet*, **2**, 332.

MARSHALL, W. J. S. (1967). Herpes simplex encephalitis treated with idoxuridine and external decompression. *Lancet*, **2**, 579.

MURRAY, K. D., HOWARTH, W. H., MOORE, B. W. & WOLANSKI, B. (1966). Herpes simplex meningo-encephalitis. *Med. J. Aust.*, **1**, 291.

OLSON, L. C., BEUSCHER, E. L., ARTENSTEIN, M. S. & PARKMAN, P. D. (1967). Herpesvirus infections of the human central nervous system. *N. Engl. J. Med.*, **277**, 1271.

PEARCE, J. M. S. & BARWICK, D. D. (1964). Recovery from presumed subacute inclusion-body encephalitis. *Brit. med. J.*, **2**, 611.

SIGURDSSON, B. (1954). Observations on three slow infections of sheep III. *Brit. vet. J.*, **110**, 307.

SMITH, M. G., LENNETTE, E. H. & REAMES, H. R. (1941). Isolation of the virus of herpes simplex and the demonstration of intranuclear inclusions in a case of acute encephalitis. *Amer. J. Path.*, **17**, 55.

TELLEZ-NAGEL, I. & HARTER, D. H. (1966). Subacute sclerosing leucoencephalitis I Clinico-pathological, electron microscopic and virological observations. *J. Neuropath. exp. Neurol.*, **25**, 560.

UPTON & GUMPERT, (1970). *Lancet*, **1**, 650.

VAN BOGAERT, L. (1945). Une leucoencéphalite sclérosante subaigüe. *J. Neurol. Neurosurg. Psychiat.*, **8**, 101.

VAN BOGAERT, L. & DE BUSSCHER, J. D. (1939). 'Sur la sclérose inflammatoire de la substance blanche des hemispheres (Spielmeyer).' *Rev. Neurol.*, **71**, 679.

WALTON, J. N. (1969). (Ed.) *Disorders of Voluntary Muscle*, 2nd edition. London: Churchill.

ZU RHEIN, G. M. & CHOU, S.-M. (1965). Particles resembling papova viruses in human cerebral demyelinating disease. *Science*, **148**, 1477.

THE PERIPHERAL NEUROPATHIES

The problem of peripheral neuropathy still presents considerable difficulties in classification, diagnosis and management. Peripheral neuropathy may present as a clinical problem in isolation or as part of many systemic disorders. It is well known as a presenting manifestation in malignant disease and occurs with increasing frequency in chronic renal failure with the increasing life expectancy of the affected persons.

Classification of the peripheral neuropathies is a matter of personal taste. It has been attempted from various points of view, notably aetiological, pathogenetic and clinical, without a completely satisfactory result ever being obtained. Simpson (1962) proposed a new classification of neuropathies on the basis of clinical similarities, including such entities as carcinomatous neuropathy, sarcoidosis and the collagenoses under the heading of "Disorders of protein metabolism". This approach to nosology is open to argument and cannot be recommended. Earl (1969) has adopted a purely clinical classification dividing the neuropathies into acute and chronic categories. which has the advantage of simplicity. The classification recommended by the World Federation of Neurology (*J. neurol. Sci.*, 1968) is the most comprehensive one recently produced. It is essentially a pathogenetic classification, reasonably logical both in its major categories and their contents. For practical purposes, however, a simple list of the commonest types probably represents the most useful classification.

We propose to discuss only a few examples in detail. Those chosen are included because of their great clinical importance and the wealth of new information which has accumulated about them in the past five years.

The Guillain-Barré syndrome

As Asbury et al. (1969) have suggested, the Guillain-Barré syndrome has replaced poliomyelitis as the most important cause of generalized paralysis in man. They also suggested that the term "idiopathic polyneuritis" should be used in preference to the host of other eponymous and descriptive terms applied to this condition in the English and American literature. There is considerable merit in this suggestion, though we have clung to the familiar eponym on this occasion because we know precisely what we mean by it. We hope the same will apply to our readers.

The clinical features of the Guillain-Barré syndrome are well known. Although most cases present with no history of an antecedent illness, a significant minority (six out of Asbury's 19 cases) give a history of a febrile episode of some kind. This ranges from a minor upper respiratory tract illness to pneumonia, usually during the three weeks preceding the onset of neurological symptoms. The condition is one of the more common neurological complications of infectious mononucleosis, it may follow Jennerian vaccination or the administration of horse serum, and has even been recorded after surgery (Arnason and Asbury, 1968.) The writers have recently seen a case in which symptoms began two weeks after the cessation of apparently successful megavoltage therapy for a thymoma. An acute peripheral neuropathy clinically indistinguishable from the Guillain-Barré syndrome has also been reported in association with bronchogenic carcinoma and with Hodgkin's disease (Currie et al., 1970).

Paralysis may develop in a few hours or over several days. Symptoms usually being in the lower limbs with rapidly ascending paralysis involving all muscle groups, often with muscle pain. Physical examination reveals partial or complete flaccid paralysis of affected muscles with absent deep tendon reflexes. The patient often complains of paraesthesiae in the extremities, though sensory testing usually demonstrates no more than very slight "glove and stocking" impairment of response to pin-prick and light touch. The extent of paralysis varies considerably from case to case, but complete flaccid quadriplegia with weakness of the diaphragm is not uncommon. In severe cases temporary bladder paralysis may occur in the early stages, and bilateral facial weakness with difficulty in swallowing is common. Extraocular palsies have been recorded on occasions (Marshall, 1963) and were seen recently in two personal cases, one of whom had complete external ophthalmo-plegia. Some cases are complicated by a persistent tachycardia, presumably due to vagal involvement, and a few develop conduction defects and eventually cardiac failure due to myocarditis (Clarke et al., 1954). The natural history of the condition is uncertain, but most cases recover spontaneously after longer or shorter periods. The commonest cause of death is respiratory paralysis, though the cardiovascular complications may be responsible in a few cases.

Diagnosis can usually be confirmed by finding a greatly raised spinal fluid protein level (often several hundred mg per 100 ml of fluid) with a normal or only slightly raised cell count. In some cases, the protein level is normal during the first few days of the illness, eventually rising to the high levels mentioned above. In such cases diagnostic difficulty may be resolved by motor nerve conduction-velocity studies. Very occasionally it may be impos-sible to distinguish the syndrome from rapidly progressive spinal cord com-pression or acute myelitis. In this situation a myelogram is imperative to avoid missing a surgically treatable compressive lesion.

The management of this condition is relatively non-controversial. The most important single factor in reducing mortality has been the application of modern methods of patient monitoring and of supporting respiration. The patient should be nursed where these techniques are available. There is no properly evaluated information about the value or otherwise of the corti-costeroids, but in spite of this we have no hesitation in recommending their exhibition in what is a potentially fatal though recoverable illness. We are convinced that they materially alter the course of the disease in some cases, though admittedly on the basis of clinical impression alone. The authors have a personal preference for the use of adreno-corticotrophic hormone by injection, though oral steroids, e.g. prednisone, are probably equally effective These drugs should be administered in high dosage until unequivocal clinical evidence of improvement is obtained. They should then be gradually tailed off to a maintenance dose since sudden withdrawal may precipitate relapse.

The pathogenesis of the syndrome remains uncertain. It is generally regarded as a non-specific allergic response to a variety of insults to the nervous system, but our knowledge of the mechanism involved is scanty. Haymaker and Kernohan (1949) emphasized the importance of oedema and dissolution of myelin as primary changes in the pathological evolution of the condition. They suggested that an inflammatory cell response was scanty and appeared late (on or after the ninth day of the illness) and this view was supported by Greenfield (1963). Recently, however, Asbury and his colleagues (1969) made a study of 19 cases, and found well-developed lymphocytic infiltrates in the spinal nerves and roots of every case examined from the first few days of illness in those who died to those making a clinical recovery. On the basis of their observations they conclude that the Guillain-Barré syndrome is closely analogous to experimental allergic neuritis (Waksman and Adams,

1955), a disease known to be due to delayed hypersensitivity mediated by specifically-sensitized lymphocytes. They suggest that the Guillain-Barré syndrome is an exactly similar process, in which peripheral nervous tissues, particularly myelin, are attacked by specifically sensitized cells. In view of this the results of lymphocyte transformation studies are awaited with interest.

Chronic progressive and relapsing forms of idiopathic polyneuropathy

In any neurological practice no cause will be found for up to 50 per cent of all neuropathies investigated. These tend to be gradually progressive or relapsing sensorimotor forms which usually involve adults in late middle life, the sexes being equally affected. Clinically similar disorders occur in infancy and early childhood and these are likely to be biologically similar to if not identical with the adult conditions. It has often been assumed that chronic or relapsing idiopathic neuropathy has an allergic basis and is in some way related to the Guillain-Barré syndrome. This assumption is based on the fact that many of these cases are steroid-responsive, though no laboratory evidence of disturbed immunological mechanism has been adduced to date. Osuntokun et al. (1966) were unable to find serum antibodies to central or peripheral nervous tissue in 15 cases of chronic idiopathic polyneuropathy, and there is as yet no reported study of cell-mediated hypersensitivity in these conditions. However, Winkler (1965) produced demyelination in cultures of foetal rat trigeminal ganglia with lymphocytes from rats with latent experimental allergic neuropathy.

Nutritional neuropathies

There has been little or no recent change in the status of nutritional neuropathy in Western European society. However, Cooke and Smith (1966) and Cooke et al. (1966) have given detailed clinical and pathological descriptions of neuropathy in adult coeliac diseases. Osuntokun (1968) has described 84 cases of what has been called "tropical ataxic neuropathy" (Montgomery et al., 1964) in the indigenous peoples of Southern Nigeria. This condition is of exceptional interest as the aetiological factors and likely pathogenetic mechanisms have already been identified. The incidence of the disease, which is usually accompanied by bilateral optic atrophy, is highest in adults of poor social and nutritional status in early middle life. The principal element in the diet of these patients was cassava, known to contain the cyanogenetic glycoside, linamarin. These subjects were shown to have abnormally high plasma cyanide and thiocyanate levels, presumably because of their diets. Osuntokun (1968) suggests that the neuropathy may be directly due to chronic cyanide intoxication, or alternatively that it may be due to low plasma levels of the sulphur-containing amino acids which are known to be involved in the detoxication of the cyanide ion (Osuntokun et al., 1968). Conditioned deficiency of vitamin B_{12}, also concerned with cyanide detoxication, may also be a factor. A therapeutic trial of hydroxocobalamin, casein and yeast has been instituted.

Porphyria

Acute intermittent porphyria, the commonest form of porphyria in north-western Europe, has always excited considerable interest both as a clinical and metabolic problem. Interest has been further stimulated of late because of its incrimination as one of the causes of British colonial problems in the eighteenth century (McAlpine and Hunter, 1966). In an admirable review of the problem Ridley (1969) has recently described the course and outcome of the disease in 25 subjects in the hope of shedding further light on its natural history. It is important to remember that although the psychiatric and abdominal manifestations may be dramatic and may occasion the affected subject great distress and disability, it is the neuropathy of porphyria which threatens life. Ridley's patients were all in young and middle adult life (age range 18 to 58 years), there was a slight preponderance of females, and the onset of neuropathy was most common during the third and fourth decades, the period when most attacks of acute porphyria occur (Goldberg, 1959). The first manifestation of the disease is usually an abdominal crisis or psychiatric breakdown. Only in a minority is the onset of the disease heralded by an episode of neuropathy. However, Ridley (1969) found that severe constipation was a common concomitant of both the abdominal and neuro-pathic crises and that it often preceded the latter. He also found that tachy-cardia frequently accompanied constipation, an association not previously noted, although Ridley et al. (1968) had described tachycardia as a fore-runner of neuropathic crises. These manifestations are presumably due to autonomic neuropathy. The neuropathy itself is predominantly motor and usually symmetrical, although strikingly asymmetrical and even proximal involvement is occasionally noted. A few patients also develop severe sensory symptoms, sometimes before the onset of muscle weakness. In most cases of neuropathy the deep reflexes are absent. Cranial nerve involvement is common, the seventh and tenth being most often involved, usually uni-laterally. Psychiatric symptoms and sphincter disturbances (retention of urine, faecal incontinence) are common in the neuropathic crises, and respiratory failure is an inevitable accompaniment of severe and fatal cases. Ridley (1969) was able to identify a heterogeneous group of possible pre-cipitating factors such as respiratory tract infections and pregnancy, but concluded that the only precipitants unequivocally incriminated in his cases were the barbiturates and sulphonamides. He suggests that the initial develop-ment of neuropathy in patients known to have porphyria is often due to the ingestion of barbiturates, and stresses the importance of preventing this. A detailed account of present knowledge of the metabolic disturbances under-lying acute intermittent porphyria can be found in Ridley's paper. He discusses the possible role of δ-amino laevulinic acid synthetase, an enzyme produced in abnormal amounts during porphyric crises, and suggests that the fact that it is "induced" by barbiturates may be related to precipitation of neuropathic crises: δ-amino laevulinic acid synthetase may cause excessive tissue consumption of pyridoxal phosphate (vitamin B_6) and thus indirectly produce neuropathy (Cavanagh and Ridley, 1967). Ridley (1969) warns, however, that the clinical syndrome associated with vitamin B_6 deficiency is very different from the neuropathy of porphyria and suggests that if there is a relationship, then it is likely to be complex.

REFERENCES

ARNASON, B. G. & ASBURY, A. K. (1968). Idiopathic polyneuritis after surgery. *Arch. Neurol.*, **18**, 500.

ASBURY, A. K., ARNASON, B. G. & ADAMS, R. D. (1969). The inflammatory lesion in idiopathic polyneuritis. *Medicine (Balt.)*, **48**, 173.

CAVANAGH, J. B. & RIDLEY, A. (1967). The nature of the neuropathy complicating acute porphyria. *Lancet*, **2**, 1023.

CLARKE, E., BAYLISS, R. I. S. & COOPER, R. (1954). Landry-Guillain-Barré syndrome: cardiovascular complications. *Brit. med. J.*, **2**, 1054.

COOKE, W. T., JOHNSON, A. G. & WOOLF, A. L. (1966). Vital staining and electron microscopy of the intramuscular nerve endings in the neuropathology of adult coeliac disease. *Brain*, **89**, 663.

COOKE, W. T. & SMITH, W. T. (1966). Neurological disorders associated with adult coeliac disease. *Brain*, **89**, 683.

CURRIE, S., HENSON, R. A., MORGAN, H. G. & POOLE, H. J. (1970). The incidence of the non-metastatic neurological syndromes of obscure origin in the reticuloses. *Brain*, **93**, 629.

EARL, C. J. (1969). The polyneuropathies. In *Disorders of Voluntary Muscle*, 2nd edition, ed. J. N. Walton. London: Churchill.

GOLDBERG, A. (1959). Acute intermittent porphyria. A study of 50 cases. *Quart. J. Med.*, **28**, 183.

GREENFIELD, J. G. (1963). In *Greenfield's Neuropathology*, 2nd edition, ed. W. Blackwood, W. H. McMenemey, A. Meyer, R. M. Norman and D. S. Russell. London: Arnold.

HAYMAKER, W. & KERNOHAN, J. W. (1949). Landry-Guillain-Barré syndrome—50 fatal cases and a critique of the literature. *Medicine (Balt.)*, **28**, 59.

J. neurol. Sci. (1968), **6**, 165. Classification of the neuromuscular disorders.

MACALPINE, I. & HUNTER, R. (1966). The "insanity" of King George III. A classic case of porphyria. *Brit. med. J.*, **1**, 65.

MARSHALL, J. (1963). The Landry-Guillain-Barré syndrome. *Brain*, **86**, 55.

MONTGOMERY, R. D., CRUIKSHANK, E. K., ROBERTSON, W. B. & McMENEMEY, W. H. (1964). Clinical and pathological observations on Jamaican neuropathy. *Brain*, **87**, 425.

OSUNTOKUN, B. O. (1968). An ataxic neuropathy in Nigeria—a clinical, biochemical and electrophysiological study. *Brain*, **91**, 215.

OSUNTOKUN, B. O., DUROWOJU, J. E., McFARLANE, H. & WILSON, J. (1968). Plasma amino acids in the Nigerian nutritional ataxic neuropathy. *Brit. med. J.*, **3**, 647.

OSUNTOKUN, B. O., PRINEAS, J. W. & FIELD, E. J. (1966). Immunological study of chronic polyneuropathies of unknown cause. *J. Neurol. Neurosurg. Psychiat.*, 29, 456.

RIDLEY, A. (1969). The neuropathy of acute intermittent porphyria. *Quart. J. Med.*, 38, 307.

RIDLEY, A., HIERONS, R. & CAVANAGH, J. B. (1968). Tachycardia and the neuropathy of porphyria. *Lancet*, 2, 708.

SIMPSON, J. A. (1962). The neuropathies. In *Modern Trends in Neurology*, 3rd Series, ed. D. Williams. London: Butterworth.

STERN, G. M. (1966). Diseases of the nervous system. In *Progress in Clinical Medicine*, 5th edition, ed. R. Daley and H. Miller. London: Churchill.

WAKSMAN, B. H. & ADAMS, R. D. (1955). Allergic neuritis: an experimental disease of rabbits induced by the injection of peripheral nervous tissue and adjuvants. *J. exp. Med.*, 102, 213.

WINKLER, G. F. (1965). *In vitro* demyelination of peripheral nerve induced with sensitized cells. *Ann. N.Y. Acad. Sci.*, 122, 287.

NEUROLOGICAL COMPLICATIONS OF CHRONIC RENAL FAILURE

The frequency with which neurological disorders are encountered in both acute and chronic renal failure is increasing steadily. The principal reasons for this are doubtless the increasing survival of patients with end-stage renal failure and the various methods used to keep them alive. One of the commonest and best known is peripheral neuropathy, first described by Charcot (1873), and a host of other but more complicated conditions have been subsequently recognized, including encephalopathy, central pontine myelinolysis and myopathy. Some of these conditions are due to renal failure *per se*, some to disorders associated with renal failure, e.g. metabolic bone disease, and others to its treatment, particularly to intermittent haemodialysis.

Peripheral neuropathy

As mentioned above, this was first recognized by Charcot but was largely ignored until Marin and Tyler (1961) reported two patients with hereditary interstitial nephritis and nerve deafness (Alport's syndrome) who developed severe peripheral neuropathies. They suggested that the neuropathy was directly attributable to the renal failure, and this suggestion was supported by Asbury *et al.* (1962, 1963), who reported the clinical and pathological features of four further cases.

Uraemic neuropathy is usually a gradually progressive, symmetrical sensorimotor neuropathy affecting the lower limbs more severely than the upper limbs. Its onset may be heralded by the development of "restless legs". The first neuropathic symptom is usually burning feet, followed by peripheral paraesthesiae and numbness and eventually by weakness in the lower limbs and the hands. Physical examination reveals dense sensory loss in a glove and stocking distribution, with variable weakness in the extremities. Motor involvement may be absent or minimal, but is sometimes sufficiently severe to immobilize the patient completely. Weakness usually begins gradually but may develop explosively or rapidly during haemodialysis. Diagnosis can be confirmed by nerve conduction velocity studies, and the development of neuropathy in apparently unaffected subjects can sometimes be anticipated by these means (Preswick and Jeremy, 1964).

Pathologically, uraemic neuropathy appears to depend predominantly on non-inflammatory distal demyelination, though the axis cylinders are damaged to a greater or less extent (Tyler, 1968). The proximal parts of the nerves are usually relatively normal (Tyler, 1968) although chromatolytic changes in anterior horn cells have been described (Asbury et al., 1963). Serum protein levels in uraemic patients are generally in the normal range. In this context it is interesting that Jennekens (1969) found significantly raised spinal fluid protein levels in most of his patients with uraemic neuropathy.

The effect of intermittent haemodialysis on the course of uraemic neuropathy is uncertain. Konotey-Ahulu and colleagues (1965) showed clinical and electrophysiological evidence of improvement in 12 out of 15 patients with uraemic neuropathy on a dialysis programme. On the other hand Tyler and Gottlieb (1965) reported several cases where neuropathy had developed or progressed during the course of intermittent dialysis, and Tyler (1968) suggested that improvement with haemodialysis was likely to occur only with a predominantly sensory neuropathy and that recovery from significant weakness was rare. Tenckhoff et al. (1965) found that neuropathy could begin explosively and progress rapidly during the course of dialysis, and that existing neuropathy could progress insidiously in spite of dialysis. They ascribed the latter to inadequate dialysis and considered that the progress of neuropathy could usually be halted by more aggressive treatment. Local experience indicates that uraemic neuropathy usually improves with intermittent dialysis, though we have recently seen a patient who developed rapidly progressive motor neuropathy during the course of intermittent dialysis, who was found to have a spinal fluid protein of 125 mg and who improved after treatment with prednisone. This suggests that some neuropathies of this kind occurring during dialysis may be akin to the Guillain-Barré syndrome.

Encephalopathy

Deterioration in personality, memory and intellectual function is common in chronic renal failure, the severity of these changes usually being directly related to the severity of the underlying metabolic disturbance and the rate at which it develops. In severe cases psychotic breakdown, epileptic manifestations of various kinds, and eventually impairment of consciousness are likely to occur. These disturbances are usually attended by generalized muscular twitching, myoclonic jerks, and tremors of various kinds and particularly *asterixis* or flapping tremor of the hands (Tyler, 1964, 1968). Tyler (1968) regards the latter as being a characteristic feature of uraemic as well as portacaval encephalopathies and suggests that the underlying physiological defect may be a periodic inhibition of muscle contraction in a single limb. Electroencephalographic abnormalities ranging from occasional short-lived runs of rhythmical slow wave activity to frank epileptic discharges can accompany any of these disturbances. The pathogenesis of these disturbances is almost certainly multifactorial, but spinal fluid pH (Posner and Plum, 1967), calcium ion concentration and water and electrolyte shifts are likely to be of considerable importance.

Intermittent haemodialysis has increased the risk of acute encephalopathic disturbances complicating the course of chronic renal failure. Minor EEG abnormalities are commonly encountered during the course of dialysis (Kerr and Osselton, 1967), but some patients may develop more serious neurological disturbances including recurrent major epileptic seizures and coma of sudden onset. In some fatal cases autopsy shows that these have been due to vascular accidents, particularly intracerebral haemorrhage. In others the cause is a sudden change in osmotic equilibrium across the blood-brain barrier, the so-called dialysis disequilibrium syndrome (Dinapoli and Johnson, 1968). This was first described by Kennedy *et al.* (1962) and by Peterson and Swanson (1964), who showed that sudden changes in consciousness occurring during dialysis not due to focal lesions such as haemorrhage were accompanied by the appearance of generalized high-voltage slow wave activity in the EEG. This, they found, was due to delayed removal of urea from the nervous system through the blood-brain barrier, a consequent rise in the osmotic pressure of the tissue fluid in the nervous system, and an abrupt ingress of water to lower this with the development of acute cerebral oedema. This problem can usually be avoided by using bathing fluids of high osmolality (containing large concentrations of glucose) in the dialyser.

Cerebral vascular accidents

Predictably, cerebral haemorrhage and infarction are common in chronic renal failure for a number of reasons, notably hypertension and a bleeding tendency. The risk of intracerebral haemorrhage is unavoidably heightened in those hypertensive subjects undergoing intermittent dialysis who are heparinized during the individual dialysis sessions or, worse still, have to take long-term oral anticoagulants because of clotting difficulties with their arteriovenous shunts (see Bradford Hill *et al.*, 1960). Recently Gaan and his colleagues (1969) described two cases of cerebral embolism, one fatal, in patients on haemodialysis. These occurred immediately after the patients' shunts were "declotted", and the authors suggest that great care should be taken with this procedure and that clots should be lysed with streptokinase if possible. Leonard *et al.* (1969) have reported three cases of subdural haematoma with no antecedent head injury in patients in whom neurological deterioration had been attributed to dialysis disequilibrium. In two cases the correct diagnosis was made only at autopsy, so the implications for the management of the neurological complications of dialysis are clear.

Central pontine myelinolysis

First described in chronic alcoholics after a frenetic binge (Adams, Victor and Mancall, 1959) this rare disorder is now known to occur as a terminal complication of end-stage renal failure, particularly after unsuccessful renal transplantation (Schneck, 1966). Pathologically, the condition is characterized by virtually complete non-inflammatory demyelination of the long fibre pathways, particularly the cortico-spinal tracts, in the pons and to a lesser extent elsewhere in the brain stem. Clinically the patients develop a spastic quadriplegia, dementia and eventually coma. The clinical course is usually only a few weeks at the most, the outcome inevitably fatal and the diagnosis made at autopsy.

Myopathy

There have been several recent accounts suggesting that proximal muscle weakness in chronic renal failure may in some instances be due to a primary disorder of muscle function (Serratrice *et al.*, 1967; Tyler, 1968). It is likely that this myopathy is similar to that occurring in metabolic bone disease generally (see Prineas *et al.*, 1965: Smith and Stern, 1967, 1969) since it occurs in its most severe form in those cases of chronic renal failure with secondary metabolic bone disease, especially osteomalacia (Floyd *et al.*, 1969).

REFERENCES

ADAMS, R. D., VICTOR, M. & MANCALL, E. L. (1959). Central pontine myelinolysis. A hitherto undescribed disease occurring in alcoholic and malnourished patients. *Arch. Neurol. Psychiat.*, **81**, 154.

ASBURY, A. K., VICTOR, M. & ADAMS, R. D. (1962). Uremic polyneuropathy. *Trans. Amer. neurol. Ass.*, **87**, 100.

ASBURY, A. K., VICTOR, M. & ADAMS, R. D. (1963). Uremic polyneuropathy. *Arch. Neurol.*, **8**, 413.

BRADFORD HILL, A., MARSHALL, J. & SHAW, D. A. (1960). A controlled clinical trial of long-term anticoagulant therapy in cerebrovascular disease. *Quart. J. Med.*, **29**, 597.

CHARCOT, J. M. (1873). *Des paraplégies urinaires.* Paris.

DINAPOLI, R. P. & JOHNSON, W. J. (1968). Neurological complications in chronic renal failure. *Med. Clin. N. Amer.*, **52**, 845.

FLOYD, M., AYYAR, D. R., HUDGSON, P. & KERR, D. N. S. (1969). Myopathy in chronic renal failure. In *Proc. E.D.T.A.*, Vol. 6, ed. D. N. S. Kerr. Amsterdam: Excerpta Medica Foundation.

GAAN, D., MALLICK, N. P., BREWIS, R. A. L., SEEDAT, Y. K. & MAHONEY, M. P. (1969). Cerebral damage from declotting Scribner shunts. *Lancet*, 2, 77.

JENNEKENS, F. G. I. (1969). Uremische polyneuropathie. Doctoral thesis, University of Utrecht.

KENNEDY, A. C., LINTON, A. L. & EATON, J. C. (1962). Urea levels in cerebrospinal fluid after hemodialysis. *Lancet*, 1, 410.

KERR, D. N. S. & OSSELTON, J. W. (1967). The EEG as a monitor of cerebral disturbance during fast and slow haemodialysis of patients in chronic renal failure. *Electroenceph. clin. Neurophysiol.*, 23, 488.

KONOTEY-AHULU, F. I. D., BAILLOD, R., COMTY, C. M., HERON, J. R., SHALDON, S. & THOMAS, P. K. (1965). Effects of periodic dialysis on the peripheral neuropathy of end-stage renal failure. *Brit. med. J.*, 2, 1212.

LEONARD, C. D., WEIL, E. & SCRIBNER, B. H. (1969). Subdural haematomas in patients undergoing haemodialysis. *Lancet*, 2, 239.

MARIN, O. S. M. & TYLER, H. R. (1961). Hereditary interstitial nephritis associated with polyneuropathy. *Neurology (Minneap.)*, 11, 999.

PETERSON, H. & SWANSON, A. G. (1964). Acute encephalopathy occurring during haemodialysis. *Arch. intern. Med.*, 113, 877.

POSNER, J. B. & PLUM, F. (1967). Spinal-fluid pH and neurologic symptoms in systemic acidosis. *N. Engl. J. Med.*, 277, 605.

PRESWICK, G. & JEREMY, D. (1964). Subclinical polyneuropathy in renal insufficiency. *Lancet*, 2, 731.

PRINEAS, J. W., STUART MASON, A. & HENSON, R. A. (1965). Myopathy in metabolic bone disease. *Brit. med. J.*, 1, 1034.

SCHNECK, S. A. (1966). Neuropathological features of human organ transplantation II. Central pontine myelinolysis and neuroaxonal dystrophy. *J. Neuropath. exp. Neurol.*, 25, 18.

SERRATRICE, G., TOGA, M., ROUX, H., MURISASCO, A. & DE BISSCHOP, G. (1967). Neuropathies, myopathies et neuromyopathies chez des urémiques chroniques. *Presse méd.*, 75, 1835.

SMITH, R. & STERN, G. (1967). Myopathy, osteomalacia and hyperparathyroidism. *Brain*, 90, 593.

SMITH, R. & STERN, G. (1969). Muscular weakness in osteomalacia and hyperparathyroidism. *J. neurol. Sci.*, 8, 511.

TENCKHOFF, H. A., BOEN, F. S. T., JEBSEN, R. H. & SPIEGLIER, J. H. (1965). Polyneuropathy in chronic renal insufficiency. *J. Amer. med. Ass.*, 192, 1121.

TYLER, H. R. & GOTTLIEB, A. A. (1965). Peripheral neuropathy in uremia. *Proceedingsof the 8th International Congress of Neurology*, Vienna.

TYLER, H. R. (1964). Asterixis. *J. chron. Dis.*, 18, 409.

TYLER, H. R. (1968). Neurologic disorders in renal failure. *Amer. J. Med.*, 44, 734.

NEUROLOGICAL COMPLICATIONS OF LIVER DISEASE

The neurological complications of liver disease were reviewed in earlier editions. Since then it has become apparent that the problem is not simply that of episodic encephalopathy developing acutely in patients with bio-

M

chemical liver failure and portal-systemic anastomosis, either spontaneous or surgical, after a gastro-intestinal haemorrhage. A chronic form of porta-caval encephalopathy is now recognized, and reports of myelopathy associated with chronic liver disease appear with increasing frequency. There has also been a description of an inborn error of metabolism in which the liver is unable to detoxicate ammonia. This results in chronic neurological illness from birth, with irreparable brain damage and early death. From the point of view of management, there have been important advances in the treatment of hepatic coma due to massive liver necrosis, e.g. exchange transfusion, cross-circulation perfusion. Organ transplantation as the definitive treatment of chronic liver disease seems to be on the threshhold.

Portacaval encephalopathy

The risk of an acute encephalopathy marked by psychiatric disorders, coma, flapping tremor (asterixis) and a variety of focal neurological disturbances is well recognized in patients with chronic liver disease. Episodes of this kind are usually precipitated by a sudden increase in the protein load on the gut, and particularly by gastro-intestinal haemorrhage. The precise mechanism whereby protein loading precipitates encephalopathy is not known, though it is assumed that the cerebral syndrome is determined by the nitrogenous breakdown products of protein catabolism in the gut. Episodes of encephalopathy are usually accompanied by a sharp rise in the serum ammonia level (normal 5–50 μg/100 ml), but it is unlikely that ammonia *per se* is responsible for the neurological disturbances. The principles of diagnosis and management of acute portacaval encephalopathy are now well-defined and the reader is referred to Sherlock (1958) for a detailed discussion.

It has been known for some time that the neuropsychiatric disturbances accompanying chronic liver disease may assume various forms (Pearce, 1963). It has, however, only recently been realized that these disturbances may become chronic, though Summerskill and his colleagues reported progress to a chronic state in 1956. Victor *et al.* (1965) reported a group of 27 subjects of chronic liver disease who developed a fairly stereotyped neurological illness which they termed the acquired (non-Wilsonian) type of chronic hepatocerebral degeneration. As the name implied, the authors appreciated that the disorder was not determined by an inborn error of copper metabolism although its clinical features resembled those of Wilson's disease. The patients presented with dementia of varying severity, titubation, facial dyskinesias of the kind produced by the phenothiazines, dysarthria, choreo-athetosis, and ataxia. Striatal tremors in the limbs were also commonly seen, though persistent flapping tremor was infrequent. All the patients had either abnormal fasting serum ammonia levels or abnormal ammonia tolerance, and in the cases studied at autopsy the histological changes found in the basal ganglia were characteristic of those seen in chronic hepatic failure, comprising dense gliosis and "giant" protoplasmic astrocytes (Alzheimer cells). Victor and his colleagues noted that these patients usually responded poorly to the routine treatment for acute portacaval encephalopathy, though in their review of the chronic neuropsychiatric syndromes of chronic liver disease Read *et al.* (1967) reported improvement in mental symptoms, particularly in some patients with neomycin therapy or colonic exclusion.

Portacaval myelopathy

Portacaval encephalopathy may be accompanied by clinical and pathological evidence of involvement of the spinal cord. This was first described by Zieve *et al.* (1960), and a number of workers have reported this condition subsequently. In all cases the patients developed a spastic paraparesis, with spasticity usually out of proportion to weakness and what Liversedge and Rawson (1966) described as a "puppet" gait. Sensory loss in these cases was minimal (Read *et al.*, 1967) or absent (Liversedge and Rawson, 1967; Pant *et al.*, 1968). In most cases the spastic paraparesis develops gradually although in others it may present explosively, sometimes after an acute episode of encephalopathy (Pant *et al.*, 1968). Two detailed neuropathological studies of this condition have been published, and both (Liversedge and Rawson, 1966; Pant *et al.*, 1968) agree that the only change in the spinal cord is widespread demyelination in the corticospinal tracts. Pant and his colleagues (1968) have suggested that this may be secondary to loss of the Betz cells from the motor cortex and that the condition is essentially a restricted encephalopathy, not a myelopathy. Clinical improvement in the paraparesis can be expected from protein restriction and neomycin therapy or from colonic exclusion.

Hyperammonaemia

This condition, an inborn error of metabolism due to deficiency of ornithine transcarbamylase (OTC), an enzyme of the urea cycle, was first described by Russell *et al.* (1962) and more detailed biochemical studies on the original patients have now been reported (Levin *et al.*, 1969). The metabolic error results in failure of detoxication of ammonia. The patients usually present in early infancy, though onset as late as the age of nine has been recorded. Symptoms begin when an infant is weaned from the breast and the daily protein intake exceeds 1·5 g/kg body weight, with irritability, anorexia and vomiting. The child later becomes hypotonic, develops convulsions and then passes into coma. These manifestations are accompanied by progressive enlargement of the liver, and in the two cases where autopsy studies are available, cerebral atrophy. All these cases have very high serum ammonia levels (well over 100 μg/100 ml) and the diagnosis can be confirmed by demonstrating OTC deficiency in a fresh liver biopsy sample. Treatment consists in lowering the blood ammonia to non-toxic levels by restriction of dietary protein intake to less than 1·5 g/kg body weight per day. This interesting problem is reviewed in detail in a recent *Lancet* leading article (1969).

REFERENCES

Lancet (1969), 2, 196. Hyperammonaemia (Leading article).
LEVIN, B., OBERHOLZER, V. G. & SINCLAIR, L. (1969). Biochemical investigations of hyperammonaemia. *Lancet*, 2, 170.
LIVERSEDGE, L. A. & RAWSON, M. D. (1966). Myelopathy in hepatic disease and portosystemic venous anastomosis. *Lancet*, 1, 277.
PANT, S. S., REBEIZ, J. J. & RICHARDSON, E. P. JR. (1968). Spastic paraparesis following portacaval shunts. *Neurology (Minneap.)*, 18, 134.
PEARCE, J. M. S. (1963). Focal neurological syndromes in hepatic failure. *Postgrad. med. J.*, 39, 653.
READ, A. E., SHERLOCK, S., LAIDLAW, J. & WALKER, J. G. (1967). The neuropsychiatric syndromes associated with chronic liver disease and an extensive portal-systemic collateral circulation. *Quart. J. Med.*, 36, 135.
RUSSELL, A., LEVIN, B., OBERHOLZER, V. G. & SINCLAIR, L. (1962). Hyperammonaemia. A new instance of an inborn enzymatic defect of the biosynthesis of urea. *Lancet*, 2, 699.
SHERLOCK, S. (1958). Pathogenesis and management of hepatic coma. *Amer. J. Med.*, 24, 805.
SUMMERSKILL, W. H. J., DAVIDSON, E. A., SHERLOCK, S. & STEINER, R. E. (1956). The neuropsychiatric syndromes associated with hepatic cirrhosis and an extensive portal collateral circulation. *Quart. J. Med.*, 25, 245.
VICTOR, M., ADAMS, R. D. & COLE, M. (1965). The acquired (non-Wilsonian) type of chronic hepatocerebral degeneration. *Medicine (Balt.)*, 44, 345.
ZIEVE, L., MENDELSON, D. F. & GOEPFERT, M. (1960). Shunt encephalopathy. *Ann. intern. Med.*, 53, 53.

LUMBAR CANAL STENOSIS

The concept of intermittent ischaemia of the spinal cord is an old one. It was first described by Dejerine in 1911 and was revived by Blau and Logue (1961), who described the unusual clinical presentation of a central protrusion of a single lumbar intervertebral disc. Their patient's symptoms came on after a fixed period of exercise although the arterial circulation in his lower limbs was normal. Blau and Logue (1961) accordingly applied the suggestive if semantically inappropriate name "intermittent claudication of the cauda equina" to this condition, and suggested that it was an ischaemic radiculopathy due to compression of nerve roots during exercise. It has become apparent that this syndrome can occur in the absence of significant disc protrusion (Verbiest, 1954, 1955; Joffe *et al.*, 1966). These workers described patients who presented with symptoms similar to those recorded by Blau and Logue (1961) and who had narrow lumbar canals. The stenoses in these cases were due to the presence of hypertrophic masses of bone behind the canal which were extremely difficult to remove at operation. Verbiest (1955) suggested that the bony masses may have been a developmental anomaly, whereas Joffe *et al.* (1966) felt that they were probably degenerative. Ehni (1965) has described attacks of intermittent ischaemia of the cauda equina or lower cord in elderly persons with severe degenerative changes in the lumbar spine. Posterior disc protrusions at different levels combined with hypertrophy of the ligamentum flavum effectively produce stenosis of the lumbar canal. It is theoretically possible that this syndrome could be produced by severe degenerative vascular disease in the absence of skeletal abnormalities, although ischaemia of the cord or cauda is said to be rare in this situation (Henson and Parsons, 1967).

The patients complain of attacks of pain, sensory disturbance or weakness in the lower limbs precipitated by exercise, usually walking or climbing stairs. At any one time the distance walked is likely to be fixed, though this will tend to become less with the passage of time. Distinction between intermittent ischaemia of the neuraxis and true intermittent claudication may be difficult, particularly if the peripheral pulses in the lower limbs are diminished or absent. Attacks of sensory disturbance may take any form, but in our experience patients often describe a warm feeling in one or both legs which spreads upwards towards the groins. Eventual development of a progressive neurological deficit (cauda equina syndrome) is likely without treatment, though progress in the majority is slow. Transient disturbance of sphincter control should be regarded as an indication for prompt investigation and treatment. Physical examination at rest tends to be unremarkable, though absence of one or both ankle jerks is to be expected where there is advanced degenerative disease of the lumbar intervertebral discs. Re-examination after a period of exercise comparable to that which precipitates symptoms will often reveal short-lived weakness, reflex changes or sensory loss.

The clinical diagnosis may be supported by the plain radiographic demonstration of the hypertrophic bone masses described by Verbiest (1954, 1955) or of advanced generalized lumbar spondylosis. Confirmation of the diagnosis depends on myelography, which shows narrowing of the lumbar canal from which egress of the contrast medium is delayed. The stenosis may be so severe that movement of Myodil from the canal can be held up for several days (Joffe *et al.*, 1966). In cases associated with severe lumbar spondylosis trapping of a bolus of Myodil in a loculus between two large posterior disc protrusions may give the impression that the dye has been injected subdurally. Where symptoms are incapacitating or a progressive neurological deficit has developed, surgical decompression of the lumbar canal is indicated.

REFERENCES

BLAU, J. N. & LOGUE, V. (1961). Intermittent claudication of the cauda equina. *Lancet*, **1**, 1081.

DEJERINE, J. J. (1911). La claudication intermittente de la moelle épinière. *Presse méd.*, **19**, 981.

EHNI, G. (1965). Spondylotic cauda equina radiculopathy. *Tex. St. J. Med.*, **61**, 746.

HENSON, R. A. & PARSONS, M. (1967). Ischaemic lesions of the spinal cord: an illustrated review. *Quart. J. Med.*, **36**, 205.

JOFFE, R., APPLEBY, A. & ARJONA, V. (1966). "Intermittent ischaemia" of the cauda equina due to stenosis of the lumbar canal. *J. Neurol. Neurosurg. Psychiat.*, **29**, 315.

VERBIEST, H. (1954). A radicular syndrome from developmental narrowing of the lumbar vertebral canal. *J. Bone. Jt. Surg.*, **36B**, 230.

VERBIEST, H. (1955). Further experience on the pathological influence of a developmental narrowness of the bony lumbar vertebral canal. *J. Bone Jt. Surg.*, **37B**, 576.

RECENT ADVANCES IN THE STUDY OF MUSCLE DISEASE

Classification

No classification of muscle disease will ever be completely satisfactory, although the one recently published by the Research Group of Neuromuscular Diseases of the World Federation of Neurology (*J. neurol. Sci.*, 1968) is certainly workable. It is too detailed for most neurologists, but an abbreviated version containing the more important entities should be a useful guide to the nosology of muscle disease. Amongst the important advances recognized in this new classification are a relatively benign form of X-linked recessive muscular dystrophy (Becker, 1957), the separation of the oculopharyngeal variant of ocular myopathy (Victor *et al.*, 1962) and the inclusion of a number of new metabolic myopathies. The greatly expanded list of named entities under the general heading of benign congenital myopathy points to the contribution made to the contraction of this heterogeneous group by the application of electron microscopy and histochemistry to the pathological study of muscle disease. It must be admitted that the structural changes found in conditions like nemaline myopathy (Shy *et al.*, 1961) and central core disease (Shy and Magee, 1956) are unlikely to be absolutely specific. However, these changes are not found in such profusion in other muscle disorders and the detailed study of their biochemistry and molecular biology will provide fundamental information about the disease processes, and indeed about normal muscle structure and function. These problems are discussed in detail by Hudgson and Pearce (1969).

Muscular dystrophy

Muscular dystrophy in its various forms continues to defy the efforts of those engaged in the investigation of its pathogenesis and treatment. So far as X-linked recessive progressive muscular dystrophy is concerned, it has become clear that the disease is largely "burnt out" by the time the diagnosis becomes clinically apparent, and that the most active muscle destruction occurs during the so-called preclinical phase (Pearson, 1962; Heyck *et al.*, 1966; Hudgson *et al.*, 1967a; Mastaglia *et al.*, 1969). The fundamental histopathological changes in Duchenne dystrophy are muscle necrosis and regeneration, the latter being inevitably abortive (Hudgson *et al.*, 1967a; Mastaglia *et al.*, 1969). These changes result in gross elevation of serum muscle enzymes, particularly creatine kinase (CK) in the neonatal period, and permit diagnosis by estimation of the CK level in cord blood immediately after birth (Pearce *et al.*, 1964). Muscle biopsy at this stage will reveal the histological changes described above.

Regrettably, there is no successful specific treatment for the various muscular dystrophies, although the lives of sufferers can be lengthened and made more tolerable by the provision of devices to aid mobility, adequate physiotherapy, and the prompt exhibition of antibiotics in even minor respiratory infections (Walton and Gardner-Medwin, 1969). Psychological support of the patient and his family is of the greatest importance, and with respect to the latter the increasing availability and accuracy of carrier detection and genetic counselling services may help to minimize the incidence of the X-linked recessive forms in the community. Approximately 65 per cent of all female carriers of the gene for either form of X-linked recessive dystrophy have abnormally high serum CK levels and can be identified by estimating the activity of this enzyme (Pearce *et al.*, 1964). Unfortunately the frequency of detection cannot be improved by provocative techniques such as moderate exercise (Hudgson *et al.*, 1967b) and indeed violent exercise produces a sharp rise in the serum activity of CK in *normal* subjects (Griffiths, 1966; Vejjajiva and Teasdale, 1965). However, electromyography may demonstrate patchy myopathic changes in the muscles of carriers, and the combination of serum CK measurement with quantitative electromyography (Gardner-Medwin, 1968a and b; Willison, 1968) increases the detection rate to over 90 per cent. The carrier should then be told that she has a one-in-four chance of bearing a dystrophic child, but the final decision as to whether or not to risk pregnancy clearly rests with the individual.

Spinal muscular atrophy in infancy

The prognosis in the majority of cases of X-linked recessive dystrophy is gloomy, the patients usually dying in late adolescence. In the benign (Becker) form of X-linked recessive dystrophy, and in limb-girdle dystrophy, survival into adult life is the rule though disability may be severe, and in facio-scapulo-humeral dystrophy the patient often leads a relatively normal life into middle-age. However, the problem of giving a patient an unnecessarily poor prognosis after making a mistaken diagnosis of dystrophy, first pointed out by Nattrass (1954) remains. Gardner-Medwin *et al.* (1967) reviewed a group of cases originally diagnosed as Duchenne or limb-girdle dystrophy, some of whom had survived for extraordinarily long periods. These patients were all shown to have so-called "pseudomyopathic" spinal muscular atrophy or the Kugelberg-Welander syndrome (Wohlfart *et al.*, 1955; Kugelberg and Welander, 1956) which in most cases has a significantly better outlook than any kind of muscular dystrophy. Many of these patients bore striking clinical resemblances to muscular dystrophy with similarly selective muscle wasting and weakness, and some even showed pseudohypertrophy of the calves or other muscle groups. The correct diagnosis was made in each case by finding the changes of *chronic denervation* on electromyography and in muscle biopsies; the finding underlines the importance of these two techniques in the routine assessment of clinical problems in muscle disease.

The precise nature of the spinal muscular atrophies of infancy and their possible relationship to adult motor neurone disease on the one hand and the heredofamilial ataxias on the other remains uncertain. Sibships of both the Kugelberg-Welander syndrome and Werdnig-Hoffmann disease have been described, though family histories are otherwise lacking, which suggests that these conditions may be determined by autosomal recessive genes. Gardner-Medwin *et al.* (1967) recorded one family where cases of both conditions occurred and suggested that pseudomyopathic spinal muscular atrophy was simply a slowly progressive variant of Werdnig-Hoffmann disease. The problems of genetics and nosology in the spinal muscular atrophies are further discussed by Liversedge (1969). Japanese workers (Tsukagoshi *et al.*, 1965; Araki *et al.*, 1966) have claimed that there may be an element of true myopathy in some cases of "spinal" muscular atrophy on the basis of moderate elevation in serum muscle enzymes. Other workers (Drachman *et al.*, 1967; Gardner-Medwin *et al.*, 1967), however, found that histological evidence of secondary myopathic changes was common in chronically denervated muscle, and suggested that elevation in serum muscle enzymes in spinal muscular atrophy was probably due to "leakage" from such foci.

Metabolic myopathies

Myopathies which form but one segment of a generalized metabolic or immunological disturbance are recognized with increasing frequency. Those associated with malignant disease and chronic renal failure (pp. 319–39) and collagen vascular disease certainly fall into this category, as do those associated with thyrotoxicosis, Cushing's syndrome and metabolic bone disease. Muscle weakness in a non-specific sense has long been recognized as a concomitant of conditions such as osteomalacia and hyperparathyroidism, but it is only recently that a specific myopathy has been defined in these disorders (Prineas *et al.*, 1965; Smith and Stern, 1967; Frame *et al.*, 1968; Smith and Stern, 1969). Myopathy in metabolic bone disease usually produces quite severe proximal muscle weakness, particularly in the pelvic girdles. Weakness is often accompanied by bone pain, which may be severe. Electromyography demonstrates myopathic abnormalities in most cases (Smith and Stern, 1969) though these changes are slight or absent in some patients. No characteristic pathological abnormalities have so far been found in muscle biopsy material from these patients. The serum calcium levels in those with osteomalacia and serum vitamin D levels are also likely to be low. Treatment with vitamin D is usually followed by clinical improvement (Prineas et al., 1965; Smith and Stern, 1969).

Myopathy in Cushing's syndrome is well recognized, and recently Prineas et al. (1968) reported the development of myopathy in groups of patients recently subjected to bilateral adrenalectomy for Cushing's syndrome due to adrenal hyperplasia. All these patients had greatly increased serum ACTH levels, and muscle biopsy showed that the muscle fibres which normally contained high concentrations of oxidative enzymes held much more sudanophilic lipid than control material from normal subjects (Prineas and Ng, 1967). Another possibly genetically determined defect of fat metabolism in skeletal muscle was recently described in a young woman born of a consanguineous marriage (Bradley et al., 1969). The patient presented with a severe myopathy affecting mainly the upper limbs and the cervical muscles and was shown to have enormously increased amounts of neutral fat in her muscle fibres.

The periodic paralyses

Periodic attacks of severe generalized muscle weakness with complete recovery between attacks have been recognized for may years, though it was not until 1875 that Westphal clearly separated the syndrome from hysteria. There are at least four separate forms of this disease; hypokalaemic (Biemond and Daniels, 1934); hyperkalaemic (*adynamia episodica hereditaria*) (Gamstorp, 1956); normokalaemic (Poskanzer and Kerr, 1961); and thyrotoxic. The last is particularly common in the Orient (McFadzean and Yeung, 1967). The first three varieties are familial, though occasional sporadic cases of hypokalaemic periodic paralysis occur. In the hypokalaemic and hyperkalaemic forms the attacks are characterized respectively by a rise or fall in the serum potassium level, and a fall in serum potassium is usually recorded in thyrotoxic periodic paralysis. No characteristic electrolyte changes have been found during attacks of normokalaemic periodic paralysis (Poskanzer and Kerr, 1961; Bradley, 1969). Attacks of the hypokalaemic form tend to be relatively infrequent but may be prolonged and severe, whereas in adynamia they may occur daily, but are short-lived and often do not incapacitate the patient severely. Intravenous potassium aborts attacks of hypokalaemic paralysis and precipitates attacks of adynamia and normokalaemic paralysis. Hypokalaemic attacks can be precipitated by insulin and glucose, while these agents prevent or abort attacks of adynamia. Myotonia is common in attacks of adynamia and can also occur in hypokalaemic episodes. Development of a progressive proximal myopathy in hypokalaemic periodic paralysis is well recognized (Pearson, 1964; Howes et al., 1966; Odor et al., 1967). A voluminous literature is accumulating on the water and electrolyte shifts between the extracellular and intracellular compartments (reviewed in detail by Bradley, 1969), the electrophysiological abnormalities in muscle cell membranes (McComas et al., 1968) and the pathology of the muscle cell in these conditions, though the fundamental metabolic errors underlying them have yet to be elucidated. However, individual attacks can be dealt with in the ways described above. Acetazolamide (Diamox) sometimes improves the myopathy of hypokalaemic periodic paralysis (Resnick et al., 1968) and bendrofluazide reduces the frequency and severity of attacks in adynamia (Bradley, 1969).

REFERENCES

ARAKI, S., IWASHITA, H. & YOSHIGORO, K. (1966). Atypical progressive muscular atrophy. Lancet, 2, 1362.

BECKER, P. E. (1957). Neue Ergebnisse der Genetik der Muskeldystrophien. Acta Genet. med. (Roma), 7, 303.

BIEMOND, A. & DANIELS, A. P. (1934). Familial periodic paralysis and its transition into spinal muscular atrophy. Brain, 57, 91.

BRADLEY, W. G. (1969). Adynamia episodica hereditaria. Clinical, pathological and electrophysiological studies in an affected family. Brain, 92, 345.

BRADLEY, W. G., GARDNER-MEDWIN, D., HUDGSON, P. & WALTON, J. N. (1969). Myopathy with abnormal lipid metabolism in skeletal muscle. Lancet, 1, 495.

DRACHMAN, D. B., MURPHY, S. R., NIGAM, M. P. & HILLS, J. P. (1967). "Myopathic" changes in chronically denervated muscle. Arch. Neurol., 16, 14.

FRAME, B., HEINZE, E. G., BLOCK, M. A. & MANSON, G. A. (1968). Myopathy in primary hyperparathyroidism. Ann. intern. Med., 68, 1022.

GAMSTORP, I. (1956). Adynamia episodica hereditaria. Acta. paediat. Stockh. Suppl. 108.

GARDNER-MEDWIN, D. (1968a). Some problems encountered in the use of electromyography in carrier detection. In Research in Muscular Dystrophy. Proceedings of the 4th Symposium of the Muscular Dystrophy Group of Great Britain. London: Pitman Medical Publishing Co.

GARDNER-MEDWIN, D. (1968b). Studies of the carrier state in the Duchenne type of muscular dystrophy. Part II. Quantitative electromyography as a method of carrier detection. J. Neurol. Neurosurg. Psychiat., 31, 124.

GARDNER-MEDWIN, D., HUDGSON, P. & WALTON, J. N. (1967). Benign spinal muscular atrophy arising in childhood and adolescence. J. Neurol. Sci., 5, 121.

GRIFFITHS, P. D. (1966). Serum levels of adenosine triphosphate: creatine phosphotransferase (creatine kinase). The normal range and the effect of muscular exercise. Clin. chim. Acta., 13, 413.

HEYCK, H., LÜDERS, C. J. & LAUDAHN, G. (1966). Beitrag zur Dystrophia musculorum progressiva: V Histologische befunde im präklinischen Stadium der Dystrophia musculorum progressiva Typ Duchenne. Klin. Wschr., 44, 813.

HOWES, E. L., PRICE, H. M., PEARSON, C. M. & BLUMBERG, J. M. (1966). Hypokalemic periodic paralysis: electron microscopic changes in the sarcoplasm. *Neurology (Minneap.)*, **16**, 242.

HUDGSON, P. & PEARCE, G. W. (1969). Ultramicroscopic studies of diseased muscle. In *Disorders of Voluntary Muscle*, 2nd edition. ed. J. N. Walton. London: Churchill.

HUDGSON, P., PEARCE, G. W. & WALTON, J. N. (1967a). Preclinical muscular dystrophy: histopathological changes observed on muscle biopsy. *Brain*, **90**, 565.

HUDGSON, P., GARDNER-MEDWIN, D., PENNINGTON, R. J. T. & WALTON, J. N. (1967b). Studies of the carrier state in the Duchenne type of muscular dystrophy. Part I. Effect of exercise on serum creatine kinase activity. *J. Neurol. Neurosurg. Psychiat.*, **30**, 416.

J. neurol. Sci. (1968), **6**, 165. Classification of the neuromuscular disorders.

KUGELBERG, E. & WELANDER, L. (1956). Heredofamilial juvenile muscular atrophy simulating muscular dystrophy. *Arch. Neurol. Psychiat. (Chic.)*, **75**, 500.

LIVERSEDGE, L. A. (1969). The central neuronal muscular atrophies and other dysfunctions of the anterior horn cells. In *Disorders of Voluntary Muscle*, 2nd edition. ed. J. N. Walton. London: Churchill.

ODOR, D. L., PATEL, A. N. & PEARCE, L. A. (1967). Familial periodic paralysis with permanent myopathy. A clinical and ultrastructural study. *J. Neuropath. exp. Neurol.*, **26**, 98.

McCOMAS, A. J., MROŻEK, K. & BRADLEY, W. G. (1968). The nature of the electrophysiological disorder in adynamia episodica. *J. Neurol. Neurosurg. Psychiat.*, **31**, 448.

McFADZEAN, A. J. S. & YEUNG, R. (1967). Periodic paralysis complicating thyrotoxicosis in Chinese. *Brit. med. J.*, **1**, 451.

MASTAGLIA, F. L., PAPADIMITRIOU, J. M. & KAKULAS, B. A. (1969). Regeneration in Duchenne muscular dystrophy—A histological, ultrastructural and histochemical study. *Proc. Aust. Ass. Neurol.*, **6**, 93.

NATTRASS, F. J. (1954). Recovery from "muscular dystrophy". *Brain*, **77**, 549.

PEARCE, J. M. S., PENNINGTON, R. J. T. & WALTON, J. N. (1964). Serum enzyme studies in muscle disease. Part III. Serum creatine kinase activity in relatives of patients with Duchenne type of muscular dystrophy. *J. Neurol. Neurosurg. Psychiat.*, **27**, 181.

PEARSON, C. M. (1962). Histopathological features of muscle in the preclinical stage of muscular dystrophy. *Brain*, **85**, 109.

PEARSON, C. M. (1964). The periodic paralyses: differential features and pathological observations in permanent myopathic weakness. *Brain*, **87**, 341.

POSKANZER, D. C. & KERR, D. N. S. (1961). A third type of periodic paralysis with normokalaemia and favourable response to sodium chloride. *Amer. J. Med.*, **31**, 328.

PRINEAS, J. W. & NG, R. C. Y. (1967). Ultrastructural features of intracellular lipid in normal human muscle. *Neurology (Minneap.)*, **17**, 1092.

PRINEAS, J. W., HALL, R., BARWICK, D. D. & WATSON, A. J. (1968). Myopathy associated with pigmentation following adrenalectomy for Cushing's syndrome. *Quart. J. Med.*, **37**, 63.

PRINEAS, J. W., STUART MASON, A. & HENSON, R. A. (1965). Myopathy in metabolic bone disease. *Brit. med. J.*, **1**, 1034.

RESNICK, J. S., ENGEL, W. K., GRIGGS, R. C. & STAM, A. C. (1968). Acetazolamide prophylaxis in hypokalaemic periodic paralysis. *N. Engl. J. Med.*, **278**, 582.

SHY, G. M., ENGEL, W. K., SOMERS, J. E. & WANKO, T. (1963). Nemaline myopathy: a new congenital myopathy. *Brain*, **86**, 793.

SHY, G. M. & MAGEE, K. R. (1956). A new non-progressive myopathy. *Brain*, 79, 610.

SMITH, R. & STERN, G. M. (1967). Myopathy, osteomalacia and hyperparathyroidism. *Brain*, **90**, 593.

SMITH, R. & STERN, G. M. (1969). Muscular weakness in osteomalacia and hyperparathyroidism. *J. neurol. Sci.*, **8**, 511.

TSUKAGOSHI, H., NAKANISKI, T., KONDO, K. & TSUBAKE, T. (1965). Hereditary proximal neurogenic muscular atrophy in adult. *Arch. Neurol.*, **12**, 597.

VEJJAJIVA, A. & TEASDALE, G. M. (1965). Serum creatine kinase and physical exercise. *Brit. med. J.*, **1**, 1653.

VICTOR, M., HAYES, R. & ADAMS, R. D. (1962). Oculopharyngeal muscular dystrophy. A familial disease of late life characterised by dysphagia and progressive ptosis of the eyelids. *N. Eng. J. Med.*, **267**, 1267.

WALTON, J. N. & GARDNER-MEDWIN, D. (1969). Progressive muscular dystrophy. In *Disorders of Voluntary Muscle*, 2nd edition. ed. J. N. Walton. London: Churchill.

WESTPHAL, C. (1885). Über einen merkururdigen Fall von periodischer Lähmung aller veer Extremitäten mit gleichzeitigem Erloxchen der electrichen Erregbarkeit während der Lähmung. *Berl. klin. Wschr.*, **22**, 489.

WILLISON, R. G. (1968). The problem of detecting carriers of Duchenne muscular dystrophy by quantitative electromyography. In *Research in Muscular Dystrophy*. Proceedings of the 4th symposium of the Muscular Dystrophy Group of Great Britain. London: Pitman Medical Publishing Co.

WOHLFART, G., FEX, J. & ELIASSON, S. (1955). Hereditary proximal spinal muscular atrophy—a clinical entity simulating progressive muscular dystrophy. *Acta psychiat. (Kbh)*, **30**, 395.

11 The Chromosomes of Man

C. A. CLARKE

INTRODUCTION. DEFINITION OF TERMS. DESOXYRIBONUCLEIC ACID. TECHNIQUES AND NOMENCLATURE. NON-DISJUNCTION IN THE SEX CHROMOSOMES. THE LYON HYPOTHESIS. NON-DISJUNCTION IN THE AUTOSOMES. TRANSLOCATION. CHROMOSOMES AND ABORTIONS. CHROMOSOMES AND LEUKAEMIA. THE MAPPING OF CHROMOSOMES. GENETIC COUNSELLING.

INTRODUCTION

IT would be idle to pretend that chromosomal abnormalities account for more than a fraction of human pathology, and it is unnecessary for a clinician to be acquainted with every newly published set of marionettes. Nevertheless, chromosomes are coming closer to ordinary medicine and some knowledge of them is desirable—the information is basic and in a few cases can be most helpful in accurate diagnosis and prognosis.

Before discussing the clinical aspects of the discipline it is important to learn (or re-learn) some of the terminology.

DEFINITION OF TERMS

Karyotype. This is the term used to mean the whole chromosomal picture of *somatic* cells and normally, no matter what organ is examined, there are 22 pairs of autosomes and one pair of sex chromosomes, X and Y in the male and X and X in the female. It is important to remember that genes only exert their effect in appropriate tissues; for example, the sex chromosomes are inert as regards sex, except in the cells of the reproductive organs where they become responsible for the differentiation of the gonads.

Mitosis. This is the process which occurs when somatic nuclei divide. Each chromosome duplicates (*syn*. replicates) itself, so that two chromatids are formed; one of these passes to one pole of the nucleus and the other to the opposite one. The nucleus and the cell then also divide and form two new daughter cells, each of which carries an exactly similar complement of genes to the mother cell. The other features to be remembered about mitosis are: (1) that the homologous chromosomes do not pair (cf. meiosis) and (2) that the chromatids are held together for a short time by the centromere and it is then that further division can be halted by colchicine and the chromosomes examined and photographed (see Fig. 11.3). The position of the centromere is constant for any given chromosome and is normally situated anywhere except at the extreme end.

Meiosis. This type of division occurs only in the testes and ovaries, the process taking place in many precursors of the spermatozoa (spermatocytes) simultaneously but only in one oöcyte at a time. Though there are many steps in meiosis there are only two essentials to remember: (i) in each ovum and spermatozoon the chromosome number is halved, so that it becomes haploid instead of diploid; (ii) genetic interchange (crossing-over or recombination) occurs at the stage when the homologous chromosomes (one of which is paternal and one maternal) pair, which they do before they separate.

Crossing-over or recombination. It is uncertain as to precisely what happens during crossing-over. Most descriptions suggest that the exchange of genetic material is brought about by breakage and rejoining of parts of the two chromatids. However, the old explanation of Belling (1933) is more in keeping with the chemistry of DNA. He suggested that the duplication of the chromosomes takes place irregularly so that the connecting fibres join up groups of genes from both paternal and maternal chromatids. Figure 11.1 explains this in more detail.

Non-disjunction. If a pair of homologous autosomes or the sex chromosomes stay together instead of separating at meiosis, non-disjunction is said to have occurred. The resulting spermatozoon or ovum then receives either *two* of the particular chromosome involved or *none*, though in all other respects the gamete will have the normal chromosome complement. On fertilization with a normal gamete, the zygote will either be trisomic or monosomic for the particular pair of chromosomes in which non-disjunction has occurred. Non-disjunction can also occur at mitosis, after which mosaicism (q.v.) results. Mongolism is usually due to trisomy of chromosome 21, and Klinefelter's syndrome (XXY) and some forms of Turner's syndrome (XO) are examples of trisomy and monosomy respectively involving the sex chromosomes (but see German (1970) for recent views on Turner's syndrome).

Isochromosome. The simplest way to understand this is to take a specific instance; for example, Turner's syndrome. Most women who suffer from this are chromosomally XO, but sometimes they are XX, and in this case one of the Xs is often abnormal (an isochromosome). This is produced as follows: normally the X chromosome divides longitudinally (down the

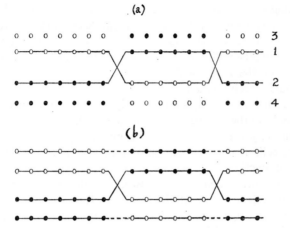

FIG. 11.1. The diagram shows how the duplication of chromosomes and crossing-over may take place at meiosis. In (a) two
chromosomes (1, 2) are shown wound round each other and
replication has taken place (3, 4). In (b) the new connecting fibres
have joined up replicated groups of genes from *both* chromosomes
so that the two new chromatids, instead of being exact copies of
the old, contain some maternal and some paternal genes, (Belling,
1933).

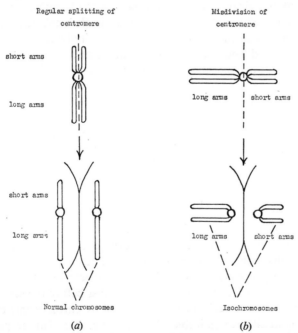

FIG. 11.2. The origin of an isochromosome through misdivision
of the centromere during mitotic division. (By courtesy of Dr W. G.
Harnden and Messrs Heinemann.)

middle) so that each daughter cell receives both the long and the short arms of the chromosome with all their genes. If the X chromosome divides *across* (see Fig. 11.2b) there results either an isochromosome made up of two long arms of the X, which will contain two sets of the genes on the long arm but none of those on the short, or *vice versa*. Isochromosomes are also probably formed, though rarely, as a result of abnormal division of the autosomes.

Barr body. This is a densely staining body just inside the nuclear membrane which is present in the somatic cells of females (who are said to be chromatin positive) but only rarely in males (chromatin negative), and it is usually tested for in cells from a buccal smear (see Fig. 11.5). It almost certainly represents the inactive X chromosome (see Lyon hypothesis, p. 369).

Another structure which helps to distinguish the sexes cytologically is the drumstick appendage (see Fig. 11.6) which is found in about 3 per cent of the neutrophil leucocytes of females, but is absent in males. The incidence of the trait is influenced by the degree of lobing of the nucleus, the more highly lobed cells having a greater incidence of drumsticks (Mittwoch, 1967).

Translocation. In a translocation two non-homologous chromosomes have joined together (a small piece from each being lost in the process). As a result, when the chromosomes are arranged in pairs, it is found that one each of two different pairs, e.g. one of the number 13s and one of the number 15s is missing, and in their place is an abnormally large chromosome. The important thing to remember when this happens is that the total amount of chromatin remains normal (or nearly so); the individuals concerned are therefore unaffected and are known as translocation carriers. It is in the succeeding generation that abnormalities may occur. Ford and Clegg (1969) give an up-to-date account of a particular type of translocation (i.e. where there is exchange of terminal segments between non-homologous chromosomes).

Deletion. A deficiency of part of a chromosome. The small abnormal chromosome (Ph_1) often present in myeloid leukaemia is thought to be the result of a deletion, probably in chromsome 21.

The *cri du chat* syndrome (see p. 379) is caused by a deletion of part of a chromosome No. 5.

Mosaicism. Individuals who are mosaics have tissues some of which are of one chromosomal constitution and some of another; for example, a proportion of patients with Turner's syndrome are XO/XX mosaics. The condition results either from non-disjunction (q.v.) occurring at mitosis or because of *anaphase lag*, where a chromosome gets lost at the stage during which the duplicated chromosomes pull apart just before the separation into two daughter cells. Mosaicism can be detected by chromosome culture, but it is also potentially recognizable clinically, e.g. if a Turner patient were colour-blind in one eye and not in the other. Mongol mosaicism, e.g. 46/47, is being increasingly recognized (see p. 373). A mosaic differs from a

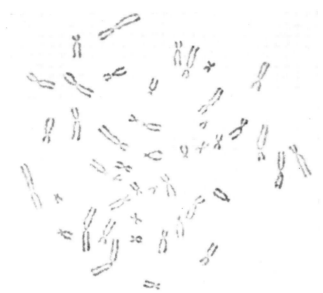

Fig. 11.3. This shows the 46 chromosomes from a single somatic male cell undergoing mitosis. The chromosomes have doubled but are still held together by their centromeres. (By courtesy of Dr S. Walker and Messrs Blackwell.)

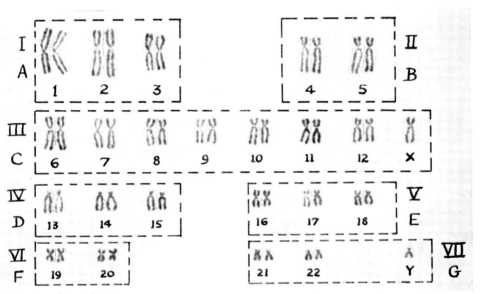

Fig. 11.4. This shows the same 46 doubled chromosomes as in Fig. 11.3. The autosomes are arranged in decreasing order of size and numbered from 1 to 22. The X and Y are not numbered. The seven groups of the Denver and Patau classifications are indicated by the Roman numerals and appropriate letters. (By courtesy of Dr S. Walker and Messrs Blackwell.)

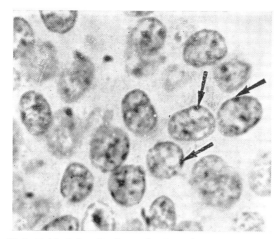

Fig. 11.5. Epithelial cells from the buccal mucosa of a female patient showing Barr bodies in the nuclei ("chromatin positive"). (By courtesy of Dr Winston Evans, David Lewis Northern Hospital, Liverpool.)

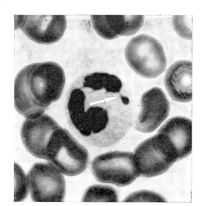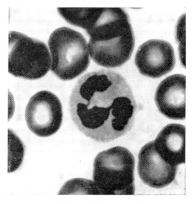

Fig. 11.6. *Left:* Neutrophil leucocyte, a drumstick nuclear appendage, in a blood film from a normal female. Giemsa stain. Mag. × 1800.
Right: A neutrophil leucocyte from a normal male, in which cells with drumstick appendages are lacking. This cell would, equally well, illustrate over 90 per cent of neutrophils of females. Giemsa stain. Mag. × 1800.

chimaera in that a mosaic is formed of the cells of a single zygote lineage while a chimaera has cells which derive from two or more distinct zygote lineages (see Ford (1969) for a full account of this).

Locus. This is the site on a chromosome occupied by a particular gene or a member of a particular allelomorphic series.

Linkage. Genes, or more accurately the loci which they occupy, which are situated on the same chromosome are said to be linked and are inherited together, except when crossing-over occurs. The loci for the nail-patella syndrome and for the ABO blood group alleles are an example of this in man. The closer together the genes, the less likely is crossing-over to occur, and some genes are so close together that they have never been observed to become separated. Those comprising the Rh blood group complex, for instance, are inherited as a unit, though there must have been occasional crossing-over *within* the complex (which is an example of a supergene) in order to give rise to some of the rarer Rh genotypes.

Phenocopy. An exact replica of an inherited character, but produced environmentally. The deaf-mutism in the offspring of mothers who have had rubella in the first three months of pregnancy is indistinguishable from the inherited type.

REFERENCES

BELLING, J. (1933). Crossing-over and gene rearrangements in flowering plants. *Genetics*, **18**, 388.

FORD, C. E. (1969). Mosaics and chimaeras. *Brit. med. Bull.*, **25**, No. 1, 104.

FORD, C. E. & CLEGG, H. M. (1969). Reciprocal translocation. *Brit. med. Bull.*, **25**, No. 1, 110.

GERMAN, J. (1970). A unifying concept in relation to the gonadal dysgeneses. *Clin. Genetics*, Vol. I, No. 1, pp. 15–27.

HARNDEN, D. G. (1962). In *Chromosomes in Medicine*, ed. Hamerton, Heinemann Ltd.

MITTWOCH, URSULA (1967). *Sex Chromosomes*. New York and London: Academic Press.

DESOXYRIBONUCLEIC ACID (DNA)

Chromosomes are composed of desoxyribonucleic acid (DNA) and a molecule of this consists of two chains, each made up of a desoxyribose phosphate backbone and a series of purine and pyrimidine bases which pair with those on the opposite chain. The molecule is constructed like a double spiral staircase of which the phosphate backbones form the "bannisters" and the nitrogenous bases the "steps". The pyrimidine bases forming these "steps" are cytosine and thymine, and the purines adenine and guanine. Thymine normally pairs with adenine (mnemonic "t s and a s") and guanine with cytosine (mnemonic "Gc"). Figures 11.7 and 11.8 illustrate these points. A single molecule of DNA may have as many as 10,000 purine-pyrimidine pairs and its molecular weight is about 6,000,000. The original

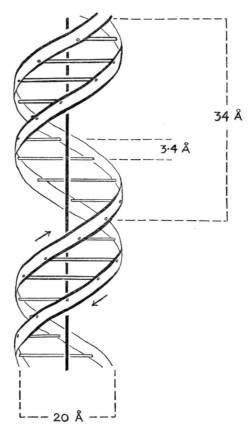

34 Å

3·4 Å

20 Å

Fig. 11.7. Diagram representing the double spiral "staircase" of the DNA molecule, giving dimensions in Ångstrom (one hundred millionth of a centimetre) units. The outer bands represent the phosphate-sugar chains and the horizontal rods the paths of the bases holding the chains together. The arrows indicate that the sequence of bases goes one way in one chain and the opposite way in the other. The vertical line represents the axis of the molecule.

paper on the structure of DNA (Watson and Crick, 1953) is readily comprehensible to any physician and no later work has contradicted it.

Replication. It is worth considering how the replication of DNA is effected. It is probable that its two chains, which are wound round each other, separate and then each single chain will have a series of bases needing new partners. These are taken from the nucleotide pool and the appropriate freshly synthesized nucleotide bonds itself to the right base on the old chain (guanine plus its sugar and phosphate if cytosine is needing a new partner, adenine plus its sugar and phosphate if thymine is needing one, and so on). This mode of replication is called "semi-conservative" since each new double chain consists of one old and one new chain and is consistent with the Belling hypothesis of the events occurring at meiosis (see Fig. 11.1).

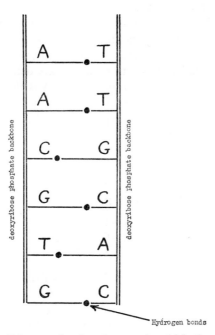

FIG. 11.8. Diagram showing the way in which the nitrogenous bases of DNA are paired, facing inwards from the phosphate-sugar chain and joined together by hydrogen bonds.

Supporting evidence that this hypothesis of replication is correct came from the work of Meselson and Stahl (1958). These workers grew *E. coli* for many generations in a medium of which the nitrogen consisted entirely of the radio-active isotope N^{15}. Eventually, therefore, this constituent of the DNA molecule was all in the labelled and readily identifiable form. The bacteria were then transferred to a medium where the nitrogen was of the ordinary form (N^{14}), and after one generation all the molecules were found to be hybrid, containing equal amounts of N^{14} and N^{15}. In the next generation the number of hybrid molecules remained the same, but an equal number of pure N^{14} molecules had appeared, and these continued to increase in subsequent generations.

More recently there has been a remarkable advance in that DNA has been synthesized *in vitro*. Goulian, Kornberg and Sinsheimer (1967) put the

DNA of a pigmy virus (Phi X174), labelled with tritium, in a test-tube together with the bases adenine, guanine, cytosine, and, instead of thymine, bromouracil. The addition of the enzyme polymerase caused a circle of artificial DNA to be formed from the bases around that of the natural DNA. The two circles could be separated, because bromouracil is heavier than thymine. This artificial DNA was found to be able to reproduce itself just as if it were natural DNA, and so, moreover, was a second generation artificial DNA which these workers formed from their first artificial DNA. The authors feel that it might in the future be possible to attach a particular gene to harmless viral DNA and use this virus as a vehicle for delivering the gene to the cells of a patient who has an hereditary defect.

The genetic code. The vital importance of DNA is that it can initiate the transmission of information to the amino-acids in the cytoplasm so that they can form correct polypeptide sequences and hence the right proteins. For example,

$$G—C$$
$$C—G$$
$$A—T$$

would carry a different message from that of:

$$A—T$$
$$G—C$$
$$T—A$$

Although the information arises in the DNA of the nucleus, the proteins are manufactured in small particles in the cytoplasm called ribosomes. An intermediate step is to transmit the information to the ribosomes by "messenger" RNA, which is similar to DNA but has only one chain. It is slightly different in constitution, having uracil instead of thymine, and presumably when the DNA "says" adenine-thymine, the RNA (having only one chain) translates this into adenine-uracil.

The deciphering of the genetic code. It is known experimentally that a sequence of uracil in the RNA ensures that a chain of the amino-acid phenylalanine results, whereas a cytosine sequence produces proline, but how many bases form the code word determining one specific amino-acid sequence? Crick *et al.* (1961) have shown that (for bacteriophage anyway) the answer is *three*, and the reasoning for this is as follows:

First, if the coding were of four bases there would only be 16 combinations (4×4) which would not be enough to code the 20 or more essential amino-acids. However, using three of the four bases there are 64 $(4 \times 4 \times 4)$ different groupings which is more than adequate and it seems probable that more than one triplet codes the same amino-acid. Secondly, Crick and his colleagues (1961) have performed some critical experiments with the bacteriophage, T4. This phage will normally grow on two different strains of *E. coli*, but when a mutation consisting of the addition of a purine or pyrimidine base takes place in the DNA of the phage, it puts wrong the coding which follows the mutation, and then the phage is only able to grow on one of the strains of the bacterium. When, however, a second mutation consisting of a deletion of a base takes place close to the first one, the original order is restored in subsequent bases and the phage will then grow on both strains of *E. coli*. This could occur, however, if many bases formed the codeword, but the triplet hypothesis is shown to be true by the fact that two more additions besides the first one—that is three additional bases in all—will restore the subsequent bases to their original and correct order. This would only be the case if the code consisted of a word of three or a multiple of three letters.

That the three bases are only read once and that the code does not overlap is proved by the fact that a mutation in the sense of alteration (not deletion or addition) of a base only alters one amino-acid. It does *not* alter the amino-acids controlled by the "words" on each side of the mutated "word".

It is probable that what happens in bacteriophage is applicable to man. In sickle-cell haemoglobin, for example, the single substitution of the amino-acid valine for glutamic acid is sufficient to change Hb A to Hb S, and this could be explained by a mistake in the pairing of the DNA bases. Thus if adenine were temporarily to occur as its isomer at the moment of replication. it might pair with cytosine instead of thymine. At the next replication, however, adenine, having reverted to its usual form, would pair normally with thymine and cytosine with guanine. There would, however, have been one change in the sequence of bases and this would be reproduced indefinitely.

It must be emphasized that what has been discussed is at the molecular level, whereas what follows mainly concerns structures visible under the microscope.

REFERENCES

CRICK, F. H. C., BARNETT, L., BRENNER, S. & WATTS-TOBIN, R. J. (1961). General nature of the genetic code for proteins. *Nature*, **192**, 1227.

GOULIAN, M., KORNBERG, A. & SINSHEIMER, R. L. (1967). Enzymatic synthesis of DNA. *Proc. Nat. Acad. Sci., U.S.A.*, **58**, 2321.

MESELSON, M. & STAHL, F. W. (1958). The replication of DNA in *Escherichia coli*. *Proc. Nat. Acad. Sci. U.S.A.*, **44**, 671.

WATSON, J. D. & CRICK, F. H. C. (1953). The structure of DNA. Cold Spring Harbor Symposium. *Quant. Biol.*, **18**, 123.

TECHNIQUES AND NOMENCLATURE

Chromosomes can only be seen in actively dividing cells, and it is therefore usually bone marrow, peripheral blood and skin which are investigated.

Bone marrow

This is most often looked at in leukaemia and therefore the cells are examined without culture in order to obviate normal cells overgrowing the leukaemic ones. A few drops of marrow only are necessary and the technique is given by Dyke (1968).

Peripheral blood

An ideal volume is 10 ml. This is a large amount to take from a child (though experts can get it either from the jugular vein or the fontanelle), but Arakaki and Sparkes (1963) have described a method for making preparations from small volumes (0·05–2 ml) of blood obtainable from skin puncture. With adults, however, the larger amount of blood is readily available. The blood is incubated in a medium containing amino-acids and vitamins, and the interval before preparations can be made is two or three days. With blood it is the lymphocytes which are studied, many of the polymorphs being "old", and mature red cells always without nuclei. Whole blood is used in micro-techniques, and leucocytes only in the macro-method.

Skin

A very thin slice is taken off with a sharp scalpel. It is at least one and sometimes several weeks before chromosome preparations can be made, and the culture is grown in TC 199 and foetal calf serum.

With all three types of culture, colchicine is added after the requisite incubation time, and this halts the process of cell division so that the chromatids remain attached by the centromere. The cells are next caused to swell by exposure to a hypotonic solution, and this enables the chromosomes to spread out so that they are more readily analysable. They are next fixed and stained.

It is then necessary to count and identify the chromosomes accurately, and for this many cells from one culture must be examined, because breakages and other accidents lead to difficulties.

A chromosome is described and classified according to three criteria: (a) its length, (b) the position of the centromere, and (c) distinguishing features such as the presence of satellites (though the diagnostic value of these is less than was originally thought (Ford, 1962)) and (d) by the use of autoradiography (see below).

In Fig. 11.4 it is shown how, by convention, the 22 pairs of autosomes are arranged and numbered in decreasing order of size. The X and Y are not numbered. The largest chromosome is about five times as long as the

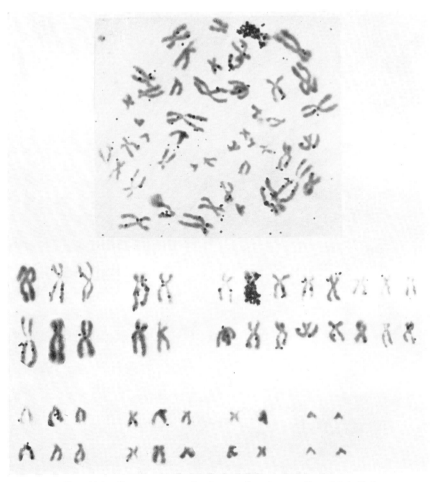

FIG. 11.9. Chromosomes of a human female somatic cell labelled with tritiated thymidine, showing the heavy labelling of one of the Xs. (see p. 363). (By courtesy of Gilbert *et al.*, and the Editor of *Nature*.)

smallest, and the centromere varies in position from median to almost terminal.

Any chromosome pair can be allotted to one of seven groups (the Denver classification) and sometimes, but not always, it is possible to differentiate the chromosomes within these groups. The groups are: 1 to 3, 4 to 5, 6 to 12 including X, 13 to 15, 16 to 18, 19 to 20 and 21 to 22 including Y. An alternative classification, that of Patau, labels the seven groups with the letters A to G.

As regards identification, it is generally considered that the chromosome pairs 1, 2, 3 and 16 can be recognized on sight alone. The following pairs are difficult to distinguish from each other: 4 and 5, the whole group 6 to 12, including X, the 13 to 15 group, 17 and 18, 19 and 20, and 21, 22 and Y. Autoradiography helps to separate 4 and 5, 13, 14 and 15, and 21 and 22 from Y by patterns of late labelling. It also clearly labels any X chromosome over and above a single complement. The Y is usually distinguished by its morphology, the chromatids lying parallel to one another and having no satellites, but it can now also be recognized by a simple fluorescent staining technique (Pearson et al. (1970) and George (1970)).

By means of labelling the chromosomes with tritiated thymidine it is possible to observe the rate of synthesis of DNA, and Fig. 11.9 shows the chromosomes of a human female cell thus treated. The subject will be returned to in the section on the Lyon hypothesis (see p. 369).

REFERENCES

ARAKAKI, D. T. & SPARKES, R. S. (1963). Microtechnique for culturing leukocytes from whole blood. *Cytogenetics*, **2**, 57–60.

DYKE, S. C. (1968). *Recent Advances in Clinical Pathology*, Series V. London: Churchill.

FORD, C. E. (1962). In *Chromosomes in Medicine*. ed. J. L. Hamerton. London: Heinemann, p. 56.

GEORGE, K. P. (1970). Cytochemical differentiation along human chromosomes. *Nature*, **236**, 80–81.

PEARSON, P. L., BOBROW, M. & VOSA, C. G. (1970). Technique for identifying Y chromosomes in human interflux nuclei. *Nature*, **226**, 78–80.

NON-DISJUNCTION IN THE SEX CHROMOSOMES

It will be evident that non-disjunction can be either maternal or paternal, and Figures 11.10 and 11.11 show that the consequences are different, YO and XXX being possibilities if the female gametes are at fault. Although it is

clinically immaterial which partner is responsible, it is interesting to know
that this point can sometimes be decided, and two methods are available:

Detection by means of colour vision studies

Red-green colour blindness is, like haemophilia, inherited as a sex-linked
recessive and XO individuals have the same incidence (about 8 per cent) of
the disability as do normal men (XY). If a non-colour-blind patient with

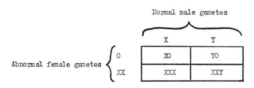

		X	Y
Abnormal female gametes	0	XO	YO
	XX	XXX	XXY

XO   Abnormal female (Turner's syndrome)

YO   Almost certainly inviable

XXX   Abnormal female (triple X, formerly called 'super-female')

XXY   Abnormal male (Klinefelter's syndrome)

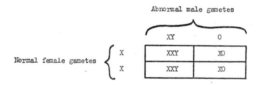

Abnormal male gametes

		XY	O
Normal female gametes	X	XXY	XO
	X	XXY	XO

XXY   Klinefelter's syndrome

XO   Turner's syndrome

FIGS. 11.10 and 11.11. Showing the effects of non-disjunction in
the sex chromosomes. These abnormal gametes are produced if the
non-disjunction occurs at the *first* meiotic division. If it occurs at
the second meiotic division as well, XX and YY sperm could also
be produced, and four different types of abnormal offspring could
result, XXY, XO and XXX as above and also XYY. Males with
this last chromosome constitution, XYY (produced by non-
disjunction in a Y-bearing sperm) are described below (p. 367).

Turner's syndrome had a colour-blind mother and a normal father we should
know that she must have received her single X chromosome from her
father, and, since she is XO, non-disjunction must have taken place in the
mother. Incidentally, we should also know that it is possible for an O egg
(i.e. one without an X chromosome) to become fertilized.

Detection by means of the Xg^a antibody. Mann and his colleagues (1962)
made the important discovery that there was an X-linked blood-group
system which they called Xg. Because it is X-linked, males can only be either
Xg^a or Xg, whereas in women there are three possibilities—Xg^{a}Xg^a (homozygous positive), XgXg (homozygous negative) and Xg^{a}Xg (the heterozygote.)

Since the frequency of the heterozygote is as high as 46 per cent in Europe, many families will segregate for Xg[a] and Xg. Using this blood group (as well as colour vision studies) it has been shown that in Turner's syndrome the single X is maternal in about 74 per cent of cases, whereas in only 26 per cent of cases it is derived from the father, the non-disjunction therefore more usually being paternal (Race and Sanger, 1969). An example of the type of family which gives information is one where an XO child is found to be Xg[a], and she has an Xg mother and an Xg[a] father. The antigen could not therefore have come from the mother—and nor could the X, so both must have come from the Xg[a] father, and in this case the non-disjunction has occurred in the mother.

The same method can also be used to find out the origin of the non-disjunction in the parents of cases with Klinefelter's syndrome (see below). Here the non-disjunction has taken place in the father in about 40 per cent of cases.

Turner's syndrome

The characteristic picture is of a girl of very short stature, lacking secondary sexual characteristics and having primary amenorrhoea. There is an increased, i.e. more female-like (not directly related to the missing X-chromosome) carrying angle to the forearm, and webbing of the neck is frequently present. Where this last is found the incidence of associated malformations (congenital heart disease, renal anomalies and intellectual subnormality) is higher than where it is absent. The diagnosis of ovarian maldevelopment is usually indirect and based on the lack of secondary sex characters, the excess (after puberty) of pituitary gonadotrophins and the results of nuclear sexing. Though ovarian follicles are usually absent they occasionally occur, and some patients with the syndrome have been known to menstruate. There is even one record of a chromatin-negative XO Turner female producing a normal offspring (Bahner et al., 1960).

On skin sexing most patients with Turner's syndrome are chromatin negative and most have 45 chromosomes (particularly those with webbing of the neck) and the missing one is an X. However, about one-fifth of patients are chromatin positive and the explanation for this may be that they are (a) mosaics, e.g. XO/XX, (b) possessors of a normal X and an isochromosome of the long arm of the X (see p. 356), or (c) carriers of a normal X and part of the second one ("fragmented X"). The review by Jacobs (1969) should be consulted for a full account of abnormalities of the sex chromosomes, and that of German (1970) for Turner's syndrome in particular.

The shortness of stature and the other somatic abnormalities frequently associated with an XO sex chromosome complement are not present in females who have a normal X and an isochromosome of the short arm of the X; they are present, however, when the isochromosome is formed of the two long arms. It appears, therefore, that the genes influencing the development of stature, and of the other somatic characters frequently abnormal in XO females, are situated on the short arm of the X chromosome, and that for normal development of these characters in the female the short arms of two X chromosomes should be present. It would seem that genes present on the long *and* short arms of *both* X chromosomes are necessary for the development of a functioning ovary, and that masculinizing genes are situated on the short arm of the Y chromosome and close to the centromere (Jacobs, 1969).

Though nothing basic can be altered, it is important to recognize Turner's syndrome, since after the age of 12 oestrogens can be administered to bring about spurious menstruation, helpful for psychological reasons. Furthermore, a definite diagnosis also enables a prognosis of permanent infertility to be given with almost complete certainty.

In practice the clinical features are sometimes bizarre, and there is no hard and fast correspondence between them and the chromosomal complement. Patients with only minor abnormalities may be found and sometimes both male and female sexual characteristics are present. So-called "male Turner" cases occur, their features being webbing of the neck, stunting and abnormal testicular development. Such individuals may have the normal XY constitution, but XX/XY has been reported (the patient in this case being tall). From the point of view of memorizing the basic situation in Turner's syndrome it is probably better to forget about male cases, but to remember that in practice very unusual combinations can occur and for discussion of these the reader is referred to Miller (1961), Hamerton (1962) and Ford (1969) and for a reappraisal of the genetic situation to the review of German (1970).

Klinefelter's syndrome

These patients look and behave like males and it is highly probable that many of them go through life without ever consulting a physician—particularly when there is no National Service—since it is the gynaecomastia which often attracts attention in the Services. The facies is smooth, the voice often more highly pitched than normal and the general habitus eunuchoid. Some patients are married and consummation can be legally effected. Though there is a liability to mental defect many patients have normal intelligence· The outstanding clinical feature is the presence of small testes and this is generally detected only after puberty when the normal enlargement fails to occur. Investigations show that spermatogenesis is always absent but erections can be obtained and ejaculations occur, the fluid being derived from the prostate (a very small organ in this condition) and accessory glands. There is a high urinary excretion of gonadotrophins and a low one of 17-ketosteroids.

Chromosomally the majority of patients are XXY (and therefore chromatin positive) and, as would be expected, have a low incidence of colour blindness, comparable to that found in normal women. Some cases are mosaics, e.g. XY/XXY, but those which have been described do not appear to be less affected than those in whom all the cells are XXY. Some chromatin positive Klinefelter cases are XX (probably due to genetic interchange between the X and the Y) and for a discussion on this point the reader is referred to Ferguson-Smith (1966). A few patients, for unknown reasons, are chromatin negative and have the normal complement of 46 chromosomes with an XY sex pair.

Chromatin-positive patients with multiple Barr bodies sometimes occur. These may be the result of non-disjunction occurring not only at the reduction division of meiosis but at the "second meiotic division" which follows it. Fertilization may then give rise to individuals who are XXXY and XXXXY and the clinical features of both these include mental deficiency, webbing of the neck and small testes. The details of non-disjunction occurring at the first and second meiotic division are complicated and the reader is referred to Hamerton (1962).

Theoretically, if non-disjunction took place with equal frequency in male and female parents, if the zygotes were all equally viable and if there were no other cause for the two syndromes, one would expect equal numbers of Turner and Klinefelter cases. However, XO, partly on account of congenital heart disease, is less viable than XXY, and in fact there are many fewer Turner patients. Moore (1959) found none (at any rate those who were XO) in 1804 newborn babies who were apparently female, whereas Court-Brown and Smith (1969) report an incidence of chromatin-positive males of 1·7 per 1000 in a population survey of more than 41,000 consecutive live male births. A clinician obtains quite a different idea, since the amenorrhoea of the Turner cases always brings the patient to a doctor, whereas the disabilities of the Klinefelter very often do not.

Turner and Klinefelter patients can legitimately be included under the term "congenital abnormalities", using the U.S.A. definition of such an abnormality as one which is capable of being recognized at birth. Under the English definition they could not be so included, since they are not generally recognizable macroscopically but only by nuclear sexing.

The XYY syndrome

In 1961, Sandberg and his colleagues discovered the first male with an XYY chromosome complement. By 1965, 12 such males had been described and in that year Jacobs and her colleagues showed, from their study of men in the maximum security hospital at Carstairs in Scotland, that there were more men there with a 47/XYY complement than could reasonably be attributed to chance. These men showed no consistent physical abnormality and in none was there evidence of impaired sexual development (Price *et al.*,

1966). The heights of these males were on average about 15 cm greater than those of 46/XY males from the same hospital. Subsequently, Casey and his colleagues (1966) examined the tall men at the English maximum security hospitals of Rampton, Moss Side and Broadmoor, and confirmed the findings of Jacobs *et al.* (1965) that there must be unusual numbers of these men in the maximum security hospitals with a 47/XYY complement. Finally, Price and Whatmore (1967a, b) examining in detail the records and family backgrounds of the 47/XYY males from Carstairs, adduced evidence which strongly supported the idea that the behavioural disturbances of these men were primarily determined by their abnormal genotype—but not all XYY men are tall or criminal. Court-Brown (1968) reviews this very interesting and important subject in detail (see also Court-Brown, 1967).

The "Triple-X" female (XXX)

A few of these patients have been described, and the surprising thing is that they show very little physical abnormality and are sometimes fertile. It may be that as only one X chromosome per cell needs to be working (see Lyon hypothesis, p. 369) an extra non-working X does not much interfere with normal function. The first two cases reported had both menstruated, the first irregularly and the second quite normally. Although the second was mentally abnormal it is uncertain how far this was associated with her chromosome defect since she was ascertained during routine screening for nuclear sex in an institution. The nuclear sex findings are of interest. In the buccal mucosa a higher proportion of chromatin-positive cells is found than in normal women or in chromatin-positive males with Klinefelter's syndrome and, as would be expected, a high proportion of the triple-X females have two sex chromatin masses. The chromosome number is 47 and the sex formula is that of XXX. Two patients studied by Barr have had offspring, some of them girls (see Polani, 1962). These children appear normal and in those who have had their nuclear sex investigated there has been no discrepancy between this and the phenotype, though it would be expected that fertile triple-X females would produce some chromosomally abnormal offspring, on an average half their sons being XXY and half their daughters XXX. Whether this will be so is so far unknown. The frequency of the triple-X condition, as judged from surveys of patients in institutions for the mentally defective, would appear to be slightly less than, but of the same order as, that of the chromatin-positive Klinefelter's syndrome (Fraser *et al.*, 1961).

REFERENCES

BAHNER, F., SCHWARZ, G., HARNDEN, D. G., JACOBS, P. A., HEINZ, H. A. & WALTER, K. (1960). A fertile female with XO chromosome constitution. *Lancet*, **2**, 100.

CASEY, M. D., SEGALL, L. J., STREET, D. R. K. & BLANK, C. E. (1966). Sex chromosome abnormalities in two state hospitals for patients requiring special security. *Nature, (Lond.),* **209**, 641–642.

COURT-BROWN, W. M. (1967). *Human Population Genetics.* Amsterdam: North Holland.

COURT-BROWN, W. M. (1968). Males with an XYY sex chromosome complement. *J. med. Genet.,* **5**, 341–359.

COURT-BROWN, W. M. & SMITH, P. G. (1969). Human population genetics. *Brit. med. Bull.,* **25**, No. 1, 74.

FERGUSON-SMITH, M. A. (1966). X-Y chromosome interchange in the aetiology of true hermaphroditism and of XX Klinefelter's syndrome. *Lancet,* **2**, 475.

FORD, C. E. (1969). Mosaics and chimaeras. *Brit. med. Bull.* **25**, No. 1, 104.

FRASER, JEAN H., BOYD, E., LENNOX, B. & DENNISON, W. M. A. (1961). A case of Klinefelter's syndrome. *Lancet,* **2**, 1064.

GERMAN J. (1970). A unifying concept in relation to the gonadal dysgeneses. *Clin. Genetics,* Vol. 1, No. 1, pp. 15-27.

HAMERTON, J. L. (1962). *Chromosomes in Medicine.* London: Heinemann.

JACOBS, P. A. (1969). Structural abnormalities of the sex chromosomes. *Brit. med. Bull.,* **25**, No. 1, 94.

JACOBS, P. A., BRINTON, M., MELVILLE, M. M., BRITTAIN, R. P. & McCLEMONT, W. F. (1965). Aggressive behaviour, mental subnormality and the XYY male. *Nature (Lond.),* **208**, 1351.

MANN, J. D., CAHAN, A., GELB, A. G., FISHER, N., HAMPER, J., TIPPETT, P., SANGER, R. & RACE, R. R. (1962). A sex-linked blood group. *Lancet,* **1**, 8.

MILLER, O. J. (1961). Developmental sex abnormalities. In *Recent Advances in Human Genetics.* ed. L. S. Penrose. London: Churchill.

MOORE, K. L. (1959). Sex reversal in newborn babies. *Lancet,* **1**, 217.

POLANI, P. E. (1962). Sex chromosome anomalies in Man. In *Chromosomes in Medicine.* ed. J. L. Hamerton. London: Heinemann, p. 102.

PRICE, W. H., STRONG, J. A., WHATMORE, P. B. & McCLEMONT, W. F. (1966). Criminal patients with XYY chromosome complement. *Lancet,* **1**, 565.

PRICE, W. H. & WHATMORE, P. B. (1967a). Behaviour disorders and pattern of crime among XYY males identified at a maximum security hospital. *Brit. med. J.* **1**, 533.

PRICE, W. H. & WHATMORE, P. B. (1967b). Criminal behaviour and the XYY male. *Nature (Lond.),* **213**, 815.

RACE, R. R. & SANGER, R. (1969). Xg and sex chromosome abnormalities. *Brit. med. Bull.,* **25**, No. 1, 99.

SANDBERG, A. A., KOEPF, G. F., ISHIHARA, T. & HANSAHKA, T. S. (1961). An XYY human male. *Lancet,* **2**, 488.

THE LYON HYPOTHESIS

It will be remembered that mosaicism was frequently referred to in the last section, and that its definition is set out in the glossary of terms. In the examples given, the individuals mentioned have always been abnormal, but in the Lyon hypothesis it is suggested that *all* women are mosaics with regard to their two X chromosomes. This is an important concept and well worth serious consideration.

Though all female somatic cells look chromosomally similar under the microscope, Lyon (1961) postulates that at about the twelfth day after fertilization one of the X chromosomes in every cell of the female foetus becomes inactive. *Which* of the two Xs becomes inactive is decided at random for every cell, but once it is decided, all the descendants of that cell follow the same pattern. The result is that about half the somatic cells of the female will have an inactive maternal X chromosome and the paternal one will be "working" whereas the opposite will be the case in the remaining 50 per cent. In men the single X will always be working in all the cells. Lyon showed that this did in fact seem to be the case in mice, as female animals which were carrying a dominant gene for coat colour on their maternal X and a recessive allele on their paternal one did show patchiness of coat colour—just what would be expected if sometimes the dominant gene was in action and sometimes the recessive one. The tortoiseshell cat is also elegantly explained, since such animals (which are almost invariably female) are heterozygous for an X-linked gene controlling coat colour, and in some cell lines the X carrying one gene is inactivated and in some that carrying the other. This fits in with the fact that some of the rarely occurring tortoiseshell *males* have been found to have an abnormal XXY chromosome complement.

It will be remembered (see p. 356) that in man the X chromosome forming the Barr body is recognizable because it stains deeply (the DNA being tightly coiled) and it is thought to be the non-working X, this meaning that it is genetically inactive though it can and does replicate. The tight coiling may prevent the production and release of messenger RNA which transmits the chemical instructions from the genes. Labelling with tritiated thymidine shows that it is the Barr body X which synthesizes DNA later than the working one (see Fig. 11.9).

The Lyon hypothesis explains why too much or too little chromatin does not greatly upset the mental or physical development of individuals where an X chromosome is concerned, whereas trisomy or monosomy for any of the autosomes is highly damaging. The hypothesis also explains why women are in many ways so little different from men—if both their X chromosomes were active they would have twice as many X-linked genes as males, which they do not. This can actually be tested when a dosage effect is present, for example in glucose-6-phosphate dehydrogenase production where it is found that normal women do not make twice as much as do normal men. Furthermore, where this enzyme is deficient the hypothesis is also supported, since women known from family studies to be heterozygous for G-6-PD deficiency can be shown to have two races of red cells, one producing the enzyme and the other not, according to whether the normal or the abnormal X was the "working" one in the nucleated precursor. Moreover, G-6-PD production has been observed to be variable in heterozygous women, and this would be explained if the two lines of cell were not always present in precisely a 50 : 50 ratio (Beutler *et al.*, 1962).

Not all the evidence, however, supports Mary Lyon, and one difficulty concerns the new X-linked Xg blood group system. Women who are heterozygous Xg^a/Xg, having received Xg^a from one parent and Xg from the other, ought on the Lyon hypothesis to have two races of red blood cells, one possessing the Xg^a antigen and the other not. Reed and his colleagues (1963) have shown, however, that this is not so—they have the antigen on *all* their red cells. The explanation for this may well be that the non-working X is not inactive over the whole of its length (see Russell, 1963).

Another interesting argument against the hypothesis is based on the study of isochromosomes. Some patients, as has been seen above (p. 365) possess an isochromosome of the long arm of the X together with a normal chromosome, and show the clinical features of Turner's syndrome though they are not XO. The point is that here the two XXs can be morphologically distinguished and the Lyon hypothesis therefore rigorously tested. If roughly half the cells had a deeply staining isochromosome and the other half a deeply staining normal chromosome, the theory would be powerfully upheld. In fact, the Barr body is always found to be the isochromosome (Muldal *et al.*, 1963). This objection, strong as it is, has been countered by Gartler and Sparkes (1963). They point out that in the embryo about half the normal X chromosomes will be inactive. These, when paired with the isochromosome of the long arm of the X, will be effectively homozygous for the deficiency of the short arm, and this combination will probably be lethal. If this were so, all the cells containing an inactive X would be eliminated, leaving only those containing an inactive isochromosome (and in which the normal X was working) and this is why the inactive iso-X would form the Barr body in all the cells. This explanation does not, however, satisfy everyone, and the matter is still very much disputed (Lyon, 1963; Rhode and Berman, 1963). Grüneberg (1967) presents other arguments against the hypothesis, but it is in essence generally accepted.

Further information of a general nature on the Lyon hypothesis can be found in three leading articles, in the *Lancet* (1963) the *British Medical Journal* (1963) and the *Lancet* (1970).

REFERENCES

BEUTLER, E., YEH, M. & FAIRBANKS, V. F. (1962). The normal human female as a mosaic of X chromosome activity: studies using the gene for G-6-PD deficiency as a marker. *Proc. Nat. Acad. Sci.*, **48**, 9.

Brit. med. J., **2**, 1215 (1963). The Lyon hypothesis.

GARTLER, S. M. & SPARKES, R. S. (1963). The Lyon Beutler hypothesis and isochromosome X patients with the Turner syndrome. *Lancet*, **2**, 411.

GRÜNEBERG, H. (1967). Sex-linked genes in Man and the Lyon hypothesis. *Ann. hum. Genet.*, **30**, 239.

Lancet, **2**, 759 (1963). Lyonisation of the X-chromosome.

Lancet, **2**, 29 (1970). Is Lyonisation total in Man?

LYON, MARY, F. (1961). Gene action in the X-chromosome of the mouse (*Mus musculus L.*). *Nature*, **190**, 372.

LYON, MARY F. (1963). Lyonisation of the X-chromosome. *Lancet*, **2**, 1120.

MULDAL, S., GILBERT, C. W., LAJTHA, L. G., LINDSTEN, J., ROWLEY, J. & FRACCARO, M. (1963). Tritiated thymidine incorporation in an isochromosome for the long arm of the X chromosome in Man. *Lancet*, **1**, 861.

REED, T. E., SIMPSON, N. E. & CHOWN, B. (1963). The Lyon hypothesis. *Lancet*, **2**, 467.

RHODE, R. A. & BERMAN, N. (1963). The Lyon hypothesis and further malformation postulates in the chromosome syndromes. *Lancet*, **2**, 1169.

RUSSELL, LIANE B. (1963). Evidence from six X-chromosome translocations bearing on the single active X hypothesis. Paper read at XI Internat. Cong. Genet., The Hague.

NON-DISJUNCTION IN THE AUTOSOMES

Clinical features and mechanism of production of the various syndromes

21 Trisomy, i.e. mongolism or Down's syndrome

This is by far the commonest congenital abnormality caused by a chromosomal aberration and the usual ("regular") type is caused by non-disjunction in the small acrocentric chromosome pair No. 21 (Lejeune *et al.*, 1959; Jacobs *et al.*, 1959). These patients therefore have 47 chromosomes. (As will be explained later, the same clinical picture can be produced by a translocation also involving chromosome 21, but in both cases the patient is either actually or effectively trisomic for this chromosome.)

The following points are worth emphasizing:

(1) Most European populations have a mongol frequency of one in 636 to one in 776 at birth in maternity hospitals, and the relationship of the condition to maternal age, together with the risks of recurrence, is shown in Table 11.1.

TABLE 11.1

Relationship of maternal age to Trisomy 21

Maternal age	Risk of occurrence	Risk of recurrence
20–30	1 : 1500	1 : 500
30–35	1 : 750	1 : 250
35–40	1 : 600	1 : 200
40–45	1 : 300	1 : 100
45–up	1 : 60	1 : 20

Redding and Hirschhorn (1968), by courtesy of the authors and the editor of the *March of Dimes*.

The fact that the trait is often associated with increasing maternal age and that the mongol child resembles its mother in blood group more than would be expected by chance make it probable that the non-disjunction causing the condition usually takes place in the mother (Penrose, 1961).

(2) At birth and in the neonatal period the mongol child has a head which tends to be small and globular. The ears are set low on the scalp and are oval with small lobules. The eyes slant slightly upward and outward because of an epicanthal fold, which covers the medial angle of the palpebral fissure. The forehead is less receding than that of a normal baby, the bridge of the nose generally absent or poorly developed and the crest of the nose small. The mouth tends to hang open, and the tongue is usually enlarged, heavily fissured and protruding. Grey-white spots of depigmentation are seen in the iris (Brushfield's spots). The little fingers are short and curved, owing to a hypoplastic middle phalanx. The hands are broad and simian-like, *with a single transverse palmar crease*—this last feature being of great diagnostic value. The big toe is offset from its fellows. Congenital heart lesions are found in some cases. At birth the mongoloid child is of average size, but at later periods of life he is characteristically small. It is estimated that the average adult person with mongolism, of whom there are many, never exceeds the stature of a ten-year-old boy. The resemblance to the Oriental is at most superficial; in fact, the differences from normal are so striking that it is quite easy to recognize the condition in those of Oriental heritage (Harrison, 1962). Since mongolism can be recognized at birth, it is a congenital abnormality by the British definition.

Sometimes non-disjunction has occurred in chromosome 21 *and* in the sex chromosomes as well. Thus Ford and his colleagues (1959) described a patient who had the combined features of Klinefelter's syndrome *and* mongolism. The bone-marrow cells each contained 48 chromosomes, one of the extra ones being an X and the other the small additional chromosome 21.

Mongol mosaicism

The non-disjunction of which we have been writing is *meiotic* non-disjunction because it takes place at meiosis, with the result that all the cells are abnormal and this will give rise to a zygote having a uniformly abnormal number of chromosomes. Sometimes, however, non-disjunction occurs after the zygote has been formed and it is then mitotic and errors may occur at any of the divisions, so that two or more cell lines may be established. This is known as *chromosomal mosaicism*. The diagram (Fig 11.12) shows how two and three cell lines respectively are formed. Of particular interest to the clinician is mosaicism in mongolism, since not infrequently one sees individuals who, though perfectly normal mentally, have some of the other physical stigmata of the disorder—i.e. abnormal palm print patterns.

N

Clarke *et al.* (1961) report in detail such a case, who had a mongoloid facies and the characteristic palm print pattern, but the I.Q. at two years and three months was 100. She was found to be a 21-trisomic/normal mosaic.

Mosaicism may also explain the occurrence of more than one mongol in a family when this is not due to a translocation. It is then assumed that some of the gametes, either maternal or paternal, have 24 chromosomes, the extra one being a second chromosome 21.

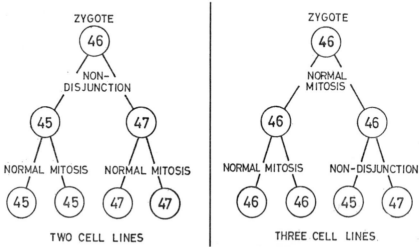

Fig. 11.12. The production of chromosome mosaics by mitotic non-disjunction after the formation of a normal zygote. (By courtesy of Dr D. G. Harnden and Messrs Heinemann.)

Dermatoglyphic patterns (the lines and ridges of the hands) have been particularly studied in mongol mosaics and the patterns found to deviate from the normal more than half-way in the direction of mongolism; the ridges are therefore regarded as a sensitive index of the presence of trisomic cells but the correlation between the proportion of these and the tendency of the patterns to resemble the mongol type is poor.

Since Penrose (1963) thinks that the data suggest that as many as 10 per cent of the mothers of mongols may be mosaics, it is important that the usefulness of dermatoglyphics should be more widely known. For a recent survey on this topic the reader should consult a paper by Holt (1964).

17–18 Trisomy

Non-disjunction for chromosome No. 17 (possibly any of the 16–18 group) leading to trisomy for one of these was first described by Edwards *et al.* (1960) and the clinical picture is now fairly well-defined. Affected infants have the following characteristics: mental retardation, a peculiar shaped skull (small mandible and prominent occiput), low-set and malformed ears, a receding chin and stubby tightly flexed fingers, with the index commonly overlapping the medius. The feet are of rocker-bottom type. Ventricular septal defect is often present. Gottlieb *et al.* (1962) report three cases of the syndrome and review the literature, and Rosenfield *et al.* (1962) compare the syndrome with that of the 13–15 trisomy. In one of their 17–18 trisomy cases "medial" arteriosclerosis was present and the authors conjecture that genes on chromosomes 17–18 may be connected with the integrity of the internal elastic lamina.

13—15 Trisomy

This syndrome was first described by Patau *et al.* (1960). Again the infants are mentally backward and have multiple abnormalities, with much in common with the preceding syndrome. However, eye defects such as colobomata or anophthalmia are found much more often, and there are neurological features such as fits and hypotonia. Cleft palate and harelip are described and sometimes capillary haemangiomata are present. The fingers are flexed but the medius overlaps the index (cf. 17–18 trisomy). Congenital heart disease is characteristic. It is of interest that mental deficiency is a feature of mongolism, trisomy 17 and trisomy 13–15 and it is likely that any major increase in chromatin causes this and that it is not specific for trisomy of any particular chromosome. (See Polani (1969) for further discussion of 17–18 and 13–15 trisomy.)

REFERENCES

CLARKE, C. M., EDWARDS, J. H. & SMALLPEICE, V. (1961). 21-trisomy/normal mosaicism. *Lancet*, **1**, 1028.

EDWARDS, J. H., HARNDEN, D. G., CAMERON, A. H., CROSSE, V. M. & WOLFF, O. N. (1960). A new trisomic syndrome. *Lancet*, **1**, 787.

FORD, C. E., JONES, K. W., MILLER, O. H., MITTWOCH, U., PENROSE, L. S., RIDLER, M. & SHAPIRO, A. (1959). The chromosomes in a patient showing both mongolism and the Klinefelter syndrome. *Lancet*, **1**, 709–710.

GOTTLIEB, M. I., HIRSCHHORN, K., COOPER, H. I., LUSSKIN, N., MOLLOSHOK, R. E. & HODES, H. L. (1962). Trisomy-17 syndrome. *Amer. J. Med.*, **33**, 763–773.

HARNDEN, D. G. (1962). *Chromosomes in Medicine*. ed. Hamerton. London: Heinemann.

HARRISON, T. R. (1962). *Principles of Internal Medicine*, 4th edit. New York: McGraw-Hill.

HOLT, SARAH B. (1964). Finger-print patterns in mongolism. *Ann. Hum. Genet. Lond.*, **27**, 279–282.

JACOBS, P. A., BAIKIE, A. G., COURT-BROWN, W. M. & STRONG, J. A. (1959). The somatic chromosomes in mongolism. *Lancet*, **1**, 710.

LEJEUNE, J., GAUTHIER, M. & TURPIN, R. (1959). Les chromosomes humains en culture de tissus. *C.R. Acad. Sci. (Paris)*, **248**, 602.

PATAU, K., SMITH, D. W., THERMAN, E., INHORN, S. L. & WAGNER, H. P. (1960). Multiple congenital anomaly caused by an extra autosome. *Lancet*, **1**, 790.

PENROSE, L. S. (1961). Mongolism. *Brit. med. Bull.*, **17**, 184.

PENROSE, L. S. (1963). Dermatoglyphs in mosaic mongolism and allied conditions. Paper read at XI Internat. Cong. Genet., The Hague.

POLANI, P. E. (1969). Autosomal imbalance and its syndromes, excluding Down's. *Brit. med. Bull.*, **25**, No. 1, 81.

REDDING, A. & HIRSCHHORN, K. (1968). Guide to human chromosome defects. Birth Defects, Original Article series. *March of Dimes*, vol. IV, No. 4, pp. 1–16.

ROSENFIELD, R. L., BREIBART, S., ISAACS, H., KLAVIT, H. D. & MELLMANN, W. J. (1962). Trisomy of chromosomes 13–15 and 17–18: its association with infantile arteriosclerosis. *Amer. J. med. Sci.*, **244**, 763.

TRANSLOCATION IN THE AUTOSOMES

15—21 translocation as a cause of mongolism

Although the majority of cases of mongolism are due to non-disjunction, occasionally no additional chromosome is present but simply extra chromatin resulting from an exchange of parts from one chromosome to another non-homologous one—that is a translocation. Carter *et al.* (1960) were the first to recognize this cause of mongolism.

It is now clear that wherever there is a family history of mongolism in relatives, or where a young mother has already given birth to a mongol and is likely to have more children, the maternal and paternal chromosomes should be examined. Figure 11.13 shows diagrammatically the various types of gamete that a translocation carrier can make. Some are more likely to be formed than others because the presence of the translocated chromosome upsets normal pairing at meiosis; and like centromeres repel one another and will not usually pass into the same gamete (see Fig. 11.13, *f* and *g*).

It must be emphasized that Figure 11.13 demonstrates gametes and that they will be joined in the zygote by normal gametes from the normal parent. Those gametes therefore which contain the translocated chromosome *and* a chromosome 15 or a chromosome 21, or both (Fig. 11.13, *c, f* or *g*) will, when the normal parent's chromosome 15 and 21 are added to them at fertilization, give rise to an individual with too much chromatin; further-more, those individuals who are effectively trisomic for chromosome 21 will be mongols. The offspring arising from a gamete containing the trans-located chromosome only (Fig. 11.13, *b*) will have almost exactly the normal amount of chromatin and will therefore be normal, though a carrier. An individual arising from the normal gamete (Fig. 11.13, *d*), and paired with a normal one from the other parent, will be normal and have normal offspring. The combination with (*e*), (*h*) and (*i*) would be lethal.

It is therefore very helpful, in assessing the probability of relatives of mongols giving birth to mongols, to know whether the condition is caused by a translocation or by non-disjunction in a parent. In the case of the

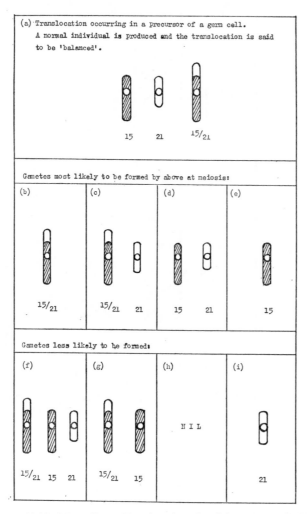

FIG. 11.13. Mongolism. Translocation involving 15 and 21. N.B. From (b) to (c) are gametes which will be joined at fertilization by a normal 15 and a normal 21 chromosome from the other parent.

translocation one parent (probably the mother) will be a carrier, and about one in four of her subsequent children are likely to be mongols, as are about one in four of the children of any member of a family who is carrying the translocation.

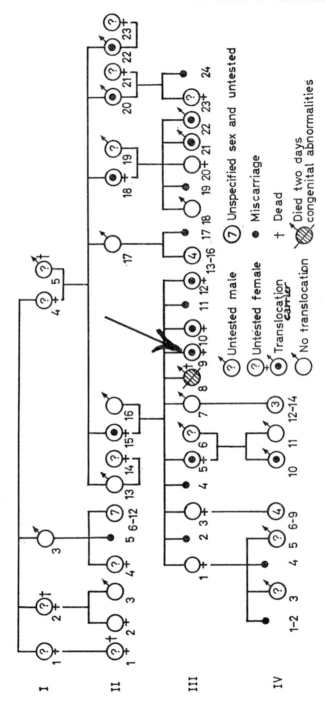

Fig. 11.14. Pedigree 1. Showing inheritance of a 13–15 translocation. The proposita is indicated by an arrow.
N.B. The point about the pedigree is that in it there are a large number of individuals who are carriers of the translocation but none who are definitely trisomic—though III, 8 may have been. The inheritance of the translocation is seen through three generations (see page 379). (By courtesy of Drs S. Walker and R. Harris and the Editor of *Annals of Human Genetics*.)

Translocation in the 13–15 group

Here, in precisely the same way that a portion of chromosome 21 can be translocated on to 15, so a piece of chromosome 13 can be translocated on to 15. One would expect—and indeed it has been found—that when this occurs both translocation carriers and trisomics result, the latter having the features shown on p. 375. A Liverpool family pedigree in which we have been particularly interested (Walker and Harris, 1962) consisted of individuals in which a 13–15 translocation had occurred, but in which there were no known trisomics. The translocation carriers have, of course, 45 chromosomes instead of 46 (as in the mongol translocation carriers) and they are normal (or such abnormalities as are present are not considered to be due to the translocation) and this is because the total chromatin is almost normal. It will be seen from Fig. 11.14 that the ratio of translocation carriers to non-carriers is about 1 : 1 but there is not, as in the mongol families, one trisomic in four children. The reason for the difference between the two types of translocation may be that there is increased lethality in the 13–15 abnormality because here the trisomic would receive a considerable quantity of extra chromatin, chromosomes 13 and 15 being bigger than 21.

For a full account of autosomal imbalance and its syndromes (excluding Down's) see Polani (1969).

REFERENCES

CARTER, C. O., HAMERTON, J. L., POLANI, P. E., GUNALP, A. & WELLER, S. D. V. (1960). Chromosome translocation as a cause of familial mongolism. *Lancet*, **2**, 678.

POLANI, P. E. (1969). Autosomal imbalance and its syndromes excluding Down's. *Brit. med. Bull.*, **29**, No. 1, 81.

WALKER, S. & HARRIS, R. (1962). Familial transmission of a translocation between two chromosomes of the 13–15 group. *Ann. Hum. Genet.*, *(Lond.)*, **26**, 151.

Deletion

The cri du chat syndrome

This abnormality was discovered by Lejeune and his colleagues (1963), who found that it was caused by a deletion of the short arm of chromosome 5. The main characteristic of the syndrome is the curious mewing cry, which is due to weakness and under-development in the upper part of the larynx; cardiovascular anomalies are frequent, but other abnormalities like coloboma of the iris or cleft lip and palate have been rarely observed (see also p. 385).

REFERENCE

LEJEUNE, J., LAFOURCADE, J., BERGER, R., VIALETTE, J., SERINGE, P. & TURPIN, R. (1963). Trois cas de délétion partielle du bras court d'un chromosome 5. *CR. Acad. Sci. Paris*, **257**, 3098.

CHROMOSOMES AND ABORTIONS

Spontaneous abortions contain a high proportion of gross chromosomal abnormalities, and a survey of 548 cases showed that 132 had abnormal karyotypes, i.e. about 24 per cent. The incidence, however, depends on the age of the foetuses, ranging from about 65 per cent in first trimester cases to approximately 10 per cent in those which were studied later. In contrast to this the karyotypes of (legally) induced abortuses, i.e. not spontaneous ones, show an incidence of around 2 per cent only. A large proportion of spontaneously aborted foetuses cannot be successfully cultured and karyotyped, mainly because much of the material is necrotic having been dead *in utero* for some length of time, but indirect evidence suggests that both successful and failed cultures have the same frequency of chromosomally abnormal abortuses.

Table 11.2 indicates the distribution of chromosome abnormalities in 120 karyotypes from spontaneous abortions, of which 50 are from the large series of Carr (1967).

TABLE 11.2

Distribution of chromosome abnormalities in spontaneous abortions

	Abnormality	No. of abortuses	Total	Percentage
Monosomy	XO	24		
	Double Monosomy (XO + autosome)	2	26	21·7
Trisomy	A (1–3)	5		
	B (4–5)	2		
	C (6–12)	7		
	D (13–15)	9		
	E (16–18)	21	64	53·3
	F (19–20)	2		
	G (21–22)	15		
	Double trisomy	3		
Triploidy*	XXY	15		
	XXX	6	23	19·2
	XYY	2		
Tetraploidy:		3	3	2·5
Mosaicism and others		4	4	3·3
		120	120	

* That is 3 sets of autosomes and 3 sex chromosomes.

The very high incidence of autosomal trisomy (53·3 per cent) represents about 13 per cent of all recognized spontaneous abortions and probably about 1·3 per cent of all conceptions. This contrasts markedly with the estimated frequency of 0·2 per cent for autosomal trisomy in live births and indicates that such trisomy usually ends in abortion. On the other hand trisomy of the sex chromosomes (XXX, XXY, XYY), well known in the general population, has not as yet been seen in abortuses. The only autosomal trisomic conditions which are known to be at all compatible with life are those for members of the D, E and G groups but it is of interest that a high proportion of the trisomy E cases were apparently trisomic for No. 16 chromosome, this never having been found in a live birth. Equally of interest is the high incidence of triploidy, for again triploid embryos almost invariably fail to reach full term (except as mosaics) even though the gross anomalies appear to be less than those associated with trisomy. One triploid embryo from Liverpool is known to have reached 38 weeks' gestation and died only during parturition.

Monosomy (mainly XO) also has a high incidence, but surprisingly few abortuses are recognized with autosomal deficiencies, probably because they are lethal at such an early age that they have not been investigated. The high frequency of XO abortions is somewhat unexpected since individuals with Turner's syndrome can lead a reasonably normal though sterile life. The data in fact suggest that the XO condition at conception may be as high as 0·7 per cent and that approximately 98 per cent of the resulting foetuses are aborted (Polani, 1966). Polani suggests that the reason for this heavy loss may be due to lethal factors in the mother interacting with the environment, since the zygote itself appears not to be grossly imbalanced.

The trisomic conditions, particularly Down's syndrome, are known to be closely associated with increasing maternal age. From existing data there is evidence that D and G trisomic abortuses also show this maternal-age effect while XO abortuses do not, this being similar to what is found in live births. Triploidy and trisomy E (16–18) abortuses also do not show any increase in frequency with maternal age.

None of the spontaneous abortuses in Table 11.2 were found to be chromosomally unbalanced due to a translocation. Such abnormalities are more likely to occur in families with a history of repeated abortions and with this in view Wilson (1969) studied 50 couples and eight abortuses. His criteria were a history of two or more spontaneous abortions and of fewer surviving children than abortions. Two of his mothers were found to be carrying balanced translocations (one a D/D and the other an A/G) and there were also four other possible small translocation carriers. None of the aborted foetuses, all of which happened to be from chromosomally normal parents, were found to have an abnormal karyotype.

Cytogenetic investigation of abortions is a field which has already produced valuable information, and there is no doubt that much is still to be gained by further studies, providing particular care is taken in the method of selection of the material (see Geneva Conference, 1966).

REFERENCES

CARR, D. H. (1967). Chromosome abnormalities as a cause of spontaneous abortion. *Amer. J. Obstet. Gynec.*, **97**, 283.

GENEVA CONFERENCE (1966). Standardisation of procedures for chromosome studies in abortion. *Bull. Wld. Hlth. Org.*, **34**, 765.

POLANI, P. E. (1966). Chromosome anomalies and abortions. *Develop. Med. Child Neurol.*, **8**, 67.

WALKER, S. (1969). *Selected Topics in Medical Genetics.* ed. C. A. Clarke. Oxford University Press, p. 234.

WILSON, J. A. (1969). A prospective, cytogenetic study of recurrent abortion. *J. med. Genet.*, **6**, No. 1, 5.

CHROMOSOMES AND LEUKAEMIA

The Ph_1 chromosome and chronic myeloid leukaemia

The Philadelphia (Ph_1) chromosome (Nowell and Hungerford, 1960) is the typical karyotype abnormality found in the majority of cases of chronic granulocytic leukaemia, and results from the partial deletion of the long arms of one of the G group of chromosomes (probably 21) (see Fig. 11.4). It can be found in the marrow cells and in peripheral blood cultures when immature granulocytes are present, but during haematological remissions, following chemotherapy or radiotherapy, the Ph_1 cell line disappears from the blood though it persists in the marrow. It has been detected only in the immature granulocytes, erythroblasts, and megakaryocytes suggesting a possible common stem cell origin for these, since other tissues do not show the abnormality.

Of special interest are the cases of diagnosed chronic granulocytic leukaemia whose myeloid cells do *not* show the Ph_1 chromosome (Ph_1 negative). In childhood, under 15 years of age, the disease appears in two forms, a juvenile and an "adult" type, and the presence or absence of the Ph_1 chromosome provides the most certain method of distinguishing them, though they also differ in their haematological and clinical features. The juvenile form is Ph_1 negative, with thrombocytopenia usually present and the total white cell count not as high (rarely over 100,000/mm) as in the "adult" form which is Ph_1 positive. Another striking difference is the increased level of Hb F (from 15 to 55 per cent) in the juvenile form, whereas no such increase was noted in a Ph_1 positive case only eight months old. The juvenile type has a poorer response to chemotherapy than the "adult" form, the mean survival time after diagnosis being much reduced.

It is uncertain whether the Ph$_1$ finding is a sequel to the disease or precedes it, but studies on two pairs of identical twins, one with chronic granulocytic leukaemia and Ph$_1$ positive and the other normal and lacking the Ph$_1$ chromosome, suggest that it may be acquired rather than inherited. On the other hand it has also been demonstrated in the blood and marrow of two patients before clinical symptoms developed.

Chromosomes and acute leukaemia

(a) *General*. There is good correlation between the cytogenetic data and the state of remission or relapse. Thus aneuploidy was demonstrable in one series from samples of marrow in untreated acute leukaemia and in relapse, whereas in remission the normal diploid mode was restored. This contrasts markedly with chronic granulocytic leukaemia, where the aberrant Ph$_1$ chromosome remains persistent in the marrow throughout relapse and remission phases, and it is probable that the numerous chromosomal changes discovered in acute leukaemia are secondary effects.

(b) *In mongolism* (*Down's syndrome*). Mongols are known to be particularly liable to develop acute leukaemia, the incidence being about 15 times as high as in the general population. This liability may be related to the primitive lobulation known to be present in their polymorphonuclear leucocytes and this in turn to the trisomic condition of chromosome 21. An abnormality in the opposite direction makes the matter puzzling, for in acute myeloblastic leukaemia cell lines have been observed which are monosomic for chromosome 21. Miller (1966) also suggests an increased risk with Klinefelter's syndrome and other congenital aneuploid anomalies, but the evidence is still slight.

(c) *In other diseases*. There is an apparent increase in the incidence of leukaemia in patients with Fanconi's aplastic anaemia. This is characterized by pancytopenia appearing during the first few years of life and by congenital abnormalities of the hands and kidneys. The leukaemia increase may be related to the high frequency of chromatid aberrations observed in cultured lymphocytes, though these are not so readily seen in marrow cells. Similar chromosome damage has been reported in Bloom's syndrome (characterized by dwarfism and light sensitivity) inherited as an autosomal recessive.

Irradiation and leukaemia

As is well known, there is an increased risk of leukaemia in the Hiroshima and Nagasaki survivors, in patients after radiotherapy for ankylosing spondylitis, and after radio-active phosphorus therapy for polycythaemia vera. Of particular interest, because of the possibility of future developments, is the report by Goh (1966) in which three apparently normal patients previously exposed to whole body radiation showed an abnormally small chromosome, indistinguishable from a Ph$_1$, in both marrow and peripheral blood cells.

Drugs and leukaemia

Benzene is leukaemogenic and, correspondingly, chromosome aberrations have been described in persons previously exposed to the drug. Recent investigations on users of lysergic acid diethylamine (LSD) suggest that this drug may have severe cytogenetic effects, causing chromosome damage not only in the users themselves but also in children born to mothers who took LSD while pregnant.

REFERENCES

GOH, L. (1966). Smaller G chromosome in irradiated Man. *Lancet*, **1**, 659.

MILLER, R. W. (1966). Relation between cancer and congenital defects in Man. *New Engl. J. Med.*, **275**, 87.

NOWELL, P. C. & HUNGERFORD, D. A. (1960). A minute chromosome in human granulocytic leukaemia. *Science*, **132**, 1497.

WALKER, S. (1969). Chromosomes and Leukaemia. In *Selected Topics in Medical Genetics*. ed. C. A. Clarke. Oxford University Press, p. 239.

The complete references for chromosomes in abortions and chromosomes and leukaemia will be found in the sections written on these subjects by Dr S. Walker in *Selected Topics in Medical Genetics* (Oxford University Press, 1969, ed. C. A. Clarke) from which much of the present account is drawn.

THE MAPPING OF CHROMOSOMES

Genes, or the loci controlling them, situated on the same chromosome are said to be linked, and except when crossing-over occurs they are inherited together. The first autosomal linkages discovered in man were: the genes controlling the secretor character and the Lutheran blood group system (Mohr, 1951); the nail-patella syndrome and the ABO blood groups (Renwick and Lawler, 1955); elliptocytosis and the Rh blood group system (Lawler and Sandler, 1954); and pulverulent cataract and the Duffy blood group system (Renwick and Lawler, 1963). For an up-to-date list and assessment of the closeness of the linkages see Renwick (1969).

In none of these cases do we know *which* chromosome is involved. If, however, we find an abnormality to be associated with a particular autosome as in mongolism, then the possibility of mapping arises. For example, if a trisomic mongol were found to be of blood group AB and to have one group AB and one group O parent, we should know that the ABO blood group locus was situated on chromosome 21 (Renwick, 1961).

Suggested localization of the gene controlling cystic fibrosis of the pancreas on the short arm of chromosome 5

This has never been established, but the method of investigation is ingenious, and a good example of the application of logic to a genetic situation with which a physician might be confronted.

Cystic fibrosis of the pancreas is controlled by an autosomal recessive gene. The *cri du chat* syndrome, characterized by mental deficiency and a curious mewing cry due to weakness and under-development of the upper part of the larynx, is caused by a deletion of the short arm of chromosome 5. (Lejeune *et al.*, 1963).

A baby with fibrocystic disease of the pancreas was found to have the *cri du chat* syndrome (Smith *et al.*, 1968) and these authors investigated the child's parents, by means of the Spock test, for heterozygosity for fibrocystic disease of the pancreas (Spock *et al.*, 1967). Spock and his colleagues found that a euglobulin serum fraction causes a disorganized rhythm of cilial movement in rabbit respiratory tract explants both in patients with fibrocystic disease and in their parents (obligatory heterozygotes). Since the disease is a recessive, both parents should have been heterozygous, but they found that (according to the test results) only the mother was a carrier, the father being normal. They inferred that because of the deletion the child had not received the normal allele from her father, and therefore that the gene controlling fibrocystic disease might be on the missing short arm of chromosome 5. The hypothesis rests entirely on the reliability of the Spock test for heterozygosity for fibrocystic disease, and more recent work throws considerable doubt on the theory. It remains, however, a useful example of one way to tackle a genetic problem.

Linkage studies by means of hybrid cell culture

This is quite a new approach, the procedure being to mix animal cells from two different species and to grow them in culture. When this is done, a few hybrid cells are formed. Weiss and Green (1967) cultivated together a normal human diploid cell strain and a mouse cell line deficient in thymidine kinase. Hybrid cell lines were formed, and these were isolated in a medium containing hypoxanthine, aminopterin and thymidine (HAT). The hybrid cell lines contained almost all the mouse chromosomes but a very much reduced number of the human ones. The human gene for thymidine kinase permits the hybrid cell line to survive in this HAT medium, in which the mouse cell line alone would have been killed. An attempt was made to correlate thymidine kinase activity with the presence of a specific human chromosome, and it was found that though many human chromosomes were lost, all the cell lines which were able to survive in the HAT medium possessed at least one human chromosome of the 6-12 and X group.

When certain chromosomes are lost, and the markers are also lost, is one justified in assigning these markers to the lost chromosomes? The authors tested this by adding to the culture 5-chromodeoxyuridine (BUdR), a substance to which thymidine kinase deficient cells are resistant but which kills those containing the gene. Human chromosomes of the 6-12-X group

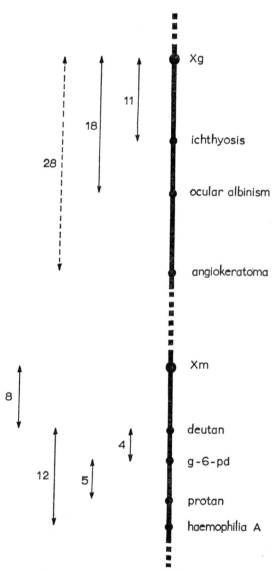

FIG. 11.15. Tentative map of the human X chromosome with the best guess at present of the location of the Xm locus in relation to previously known loci. Distances are in map units. (Berg (1967)).

were rare in the former group but more frequent in the latter. Gene mutation at the kinase locus was ruled out and the authors suggest that a chromosome of the 6-12-X group in man contains the thymidine kinase gene.

Sex linkage

In sex linkage the situation is different. Numerous genes, e.g. those controlling the Xg blood group system, glucose-6-phosphate dehydrogenase production, colour blindness, haemophilia, the Duchenne type of muscular dystrophy, agammaglobulinaemia and the Xm serum protein are sex-linked —that is, they are known to be situated on the X chromosome. By studying pedigrees in which two of the characters segregate (the Xg blood group system is often used as one), it is possible to infer from the frequency of crossing-over how closely the various genes are linked on the X chromosome. Figure 11.15 shows that there are two clusters of genes on the X which have been reliably mapped in relation to one another, but there is an unmapped section of unknown length between them. Search is continuously being made for an X-linked character which is at a measurable distance from *both* clusters and can therefore bridge this gap. New genes (not referred to here) are constantly being located but all have so far belonged to one of the two clusters.

REFERENCES

BERG, K. (1967). Practical possibilities of mapping the X chromosome as given by available markers. *Bull. Europ. Soc. Hum. Genet.*, **1**, 46.

LAWLER, SYLVIA D. & SANDLER, M. (1954). Data on linkage in Man: elliptocytosis and blood groups. IV—Families 5, 6 and 7. *Ann. Eugen.*, **18**, 328.

LEJEUNE, J., LAFOURCADE, J., BENGER, R., VIALETTE, J., SERINGE, P. & TURPIN, R. (1963). Trois cas de délétion partielle du bras court d'un chromosome 5. *C.R. Acad. Sci., Paris*, **257**, 3098.

MELLMAN, W. J., OSKI, F. A., TEDESCO, T. A., MACIERA-COELHO, A. & HARRIS, H. (1964). Leucocyte enzymes in Down's syndrome. *Lancet*, **2**, 674.

MOHR, J. (1951). *A Study of Linkage in Man*. Copenhagen: Munksgaard.

RENWICK, J. H. (1961). Elucidation of gene order. In *Recent Advances in Human Genetics*. ed. L. S. Penrose. London: Churchill.

RENWICK, J. H. (1969). Progress in mapping human autosomes. *Brit. med. Bull.*, **25**, No. 1, 65.

RENWICK, J. H. & LAWLER, SYLVIA D. (1955). Genetical linkage between the ABO blood groups and nail-patella loci. *Ann. Eugen.*, **19**, 312.

RENWICK, J. H. & LAWLER, SYLVIA D. (1963). Probable linkage between a congenital cataract locus and the Duffy blood group locus. *Ann. hum. Genet.*, **27**, 67.

SMITH, D. W., DOCTER, J. M., FERRIER, P. E., FRAIS, J. L. & SPOCK, A. (1968). Possible localisation of the gene for cystic fibrosis of the pancreas to the short arm of chromosome 5. *Lancet*, **2**, 309.

388 PROGRESS IN CLINICAL MEDICINE

SPOCK, A., HEICK, H. M. C., CRESS, H. & LOGAN, W. S. (1967). *Paediat. Res.*, **1**, 173.

WEISS, M. C. & GREEN, H. (1967). Human-mouse hybrid cell lines containing partial complements of human chromosomes and functioning human genes. *Proc. U.S. Nat. Sci.*, **58**, 1104.

GENETIC COUNSELLING

With the spread of medical knowledge there is an increasing desire among the public to read the future, and the commonest request is for information about risks to subsequent children when one has already been born with an abnormality. Alternatively, parents knowing of a skeleton in the family cupboard, may ask about the chances of its turning up in their grandchildren—though not infrequently what they really want is medical backing against a union they dislike on other grounds. Least common of all, individuals about to get married may seek advice about risks to offspring, but couples who do this are often obsessional—most young people who have decided to get married pay no attention to what a doctor says, and in general this is probably a healthy type of reaction.

Advice on genetic matters should always be given in terms of probability never certainty, and in these days of football pools patients readily understand odds. A helpful yardstick is that about one pregnancy in 30 will produce either a marked congenital malformation or a serious developmental abnormality which appears early in life (Fraser Roberts, 1970).

Fairly precise information can only be given in the minority of cases, i.e. those which show clear-cut Mendelian inheritance, and this may necessitate the study of many pedigrees. When it is found, the risks to subsequent offspring are too high to be acceptable to most people. Some examples follow:

(1) In the translocation causing mongolism there is about a one in four chance that a child of a carrier will be a mongol (see p. 376).

(2) In a disorder controlled by an autosomal dominant gene (e.g. most cases of facio-scapulo-humeral dystrophy or Huntington's chorea) the chance of any given offspring having the disease if one parent be affected is one in two, and the risk is similar for subsequent siblings.

(3) If a child is born with a recessive trait (e.g. albinism or phenylketonuria) the risk of subsequent offspring being affected is one in four. Phenylketonuria, however, requires further comment. With treatment, affected girls may survive, marry (in most cases) normal men and produce children who, though heterozygous, would all be expected to be phenotypically normal. However, it has been shown that phenylalanine from the affected mother (who often relaxes the strictness of her diet in pregnancy) can cross the placental barrier and render *all* the children mentally defective

Lancet, 1964). This is a loose example of what is known as a phenocopy, (see glossary). For information on genetic heterogeneity and the response to treatment in phenylketonuria the reader is referred to Clayton (1971).

(4) If the disease is due to a sex-linked recessive gene on the non-pairing part of the X chromosome (e.g. most forms of haemophilia and the Duchenne type of dystrophy), then an affected male married to a normal woman will have all carrier daughters but all his sons will be unaffected. Of the daughters of a carrier female half will be normal and half carriers, and of her sons half will be affected and half normal. This is well known, but in a disease such as haemophilia, if there is no family history, it is very important not to give the rather bad prognosis for relatives until one has considered the possibility of a mutation. If this has occurred in the patient then none of his sisters would be carriers. It may be very difficult to decide the point but enquiries about the disease in maternal uncles and great-uncles is important.

In many common conditions it often appears from the family history that there is a genetic component to the illness but that this is not transmitted in any clear-cut way. This may be because (1) the disorder is controlled by many genes (multifactorial inheritance), (2) the environment is also partly responsible and (3) there is heterogeneity with differing aetiologies in the various sub-groups of the disease.

In such situations the risks are empirical, the definition of this term being "the probability of occurrence of a specified event based upon prior experience and observation rather than on prediction by a general theory" (Herndon 1962).

Table 11.3 gives the empirical risk figures for some common conditions which are not inherited in any simple manner.

Detection of carriers

Another important aspect of counselling is the detection of carriers in genetic conditions. As far as the autosomes are concerned there are only two (thalassaemia and fibrocystic disease) which are of importance, since most recessive diseases are extremely rare. In thalassaemia (frequency as high as 5 to 15 per cent in some parts of Italy and in Thailand) the saline osmotic fragility of the red blood cells is invariably reduced in the heterozygotes, and this is the best screening test for detecting carriers (Weatherall, 1965). In cystic fibrosis of the pancreas (frequency about one in 2000 live births) skin fibroblast cultures show cytoplasmic metachromasia not only in the affected children but also in their parents who are obligatory heterozygotes (Danes and Bearn, 1968).

The detection of the carrier state is of much more importance in the commoner X-linked conditions (for example in counselling the sister of a man with haemophilia), and in general the assessments are made by biochemical methods. Table 11.4 lists some of the diseases for which tests are

TABLE 11.3

Empiric Risks for Some Common Disorders (in per cent)

Condition	Normal parents having an affected child	Normal parents having a second affected child	Affected parent having an affected child
Congenital hip dislocation	0·07 (1M : 6F)	5	5
Pyloric stenosis	0·3 (5M : 1F)	4	6
Hare lip with or without cleft palate	0·1 (2M : 1F)	4	4
Cleft palate only	0·04	2	7
Epilepsy	0·5	10	5
Clubfoot	0·1 (2M : 1F)	5	7
Anencephaly	0·2 (1M : 3F)		
Spina bifida	0·3 ≃	5	—
Hydrocephalus	0·2		—
Schizophrenia	1·0	14	16
Mental retardation (non-specific types)	1·0	15	35

Emery (1968). By courtesy of the author and Messrs E. & S. Livingstone

TABLE 11.4

Trait	Test	Percent detectable
Hemophilia A (classical)	plasma factor VIII	85
Hemophilia B (Christmas disease)	plasma factor IX	90
Gargoylism (Hunter's syndrome)	granules in skin fibroblasts	100 (possibly)
Vit. D resistant rickets (Hypophosphatemia)	serum phosphorus	100 (probably)
G6PD deficiency	erythrocyte G6PD	75
Muscular dystrophy (severe, Duchenne type)	serum creatine kinase	70
Muscular dystrophy (mild Becker type)	serum creatine kinase	50
Diabetes insipidus (nephrogenic)	urine concentration	80

Emery (1968). By courtesy of the author and Messrs E. & S. Livingstone available and the approximate proportions of detectable heterozygotes are given.

There is much more to counselling than what has been written here, and readers are referred to Emery (1968). As he says, "Medical genetics seems likely to become the preventive medicine of the future".

REFERENCES

CLAYTON, BARBARA E. (1971). Annotation, Phenylketonuria. *J. med. Gerat.*, **8**, 37.

DANES, B. S. & BEARN, A. G. (1968). A genetic cell marker in cystic fibrosis of the pancreas. *Lancet*, **1**, 1061.

EMERY, A. E. H. (1968). *Elements of Medical Genetics*. Edinburgh and London: Livingstone.

FRASER ROBERTS, J. A. (1970). *An Introduction to Medical Genetics*, 5th ed. Oxford University Press.

HERNDON, C. N. (1962). Empiric risks. In *Methodology in Human Genetics*. ed. Burdette. San Francisco: Holden-Day, pp. 144–155.

Lancet, **1**, 598 (1964). Maternal phenylketonuria.

WEATHERALL, D. J. (1965). *The Thalassaemia Syndromes*. Oxford: Blackwell Scientific Publications.

12 Organ Transplantation

R. Y. CALNE

IMMUNOLOGICAL FACTORS. EXPERIMENTAL RENAL TRANS-
PLANTS. RENAL TRANSPLANTATION BETWEEN IDENTICAL
TWINS. HETEROLOGOUS AND HOMOLOGOUS RENAL TRANS-
PLANTATION IN MAN. TRANSPLANTS FROM PRIMATES. SELEC-
TION AND MANAGEMENT OF PATIENTS FOR TRANSPLANTA-
TION. ORGAN STORAGE. COMPLICATIONS OF RENAL TRANS-
PLANTATION. TRANSPLANTATION OF THE HEART, LIVER AND
LUNGS. ETHICAL CONSIDERATIONS. THE PRESENT POSITION.

ORGAN transplantation is a serious therapeutic effort to restore to normal life people dying of fatal disease of an organ which could not otherwise be treated. The clinical efforts are backed by sound experimental work. The medical objectives are no different in principle from those of traditional surgical practice. The extraordinary publicity that followed clinical heart transplantations rather obscured these simple observations. The only new factor of principle in organ transplantation is where organs are taken from cadavers, since to be of value the organ must be cooled and removed shortly after death. I would maintain, however, that even in this highly emotive aspect of organ transplantation it is possible for the procedure to be conducted without in any way interfering with traditional medical ethics.

It is in the field of renal transplantation that the clinical need is most evident. In England and Wales approximately 7000 people die every year from chronic bilateral kidney disease, and approximately half of these are between the ages of five and 55 and would therefore be potential beneficiaries from renal transplants.

The biological factors that apply to any tissue transplanted from one individual to another will be considered in the first section, followed by a summary of the results of renal transplantation throughout the world and a discussion of the selection of patients and their management for renal transplantation. There then follows a short section on transplantation of the heart, liver and lungs and finally some observations on the ethics of transplantation.

It has been known for many years that free grafts of skin could be used from one part of an individual's body to another and would "take" successfully provided the grafts were undamaged and thin enough to achieve revascularization. It has also been shown that skin grafts can be transplanted from one identical twin to another and will also take satisfactorily. However, skin grafts from one member of any species to another unrelated member of the same species have been universally unsuccessful. The mechanism of the rejection of the transplanted tissue was clarified by the work of Medawar and his colleagues in the 1940s (Medawar, 1944, 1945). Their work showed the process to be immunological in nature.

IMMUNOLOGICAL FACTORS

In the case of homologous skin grafts the initial behaviour is the same as with an autograft. However, from the fifth or sixth day onward changes occur which lead to the progressive destruction of the graft. Salient features of these changes are mononuclear cellular infiltration of the graft and eventual cessation of blood flow with resulting necrosis. Medawar (1944, 1945) clearly demonstrated that the character of the rejection process is immunological.

The term "immunological" requires an antigenic afferent stimulating factor, a recognition and reaction centre, and an effector mechanism.

Antigen

Most studies of transplantation antigen have been made by injecting various tissue extracts into animals and subsequently determining whether they have been specifically sensitized. Thus, accelerated breakdown of skin grafts would suggest that the tissue fraction contained transplant antigen. There is now much evidence in favour of the antigen being a glycoprotein present in cell membrane. However, the precise chemical nature of transplant antigen is unknown.

Recognition and reacting centre

Mitchison has shown that lymph-node cells have the property of recognizing grafted tissue as foreign and reacting against it (Mitchison, 1953; Mitchison and Dube, 1955). It is probable that lymphoid cells in other parts of the reticulo-endothelial system also possess this property. Work by Gowans and his colleagues (1962) has shown that for a given antigenic stimulus a small proportion of small lymphocytes become activated and give rise by differentiation to a population of pyronin-postive cells. These in turn produce a further series of small lymphocytes, which may well be specifically active against the graft.

Effector mechanism

There is now much evidence that both humoral antibodies and cellular immune mechanisms may destroy a graft. It is likely that cellular immune mechanisms predominate in first-set graft destruction, whilst circulating antibodies can play an important part in the destruction of second-set grafts in sensitized hosts. It seems that in certain situations both these elements of the effector system might work synergistically in destroying transplanted tissue. Circulating antibody can however also protect a graft from destruction. This interesting phenomenon, called "enhancement", is not well understood. It can most easily be demonstrated with transplanted tumours.

Immunological tolerance

To survive in an environment where exposure to virulent micro-organisms is commonplace the possession of a lymphoid system that can recognize and react specifically against exogenous material is an obvious advantage. There must be a safeguarding mechanism to prevent reaction against the organism's own body constituents, but there is no apparent biological reason why the recognition system should be selective in its reaction against exogenous material, attending to the destruction of harmful bacterial antigens yet accepting homografts. Thus the ability to accept homografts has never been of survival advantage in evolutionary selection.

In 1945 Owen observed that most dizygotic cattle twins are red blood cell chimeras, each twin having both its own and its partner's red blood cell antigens. Such twins are synchorial and therefore exchange foetal blood.

Anderson *et al.* (1951) attempted to distinguish monozygotic from dizygotic cattle twins by skin grafting. They had no success, for they found that dizygotic cattle twins accepted skin from their respective partners. This finding led to a series of experiments which revealed a new approach to problems of tissue transplantation and amply fulfilled the prophecies of Burnet and Fenner (1949), who suggested that in embryonic life the reticulo-endothelial system must learn to distinguish "self" from "non-self" constituents and that native factors would have a protective "self marker". If the embryo is presented with foreign material before it has developed the ability to make the distinction it will accept this material as if it were its own and will not subsequently be able to react against it. The naturally produced tolerance to dizygotic twin tissue is highly specific and applies only to the twin in question, the ability to react against homografts from siblings other than the twin partner being retained.

Experimental production of immunological tolerance fully confirmed this interpretation of the phenomenon in dizygotic calf twins. Billingham *et al.* (1954) produced lasting and specific immunological tolerance in mice by injecting embryos of one highly inbred strain with living cells of another inbred strain and subsequently challenging the injected animals after birth with skin grafts from the original donor strain. This homologous tissue often survived permanently. If the initial injection of tissue was delayed until the day of birth, tolerance could still be produced (Billingham and Brent, 1957), but injection between 24 and 72 hours after birth, the so-called "neutral" period, produced no effect. After this period injection merely produced immunity with an aggravated second set rejection. An initial injection of spleen or kidney cells produced tolerance to skin, indicating a tolerance to the organisms in question with no evidence of tissue specificity. Tolerance was sometimes only partial, the second challenging grafts being rejected after a delay.

Felton (1949) showed that very large doses of pneumococcal polysaccharide prevented adult mice from acting against pneumococci. This "immunological paralysis" was specific for the antigen in question. It was long-lasting and directly related to the antigenic dose. Work by Dresser (1960) suggest that this phenomenon may be related to immunological tolerance. Certainly increasing doses of antigen can postpone the "neutral" period in neonatal mice.

It was found that porcine liver allografts may survive considerable periods without rejection (Peacock and Terblanche, 1967; Calne et al., 1967). In marked contrast to the liver, skin, kidney and heart allografts are usually rapidly rejected by the pig. Orthotopic liver allografts will protect donor specific skin and kidney grafts from rejection while previously sensitized pigs can reject liver allografts aggressively (Calne et al., 1969). Further experiments suggested that the mechanism of immunosuppression produced by liver allografts in the pig was in fact immunological tolerance which occurred in animals which were nevertheless immunologically mature. It was felt that the most likely explanation was that the liver graft in the pig releases histocompatibility antigens in a toleragenic form and that these antigens can induce partial immunological tolerance. The immunological effects of pig liver allografts are profound and non-toxic. Some animals achieved an eight-fold gain in weight and thrived. One sow became pregnant and delivered nine normal piglets (Fig. 12.1).

Reaction of graft against host

Dempster (1953) first suggested that a homograft containing immunologically competent cells might react against the recipient.

If adult lymphoid cells are injected into unrelated animals to produce immunological tolerance, or to repopulate the marrow of irradiated animals, the recipients in either case are unable to react against the injected cells, and the stage is set for a graft-versus-host reaction. This is probably the explanation of "runt" disease in tolerant mice (Billingham and Brent, 1959) and "homologous" or "secondary" disease in irradiated animals (Trentin, 1956). Mice with runt disease fail to thrive and are susceptible to infection. A similar disease can affect tolerant chickens; such animals often develop gross splenomegaly (Simonsen, 1957). A proportion of irradiated and marrow-grafted animals suffer from diarrhoea and wasting (Graber et al., 1958). There may also be a haemolytic process involved (Porter, 1960; Piomelli and Brooke, 1960).

The observation that foetal lymphoid tissue, which can presumably become tolerant to host antigens, does not produce these syndromes is evidence in favour of the above interpretation of these diseases (Barnes et al., 1958; Uphoff, 1958; Porter, 1959).

Any attempts to utilize immunological tolerance or irradiation and marrow grafting for clinical purposes would raise the theoretical possibility of a graft-versus-host reaction unless only immunologically incompetent or foetal cells were used as grafts.

Genetic factors

By various manipulations with inbred strains of mice, Gorer (1956) and Snell (1953) were able to clarify the inheritance of tissue transplantation or histocompatibility factors. These factors have independent actions so that permanent survival of a graft requires that the recipient possesses all the dominant genes of the donor.

The individual inbred strains are homozygous, but when individuals of different strains are used, the F_1 hybrids will be heterozygous; thus each F_1 individual will have an identical genetic make-up and will accept sibling grafts, and will also accept grafts from individuals of either parent strain. However, grafts in the other direction, from the F_1 hybrid to the parent strain, will be rejected.

In mice one important locus has been extensively studied. This H-2 locus may contain 12 alleles, and in the mouse there are probably another 14 loci where antigenic properties can be referred. It is of interest that the male mouse had an additional weak factor not present in the female. This presumably resides on the Y chromosome.

As a result of much work on this subject the rudiments of transplantation genetics in the mouse are known. It is presumed that similar mechanisms operate in other mammals, and there is evidence that this is the case in man. Although the histocompatibility factors and red blood cell groups are linked genetically in mice they do not appear to be so in other species.

The principles outlined are probably applicable to most tissue grafts. Notable exceptions are cornea, the anterior chamber of the eye, and cartilage, where the effector mechanism lacks access; grafts in the brain, from which it seems that antigen cannot reach the reacting centre; and non-living structural grafts such as arteries. The ovary and to a less extent other endocrine glands seem to be less antigenic than most other tissues, and may survive for long periods in homologous hosts. In the kidney typical rejection occurs.

REFERENCES

ANDERSON, D., BILLINGHAM, R. E., LAMPKIN, G. H. & MEDAWAR, P. B. (1951). The use of skin grafting to distinguish between monozygotic and dizygotic twins in cattle. *Heredity*, **5**, 379.

BARNES, D. W. H., ILBERY, P. L. T. & LOUTIT, J. F. (1958). Avoidance of secondary disease in radiation chimeras. *Nature, Lond.*, **181**, 488.

BILLINGHAM, R. E. & BRENT, L. (1957). A simple method for inducing tolerance of skin homografts in mice. *Transplant. Bull.*, **4**, 67.

BILLINGHAM, R. E. & BRENT, L. (1959). Quantitative studies on tissue transplantation immunity. IV. Induction of tolerance in newborn mice and studies on the phenomenon of Runt disease. *Phil. Trans.*, B, **242**, 439.

BILLINGHAM, R. E., BRENT, L., MEDAWAR, P. B. & SPARROW, E. H. (1954). Quantitative studies on tissue transplantation immunity. I. The survival times of skin homografts exchanged between members of different inbred strains of mice. *Proc. roy. Soc.*, B, **143**, 43.

BURNET, F. M. & FENNER, F. (1949). *The Production of Antibodies*. Melbourne: MacMillan.

CALNE, R. Y., WHITE, H. J. O., YOFFA, D. E., MAGINN, R. R., BINNS, R. M., SAMUEL, J. R. & MOLINA, V. P. (1967). Observations of orthoptic liver transplantation in the pig. *Brit. med. J.*, **2**, 478.

CALNE, R. Y., WHITE, H. J. O., BINNS, R. M., HERBERTSON, B. M., MILLARD, P. R., PENA, J. R., SALAMAN, J. R., SAMUEL, J. R. & DAVIS, D. R. (1969). Immunosuppressive effects of the orthoptically transplanted porcine liver. *Trans. Proc.*, **1**, 321.

DEMPSTER, W. J. (1953). Kidney homotransplantation. *Brit. J. Surg.*, **40**, 447.

DRESSER, D. W. (1960). A study of immunological mechanisms in mice. Ph.D. Thesis, University of Edinburgh.

FELTON, L. D. (1949). The significance of antigen in normal tissues. *J. Immunol.*, **61**, 107.

GORER, P. A. (1956). Some recent work on tumour immunity. *Advances in Cancer Research* (Academic Press), **4**, 149.

GRABER, P., COURCON, J., MERRILL, J. P., ILBERY, P. L. T. & LOUTIT, J. F. (1958). Immuno-electrophoretic study on the serum of mice irradiated by lethal doses of X-ray and protected by rat bone marrow. *Transplant. Bull.*, **5**, 58.

MEDAWAR, P. B. (1944). The behaviour and fate of skin autografts and skin homografts in rabbits. *J. Anat.*, **78**, 176.

MEDAWAR, P. B. (1945). A second study of the behaviour and fate of skin homografts in rabbits. *J. Anat.*, **79**, 157.

MITCHISON, N. A. (1953). Passive transfer of transplantation immunity. *Nature, Lond.*, **171**, 267.

MITCHISON, N. A. & DUBE, O. L. (1955). Studies on the immunological response to foreign tumour transplants in the mouse. II. The relation between haemagglutinating antibody and graft resistance in the normal mouse and mice pretreated with tissue preparation. *J. exp. Med.*, **102**, 179.

OWEN, R. D. (1945). Immunogenetic consequences of vascular anastomoses between bovine twins. *Science*, **102**, 400.

PIOMELLI, S. & BROOKE, M. S. (1960). Erythrocytes as a tool in studies on rabbit radiation chimeras and secondary disease. *Ann. N.Y. Acad. Sci.*, **87**, 472.

PORTER, K. A. (1960). Immune hemolysis: a feature of secondary disease and runt disease in the rabbit. *Ann. N.Y. Acad. Sci.*, **87**, 391.

PORTER, K. A. (1959). Use of foetal haemopoietic tissue to prevent late deaths in rabbit chimeras. *Brit. J. exp. Path.*, **40**, 273.

SIMONSEN, M. (1957). The impact on the developing embryo and newborn animal of adult homologous cells. *Acta path. microbiol., Scand.*, **40**, 480.

SNELL, G. D. (1953). *Physiopathology of Cancer*. New York: Hoeber.

TERBLANCHE, J., PEACOCK, J. H., HOBBS, K. E. F., HUNT, A. C., BOWES, J., TIERRIS, E. J., PALMER, D. B. & BLECHER, T. E. (1968). Orthoptic liver homotransplantation. An experimental study in the unmodified pig. *S. Afr. med. J.*, **42**, 486.

TRENTIN, J. J. (1956). Mortality and skin transplantability in X-irradiated mice receiving isologous, homologous or heterologous bone marrow. *Proc. Soc. exp. biol.*, **92**, 688.

UPHOFF, D. E. (1958). Preclusions of secondary phase of the radiation syndrome by inoculation of fetal hematopoetic tissue following lethal total body X-irradiation. *J. nat. Cancer Inst.*, **20**, 625.

EXPERIMENTAL RENAL TRANSPLANTS

There is now a large amount of literature on the fate of homologous kidney grafts in untreated dogs. The findings of Dempster (1953) and Simonsen *et al.* (1953) have been amply confirmed by other workers. In brief, canine renal transplants usually cease to function five to eight days after operation. Very occasionally a transplant functions for 14 days. From the third day after transplantation the renal cortex becomes progressively infiltrated with lymphoid cells, many of which take up pyronin stains and have the appearance of immature plasma cells (Fig. 12.2). The infiltration begins round small blood vessels and in the periglomerular interstitial tissues. *Pari passu* with the cellular infiltration, the kidney becomes enlarged and oedematous, and tubular function deteriorates. The endothelium of the blood vessels becomes reduplicated, renal blood flow is reduced, renal function is rapidly depressed and finally there is anuria.

A second kidney from the same donor to the same recipient will function for a shorter period than the first kidney, whilst a second kidney from a different donor usually behaves like a "first-set" kidney. The accelerated rejection of a "second-set" kidney may occur with little cellular infiltration, the main histological change being acute interstitial cortical haemorrhage (Fig. 12.3).

The above findings are consistent with the present picture of tissue transplantation in general.

The discrete mechanism of destruction of a "first-set" unmodified renal transplant in the dog has been studied by electron microscopy by Kountz *et al.* (1963), who considered that the initial damage in the kidney occurs in

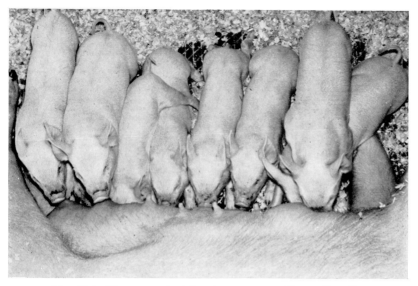

FIG. 12.1. Nine normal piglets born to sow 18 months after orthotopic liver allografting. No immunosuppressive treatment was given. (By courtesy of *Nature*.)

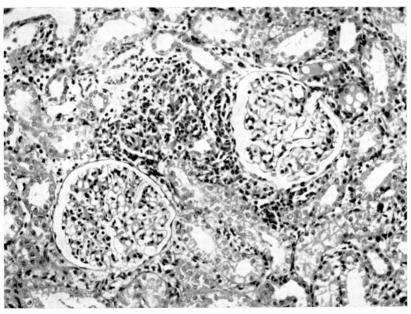

FIG. 12.2. Section of first-set homograft reaction showing interstitial infiltrate of lymphoid cells (Porter and Calne, 1960).

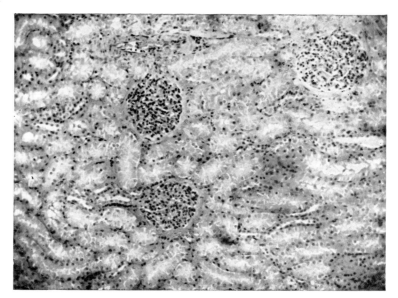

FIG. 12.3. Section of second-set renal transplant showing extensive interstitial haemorrhage in the cortex.

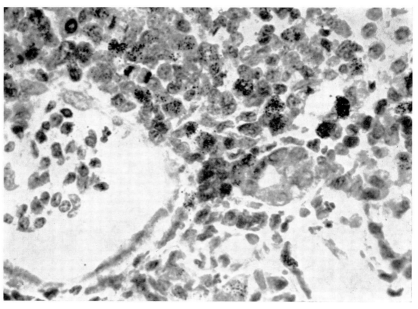

FIG. 12.4. Autoradiograph of a canine kidney 4 days after homo-transplantation. Half an hour previously 450 μc^3 H-thymidine had been infused into the renal artery of the homograft. An area in which many of the infiltrating cells are heavily labelled is shown. Two unlabelled cells in mitosis lie above the glomerulus in the upper left of the picture. Haematoxylin and eosin $\times 450$.

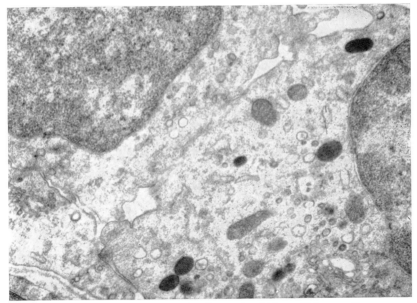

FIG. 12.5. Electromicrograph of a canine kidney 48 hours after homotransplantation. There is intimate association between an infiltrating "monocyte-like" host cell (on right of picture) and an endothelial cell lining one of the peritubular capillaries. At two points there is apparently breakdown of the membranes and fusion of the cytoplasm of the cells. × 32,000. (Porter *et al.*, 1964.)

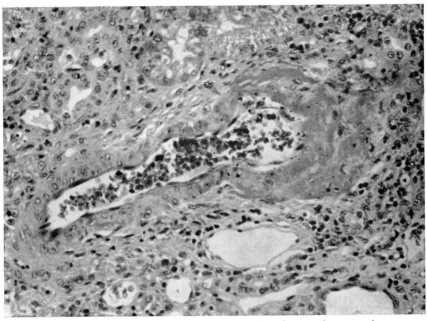

FIG. 12.6. Renal homotransplant at 24 days from a dog treated with 6-mercaptopurine. Part of the wall of an interlobular artery is affected by fibrinoid necrosis. There is some cellular infiltration in the surrounding interstitium. H. & E. × 160. (Porter *et al.*, 1964.)

the peritubular venules which disrupt, and that the renal damage is a result of the ischaemia produced by vascular disorganization. Porter *et al.* (1964) have studied the same phenomenon both with electron microscopical techniques and also by labelling recipient thoracic duct lymphocytes and the lymphoid cells from the spleen and the cells infiltrating renal transplants. The fate of these cells has been followed by autoradiography. Lymphoid cells from the spleen and thoracic duct enter the blood stream and infiltrate the cortex of transplants undergoing rejection. Following renal transplantation, lymphoid follicles both in the spleen and lymph nodes show marked hyperplasia with a predominance of pyronin-positive cells.

Lymphoid cells in rejecting transplants proliferate in the renal interstitium subdividing every 12 hours (Fig. 12.4 autoradiograph). The damage to the peritubular venules appears to follow actual contact of lymphoid cells with the endothelium wall (Fig 12.5), which is in agreement with findings of Kountz *et al.* (1963). Fibrinoid necrosis of arteries and arterioles is found as the terminal event in a small number of transplants during rejection (Fig. 12.6).

It is obvious from the above summary that there is little understanding of the discrete biochemical factors concerned in the rejection of transplanted tissue, and we have only a very indistinct conception of the gross morphological changes that occur in this process. With so little data available, the surgeon wishing to prevent rejection of transplanted organs is faced with a problem that cannot at present be solved in a deductive manner.

Ways of preventing rejection of homologous tissue

It has not been possible to prevent antigen release from the kidney or access to the kidney of antibody mechanisms. Two main categories of procedures have been investigated experimentally to prevent rejection of kidney transplants.

1. Attempts to produce specific immunosuppression using donor antigen:
    (*a*) Neonatal immunological tolerance
    (*b*) Immune paralysis with large doses of antigen
    (*c*) Enhancement with specific antibody.

2. Reduction of the lymphoid cell population or damage to the lymphoid cells:
    (*a*) Total body irradiation
    (*b*) Splenectomy
    (*c*) Thymectomy
    (*d*) Thoracic duct lymph drainage
    (*e*) Irradiation of the blood and kidney
    (*f*) Anti-lymphocyte serum
    (*g*) Antimetabolite and cytotoxic drugs
    (*h*) Corticosteroids.

It is obvious that the eventual goal of immunosuppression is to obtain a completely specific effect in relation to the kidney without any toxicity. There is evidence, to be discussed later, that the longer an organ transplant can be shielded from immune attack the greater is its likelihood of long-term survival, no matter what method is used to produce the initial immunosuppression. Eventually some specificity of control of the immune system appears to result from the presence of the transplant. Natural and experimental tolerance has been investigated in experimental kidney grafts (Simonsen, 1955; Calne, 1961; Puza and Gombos, 1958) and it has already been mentioned that liver allografts in the pig seem able to produce specific immunological tolerance and protection of renal allografts from the same donor source as the liver. Zimmerman, Stuart and Wilson (1965) produced prolonged survival of dogs treated with subcellular donor material. They felt that this was probably due to enhancement. A combination of cellular antigen and antibody treatment has resulted in specific immunological suppression of rejection of renal allografts in rats (Stuart *et al.*, 1968).

There is evidence that a phenomenon that may be interpreted in terms of enhancement occurs in long-tolerated transplants. Murray *et al.* (1964) have reported the results of some very interesting experiments in dogs with renal transplants treated with immunosuppressive agents.

1. A dog living more than nine months after a renal transplant rejected the second kidney from the same donor within 23 days while the first kidney thrived and continued to function.
2. Two well-tolerated canine renal homografts were transplanted back to the original donors at 269 and 554 days after homotransplantation. The kidneys continued to function and maintain life with no evidence of rejection.
3. Three long-surviving transplants were grafted into unrelated indifferent animals. They were promptly rejected, indicating retention of antigenicity.

Thus a recipient tolerating a renal homograft may not have complete central immune inhibition for all the antigens of the transplant, since a second kidney from the same source can be rejected. Therefore a change must have occurred in the first transplanted kidney, which does not involve an addition of new antigens because the kidney could be returned to the original donor without being rejected. It would seem likely that those antigens on the donor kidney which differed from the recipient's were specifically deleted, and this could well have been due to a blocking type of circulating antibody. It would be reasonable to describe this phenomenon as enhancement.

Several effective procedures probably act directly on the lymphoid tissue; first, *total body X-irradiation*. To prevent rejection of homologous tissue a very high dose of X-rays is necessary. In fact, in order to inhibit renal homograft rejection experimentally it is necessary to destroy the haematopoietic tissue in the bone marrow. Thus below 1000 r total body X-irradiation typical rejection occurs (Hume *et al.*, 1960), whilst above 1300 r rejection is inhibited, but only one dog has survived more than a few days. This animal, which received a marrow graft and a kidney from the same donor, died from pneumonia 49 days after renal transplantation (Mannick *et al.*, 1959).

Splenectomy and *thymectomy* have been disappointing procedures so far as their immunosuppressive effect is concerned in adult outbred animals receiving kidney grafts (Veith, Luck and Murray, 1963; Kountz and Cohn, 1962; Calne, 1963).

Thoracic duct lymph drainage

McGregor and Gowans (1963) showed that rats depleted of lymphocytes by chronic drainage from the thoracic duct were unable to produce normal antibody responses, and the rejection of skin grafts was delayed. In dogs with thoracic duct fistulae Samuelson, Fisher and Fisher (1963) found that homologous skin grafts survived twice as long as controls.

Selective irradiation

Kauffman *et al.* (1965) found that local irradiation of experimental renal transplants in dogs produced a modest increase in their functional survival. They felt that one possible explanation of the results was that the irradiation was destroying or damaging immunologically competent cells which had infiltrated the graft. Cronkite *et al.* (1962) showed that prolonged irradiation of extracorporeally shunted blood produced a marked lymphopenia. Wolf *et al.* (1966) studied yttrium implants suspended intra-arterially in dogs, and this produced modest prolongation of functional survival of kidney transplants.

Intra-lymphatic irradiation of the lymphoid system has been used as an immunosuppressive treatment. It certainly produces marked lymphopenia and destruction of lymph nodes, and in addition there is some prolongation of kidney graft survival (Wheeler, White and Calne, 1965).

Antilymphocyte serum

In 1899 Metchnikoff produced an antiserum in guinea-pigs against rabbit lymph-node cells, and in 1937 Chew and Lawrence injected guinea-pig lymph-node cells into rabbits and produced an antiserum which caused reduction in circulating lymphocytes in guinea-pigs. A similar antiserum was prepared by Cruikshank in 1941 in rabbits against rat lymph-node cells. Woodruff (1960) reported experiments performed in the early 1950s with rabbit-anti-rat lymphocyte serum which caused marked lowering of the numbers of circulating lymphocytes within two hours of injecting the serum.

However, this serum did not prolong survival of homografts of skin, ovary and adrenal, and despite daily injections of antiserum the lymphocyte count rose to the pre-treatment level by the tenth day. In 1963, Woodruff and Anderson succeeded in producing long-term survival of skin grafts in rats using rabbit-anti-rat anti-lymphocyte serum raised in the rabbits by injection of thoracic duct lymphocytes collected from the rats. They found that thoracic duct drainage prior to antiserum administration and grafting improved the long-term survival. Similar results were produced in mice by Gray, Monaco and Russell (1964). Jeejeebhoy (1965) thymectomized adult rats which were given rabbit-anti-rat lymphocyte serum. He found augmentation of immuno-suppression in relation to skin homografts. Similar results were found in mice by Monaco, Wood and Russell (1965). They felt that thymectomy performed prior to serum treatment inhibited recovery from immunological depression produced by the anti-lymphocyte serum.

Levy and Medawar (1966a) found that an anti-lymphocyte serum prepared in rabbits against murine thymocytes was very effective in prolonging skin graft survival, particularly when the serum was given after grafting. However, these workers did not observe any additional benefit from thymectomy (Levy and Medawar, 1966b). Application of anti-lymphocyte serum to prolongation of renal homograft survival in dogs has been studied by Abaza (1966) and Abaza et al. (1966). He produced anti-lymphocyte serum against canine thoracic duct lymphocytes injected into sheep and horses. That produced by the sheep was ineffective in prolonging renal homograft survival and reacted weakly in vitro. However, the horse-anti-dog lymphocyte serum appreciably prolonged renal homograft survival. It was administered one day before renal transplantation and continued daily for 60 days in a dose of 3 ml/kg body weight per day. The dose was then halved for a further 20 days. A single intravenous injection markedly depressed the circulating lymphocytes, but the daily administration produced only a moderate lympho-penia. There was lymphocyte depletion in the lymph nodes and spleen. The grafted kidneys functioned for more than 21 days in 87 per cent of the antiserum-treated dogs. Infection manifested as distemper, hepatitis, or pneumonia caused death in 50 per cent of the antiserum-treated dogs. The complications of the anti-lymphocyte serum besides the liability to infection were serum sickness and hepatotoxicity. In vitro the serum produced a com-plement-dependent cytotoxic effect on canine lymphocytes and lymphocyte agglutination which did not require complement.

The mode of action of anti-lymphocyte serum is not understood; it is unlikely that it is solely due to destruction of or damage to circulating and tissue lymphoid cells. The antiserum is absorbed with canine red cells before use to prevent haemolytic responses, but nevertheless the serum must contain a large number of antibodies against a variety of tissue components, and the serum itself is likely to be antigenic. However, it is of interest that Abaza

(1966) found that anti-lymphocyte serum was less antigenic than normal horse serum, and it is possible that the anti-lymphocyte serum inhibits allergic reactions against horse antigens. Levy and Medawar (1966a) observed that anti-lymphocyte serum inhibited the second-set response to skin grafts and it was very effective in prolonging skin graft survival between widely disparate strains of mice. This observation was in contrast to all other immunosuppressive measures. They discuss the possibility that the serum was coating lymphocytes and "blindfolding" them. However, further work by these authors (Levy and Medawar, 1966b) suggested that the anti-lymphocyte serum might be acting as a stimulant to lymphoid cells, rather like phytohaemagglutinin, committing them to activity which prevented them from participating in a normal manner in immune reactions. They suggested the term "sterile activation" for this process. Unlike other workers, Levy and Medawar observed hypertrophy of lymphoid tissue following treatment with anti-lymphocyte serum; large blast cells appeared in the lymphoid follicles. They point out that anti-lymphocyte serum is not producing immunological tolerance since tolerance, by definition, must be produced by a specific antigen, whereas anti-lymphocyte serum is entirely non-specific in its immunosuppressive action. The evidence to date would suggest that anti-lymphocyte serum is not yet an ideal immunosuppressive agent, disadvantages being liability to allergic reactions from the serum itself, possible nephrotoxicity and hepatotoxicity, and a non-specific impairment of resistance to infection. The main active fraction appears to lie in the gamma G protein (Iwasaki et al., 1967). There is at present difficulty in assaying and comparing anti-lymphocyte sera. In vitro agglutinating or cytotoxicity titres are not necessarily related to the immunosuppressive activity. There are conflicting opinions about how the most efficacious serum can be produced and also how it should be given, and how long treatment with anti-lympho-cyte serum must be continued after the grafting operation in order to maintain the immunosuppressive effect. There is also marked species difference, and the most potent serum so far produced is that of the rabbit against the mouse. It is not yet known which species will produce the best sera for therapeutic use in man. There is a great deal of work to be done before we will know the full potentialities of anti-lymphocyte serum. Further progress in the use of anti-lymphocyte serum is to be expected; in particular, more powerful and specific sera are likely to be produced, and it is probable that more purified components will be isolated.

The effect of anti-metabolite drugs on the survival of canine renal homo-transplants

Schwartz and Damashek (1959) found that 6-mercaptopurine given to rabbits at the same time as an homologous protein antigen (human serum albumin) rendered the animals specifically tolerant to further doses of the antigen, even after the drug had been stopped (Fig. 12.7). Treatment of recipient animals with 6-mercaptopurine was shown to prolong functional survival of canine renal transplants (Calne, 1960, 1961a; Zukoski *et al.*, 1961), and other thiopurines have recently been shown to be active, the most potent and consistent suppression of the rejection process being produced by a combination of Actinomycin C and imidazolyl thiopurine, azathioprine (Imuran—BW 57–322) (Calne, 1961b; Calne and Murray, 1961; Calne

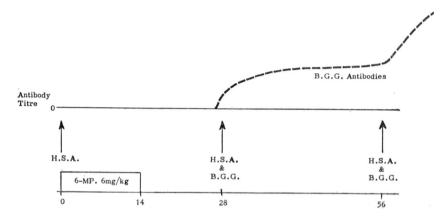

Specific Antigen + thiopurine in large doses during <u>inductive phase</u> of antibody synthesis
——▶ specific "tolerance" after drug stopped.

FIG. 12.7. Schematic diagram of the experiments reported by Schwartz and Dameshek (1959). Shows a specific drug induced immunological tolerance to the antigen, human serum albumin (H.S.A.) produced by 14 days' treatment with 6-mercaptopurine. Effect persisted after cessation of drug treatment. However, the rabbits were able to produce antibodies against antigen, bovine gammaglobulin (B.G.G.). (Calne, 1963.)

et al., 1962). The thiopurines alone or in combination with other agents studied all lack consistency of action in non-toxic doses; nevertheless, nine out of 104 bilaterally nephrectomized dogs with renal transplants survived more than three months with good renal function and three of these survived six months. It will be remembered that in untreated animals rejection usually occurs within four to eight days.

Although the thiopurines probably impair resistance to infection, both by their effects on immune competence and by depression of the bone marrow, some degree of specificity similar to that discussed in Schwartz's and Dameshek's experiments (1959) is probably determined by giving the drug during the inductive phase of the immune response to the antigen in question, namely the homologous kidney.

The effect of steroid drugs

Goodwin *et al.* (1963) reported marked amelioration of a homograft reaction in a patient with a renal transplant when large doses of prednisone were administered. Zukoski, Callaway and Rhea (1965) reported two very long-surviving bilateral nephrectomized dogs with renal transplants where immunosuppression had been achieved by administration of 30 mg prednisolone daily starting two days before operation. Both dogs were still alive at the time of the report, one at 1177 days and the other at 477 days. The first dog had been given prednisolone for 428 days and then no further medication. Marchioro *et al.* (1964) produced clear evidence of reversal of rejection by prednisolone in dogs with renal transplants treated with Azathioprine; seven of the eight animals had a favourable response shown by a falling blood urea nitrogen, increase in urine output and decrease in proteinuria. However, gastro-intestinal bleeding was a complication observed in six of the eight animals. Prednisolone was started soon after it became certain that the process of rejection had begun.

REFERENCES

ABAZA, H. M. (1966). The effect of antilymphocyte antiserum on the immune response to kidney homografts. Ph.D. thesis, University of Edinburgh.

ABAZA, H. M., NOLAN, B., WATT, J. G. & WOODRUFF, M. F. A. (1966). *Transplantation*, **4**, 618.

CALNE, R. Y. (1961). *Brit. J. Surg.*, **48**, 384.

CALNE, R. Y. (1963). *Nature (Lond.)*, **199**, 388.

CALNE, R. Y. (1960). *Lancet*, **1**, 417.

CALNE, R. Y. (1961a). *Brit. J. Surg.*, **48**, 384.

CALNE, R. Y. (1961b). *Transplant. Bull.*, **28**, 65.

CALNE, R. Y. & MURRAY, J. E. (1961). *Surg. Forum*, **12**, 118.

CALNE, R. Y., ALEXANDRE, G. P. J. & MURRAY, J. E. (1962).

CHEW, W. B. & LAWRENCE, J. S. (1937). *J. Immunol.*, **33**, 271.

CRONKITE, E. P., JANSEN, C. R., MATHER, G. C., NIELSEN, W. O., USENIK, E. A. & SNIPE, C. R. (1962). *Blood*, **20**, 203.

CRUIKSHANK, A. H. (1941). *Brit. exp. Path.*, **22**, 126.

GOODWIN, W. E., KAUFMAN, J. J., MIMS, M. M., TURNER, R. D., GLASSOCK, R., GOLDMAN, R. & MAXWELL, M. M. (1963). *J. Urol.*, **89**, 13.

GRAY, J. F., MONACO, A. P. & RUSSELL, P. S. (1964). *Surg. Forum*, **15**, 142.

IWASAKI, Y., PORTER, K. A., AMEND, J. R., MARCHIORO, T. L., ZUHLKE, V. & STARZL, T. E. (1967). *Surg. Gynec. Obstet.*, **124**, 1.

JEEJEEBHOY, H. F. (1965). *Immunology*, **9**, 417.

KAUFFMAN, H. M., CLEVELAND, R. J., DWYER, J. J., LEE, H. M. & HUME, D. M. (1965). *Surg. Gynec. Obstet.*, **120**, 49.

KOUNTZ, S. L. & COHN, R. (1962). *Surg. Forum*, **13**, 59.

LEVY, R. H. & MEDAWAR, P. B. (1966a). *Ann. N.Y. Acad. Sci.*, **129**, 164.

LEVY, R. H. & MEDAWAR, P. B. (1966b). *Proc. nat. Acad. Sci. (Wash.)*, **56**, 1130.

MCGREGOR, D. & GOWANS, J. L. (1963). *J. exp. Med.*, **117**, 303.

MARCHIORO, T. L., AXTELL, H. K., LQVIA, M. F., WADDELL, W. R. & STARXL, T. E. (1964). *Surgery*, **55**, 412.

METCHNIKOFF, E. (1899). *Ann. Inst. Pasteur*, **13**, 737.

MONACO, A. P., WOOD, M. L. & RUSSELL, P. S. (1965). *Science*, **149**, 432.

MURRAY, J. E., SHIEL, A. G. R., MOSELEY, R., KNIGHT, P., McGAVIE, J. D. & DAMMIN, G. J. (1964). *Ann. Surg.*, **160**, 449.

PUZA, A. & GOMBOS, A. (1958). *Transplant. Bull.*, **5**, 30.

SAMUELSON, J. S., FISHER, B. & FISHER, E. R. (1963). *Surg. Forum*, **14**, 192.

SCHWARTZ, R. & DAMASHEK, W. (1959). *Nature (Lond.)*, **183**, 1682.

SIMONSON, M. (1955). *Ann. N.Y. Acad. Sci.*, **59**, 488.

STUART, F. P., SAITOH, T. & FITCH, F. W. (1968). *Science*, **160**, 1463.

VIETH, E. J., LUCK, R. J. & MURRAY, J. E. (1963). *Surg. Gynec. Obstet.*, **121**, 299.

WHEELER, J. R., WHITE, W. F. & CALNE, R. Y. (1965). *Brit. med. J.*, **2**, 339.

WOLF, J. S., O'FOLGHLUDHA, F. T., KAUFFMAN, H. M. & HUME, D. M. (1966). *Surg. Gynec. Obstet.*, **122**, 262.

WOODRUFF, M. F. A. (1960). *The Transplantation of Tissues and Organs.* Springfield, Ill.: Charles C. Thomas.

WOODRUFF, M. F. A. & ANDERSON, N. F. (1963). *Nature*, **200**, 702.

ZIMMERMAN, C. E., STUART, F. O. & WILSON, R. E. (1965). *Surg. Forum*, **16**, 267.

ZUKOSKI, C. F., LEE, H. M. & HUME, D. M. (1961). *Surg. Gynec. Obstet.*, **112**, 707.

ZUKOSKI, C. F., GALLAWAY, J. M. & RHEA, W. G. (1965). *Transplantation*, **3**, 380.

RENAL TRANSPLANTATION BETWEEN IDENTICAL TWINS

The debt that man owes directly to animal experimentation is clearly shown in the identical twin cases of renal transplantation. More than one year after transplantation two dogs survived, with life-sustaining renal autotransplants, in the surgical laboratory of Harvard Medical School. Murray and his colleagues in Boston were so impressed with the excellent general condition and renal function of these animals that they decided to embark on a programme of renal transplantation between human identical twins. The problems they faced included those of surgical technique, as well as others concerned with the management of an extremely ill patient after a major operation, and the ethical problems raised by the removal of a normal kidney from a healthy donor (Merrill *et al.*, 1956).

The success of renal transplantation between identical twins has demonstrated that, with satisfactory technique, excellent results can be obtained in man (Murray *et al.*, 1958). Functional studies of the transplant in a bilaterally nephrectomized patient, compared with his unilaterally nephrectomized donor twin, showed very similar filtration, concentration, dilution, acidification and alkalinization, in spite of the period of ischaemia and complete denervation that the transplant had suffered (Bricker *et al.*, 1965).

Of the seven pairs of identical twins with renal transplants described in the study mentioned, two recipients have since died with transplants which had developed the same disease as that in the originally affected kidney. It has been suggested by Murray *et al.* (1958) that removal of the recipient's own diseased kidneys prior to transplantation might prevent this complication, but this has not been confirmed in practice. Glomerulonephritis developing

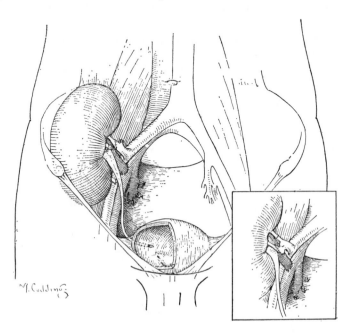

FIG. 12.8. Gross-topography of transplanted kidney. Renal vessels anastomosed to iliac vessels and ureter implanted into the bladder. (Murray *et al.*, 1958.)

in the transplant has been the main cause of failure in transplants between identical twins. A very satisfactory aspect of successful renal transplantation and bilateral nephrectomy has been the total disappearance of all the stigmata of malignant hypertension (Merrill, 1959). It is difficult to assess accurately numbers of patients in a given population who might benefit from renal transplantation. The numbers, however, are considerable. The Statistical Review of England and Wales for the year 1959 (Registrar-General, 1961) shows that between 6000 and 7000 patients die from renal disease each year out of a population of about 45 millions. Uraemia is therefore responsible for about 1 per cent of all deaths (for comparison, carcinoma of the stomach accounts for 2 per cent of deaths). These figures give no indications of the numbers suitable for operation. However, 40 per cent of deaths from nephritis and nephrosis in England and Wales occurred between the ages of five and 55 years.

Now, the incidence of twinning in the general population is approximately one out of 90 pregnancies and one pair out of three is identical (Gates, 1946). Since renal disease is not known to be more or less common in twins than in the population in general, there is slightly more than one chance in 300 that a patient with renal failure suitable for transplantation will have an identical twin. The figures above would suggest that perhaps 3000 patients a year in England and Wales would be potential beneficiaries from renal transplantation, and some ten of these would be one of identical twins. However, no renal transplants between identical twins have been reported in England and Wales to date. It would seem that either the statistics quoted are completely erroneous or that the possibility of renal transplantation between identical twins in England and Wales has not been considered. The 25 transplants between twins already mentioned would be expected to be derived from 7500 (25 × 300) cases of renal failure suitable for transplantation. The figures given above suggest that this would be the expected annual incidence in a population of 100 million persons. It would appear that a number of identical twins with terminal renal failure are dying without the offer of renal transplantation.

The principles of the surgery of renal transplantation have been fully established. They were first developed by Kuss *et al.* (1961) and are shown diagrammatically in Fig. 12.8. The main difficulty has been with urinary drainage. Most surgeons prefer to implant the ureter directly to the bladder but when the patients' own ureters are normal an alternative is to anastomose the pelvis of the transplant to the recipient's own ureter. Details of surgical technique will not be discussed further.

REFERENCES

Bricker, N. S., Guild, W. R., Reardon, J. B. & Merrill, J. P. (1965). Studies on the functional capacity of a denervated homotransplanted kidney in an identical twin with parallel observations in the donor. *J. clin. Invest.*, 35, 1364.

Gates, R. R. (1946). *Human Genetics.* New York: MacMillan.

Kuss, R., Teinutier, J. & Milliez, P. (1961). Quelques essais de greffes du rein chez l'homme. *Mém. Acad. Chir.*, 77, 755.

Merrill, J. P. (1959). Mechanisms of immunity in the rejection of transplanted tissue. *Trans. Amer. Clin. Climat. Ass.*, 71, 1.

Merrill, J. P., Murray, J. E., Harrison, J. H. & Guild, W. R. (1956). Successful homotransplantation of the human kidney between identical twins. *J. Amer. med. Ass.*, 160, 277.

Murray, J. E., Merrill, J. P. & Harrison, J. H. (1958). Kidney transplantation between seven pairs of identical twins. *Ann. Surg.*, 148, 343.

HETEROLOGOUS AND HOMOLOGOUS RENAL
TRANSPLANTATION IN MAN

Renal transplants to human recipients from pig and goat (Jaboulay, 1906), ape (Unger, 1910) and monkey (Schonstadt, 1913) have been attempted, but none has functioned. Following these ill-fated heterotransplants, several attempts were made to perform renal homotransplantation in man, but significant useful function was not obtained in a transplant until 1952, when Hume *et al.* reported on six transplants, three of which functioned for more than a month. In 1955 further cases were recorded by the same authors (Hume *et al.*) and their total experience of nine cases was discussed. The kidneys were transplanted to the thigh, the renal vessels were anastomosed to the femoral vessels, and the ureter was brought out through the skin. Four transplants functioned for between 37 and 157 days. Three of these kidneys were taken from cadavers, the fourth from a child at operation to relieve hydrocephalus. In all four cases the red blood cells of donor and recipient were compatible with each other's serum. All four recipients were in the terminal phase of chronic uraemia. The period of anoxia during the transplantation operation ranged from 55 to 200 minutes. Diuresis did not occur in the transplants immediately; there was a delay after the operation of 9 to 19 days before satisfactory flows of urine took place. The first three functioning transplants became infected. The fourth showed acute ischaemic tubular damage, interstitial oedema, and focal plasma-cell infiltration 176 days after transplantation. There was severe endothelial thickening of the intrinsic renal blood vessels. Three of the patients with functioning renal transplants were given adrenocorticotrophic hormone or cortisone. The authors suggested that blood-group compatibility between donor and recipient was desirable, but that adrenocorticotrophic hormone and cortisone probably did not contribute to the prolonged survival of these transplants. It was felt that chronic uraemia had inhibited the reticulo-endothelial systems of these patients and had resulted in the renal homotransplants being tolerated for far longer than could be achieved with renal homo-transplants in dogs.

In 1953 Michon and others reported renal transplantation from a mother to her son, who was acutely uraemic after surgical removal of a single traumatized kidney. The transplanted kidney was ischaemic for 55 minutes, it was placed in the pelvis, the renal vessels were anastomosed to the iliac vessels of the recipient, the ureter was anastomosed to the recipient's own ureter. The red blood cells of the donor and the recipient were compatible with each other's serum. Two hours after operation the transplanted kidney produced urine and the patient's uraemic state gradually improved. However, 23 days after operation, function suddenly ceased; this was preceded by a few days' proteinuria. The kidney was found to be enlarged and ecchymotic, and microscopic examination showed severe tubular degeneration and a mononuclear cellular infiltration in the renal cortex very similar to that seen in experimental renal homografts in dogs (Darmady *et al.*, 1955).

Thus, although homograft rejection in acute uraemia takes longer in man than in the dog, the process would appear to be essentially similar.

In 1957 Dammin *et al.* found that skin homografts survived very much longer in patients with chronic uraemia than in normal people. In three cases skin homografts survived 64, 115 and 115 days. The blood groups of donor and recipient did not seem to bear any relationship to the prolonged skin-graft survival. Mannick *et al.* (1960) performed renal transplants in dogs with experimentally produced uraemia. These kidneys ceased to function between 15 and 23 days later, a prolongation of two to three times the period of function of transplants in normal dogs. The mechanism whereby uraemia retards the rejection process is not known. No specific metabolite has so far been implicated.

This summary of the fate of renal homografts in unmodified human recipients provides a very inadequate background against which to assess attempts to modify the rejection process.

A microscopical rejection process similar to that observed in dogs is known to occur in man. However, the time of onset of functional arrest has varied greatly from within three weeks to more than five months. The thigh site for transplantation used by Hume and his colleagues (1955) was complicated by a high incidence of infection. The renal vascular occlusion occurring after the third day in the Group A patient with an O transplant may have been due to infection, technical factors, blood-group incompatibility or diminished blood flow associated with a homograft reaction. However, the timing is similar to the "acute functional arrest" described in man by other workers, which will be considered more fully later.

As with transplants between identical twins, homologous transplants can also develop glomerulonephritis. It remains to be seen whether or not prior bilateral nephrectomy of the recipient will prevent this disaster.

Porter and his colleagues (1963) discussed the arterial lesions occurring in four out of 17 human renal transplants. The lesions closely resemble those of polyarteritis nodosa, with fragmentation of the internal elastic lamina and marked fibrosis of the endothelium which sometimes blocks the lumen. Although increased blood pressure might aggravate such lesions, Porter and his colleagues felt that most of the damage is probably immunological. Similar changes have certainly been observed in dogs with long-term functioning transplants (Porter *et al.*, 1964).

Results of renal transplantation in man

In the last six years there has been a tremendous increase in the number of transplants performed. Thus by March 1963, 153 cases were reported, whilst in March 1965 the total had risen to 672, of which 268 transplants were still functioning; of the 672 cases, 392 transplants had been performed more than a year before March 1965. In March 1969, 2347 transplants had been reported. It is from this total collected by the Registry of Human Kidney Transplants under the direction of Dr J. E. Murray that it is possible to obtain some idea of the prognosis of renal transplantation in the different donor/recipient categories using the one year and two year survival as a measure of initial success (Table 12.1). Since histocompatibility factors are genetically determined and inherited according to Mendelian laws, it is essential to assess the results of renal transplantation in the context of the relationship between donor and recipient. Even when this pooled data is considered, and it obviously contains cases from the most experienced centres diluted with cases from centres which have only recently started renal transplantation, there can be no doubt that a large number of persons have had immense benefit from the procedure.

The remarkable improvement in the results recently reported compared with earlier experience would appear to be due to three factors. The first is the use of repeated dialysis so that moribund patients can be restored to a reasonable state of health; secondly, increasing familiarity with immuno-suppressive agents, particularly azathioprine and prednisone, which enables the physicians in charge of the patient to prevent an oscillation between violent rejection of the transplant and severe marrow depression. Use of the azathioprine is particularly difficult because serious toxic effects of a given dose may not be fully apparent until seven to ten days later. Thirdly, in the case of cadaver donors, there has been improvement in the procedures employed in removal and preservation of the kidneys. Improved results have occurred without any important conceptual advance in the immunology of transplantation or new immunosuppressive agents. The reader is referred to the following publications: Hamburger, Crosnier and Dormont (1965); Hume et al. (1964, 1966); Mowbray et al. (1965); Murray and Harrison (1963); Murray et al. (1964); Starzl (1964); Starzl et al. (1965); Straffon, Nakamoto and Kolff (1965); Calne et al. (1968).

The objective of renal transplantation is to restore moribund patients in terminal renal failure to a normal existence. When function of the transplant is satisfactory this objective is usually achieved.

As soon as good function is established in the transplant, the patient usually feels a sense of well-being even if he has previously been adequately dialysed. Patients often express an opinion that they "feel cleaner". They develop voracious appetites, and the increase in protein intake, together with the catabolism of major surgery and protein breakdown produced by steroids, may result in very large quantities of urea being excreted, often more than 40 g in 24 hours compared with the normal excretion of between 20 and 30 g in 24 hours. Uraemic peripheral neuritis may slowly improve, remain static or deteriorate during chronic intermittent dialysis. However, following renal transplantation, improvement is the rule. One of the author's patients was completely bed-ridden prior to transplantation in spite of dialysis, and now nearly four years after operation, he can walk long distances. Pericarditis will usually resolve with repeated dialysis and this resolution continues following renal transplantation. A satisfactorily functioning transplant will usually rapidly restore a raised blood pressure to normal and left ventricular failure or retinopathy regress. After the initial two to four months the dose of immunosuppressive drugs can usually be dropped. However, most workers feel it important to continue patients on immunosuppressive therapy indefinitely although in some cases prednisone can be omitted. Late rejection can occur, apparently at any time, but the longer a transplant survives without rejection the less likelihood there is of a severe acute rejection process. Nevertheless, a mild but progressive homograft reaction may occur and be difficult to diagnose. It is probably important not to change the dosage of immunosuppressive drugs rapidly in a patient whose transplant is functioning well. If the dosage of drugs is to be lowered, this should be done extremely gradually, and any evidence of impairment of renal function or other stigmata of rejection should be treated aggressively with higher drug doses. Tests of renal function may show values normal or considerably greater for one kidney. Hume *et al.* (1966) refer to studies of renal function in donor and recipients where the transplant function was described as being 200 per cent of normal, indicating marked functional hypertrophy. They also describe hypertrophy of a child's kidney transplanted to an adult.

Tissue typing

Although a variety of tests has been described to predict the results of a kidney transplant between two given individuals, it is now clear that the most useful and generally applicable method is the assessment of leucocyte groups which was pioneered by Dausset (1962). It is first of all important that there is no incompatibility of the ABO red cell groups since the transplant of an "A" kidney to a "B" recipient is liable to result in acute functional arrest. It is however permissible to transplant a kidney from a Group "O" red cell donor to a recipient of another group. In other words, the principles of blood transfusion must be followed. In patients who have had multiple pregnancies or a number of blood transfusions, or have been deliberately immunized by skin grafts or a previous organ graft, it is quite common for antibodies capable of agglutinating or destroying white cells from other individuals to appear in the serum. It is possible to determine tissue groups or histocompatibility factors in man, by testing an individual's white cells against antisera of known specificity. At present, details are not fully understood. The situation is rather analogous to red blood cell grouping before the minor groups were known. Nevertheless, even at this early stage there is definite correlation between the results of tissue typing and those of transplantation. When a match between donor and recipient is good, the likelihood of rejection is low and *vice versa*. Further progress in this field can be anticipated, and it is to be hoped that universally understood nomenclature with a clear understanding of information exchange between different tissue typing laboratories will make the organisation of transplantation much more satisfactory.

Second and subsequent transplants

When a transplant has failed, there have been numerous instances when it has been removed and a further transplant inserted. The results of Hume

TABLE 12.1

Kidney Transplant Registry, March 1969
(2347 Transplants)

	Survival		Longest surviving
	1 year	2 years	
	%	%	
Identical twin (1 per cent)	91	89	12 years
Blood relatives (48 per cent)	87	77	10 years
Cadaver (51 per cent)	42	40	5 years

et al. (1966) with successive renal transplants show that second and even third transplants can do as well or better than the first. The second transplant in one of their cases was the longest functioning cadaver transplant reported in the literature, continuing to function well at 32 months, the recipient having rejected the first transplant at two months in spite of extremely vigorous immunosuppressive therapy. A third kidney transplant in their series from a cadaver donor was functioning well at 12 months. Hume and his colleagues feel that it is important to remove the first transplant that has failed to function, and then to maintain the patient on dialysis for a minimum of 40 days before proceeding to a further transplant. They point out that the first kidney has been left *in situ* whilst a subsequent transplant has been performed. If a second kidney has been transplanted within a few days of removing the first transplant, the results have been poor. They advise that the patient should be off immunosuppression for the period between transplants.

There is, nevertheless, a serious danger that rejection of the first transplant will have sensitized the patient so that his serum is cytotoxic to a large percentage of random donors. To transplant a kidney in the presence of donor-specific cytotoxic antibodies is likely to provoke acute haemorrhagic rejection. It may be very difficult to find a compatible donor for sensitized patients, and direct cross-matching of recipient serum against potential donor lymphocytes is an essential preliminary screening procedure.

The marked improvements in results are very gratifying to those working in the field of renal transplantation. The most experienced groups are now obtaining around 90 per cent survival at one year of the transplants between close relatives who are not identical twins. The figure is probably about 50 per cent for unrelated cadaver donors. From Table 12.1 it can be seen that failures in the second year are remarkably few. The eventual fate of long-surviving transplants is unknown, but dying uraemic patients transformed to a normal existence for a number of years do not need to be convinced of the value of the procedure. The results achieved with present immuno-suppression and clinical management provide a far more optimistic view of clinical renal transplantation than would have been anticipated a few years ago.

REFERENCES

CALNE, R. Y., EVANS, D. B., HERBERTSON, B. M., JOYSEY, V., McMILLAN, R., MAGINN, R. R., MILLARD, P. R., PENA, J. R., SALAMAN, J. R., WHITE, H. J. O., WITHYCOMBE, J. F. R. & YOFFA, D. E. (1968). *Brit. med. J.*, **2**, 104.

DAMMIN, G. H., COUCH, N. P. & MURRAY, J. E. (1957). Prolonged survival of skin homografts in uremic patients. *Ann. N.Y. Acad. Sci.*, **64**, 967.

DARMADY, E. M., DEMPSTER, W. J. & STANNOCK, F. (1955). Evolution of interstitial and tubular changes in homotransplanted kidneys. *J. Path. Bact.*, **70**, 225.

HAMBURGER, J., CROSNIER, J. & DORMONT, J. (1965). *Lancet*, **1**, 985.

HUME, D. M., LEE, H. M., WILLIAMS, G. H., WHITE, H. J. O., FERRE, J., WOLFF, J. D., PROUT, G. R. JR., SLAPAK, M., O'BRIEN, J., KILPATRICK, S. J., KAUFFMAN, H. M. JR., & CLEVELAND, R. J. (1966). *Ann. Surg.*, **164**, 352.

HUME, D. M., MAGEE, J. H., PROUT, G. R., KAUFFMAN, H. M., CLEVELAND, R. J., BOWER, J. D. & LEE, (1964). *Ann. N.Y. Acad. Sci.*, **120**, 578.

HUME, D. M., MERRILL, J. P., MILLER, B. F. & THORN, G. S. (1955). Experiences with renal homotransplantation in the human: report of nine cases. *J. clin. Invest.*, **34**, 327.

HUME, D. M., MERRILL, J. P. & MILLER, B. F. (1952). Homologous transplantation of human kidneys. *J. clin. Invest.*, **31**, 640.

JABOULAY, M. (1906). Greffe de reins au pli coude par soudures artérielles et veineuses. *Lyon méd.*, **107**, 575.

MANNICK, J. A., POWERS, J. H., MITHOFER, J. & FERREBEE, J. W. (1960). Renal transplantation in azotemic dogs. *Surgery*, **47**, 340.

MICHON, L., HAMBURGER, J., OECONOMOS, N., DELINOTTE, P., RICHET, G., VAYSSE, J. & ANTOINNE, B. (1953). Une tentative de transplantation rénale chez l'homme. Aspects médicaux et biologiques. *Presse méd.*, **70**, 1419.

MOWBRAY, J. F., COHEN, S. L., DOAK, P. B., KENYON, J. R., OWEN, K., PERCIVAL, A., PORTERM, K. A. & PEART, W. S. (1965). *Brit. med. J.*, **2**, 1287.

MURRAY, J. E. & HARRISON, J. H. (1963). *Amer. J. Surg.*, **105**, 205.

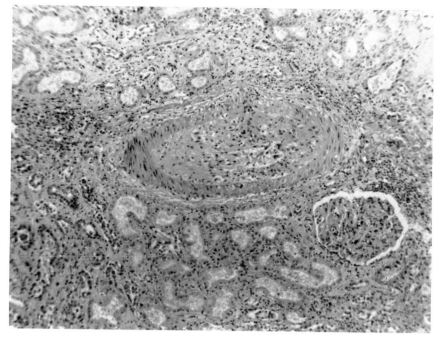

Fig. 12.9. Section of chimpanzee's kidney 8 months after transplantation into a human. There is a marked intimal thickening of the arteries but moderately well preserved cortical architecture. (By permission of Dr Reemtsma, personal communication.)

MURRAY, J. E., MERRILL, J. P., DAMMIN, G. J., HARRISON, U. H., HAGER, E. B. & WILSON, R. E. (1964). *Ann. Surg.*, **160**, 449.

PORTER, K. A., JOSEPH, N. H., RENDALL, J. M., STOLINSKI, C., HOEHN, R. J. & CALNE, R. Y. (1964). The role of lymphocytes in the rejection of canine renal homografts. *Lab. Invest.*, **13**, 1080.

PORTER, K. A., THOMSON, W. B., OWEN, K., KENYON, J. R., MOWBRAY, J. F. & PEART, W. S. (1963). Obliterative vascular changes in 4 kidney homotransplants. *Brit. med. J.*, **3**, 639.

SCHONSTADT, quoted by MOREL, L. & PAPIN, E. (1913) Les applications physiologiques et chirurgicales des transplantations rénales. *Biol. Med.*, **11**, 397.

STARZL, T. E. (1964). *Experience in Renal Transplantation*. Philadelphia and London: Saunders.

STARZL, T. E., MARCHIORO, T. L., TERASAKI, P. I., PORTER, K. A., FARIS, T. D., HERMANN, T. J., VREDVOE, D. L., HUTT, M. P., OGDEN, D. A. & WADDELL, M. D. (1965). *Ann. Surg.*, **162**, 749.

STRAFFON, R. A., NAKAMOTO, S. & KOLFF, W. J. (1965). *Brit. J. Urol.*, **38**, 370.

UNGER, E. (1910). Nierentransplantationen. *Berl. klin. Wschr.*, **47**, 573.

TRANSPLANTS FROM PRIMATES

In 1963 interesting observations on transplantation in man were made when further transplantations from primates to man were performed—from baboon to man (Hitchcock and Starzl) and from chimpanzee to man (Reemtsma). The patients were treated with the agents described above and three baboon-to-man transplants had satisfactory renal function for two months although they required very large doses of immunosuppressive agents. The kidneys were eventually rejected.

The results of transplants from chimpanzees have been more successful. Of the first six performed by Dr Reemtsma, one patient survived for eight months after transplantation. The chimpanzee kidneys which functioned satisfactorily were transplanted to the patient's right iliac fossa and the ureters were implanted into the bladder. The patient died from pneumonia.

In rejected chimpanzee kidneys the histological features have been very similar to those seen in rejected human transplants (Fig. 12.9). In view of experimental work in animals it is amazing that primate-to-man transplants have functioned at all, and almost incredible that such a transplant has supported the life of a human being for eight months. Important theoretical questions are raised concerning the phylogenetic relationship between man and primates and perhaps other species. Undoubtedly much research effort will be devoted to hetero-transplants in the hope of clarification of histocompatibility factors relevant to animals and man with an aim to eventual selection of appropriate donors. The use of animal tissue immediately removes the ethical strictures discussed later, and also provides a source of vital unpaired organs such as heart and liver which can never be taken from live human donors.

If these experiments in heterologous transplantation had been a total failure the doctors responsible would have been condemned by other workers in this field. It is fortunate that Drs Hitchcock, Reemtsma and Starzl had the courage to perform experiments, which on purely theoretical grounds seemed to have so slender a chance of success.

REFERENCES

HITCHCOCK, C. R., KISER, J. C., TELANDER, R. L. & SELJESKOG (1964). Baboon renal grafts. *J. Amer. med. Ass.*, **189**, 934.
REEMTSMA, K., McCRACKEN, B. H., SCHLEGEL, J. U., PEARL, M. A., PEARCE, C. W., DEWITT, C. W., SMITH, P. E., HEWITT, R. L., FLINNER, R. L. & CREECH, O. (1964). Renal heterotransplantation in man. *Ann. Surg.*, **160**, 384.
STARZL, T. E., MARCHIORO, T. L., PETERS, G. N., KIRKPATRICK, C. H., WILSON, W. E. C. PORTER, K. A., RIFKIND, D., OGDEN, D. A., HITCHCOCK, C. R. & WADDELL, W. R. (1964). Renal heterotransplantation from baboon to man: experience with 6 cases. *Transplantation*, **2**, 752.

SELECTION AND MANAGEMENT OF PATIENTS FOR TRANSPLANTATION

Only patients in the terminal stages of uraemia should be considered as possible candidates for renal transplantation. In general, adults are the most suitable recipients, but it is hard to define upper and lower age limits. In the very young it may be technically difficult to transplant a kidney and the multiple venepunctures, dialyses and a major operation which are formidable for an adult may well be considered unjustified in a young child. Similar considerations would apply to the elderly, who are also unlikely to withstand major surgery and the immunosuppressive regime as well as a younger person.

The commonest diseases responsible for renal failure are glomerulonephritis and polycystic kidneys. In chronic uraemia, rejection of a transplant is likely to be less aggressive than in acute uraemia, although successful transplants have been performed in patients with acute loss of renal function. Most workers believe that recipients suffering from acute immunological disorders, especially polyarteritis nodosa or disseminated lupus erythematosus, should not be candidates for renal transplantation because of the danger of these disorders occurring in the transplant. Similar arguments are raised for patients suffering from active glomerulonephritis.

Indications for dialysis

By the time the decision has been made to offer the patient a renal transplant, all conventional medical therapy will have been administered, and if he is not actually moribund the patient will be very gravely ill. The uraemia may be complicated by infection, cardiac failure and hypertensive encephalopathy. To submit a patient in this condition to a major operation and then administer toxic drugs is likely to result in a high percentage of failures, and this has in fact been the early experience of most workers. However, repeated dialysis may improve the patient's general condition to a remarkable degree (Hegstrom et al., 1962). Repeated peritoneal dialysis can produce satisfactory results, but peritoneal dialysis is liable eventually to lead to infection in the peritoneal cavity, and this may cause abscess formation after renal transplantation. Although it is more complicated and adds the further risk of sensitizing the patient with blood transfusions, most investigators feel that repeated haemodialysis is preferable. A procedure that has given encouraging results is to insert a Scribner type of arteriovenous shunt into the recipient as soon as renal transplantation has been decided upon, or alternatively to construct a suture anastomosis to produce an arteriovenous shunt (Brescia Cimeno), and then to dialyse the patient repeatedly until his general condition is satisfactory for the operation. During dialysis the complications of uraemia are likely to resolve and the blood pressure often falls to safe levels. If hypertension is not controlled by lowering the total body-sodium with dialysis, both the patient's own kidneys can be removed. This will probably result in the blood pressure falling to normal, provided dialysis is reasonably frequent. The Kiil dialyser, as used extensively by Scribner and his colleagues (Cole et al., 1963), seems to be very satisfactory for this purpose and although dialysis takes approximately 12 hours this machine requires little priming with blood and the cellophane membrane is relatively cheap.

Indications for bilateral nephrectomy

Most workers agree that the patient's own kidneys should be removed if they are grossly infected. The other indications for bilateral nephrectomy are less well established. Malignant hypertension may revert to normal levels following renal transplantation if the transplant functions well. However, this is not always the case, and if hypertension persists despite good transplant function, removal of the patient's own kidneys will probably result in a reduction of blood pressure toward normal levels.

Removal of glomerulonephritic kidneys to prevent glomerulonephritis occurring in the transplant has already been mentioned. It has however not yet been established that bilateral nephrectomy performed prior to transplantation will prevent the development of this complication in transplanted kidneys, and some transplanted kidneys have developed glomerular lesions, even when the original disease of the patient was not glomerulonephritis. Following successful renal transplantation the patient's diseased kidneys often become anuric, even if they were producing approximately one litre of urine a day prior to transplantation. The stasis in the renal pelvis and ureter predisposes to infection, and some workers feel that bilateral nephrectomy should therefore be performed to prevent this complication, though infection of the anuric kidney is not inevitable.

ORGAN STORAGE

The main difficulty in using cadaveric kidneys for renal transplantation is the ischaemic damage that the organ is likely to suffer. At present the most successful and safest way of increasing ischaemic survival is to cool the kidney. Lapchinski (1960) perfused dog kidneys and kept them at 4°C for up to 28 hours. The kidneys were then autotransplanted, and in some experiments a satisfactory return of renal function was demonstrated by subsequent removal of the undisturbed kidney, with continued survival of the animal.

Simple surface cooling with ice minimizes ischaemic damage in stored kidneys (Calne et al., 1963). Kidneys were removed from dogs and placed in a polythene bag surrounded by ice. The behaviour of these kidneys was studied after retransplantation to their original donors. It was found that this method permitted adequate function in the re-implanted kidneys after up to 12 hours of preservation, so that the animals could withstand the severe test of an immediate opposite nephrectomy. After between 12 and 17 hours of preservation, some animals survived if the opposite remaining kidney was left for a period of weeks before removal. With more than 17 hours of preservation, severe irreversible damage occurred in the kidneys and useful function was not obtained. The interstitial reaction in these kidneys after cortical damage was similar to that seen in some human cadaveric transplants, and in some kidneys a cellular infiltrate was observed with plasma cells predominating. Plasma cells have been specially implicated in the immunological rejection of homologous transplanted kidneys, and these changes in autologous transplants further complicate assessment of renal histology of grafted kidneys which have suffered ischaemic damage. It is likely that with human cadaveric transplants much of the damage occurs between the time of death and the time of removal of the kidney, before cooling can be started. Surface cooling rapidly lowers the temperature in canine kidneys, but the larger human kidney is cooled more efficiently by perfusion.

A suitable innocuous cold perfusion system to bring the temperature of the kidney down to around 10°C, when it is placed in a polythene bag surrounded by ice has been described by Brunius et al. (1968). Using this method it is possible to keep the kidney for seven hours with very little deterioration of the parenchyma. Longer methods of preservation which would allow a kidney transplantation to be done as an elective procedure rather than as an emergency require complicated perfusion apparatus. Belzer *et al.* (1967) described a perfusion apparatus which enabled a consistently good result to be obtained over a 72-hour period, after which preserved dog kidneys would function well after being reimplanted.

Although the possibility of kidney storage for an indefinite period of time may be realized in the future, little success has so far been achieved in this field, and it would be rash to predict a solution before the homograft problem is overcome.

REFERENCES

BELZER, F. O., ASHBY, B. S. & DUNPHY, J. E. (1967). *Lancet*, 2, 536.

BRUNIUS, U., BERGENTZ, S. E., EKMAN, H., GELIN, L-E. & WESTBERG, C. (1968). *Scand. J. Urol. & Nephrol.*, 2, 15.

CALNE, R. Y., PEGG, D. E., PRYSE-DAVIES, J. & LEIGH BROWN, F. (1963). Renal preservation by ice-cooling. An experimental study relating to kidney transplantation from cadavers. *Brit. med. J.*, 2, 651.

CALNE, R. Y. (1964). Renal transplantation in man: a review. *Brit. J. Surg.*, 51, 282.

COLE, J. J., POLLARD, T. L. & MURRAY, J. S. (1963). Studies on the modified polyprotylene Kiil dialyser. *Trans. Amer. Soc. Int. Organs*, 9, 67.

HEGSTROM, R. M., MURRAY, J. S., PENDRAS, J. P., BURNELL, J. M. & SCRIBNER, B. H. (1962). Two years' experience with periodic hemodialysis in the treatment of chronic uremia. *Transactions, ASAIO*, VII.

LAPCHINSKI, A. G. (1960). Recent results of experimental transplantation of preserved limbs and kidneys and possible use of this technique in clinical practice. *Ann. N.Y. Acad. Sci.*, 87, 539.

COMPLICATIONS OF RENAL TRANSPLANTATION

In the last few years, an extremely large number of complications have been reported in patients with renal transplants. Some of these complications have been in the transplanted kidney, others have been associated with the disease from which the patient originally suffered, and there has also been considerable morbidity from the use of immunosuppressive drugs. A comprehensive discussion of all the complications described would be outside the scope of this book, but the most common and important ones will be considered.

Complications can occur with surprising rapidity and their onset is particularly common in the first two months after operation. Accordingly, it is absolutely essential during this period to make the following daily observations of the patient:

1. Full clinical examination including careful palpation of the transplant.

2. Recording of temperature, pulse, respiration, blood pressure and body weight.
3. Determination of serum electrolytes and urea, urinary electrolytes, glucose and 24-hour excretion of protein and urea.
4. Examination of centrifuged deposit in the urine for lymphoid and epithelial cells.
5. Full blood picture including platelets and haemoglobin.

The following observations are performed weekly:
1. Chest X-ray.
2. X-ray of pelvis to show kidney size.
3. Urine culture.
4. Creatinine clearance.
5. Liver function tests.

In the course of the patient's care it is obvious that other investigations may be required. In particular, a renogram and scan and intravenous pyelography may be helpful, and occasionally a renal biopsy is indicated. After two months the daily observations can be changed to two or three times a week. It is probably advisable to keep the patient under the care of the transplantation centre until four months have elapsed following operation, and thereafter surveillance can be delegated to a competent physician with access to adequate laboratory facilities.

This very careful follow-up of the patient may involve him in social difficulties with regard to accommodation for himself and his family, and it may be impossible for him to return to work in the first four months. However, once he is ambulant and good renal function has been demonstrated in the transplant it is preferable for him to live out of hospital. It may be of great value to a transplant centre to have designated accommodation available for patients during this period of intensive surveillance. If the patient can find part-time employment during this time it will help his morale. Once the four-month period is past, the incidence of complications becomes less and the patient should be able to enjoy a normal life, his only restriction being the regular taking of immunosuppressive drugs by mouth and weekly attendance at hospital for follow-up as described above.

Renal complications

The most important renal complication is immunological rejection of the transplant. Sudden cessation of function of a transplant is most likely to be due to an acute rejection crisis, but there are other possibilities.

If an initial satisfactory diuresis has been established, the cause cannot be primary technical failure. It is probable that acute lesions have occurred in transplants which had never functioned and were not examined until infarction of the kidney had progressed to necrosis. Thus the operative ischaemia, especially with cadaveric donors, often causes an initial anuria due to acute tubular necrosis, and a catastrophe occurring in such a kidney, no matter what its cause, is likely to diminish the renal blood flow and predispose the main renal vessels to thrombosis. Excluding rejection, recognized causes of sudden functional arrest in a transplant are massive cortical haemorrhage, acute glomerulonephritis, thrombosis of major blood vessels, acute interstitial oedema and tubular necrosis.

Non-renal complication of kidney transplantation

Complications of azathioprine have been discussed. Hepatotoxicity seldom occurs with therapeutic doses unless the patient has impaired liver function or develops hepatitis. In such circumstances it may be dangerous to continue azathioprine. The dangers of marrow toxicity are increased liability to infection from agranulocytosis, and haemorrhage due to thrombocytopenia. If there is a rapidly falling white count, it is obviously necessary to reduce or stop the drug, but the effects of a toxic dose of azathioprine on the marrow are not manifest until 10 days afterwards, so management can be very difficult. If the total peripheral white count falls below 2000 it is advisable to nurse the patient with barrier precautions.

Treatment of both established agranulocytosis and thrombocytopenia is very unsatisfactory. Fresh blood transfusions may be of value, and prophylactic antibiotics are usually given. Haemorrhage from thrombocytopenia may occur anywhere, but the lung is particularly susceptible.

Complications of steroids

Many of these have already been mentioned; they include susceptibility to all kinds of infection. In particular, appendicitis may be confused with a rejection crisis if the transplant is in the right iliac fossa. Peptic ulceration producing perforation or haemorrhage is a very serious complication in a patient with a transplant. The effects of large doses of steroids on the skeleton can cause stunting of growth in children and spontaneous fractures. All the features of Cushing's syndrome may be produced and the diabetic state may require insulin. Pancreatitis occurring after transplantation is believed to be due to steroids (Monaco and Russell, 1966). Very high doses of steroids may produce convulsions.

Non-traumatic systemic fat embolization has been reported in a patient with a renal transplant following reduction in steroid dosage, by Jones, Engleman and Najarian (1965). They felt that the most likely source of the embolic fat was steroid-induced fatty change in the liver. Increasing levels of serum triglycerides and clinical features of systemic fat embolism followed rapid reduction of prednisone dosage from 120 mg a day. The patient became lethargic with abdominal pain, numbness and weakness in the calves and a burning sensation in the soles of the feet. Serum triglycerides rose from 795 mg/100 ml (normal was 30–150 mg/100 ml) to 1815 mg/100 ml and there was impaired renal function. The patient subsequently died and evidence of systemic fat embolization was found at autopsy. Fat embolization could be the cause of avascular bone necrosis in transplant patients.

Blood pressure changes

The anuric patient undergoing dialysis and subsequent renal transplantation provides much interesting data relating to blood pressure control. Although dialysis with removal of sodium and fluid usually controls hypertension, Hume et al. (1966) report on cases that have not been controlled with depletion of sodium and fluid to the point of shock. They have found that some of the patients could be controlled only by bilateral nephrectomy, and one of their cases could not be controlled by bilateral nephrectomy and dialysis but required a functioning renal transplant for the blood pressure to be manageable. There are other cases where even this procedure does not result in a normal blood pressure due, presumably, to structural alterations of the peripheral arteries and arterioles. Therefore, the only way a normal blood pressure can be produced is by reducing the cardiac output to a point where ischaemia of vital structures occurs.

Three types of hypertension have been described following renal transplantation:

1. Acute hypertension at the time of transplantation associated with *ischaemic damage* to the transplant (Swales and Morgan, 1965).
2. Hypertension associated with *rejection* (Starzl, 1964).
3. Hypertension due to *glomerulonephritis* affecting the transplant (Murray, Merrill and Harrison, 1958).

Transmission of malignancy

Unsuspected metastatic carcinoma in a renal transplant can subsequently grow and cause the death of the recipient. McIntosh et al. (1965) described. a case of renal transplantation in which the donor died from carcinoma of the pharynx. There was no obvious growth on inspection of the kidney at the time of operation, and initially the transplant functioned satisfactorily; however, the patient gradually developed metastases in the liver from which he died eight months later. Martin, Rubini and Rosen (1965) described a somewhat similar case. The donor died from bronchogenic carcinoma and there was no gross evidence of metastasis in the kidney at the time of transplantation. Four months after operation malignant cells were found in a biopsy of the transplant. This tumour was of the same histological appearance as that in the donor. The recipient died from widespread metastasis of the transplanted growth five months after transplantation.

This very serious complication of renal transplantation would appear to contra-indicate the use of kidneys from patients dying of malignant disease with the exception of primary cerebral tumours, which do not metastasize outside the central nervous system.

Transmission of infective diseases

Any infection present in the blood stream of the donor at the time the kidney is removed may be transmitted to the recipient, who is particularly susceptible to infection. Hepatitis occurred in six of the cases of Hume *et al.* (1966), and three staff looking after the patients also developed infective hepatitis. Of particular interest was the outcome where the two kidneys from a cadaver donor were transplanted into recipients who both developed infective hepatitis. Hood *et al.* (1965) have reported the transmission of histoplasmosis by a transplanted kidney.

Hyperparathyroidism

Secondary parathyroid hyperplasia is a common sequel to long-standing renal failure. McPhaul *et al.*, (1964) described the development of autonomous hyperparathyroidism following restoration of renal function with a transplant. After renal transplantation there was marked hypophosphataemia, phosphaturia, hypercalciuria and hypercalcaemia. The primary renal disease was glomerulonephritis. Three and a half of the four hyperplastic parathyroid glands were removed surgically and this resulted in a normal serum calcium. Similar cases were reported by Wilson *et al.* (1965); they suggested that when it is indicated subtotal parathyroidectomy should precede renal transplantation whenever possible. Hume *et al.* (1966) reported stone formation in a transplant due to autonomous hyperparathyroidism occurring after operation. It is certainly most important to assess the patient's calcium and phosphate metabolism before and after transplantation so that the transplant is not damaged by hyperparathyroidism.

Arthropathy

Arthropathy resembling gout can follow renal transplantation (Calne *et al.*, 1966). However, chemical analysis of the periarticular deposits shows high concentrations of calcium and phosphorus and a negligible reaction for urates. The joint surfaces are not involved. The lesions are probably an example of pseudo-gout, a crystal-induced arthropathy described by McCarty, Kohn and Faires (1962). It occures in patients on chronic intermittent dialysis (Caner and Decker, 1964). The calcium deposits are probably due to impaired renal function. At autopsy on the case of Calne *et al.*, there was no evidence of parathyroid hyperplasia, and the function of the transplant had been poor for two and a half years.

Splenomegaly

Hamburger, Crosnier and Dormont (1964) described splenomegaly occurring in patients with renal transplants between the third and fourteenth month after transplantation. At splenectomy in all cases they found hyperplasia of the white pulp and congestion of the red pulp with interstitial fibrosis and reticular hyperplasia. The cause of the splenomegaly has not been determined but could presumably be a manifestation of the host-against-graft reaction.

Pulmonary complications

Pneumonitis characterized by fever, hilar and lung field shadows on X-ray, but often without any pulmonary symptoms, may follow renal transplantation. When these patients are investigated the majority are found to have either pulmonary oedema associated with fluid retention, usually coinciding with a rejection episode, or alternatively infection of the lung. This may be bacterial, or due to viruses, fungi or other parasites. Cytomegalic inclusion disease, *pneumocystis carinii*, tuberculosis, monilia and aspergilla infestation have all been described. Fungal infections may be treated with amphotericin B. This drug is nephrotoxic and the dose therefore needs to be carefully regulated. Robbins *et al.* (1965) have successfully treated *pneumocystis carinii* infection in a patient with hypogammaglobulinaemia using pentamidine isocyanate. Sometimes, however, the syndrome occurs without any obvious cause being found, and it has been suggested by Hume *et al.* (1966) that circulating antibodies, perhaps directed at the transplant endothelium, can also damage the patient's own lung. They call this condition "transplant lung" and have described characteristic changes in pulmonary function. There is evidence by analogy that during rejection of canine renal homotransplants there may be some damage to the animal's own kidneys (Hager, DuPuy and Wallach, 1964; Veith *et al.*, 1965).

The pulmonary changes tend to resolve if rejection in the transplant is overcome; however, "transplant lung" may predispose the lungs to subsequent infection with any of the agents mentioned above.

Erythraemia

The relation of the kidney to the production of erythropoietin and control of erythropoiesis has been the subject of much study, and is not at present fully understood. There is much evidence that most of the erythropoietin is produced by the kidney, although it is possible that there may be additional extra-renal sites of erythropoietin production. Generally, following a successful renal transplant, the anaemia of the uraemic state resolves, due presumably to the absence of uraemic depression of the bone marrow together with restoration of erythropoietin production. However there occasionally appears to be an excess of erythropoietin production producing polycythaemia. Nies, Cohn and Schrier (1965) refer to a patient who, six weeks after renal transplantation, was found to produce a large number of nucleated red cells in the peripheral blood. The packed cell volume and red cell mass rose to abnormal levels, and urinary erythropoietin excretion during the latter portion of the phase of rapid red cell production was approximately nine times the upper limits of normal. The outpouring of nucleated red cells seemed to occur in association with rejection crisis, and there was no evidence of severe haemolysis. There was a normal plasma iron turnover and essentially normal utilization of ^{59}Fe tagged red cells. The authors felt that ischaemic damage to the transplant stimulated the production of erythropoietin. Calne *et al.* (1966) also reported erythraemia in a patient following transplantation. Prior to operation their patient was clinically anaemic and required 0·5–1 litre of blood at each haemodialysis. For six weeks following operation his haemoglobin remained in the range of 11·5 to 12·5 g/100 ml. Over the next six weeks a progressive rise occurred until the haemoglobin reached a level of 18·8 g. The white blood cell count was between 4000 and 7000 per c.mm, platelets 150,000–200,000 per c.mm, packed cell volume 54 per cent and red cell count 5·6 million cells per c.mm. A film of the blood showed a moderate degree of anisocytosis only, with a reticulocyte count of 3 to 5 per cent. The plasma erythropoietin level was markedly increased. This patient was not apparently undergoing a rejection crisis at this time, but he did develop a deep vein thrombosis and pulmonary emboli.

Pulmonary emboli

The increased incidence of pulmonary emboli in transplant cases following splenectomy has already been mentioned, and also the possible association with erythraemia. Starzl *et al.* (1964) performed a successful pulmonary embolectomy in a patient with a renal transplant. The diagnosis was made when the patient developed cardiac arrest, and the embolus was removed with the aid of cardio-pulmonary bypass. Hume *et al.* (1966) found a significant increase in the incidence of pulmonary emboli after splenectomy and have abandoned this procedure. They observed a fourfold increase in thrombo-embolic phenomena and a twofold increase in infections in splenectomized patients, with no improvement in overall survival.

Psychiatric disturbances

It is not surprising that patients subjected to chronic intermittent dialysis, renal transplantation, isolation to prevent infection, and intensive medical care, should be susceptible to psychiatric disorders. In addition, high doses of steroids may produce acute psychotic episodes. Psychiatric breakdown following renal transplantation is to be anticipated in patients with a previous history of psychiatric trouble. However, many patients who have been very depressed during uraemia before transplantation recover their normal buoyancy after operation. Secondary psychiatric abnormalities may also occur in patients with a high serum calcium due to hyperparathyroidism.

REFERENCES

CALNE, R. Y., LOUGHRIDGE, L., MacGILLIVRY, J. B. & SWALES, J. D. (1966). *Brit. med. J.*, **2**, 684.
CANER, J. E. Z. & DECKER, J. L. (1964). *Amer. J. Med.*, **36**, 571.
HAGER, E. B., DuPUY, M. P. & WALLACH, D. F. H. (1964). *Ann. N.Y. Acad. Sci.*, **120**, 447.
HAMBURGER, J., CROSNIER, J. & DORMONT, J. (1964). *Ann. N.Y. Acad. Sci.*, **120**, 558.
HOOD, A. B., INGLIS, F. G., LOWENSTEIN, L., DOSSETOR, J. B. & MacLEAN, L. D. (1965). *Canad. med. Ass. J.*, **93**, 587.
HUME, D. M., LEE, H. M., WILLIAMS, G. H., WHITE, H. J. O., FERRE, J., WOLF, J. D., PROUT, G. R. JR., SLAPAK, M., O'BRIEN, J., KILPATRICK, S. J., KAUFF-MAN, H. M. JR. & CLEVELAND, R. J. (1966). *Ann. Surg.*, **164**, 352.
JONES, J. P., ENGLEMAN, E. P. & NAJARIAN, J. S. (1965). *New Engl. J. Med.*, **273**, 1453.
McCARTY, D. J. JR., KOHN, N. N. & FAIRES, J. S. (1962). *Ann. Intern. Med.*, **56**, 711.
McINTOSH, D. A., McPHAUL, J. J., PETERSON, E. W., HARVIN, J. S., SMITH, J. R., COOK, F. E. & HUMPHREYS, J. W. (1965). *J. Amer. med. Ass.*, **192**, 143.
McPHAUL, J. J., McINTOSH, D. A., HAMMOND, W. S. & PARK, O. K. (1964). *New Engl. J. Med.*, **271**, 1342.
MARTIN, D. C., RUBINI, M. & ROSEN, V. J. (1965). *J. Amer. med. Ass.*, **192**, 752.
MONACO, A. P. & RUSSELL, P. S. (1966). *Surg. Clin. N. Amer.*, **46**, 713.
MURRAY, J. E., MERRILL, J. P. & HARRISON, J. H. (1958). *Ann. Surg.*, **148**, 343.
NIES, B. A., COHN, R. & SCHRIER, L. (1965). *New Engl. J. Med.*, **273**, 785.
ROBBINS, J. B., MILLER, R. H., AREAN, V. M. & PEARSON, H. A. (1965). Successful treatment of pneumocystic carinili pneumonitis in a patient with congenital hypogammaglobulinemia. *New Engl. J. Med.*, **272**, 708.
STARZL, T. E. (1964). *Experience in Renal Transplantation*. Philadelphia and London: Saunders.
SWALES, J. D. & MORGAN, M. N. (1965). *Lancet*, **2**, 219.
VEITH, F. J., STENZEL, K. H., THOMPSON, D. D., MARL, R. C. & RUBIN, A. I. (1965). *Surg. Forum*, **16**, 263.
WILSON, R. E., BERNSTEIN, D. S., MURRAY, J. E. & MOORE, F. E. (1965). *Amer. J. Surg.*, **110**, 384.

TRANSPLANTATION OF THE HEART, LIVER AND LUNGS

The difficulties involved in transplantation of the kidney are well known. Some of them are understood, but we have only a very superficial knowledge of the basic factors involved in the rejection of transplanted tissues. Despite our empiricism in this field, therapeutic renal transplantation is rapidly advancing, and with further development in tissue typing and new immuno-suppressive agents, continued progress is to be expected.

The experimental background to the transplantation of other organs is now extensive. It is possible to transplant successfully the liver, heart, lungs and many other organs and tissues. In general such allografts are rejected in a similar manner to the kidney, and immunosuppressive agents that prevent the rejection of renal transplants are also effective with transplants of other organs. There are, however, difficulties in the clinical application of this experimental work.

The liver and heart are unpaired vital organs, and cadavers are at present the only donor source. Both these organs deteriorate very rapidly after death, and although methods of preservation for 24 hours or more are available experimentally, we have little information as to how effective these methods would be in clinical application. Some preservation methods that are extremely effective when applied to a healthy organ which has just been removed may not be so valuable clinically. More data is required on the results of ischaemi-cally damaged organs preserved by standard methods and then transplanted. To what extent can damage be repaired during the preservation? It is obviously desirable to resuscitate an organ, and there is some evidence that this may be possible with the heart. There is nevertheless a danger that enzymes liberated during the ischaemic period will further damage the organ while it is being preserved.

Modern dialysis makes it possible to restore a patient with no renal function to excellent health, so that he is fit for major surgery. A failing heart may be assisted mechanically and cross-circulation, exchange transfusion and extra-corporeal liver perfusion can improve the condition of patients with severe hepatic diseases. However, these supporting measure are at present in no way comparable with what can be achieved by dialysis for kidney disease. Better methods of support are needed to make transplantation of these organs reasonably safe, particularly since the operations of heart and liver trans-plantation are far more extensive procedures for the patient to withstand than transplantation of a kidney. One advantage of the liver compared with the kidney is that it tends to be rejected more slowly.

Clinical transplantation of the lungs is technically easier than that of heart and liver, but the surface of the lung is subjected to the atmosphere, which is a potential source of infection. Unfortunately, pulmonary infection is one of the commonest causes of death after renal transplantation, and one would expect this to be an even more serious complication with lung transplants. Clinical transplantation of other tissues such as the pancreas and portions of the gastro-intestinal tract is possible. It is necessary to assess the dangers of immunosuppressive therapy and surgery against the expected therapeutic advantages of such transplants.

The Heart

Shumway *et al.* (1967) and Cleveland and Lower (1967) have studied orthotopic heart transplantation in the dog, and both groups have long-term survivors treated with immunosuppressive therapy. They have shown that it is possible to restore sinus rhythm to both animal and human hearts which have been ischaemic for 30 minutes at 37°C. These techniques involve coronary perfusion and defibrillation. The first transplant of a heart into man was performed by Hardy *et al.* (1966) when the donor was a chimpanzee. The heart did not function for long. Using the techniques pioneered by Shumway and Lower, Barnard (1967) performed the first much-publicized human-to-human cardiac transplant. The current status of cardiac transplantation is well known. The heart is rejected in the human body certainly as aggressively as is the kidney and there is no method of maintaining a patient whose heart is irreversibly damaged by rejection. There would appear to be correlation of the results of transplantation with tissue matching of donor and recipient. The indications for cardiac transplantation are less well understood; most cases have suffered either from chronic vascular insufficiency or cardiomyopathy.

The Liver

Liver transplantation presents a surgical challenge that was first accepted by Moore and Starzl and their colleagues in the 1950s. They showed that a reproducible technique of orthotopic liver transplantation in the dog was possible. The successfully transplanted canine liver was however subject to rejection in much the same way as a kidney; this process could be inhibited in a proportion of animals by treatment with the same immunosuppressive agents that prevent rejection of transplanted kidneys, namely azathioprine, corticosteroids and antilymphocyte serum.

Technique

The liver may be transplanted in the normal position (orthotopic transplantation). This requires preliminary hepatectomy of the recipient, but has the great advantage that the liver is easily accommodated and the vascular connections lie in a normal anatomical situation. Complications of kinking and obstruction from external pressure are unlikely to occur. Alternatively, the liver may be transplanted in an abnormal situation (heterotopic, accessory or auxiliary transplantation). The advantage with this technique is that preliminary hepatectomy is not necessary, but the disadvantages are that it may be very difficult to accommodate a large liver satisfactorily in the abdomen, and there may also be problems in providing satisfactory vascular inflow and outflow and bile drainage with the liver in an abnormal position.

The *indications* for clinical liver transplantation have not yet been fully established, but any fatal disease of the liver which is still confined to the liver is potentially suitable. Thus there are two main categories, namely primary malignant disease of the liver and non-malignant cirrhotic processes, including biliary cirrhosis and biliary atresia in infants.

The relatively common types of primary malignant disease of the liver are liver cell cancer and cholangiocarcinoma. In the United Kingdom both these diseases tend to remain localized in the liver for long periods, and metastasise locally within the liver before spreading to other situations, in particular the lungs. In many parts of Africa and Asia liver cell carcinoma metastasises rather early and is frequently associated with cirrhosis. Fatal liver disease is extremely common in Asia and Africa, but in the United Kingdom it probably accounts for only 200 deaths a year in young people, or approximately 10 per cent of deaths due to irreversible kidney disease in a similar age-group (Terblanche and Riddell, 1967). Thus it should be possible for three or four centres to cope with all those requiring liver transplantation in the United Kingdom.

Lack of satisfactory support of the patient, both before and after surgery, have been the main reason for the slowness in development of liver transplantation compared with that of the kidney. Exchange transfusion, *ex-vivo* liver perfusion, either through an animals' liver or a human cadaver's liver, or cross-circulation with man or an animal, may all temporarily improve the state of the patient in liver failure, but none of these procedures can be repeated indefinitely. Repeated exchange transfusion will utilize a vast amount of blood, and the patient may develop antibodies against blood constituents. This may also occur in *ex-vivo* perfusion and cross-circulation. There are also infective immunological and haemodynamic dangers to a human partner of cross-circulation. At their best, none of these methods compare with recurrent dialysis for renal disease.

Impaired coagulation

This is a danger in all liver transplants, particularly marked in patients with severe parenchymatous hepatic disease with jaundice. There is likely to be a defect of all clotting factors. Patients may be thrombocytopenic before operation, but if there has been operative haemorrhage, thrombocytopenia after replacement of blood may be very severe. It is essential to pay scrupulous attention to haemostasis throughout the operation. It may be advisable prior to surgery to give fresh frozen plasma and fresh blood. If there is a shortage of fresh blood during surgery we use banked blood, and at the end of surgery try to give fresh blood together with human fibrinogen. In some cases ε-aminocaproic acid has also been given. If the transplant perfuses well on restoration of the blood supply and there is good initial hepatic function, the bleeding tendency stops very quickly. In one of our cases with an accessory graft, in which the liver had been an hour at 37°C without a blood supply before it was cooled, the ischaemic damage resulted in an uncontrollable haemorrhagic state and death of the patient the following day. A similar sequel occurred in a patient with an orthotopic liver transplant. This patient was hypotensive during surgery and the shocked state resulted in poor perfusion of the graft. Both of these patients suffered from severe cirrhosis.

Results

There have been a number of clinical liver transplants performed in a variety of institutions. Patients have survived for more than a year in Denver (Starzl *et al.*, 1969). Two patients are surviving in the United Kingdom five and six months after orthotopic liver transplantation. Both patients suffered from primary cancer of the liver, one in addition having severe cirrhosis, a porto-caval shunt performed for portal hypertension, and colonic exclusion for porto-systemic encephalopathy. Both these patients are at home leading normal lives (Calne and Williams, unpublished observations).

Transplantation of the Lung

The dangers of infection after lung transplantation have already been mentioned, but a number of attempts at clinical transplantation of the lung met with little success until a young man with crippling fibrosis of both lungs requiring continuous administration of oxygen received a lung transplant in Belgium. This patient is alive and well more than six months after operation (Derom *et al.*, 1969). Thus, in spite of the dangers of sepsis, this case illustrates that infection of a transplanted lung is not inevitable.

REFERENCES

BARNARD, C. N. (1967). *S. Afr. med. J.*, **41**, 1271.

CLEVELAND, R. J. & LOWER, R. R. (1967). *Transplantation*, **5**, 904.

DEROM, FR., BARBIER, F., RINGOIR, S., ROLLY, G., VERSIEK, J., BERZSENYI, G., RAEMDONCK, R. & PIRET, J. (1969). *Tijdschr. v. Geneeskunde*, 3, 109.

HARDY, J. D., CHAVEZ, C. M., ERASLAN, S., ADKINS, J. R. & WILLIAMS, R. D. (1966). *Surgery*, **60**, 361.

MOORE, F. D., BROWNELL WHEELER, E., DEMISSIANOS, V., SMITH, L. I., BALANKURA, O., ABEL, K., GREENBERG, J. B. & DAMMIN, G. H. (1960). *Ann. Surg.*, **152**, 374.

SHUMWAY, N. E., ANGELL, W. W. & WUERFLEIN, R. D. (1967). *Transplantation*, **5**, 900.

STARZL, T. E., MARCHIORO, T. L. & PORTER, K. A. (1967). Progress in Homotransplantation of the Liver. In *Advances in Surgery*, Vol. 2, ed. C. E. Welch. Chicago: Year Book Medical Publications.

STARZL, T. E., BRETTSCHNEIDER, L., PENN, I., BELL, P., GROTH, C. G., BLANCHARD, H., KASHIWAGI, N. & PUTNAM, C. W. (1969). *Transplantation*, **1**, 216.

TERBLANCHE, J. & RIDDELL, A. G. (1967). In *The Liver* (published by A. E. A. Read). London: Butterworth.

ETHICAL CONSIDERATIONS

A surgeon proposing to remove a healthy kidney from a living donor for the purpose of transplantation accepts a considerable moral responsibility It is a tribute to human nature that relatives and friends of a dying uraemic patient so often volunteer to donate one of their own healthy kidneys if there is even an infinitesimal chance of the transplant being successful. A surgeon can only assess probabilities of success of an operation. In most surgical decisions the probability of success has only to be considered in relation to the patient. In renal transplantation from a living donor the recipient's risks remain important, but it is even more difficult for the clinician to relate these to the dangers of unilateral nephrectomy in a healthy person despite every care in ensuring that both of the donor's kidneys are functioning efficiently. The risks of nephrectomy are small but not entirely negligible; there is also the possibility that disease may occur in the donor's remaining kidney.

There is no precedent in medical ethics to guide the surgeon in this extremely difficult decision. If there is good reason to expect success and the donor is both emotionally and physically suitable, then the clinician may feel that a transplant should be performed. However, to proceed with transplantation in a situation less satisfactory than this imposes an excessive moral responsibility on the surgeon.

The problem that arises with twins under the age of 21 years requires special consideration in the matter of whether or not a child can understand the significance of the decision to donate a kidney. A point made by the Boston group (Murray, 1962) was that the psychological trauma of losing a twin would more than offset the disadvantages of a nephrectomy.

There are three main disadvantages in the use of live donors. Already some patients who have donated kidneys have suffered from severe post-operative infections and hypotension, and one identical-twin donor has developed glomerulonephritis in the remaining kidney. If the use of live donors continues it is likely that there will be fatalities. The operation is more hazardous than a routine nephrectomy, since the renal vessels have to be extensively mobilized and divided near their junctions with the aorta and cava. The surgeon must also synchronize his operation with the procedure on the recipient. Secondly, direct and indirect pressures may be exerted on the donor by his relatives without the doctor's knowledge. The donor may agree reluctantly to give his kidney or may have a sense of guilt if he refuses. The development of a satisfactory system of tissue typing might result in a "reluctant best donor" which would provide the doctor with a very difficult problem: the main value of tissue typing would be to eliminate unsatisfactory donors. Finally, it is likely that money will be offered to potential kidney donors, a distasteful and dangerous prospect.

It must be said in favour of live donors that there should be little or no ischaemic damage to the transplanted kidney and function should be better, a view which is supported by present experience. Secondly, donors can be selected from close relatives and tissue typing performed so that bad donor/ recipient combinations are avoided.

Some clinicans feel that the use of live donors is fully justified, since it gives the sick patient the best possible chance. However, present long-term results leave much to be desired and are likely to be improved only by a reliable method of tissue typing. Even with identical twins, the long-term results have not been universally successful, since at least five transplants have developed the original disease from which the patient suffered.

Most workers would agree that transplantation of cadaver organs or of kidneys that need removal for the donor's benefit—so-called "free kidneys" —is justified. However, in the case of live donors it is only with close relatives that there is at present a reasonable prospect of modest success.

There are obvious practical difficulties in transplanting a cadaveric kidney before irreversible ischaemic damage has occurred, but these are difficulties involving the goodwill of individuals and the law—and are therefore soluble. Even more susceptible to ischaemic damage than the kidney are the heart and liver, but it is possible to get excellent functioning organs following transplantation when they have been removed after traditional methods of diagnosis of death.

Much has been written concerning the removal of organs from cadaver donors, and genuine points of concern have often been distorted and exaggerated. In a civilized community most people would prefer their organs after death to help somebody else who is suffering rather than the traditional alternatives of burial or cremation. There are two prerequisites governing such a charitable donation; one, that in their last illness they will be given every possible care and there will be no modification of management in order to obtain an organ for transplantation and two, that death will have occurred beyond doubt and irreversibly. Both these points really require trust in the integrity of the profession. It is important that those looking after the dying person are not involved in the transplantation operation. The usual result of considering a patient a potential organ donor is to increase rather than decrease the efforts to save the patient. I feel that the diagnosis of death should remain absence of circulation and spontaneous respiration, since this is the traditionally accepted method of establishing death and is understood by the medical profession and laity. Moreover, it is not necessary to interfere with this definition in order to obtain organs which are suitable for transplantation. It is most important not to confuse the diagnosis of death and its relationship to removal of donor organs with the factors involved in the decision to stop resuscitative measures, in particular artificial ventilation. This decision has been taken independent of transplantation, and it depends on the diagnosis of death of the brain. It can do no good to the patient and can cause great distress to the relatives to continue mechanical ventilation in a patient who is dead. There is, however, the important safeguard if there is any chance of a mistake having been made, that when the respirator is turned cff the patient will respire spontaneously. When the decision to stop resuscitation has been made, however, this information should be made available to the transplantation team so that they can be ready to remove the organs immediately after death.

REFERENCE

MURRAY, J. E. (1962). Personal communication.

THE PRESENT POSITION

Already, patients who would otherwise be dead have survived more than a year with heart and liver transplants and more than six months with a lung transplant. There can be no doubt that advances will continue and results will improve in the transplantation of these organs. At present, however, the value of renal transplantation is fully established.

Of the 2000 to 3000 young people who die each year in England and Wales from irreversible kidney disease only 10 per cent are offered treatment in the form of transplantation or dialysis. This is a tragedy, since these two forms of treatment can restore a majority of patients to a healthy and happy existence. The reasons are complicated, but those who would argue that this country is not wealthy enough to provide treatment have a weak case, since the provision of a hospital bed at £50 a week for a patient dying of uraemia is far less economical than a kidney transplant, which can restore him to the community as a breadwinner. The cost of both transplantation and recurrent dialysis is decreasing and will continue to do so in the future. The Department of Health is in the process of establishing 25 dialysis units, each capable of treating 30 patients in the unit and of training a variable number of people for home dialysis. At the same time, renal transplantation units are being established to work in collaboration with these dialysis units, since it is now realized that the two procedures are inextricably linked and collaboration between them can treat the largest number of patients satisfactorily.

Tissue-typing facilities are improving, and there is a direct correlation of a good tissue match with the behaviour of the transplant. It is likely in the future that transplantation will be considered unethical if the match between prospective donor and recipient is shown to be poor.

A national health service should provide the best available treatment to all patients in need, but efforts to provide therapy for the large number of people who require it are doomed to failure unless there is a definite change in the attitude of the public and, even more so, the profession towards the provision of donor kidneys. The personal tragedies of those denied treatment are not fully appreciated by those who work outside dialysis and transplantation units, since they do not come into close contact with the patients and their relatives who know that treatment could be made available.

Permission and the Law

In order to be useful for transplantation, a kidney must be removed and cooled within one hour of death. Before a surgeon can remove an organ from a cadaver it is necessary—according to the present Human Tissue Act (1961)—for him to obtain permission from the relatives, unless the donor had stated in his lifetime that he wished his organs to be transplanted after death. If the donor has given permission it is not necessary to ask the relatives, though obviously they would be consulted if available. If the patient is in a terminal condition and it is clear to the relatives that the prognosis is hopeless—in spite of his receiving all possible care—then they may be approached and asked if they would give permission for removal of kidneys for transplantation after death.

According to the Human Tissue Act (1961), before organs can be removed from a cadaver it is necessary for the doctor to make "such reasonable enquiry as may be practicable" that neither the deceased nor his relatives would have objected. "Such reasonable enquiry as may be practicable" has not been clearly defined. There is only one hour after death in which to remove the kidney, so enquiries can be made only during that hour if the kidneys are to be used. The relatives are also not defined. In practice, the next of kin would seem to be the most suitable person to approach.

Many suitable donors die from causes that make them coroner's cases; therefore in addition to the relative's permission for removal of organs it is necessary to have the coroner's consent as well. The coroner alone, however, cannot give permission for organs to be removed from the body in a coroner's case, nor can organs be removed from such a body unless the coroner is agreeable; thus the coroner can forbid the removal of organs from the body.

A coroner will withhold permission if he believes that removal of organs for transplantation will interfere with his statutory duty in investigating the nature of death. Many coroners now adopt an enlightened view so as to help transplantation, which is quite possible without any interference with his duties. The coroner depends on his appointed pathologist for the necropsy report, and if the surgeon removing the organs is in contact with the pathologist then any abnormality in the organs or in the abdominal cavity will be reported to the coroner's pathologist. Of course, if the organs themselves are diseased they will not be used for transplantation. If there is any doubt, the coroner's pathologist is directly consulted.

The law is unsatisfactory, since seeking permission from the relatives who have suddenly been bereaved—particularly in the case of accidents—can cause a great deal of unnecessary distress. Moreover, in such cases there will probably be a coroner's necropsy, which is scarcely ever objected to by relatives, and objections can be overruled by the coroner. A change in the law on the lines of those recently passed in Denmark, Sweden and France is urgently required. It would be a great help in the development of transplantation if permission were automatically assumed to have been given unless active objection had been made. Safeguards would be needed so that those who do not wish their organs to be used for transplantation after death could register an objection on their own behalf and also on behalf of their children. A "contracting out" procedure on these lines would be preferable to the present "contracting in" system. Safeguards could be arranged as follows: (1) a central computer would be programmed with information of all those who objected to their organs being removed after death; this could be telephoned at any time of the day or night by the hospital; and (2) objectors could carry a card stating their views. It would still be helpful if those who actively wished their organs to be used for transplantation would carry a card stating this wish and also record their names on the computer.

Most people dying in hospital are unsuitable as organ donors because of disseminated malignancy, systemic sepsis, hypertension or renal tract disease. The most suitable cases are those of primary cerebral tumours which do not metastasize outside the skull; head injuries; cerebral haemorrhage; and myocardial infarction. The age of the donor does not seem to matter, although infant kidneys do not do well in adults. Despite the slight deterioration of renal function in old age, we have nevertheless used kidneys from donors in their seventies which have functioned satisfactorily in young recipients.

If blood is taken from the potential donor for any purpose before death, an aliquot should be sent for red cell grouping and tissue typing. Alternatively, blood can be removed immediately after death from the femoral vein or by cardiac puncture. Tissue typing takes two to three hours, but this can be done while the kidney is being removed and preserved. Since the value of tissue typing has been clearly shown and the techniques are rapidly improving, the best use of available donors to treat the maximum number of recipients and to have a good match in every case depends on collaboration between doctors covering very large densities of population. So far as the United Kingdom is concerned this will probably mean collaboration within the whole of Northern Europe.

ACKNOWLEDGEMENT

Some of the material in this article has been published by Edward Arnold (*Renal Transplantation*, 1963, R. Y. Calne). The author is grateful to Edward Arnold, Ltd, for their permission to make use of here.

13 Medical Uses of Computers

E. G. KNOX

WHAT IS A COMPUTER?

THE use of machines for calculating is not new. The etymology of the word
"calculation" reflects the original use of pebbles, and it is still a colloquialism
that we "cast up" numbers. The shop and the bank have their "counters"
where the pebbles (or coins) were cast and we still receive our change by
complementary addition, a method which uses the coins themselves as the
calculating device rather than depending upon mental arithmetic. The
scope of pebble and bead mathematics is not limited to marketing and
exchange; the Romans were successful engineers and quantity surveyors
despite a numerical notation quite unsuited to written arithmetic. We do
not need to look at a Roman abacus to know how they were used, nor to infer
what symbols were engraved at the ends of the rods or slots.

The early monopoly of pebble/bead/finger arithmetic was disturbed by
Napier's invention of the slide rule in the seventeenth century. This device
invoked two entirely new principles; first it used the addition of logarithms
in order to achieve one-step multiplication; secondly it depended upon the
use of a continuously variable attribute, length, to represent the logarithms.
The use of a continuous attribute rather than a discontinuous one such as a
pebble or a finger is the more important principle from our present point of
view, because it is the basis of the distinction between analogue computers,
which may use for their operations a variety of continuous attributes such
as resistances and capacitances, and digital computers whose operations
are based on counting.

A second disturbance in the development of arithmetic was the adaptation
of pen and paper from their primary, alphabetical tasks, but the upset is
more apparent than real. In fact, exactly as with the abacus, the basic operations of paper and pencil arithmetic are done mentally. The intermediate
and final results are simply *recorded* on the device, and the record is digital.

P

Pencil and paper methods may be seen as an extension of the abacus. The invention of the mechanical and electromechanical desk calculator added the wheel and the cog to the armamentarium of the rod and bead, the pebble, the finger, the pen and paper, and re-emphasized the dominance of digital methods.

The electric calculator introduced another technical departure. With all previous devices there was the clear distinction that the steps in the calculation were carried out in the mind of the calculator, that the device was operated according to rules held in his mind, and that the function of the device itself was purely to display intermediate and final results. The desk machine, and particularly the automatic electric machine, took upon itself the operation of some of the rules so that the person using the machine could institute a string of operations such as those involved in "multiplying" simply by pressing a button. The logical steps of such operations were specified by the mechanical arrangements within the machine. Despite this advance, most practical jobs still consisted of a *sequence* of operations, and the choice of sequence was decided, step by step, by the person operating the machine.

By contrast, the essence of a computer is that the machine controls the sequence of its own operations and is no longer (only) a device for registering the intermediate results of operations selected one at a time by its operator. It is still true that the operations are chosen and sequenced by human beings, but the entire sequence must be specified before it is started. The sequence is coded, entered into the machine and stored, and the first instruction is not obeyed until the last one has been inserted. The sequence of coded instructions is called a program, and the unique characteristic of a computer is that it is a "stored program" machine.

Although program storage is, as it were, the defining characteristic of a computer, there are four additional characteristics of great importance from the users' point of view.

The first is the high speed of operation. Computations are carried out by electronic switching circuits with no moving parts, and both the program and the data may be stored by reversing the magnetic polarity of other non-moving devices such as ferrite rings and thin films of magnetic material. Moving devices such as magnetic tape, magnetic discs and magnetic drums are also used. The non-moving devices are inertia-free, and the only limits to their switching speeds are their magnetic and electronic characteristics and the lengths of their electrical connections; operations using these devices are usually timed in microseconds (10^{-6} seconds) or even in tens and hundreds of nanoseconds (one nanosecond = 10^{-9} seconds, the time taken for light to travel one foot). Even the moving devices can transfer information at some tens of thousands of characters per second; access times to different parts of the device are more time-consuming, but high-speed drums and discs can achieve this in a few milliseconds, or some tens of milliseconds. Magnetic tapes on the other hand may take many seconds.

Data input devices such as paper-tape and punch-card readers, and data output devices such as line-printers are relatively slow, and punched tape and typewriter outputs very slow indeed by comparison. An automatic typewriter may print only ten characters per second. The range of speeds covered by these various devices is extremely wide, and a well-organized computer can intercalate a great deal of computing between the movements of its mechanical devices; a badly organized computer may be standing idle most of the time. In terms of programs, it may help to remember that speed of execution within the central processor is such that a rifle bullet may (figuratively) pursue a program down the written page and fail to overtake the point of action.

The second additional consideration is reliability. Despite the jokes about "them" computers are remarkably reliable. In practice they seldom complete a job that contains errors of operation. There may be logical errors in the program and occasionally a run may fail altogether (usually one of the inertial devices) and need to be re-run, but repeated operation of proved programs using correct data will almost always produce results containing no errors whatsoever. The error-free nature of the results is in marked contrast to almost any other form of processing information. Error saving, like time saving, is one of the main benefits of computer usage.

The third ancillary attribute is versatility. The operations of a computer are not limited to numerical operations; they operate on symbolic information of all kinds, including numbers, letters, and punctuation. Furthermore, the computer can carry out all the manipulations that are in fact logically possible. This is a large enough claim to be repeated. The computer can do with symbolic data anything which logically can be done. In less pretentious terms, however, it performs reading, writing, arithmetic and sequential logic, and it can do anything that can be specified.

The fourth ancillary consideration of a computer is its cost. Computers are very expensive. They range from about £10,000 for the smallest to about £2,000,000 for the largest; most computers for medical applications are in the range of £60,000 to £600,000. Ancillary equipment is required in addition, and staffing, maintenance, running and accommodation costs are also high. The cost in man-years of developing individual projects is often formidable, and the total expenditure on a large hospital information system during its developmental stage (e.g. the first five years) may be around £1,000,000.

To summarize, the scope of a computer is information processing; its benefits are in terms of time saving, error saving, reliability and consistency; its costs are high; it is so versatile that it can do whatever can be done with data.

Its applications to medical service and research problems must therefore be determined not so much in terms of what *can* be done but rather in terms of what *should* be done. Its overall problems are policy problems, and the decisions required are decisions about priorities. This is a point to which we shall return.

PROGRAMMING LANGUAGES

The essential fact of computing is the stored program, and before it can be read and stored by the machine it must be written, coded and prepared by a programmer. This process involves the use of two corresponding codes, the first usually a pattern of holes in cards or paper tape to be read photo-electrically by the machine, and the second a set of printed characters to be understood by the programmer. When cards are used, the printing is placed along the top edge of the card; when paper tape is used, an automatic typewriter prints the corresponding text on a separate piece of paper.

A program is a sequence of coded instructions or "statements" and each statement has a structure grammatically analogous to a sentence, with a "verb"—written in the imperative mood—and often a subject, object or indirect object or adverb. The verb, in this context, is the "operator" of a statement and the other items are "operands". Early and primitive codes were usually numeric, represented for example as a sequence of octal (nought to eight) numbers, and the internal binary patterns generated by these characters were very directly related to the elementary logical switching and addressing operations carried out electronically inside the processor.

Numerical codes such as these had stringent format requirements and were difficult to write, and manufacturers began to supply mnemonic codes both for internal addresses and for operations. The mnemonics were translated by the machine itself into "Machine Code" before they were implemented. These mnemonic languages are usually known as "User Codes" or "Assembly Languages". A further advance was made by breaking the 1 : 1 correspondence between the steps of the User Code and the Machine Code program and by constructing "Autocodes" in which one instruction could represent a more or less lengthy string of Machine Code instructions. These systems permitted a moderately complicated arithmetic operation to be expressed in a single statement instead of many, including such processes as square roots and trigonometrical conversions.

However, although the Autocodes of different machines were often related to each other, and could even be grouped into families, they offered no facility for developing a program on one kind of machine and using it on another. This requirement led to the development of "higher languages".

A "higher language" is intended in part to extend the programmer's power to specify complicated sequences in a few well-chosen symbols, as well as to achieve a form of coding capable of translation by any computer into its own individual machine code. That none has succeeded uniquely is supported by the fact that there are now dozens, if not hundreds, of such languages and translation systems. However, three languages in particular have dominated this field, namely FORTRAN, ALGOL and COBOL.

FORTRAN (FORmula TRANslation) is an American invention and is usually prepared on punch-cards. It is firmly based on the principles of reading, writing and arithmetic and it has been the most widely used of the higher languages. There is an early version called FORTRAN II and a later one called FORTRAN IV. It is a pragmatic and moderately powerful language and extremely effective for many applications. The example which follows is almost self-explanatory:

```
       PI = 3.14159
22     READ (1,20) RADIUS
20     FORMAT (F10.0)
           IF (RADIUS.LT.0.0) STOP
           VOLUME = 4./3. *PI* RADIUS **3
           WRITE (3,21) VOLUME
21     FORMAT (F15.2)
       GOTO 22
       END
```

ALGOL (ALGOrithmic Language) is a European invention. It is often prepared on paper tape and its text written in both upper and lower case. It is based on an exact grammatical analysis of the structure and syntax of mathematical (especially) and data processing operations. It is designed to stand alone as a means of expressing manipulative procedures quite apart from its use as a computer language. It is extremmly powerful in these respects and in appropriate circumstances can accomplish in a few statements what FORTRAN achieves in many, although for simpler uses there may be little to choose between them.

An example follows:

```
          begin real pi, radius, volume;
          pi: = 3·14159;
again:    radius: = read (tape reader);
          if radius < 0·0 then goto stop;
          volume: = 4/3 × pi × radius ↑3;
          write (printer, layout [a], volume);
          goto again;
stop:     end;
```

COBOL (COmmon Business Orientated Language) is usually punched into cards, and it includes essentially the FORTRAN range of arithmetic capabilities within itself. It is more "wordy" in this respect but certainly not more powerful, and it uses ADD, MULTIPLY and DIVIDE instead of +, * and /. Its main characteristic is its capability for defining file structures on magnetic storage devices and for storing records upon the files and retrieving them. It has proved the most difficult of the higher languages to implement, has not achieved a generality which adequately overcomes the variability of the filing devices used on different equipments and it is usually very time-consuming in translation. Many computer companies have eschewed it and have offered alternative "list processing languages". The special applications of COBOL and its fellows are in large-scale relatively simple file operations where the operations need to be declared explicitly and intelligibly in the language in which they are programmed.

All the higher languages incur penalties on their users in terms of machine size required, speed of operation, limits and constraints upon layout of files and results, and so on, and the "higher" and "more general" language the greater penalty. For simple jobs repeated many times, as in some commercial applications, the price may be too high. For scientific work, where a large effort of development may result in only a few runs, or in the developmental trial-and-error periods of service applications, and in any situation where generality or an early result is required, or where a detailed and explicit specification of the operation is necessary, they have much to offer.

DATA

Within the ferrite ring core-store, the processor, and the magnetic storage devices of any digital computer the data are arranged as a pattern of BITS (Binary digITS) held either in the "off" or "on" state. The bits are arranged in sets. In some computers the primary arrangement is in "characters" of six bits and the characters themselves are arranged into "words", e.g. five characters to hold an integer or ten to hold a number with a decimal point. In other machines the primary arrangement is into words of fixed length (12, or 24, or 48 bits), with the option of dividing the word into six-bit characters, half-words or other arrangements. Other machines use the "byte" which consists of eight bits and can be used either to store two numeric digits in the range 0–9 at four bits each, or a single alphabetic or punctuation character. These various arrangements offer marginal advantages or disadvantages according to the application. From the users' point of view, particularly if higher languages are employed, the internal arrangements may largely be ignored.

Data-forms for input and output, however, may not be ignored, and they are a major consideration of almost all medical data handling systems. In most applications the data presented to the machine must be prepared in character form either on paper tape or on cards. The use of paper tape or of cards for the program imposes no fundamental restriction on the form used for the data, but in practice special arrangements may have to be made to handle paper tape with FORTRAN or to handle cards with paper-tape ALGOL, and some equipment configurations, for reasons of cost, possess only one form of input.

However, the punched data are not necessarily produced by hand and digital conversions of voltage-data (e.g. electrocardiograms) may be achieved by various forms of "black box". Analogue-digital-converters (ADC devices) may work in a variety of ways. In one the input voltage is applied across a previously discharged condenser which "fills" exponentially at a rate which depends upon the voltage. The time taken is measured by switching at "full" to interrupt an electronic clock; the interrupted count is switched to a paper tape punch. The speed of a paper tape punch (e.g. 100 characters per second) limits the sampling frequency and other methods record the digital conversion to magnetic tape. Some computer configurations contain their own analogue-digital-converters and can accept varying voltage inputs directly. This is known as an on-line as opposed to an off-line system.

Most data outputs from a computer are provided in character form, and the most used device for accomplishing this is the line-printer. It is an ingenious and even improbable device in which a horizontal metal strip with an embossed set of characters moves from side to side across a paper sheet which is advanced line by line. A set of about 120 small hammers is provided, one for each print-column on the paper. The paper, the metal strip and the ink ribbon are struck together by the hammers at the precise moment when a desired character on the strip passes over a desired position on the paper. Other methods use a rotating barrel of characters instead of a strip. Speeds vary between about 100 and 1000 lines per minute. These devices are sufficiently fast to be connected on-line, although some computers operate several simultaneously. Alternative and slower forms of output are paper tape and punched cards to be used either as data storage devices, or for operating an automatic off-line typewriter. Another form of character output is the on-line tele-typewriter and another is the cathode ray (CR) oscilloscope. The "incremental graph plotter" is a useful device for non-character outputs and it draws graphs and figures using a continuous line. It may be used either on-line, or off-line through the medium of punched paper tape or magnetic tape. Oscilloscopes can also be used to present graphical results.

Despite the flexibility of computer programming methods, the operations themselves are exactly deterministic and the data specifications of a program are usually quite stringent. If errors are anticipated, they may be allowed for in the program, but it is often very difficult to correct them during the run without interrupting it. At the lowest operational level most binary character codes carry a redundant "bit" arranged so that each character is at least two bit-errors removed from every other character. Thus a single error in bit-transmission at any stage of preparing or manipulating data will result in an illegal character which stops or diverts the operation; this is known as a parity check.

At another level, the interpretation of characters and character sets often depends on their physical position on a card or disc, or on a sequence position on a paper or magnetic tape, so that a dropped duplicated or displaced character or "space" may lead to catastrophic errors. These errors may be detected fortuitously, as when the last letter of the surname is interpreted as the first number of the date of birth and subsequently defies an arithmetic instruction, but not all errors are so readily detected. Some may be found by mechanical "validation" systems in the data preparation process, and others by making exhaustive programming checks on the data after acceptance and before processing, but errors such as spelling mistakes and the inversion of the month and day of birth on a written document, which might be detected or suspected on a visual inspection, may slip without question through the most sophisticated syntactical analysis. The result may be that an identity is not recognized, but it may also be recognized incorrectly; a record may hold a valid identifier but not that of the patient for whom it was intended.

The main source of this kind of error is human intervention, particularly in copying, and for any system where uniform accuracy is essential it is necessary to eliminate these operations. If we use machines to handle information we have no option but to engineer levels of accuracy very much greater than those traditionally acceptable and commonly achieved.

OPERATING SYSTEMS

A computer which handles some hundreds of testing and production jobs each day in several languages must have an overall "master-system" for handling the variety of work which it may be offered. The combination of the master system, the "compilers" for translating higher languages, and the set of subroutines used in common by all languages are known collectively as the "software" of the computer. In practice the production of efficient and error-free software is a very exacting and difficult task, and it is as expensive to produce as the hardware. When the delivery of a new computer is delayed or its initial application unsatisfactory it is almost always a software problem which holds it up.

The art of compiler writing and the necessary investment have greatly improved in recent years. Although there are still some difficulties in providing error-free compilers for new machines, most programs can now be made to work. However, computer software facilities have recently been forced to expand greatly with the advent of time-sharing techniques, that is, methods for handling several jobs simultaneously. The difficulties of providing adequate and efficient systems for these purposes have reduced the question of compilers almost to a secondary consideration.

The development of higher languages depended largely on the increasing speed and power of computers and on a shifting "break-even" assessment as between the cost of programming time and running time. Continued improvement in power-for-cost and the need to accommodate applications which cannot wait in a queue for a day or a minute, have led to the development of clock-controlled switching systems inside a computer which divert its attention from one job to another, perhaps using different terminals in different places. A high priority terminal may be scanned every few seconds or milliseconds and the current job interrupted and postponed if the terminal comes into use. The interruption may be for a few milliseconds or microseconds while the computer responds, the previous job then progressing until the next interruption. Such a system may accommodate many terminals and give the appearance of simultaneity whilst at the same time carrying out "background" jobs inserted at the computer centre in conventional "batch" modes. These techniques are referred to as "time-sharing", and terminals with all-the-time access and short-time responses are described as "on line real time". Of course, on line real time usage may be achieved without the use of time-sharing by dedicating a small computer to a single job. Also, time-sharing methods may be used without the use of remote real time terminals and a suitable mix of file handling and arithmetical computation can proceed together with little interference of one job upon another.

Time-sharing systems are not yet fully satisfactory, and in most cases are inefficient. Most of the computing power may be used in maintaining the scanning and general housekeeping of the system rather than in running the jobs themselves. Indeed, improved efficiency will probably prove critical in determing the costs and priorities of their application.

SCIENTIFIC USES

The proper medical uses of such a versatile machine require some classification, if only to introduce some order into their arrangement. It is proposed here to do this under two general descriptive headings, *scientific* and *service*. The more customary division into *scientific* and *commercial* is rejected because it represents an outdated view of science as based essentially on numbers and arithmetic, and an equally limited view of business method as a matter only of files and accounts. In medical contexts, at any rate, the first classification is to be preferred and it is specifically a taxonomy of usages rather than of hardware or programming methods or computing careers.

It should not, however, be interpreted too rigidly because medical research, like research in any applied science, ranges from basic enquiries with no currently foreseeable application to those that are only a single step from service usage and might properly be called "developmental".

The scientific uses themselves are re-classified according to their method into "reduction" and "simulation" techniques. In the first kind we begin with data and compute a *derived* result. In the second, the approach is reversed and both the initial premises and the computational method are adjusted to produce outputs comparable to an *observed* result. In the first approach the answer to the problem is the result of the computation. In the second it consists of the method and the premises which have successfully mimicked the real situation.

Reduction Methods

Mathematical computations

The reasons for using a computer for arithmetic operations are to save time and error. The effort of developing a program for these purposes is justified either when individual calculations are lengthy and difficult, or when simple calculations are to be done frequently.

The latter situation may be met in *transforming* single values: the conversion of optical percentage transmittance to optical density, times to velocities, voltages to concentrations, test scores to IQs, point heights on spectographic traces to mg/litre, and an indefinite range of multiplication, division and linearization procedures. When digitization of instrumental results is automatic, as through an ADC device to punched paper tape, there can be considerable savings in the complexity and cost of the apparatus (e.g. a colorimeter), since calibration and linearization may be carried out in the computer instead of through the circuitry or the mechanical arrangements of the instrument.

Simple arithmetic procedures involving the reduction of more than one input variable may also be frequently repeated. Thus, dates of birth and dates of admission are converted to ages, dates of admission and discharge to duration of admission, types and quantities of food to calories, protein and carbohydrate, the dimensions of complex shapes to volumes and surface areas, combinations of clinical and biochemical findings to differential diagnosis probabilities, electrolyte levels to electrolyte requirements, radiographic co-ordinates to cardiac volumes, sequential spirometric readings to respiratory function parameters, isotope-tag readings to median cell survivals.

More complex reduction procedures are justified even when few in number. The more complicated diffusion-equilibrium equations may be classified here; also genetic linkage calculations and any problems the solutions of which depend on multiple simultaneous equations, summations of series, or integration procedures. The latter is particularly true when the integration problem is insoluble, or when the user himself cannot solve it through ordinary integral calculus. Contrary to the popular image of computer mathematical usages, it is the *non*-mathematician who may be especially assisted; he is all too likely to discover the difficult way of reaching an adequate answer, and the power of the machine may be used to overcome his lack of finesse. Integration is carried out literally by adding together a large series of very small parts. Integrations may normally be carried out mechanically in some instruments, or through special circuitry, and again there is a real possibility of savings through using the computer. Differentiation procedures may also be carried out, including those specialized forms subsumed under the term "Fourier Analysis". This is a way of analysing complex wave forms such as Electroencephalograms into spectral densities. In more than one dimension it is used to convert crystallographic interferograms into electron densities and molecular structures.

Another use of the computer is in solving the value of a variable in an equation where it has not proved possible to manipulate it so that it is on the left hand side and everything else on the right. Here one must use an iteration method, trying repeatedly with different values until the true values are found. Maximization and minimization problems may be classified here. For example, a molecular structural problem on a distended cell surface may demand a statement of the maximum area that can be covered by a complex network of linked geometrical shapes, the lengths of whose sides may be declared but whose angles may be varied.

We must include within the scope of computer mathematical manipulations not only the arithmetic and algebra of numbers but also that pertaining to "logical" or "boolean" values. Indeed, most computer programs are a mixture of arithmetic and boolean operations. Just as a number-variable, x, can "contain" any number, so a boolean variable, b, can contain any boolean value. However, there are only two boolean values, namely *true* and *false*. Just as different numbers can be manipulated through the use of arithmetic operators, $-$, $+$, $\times$, $/$, so the logical variables can be manipulated by their own appropriate operators, *and, or, not*. It is not appropriate here to digress into a discussion of boolean algebra, but it is clear that these operations are necessary to all iteration procedures including the study of pattern-syntaxes and pattern-matching computations. These are relevant in the study of chromosomes, cytological patterns, ECGs, DNA and RNA code studies, protein amino-acid-sequence analyses, and studies of the relationship between pharmacological activities and the three-dimensional structural patterns of drugs. Although the individual steps of boolean operations are simple, the structure of the full sequence in analyses such as these can be extremely complicated, so that a computer implementation is the only practical way of performing them.

For the general range of mathematical computations carried out in scientific work much of the programming has already been done. Most computing laboratories handling such work carry a library of programs, or at least of subroutines which can constitute the major part of the program. There are also several libraries and indexes open to wider access. The simpler functions, such as trigonometrical conversions, logs, and square roots, are of course intrinsic to FORTRAN, ALGOL and similar programming languages.

Statistical analysis

All statistical tests and reductions based upon tabular material are readily carried out on a computer. This includes sums, means, percentages, standard deviations, standard errors, percentiles, regression coefficients and equations, chi-square, t-test and analysis of variance. The programs are easily written and in any case can be found in many subroutine libraries. When a computer is easily to hand the need for a sophisticated desk machine is greatly reduced.

However, the particular advantage of a computer in such work is that as well as carrying out calculations upon tables, it can also prepare the tables, avoiding the need for card operations on a counter-sorter, with their relative mechanical unreliability. Hand copying and typing errors are also eliminated. The computer performs the statistical calculations on the data *prior* to tabulation, thus avoiding the loss of information inherent in the classification of values for purposes of their entry to the rows and columns of the table.

Technically, the development of satisfactory systems of preparing files of statistical material and preparing tabulations from the files has proved a much more difficult task than the programming of statistical arithmetic. It is not too difficult to write a program for a specific job, but it is hard to write a generalized program for a library and one which is suitable for the majority of jobs. Extended options of data format and of table size must be provided, and a flexible choice of row and column definitions, together with labelling and title facilities. Quite complicated preliminary transformations of single variables may be required by a user before they are tabulated, and he may also require arithmetic procedures upon combinations of variables (e.g. $3\sqrt{\text{weight/height}}$), and complex logical decisions may be required in order to decide whether a case is entered into a table in the first place (e.g. "include the boys only, exclude the twins, or if dead before 15, or if IQ not recorded"). It is necessary also to cope simultaneously with qualitative and quantitative variables in different combinations.

In fact, a number of generalized survey programs have been written.

None is so widely used as to have dominated all others, none is perfect or completely general, and most require large machines. It is more practical currently to generalize statistical programming systems at the level of providing "subroutines" in the higher languages rather than whole programs. A limited amount of additional programming is necessary to assemble a selection of subroutines appropriate to a particular job.

Computer usage in statistical analysis permits the carrying out of large scale calculations which previously would not have been practicable or would have required very stringent justification. Notably this has included multiple regression analyses in which an equation is derived, in the form below, for detecting the best way in which one of the variables (y) can be predicted in terms of weighted sums of a large number of others (x_1 to x_n).

$$y = a + b_1x_1 + b_2x_2 \ldots + b_nx_n.$$

Unfortunately, the computer provides the capacity to shoot first and ask questions afterwards and this carries the corollary that the questions may not be asked at all; misinterpreted results of such analyses have resulted in widespread expressions of regret that the computer was used in the first place. The technique of analysis known as "numerical taxonomy" is another method made possible because of computers and is therefore widely accessible to misuse. With both techniques it is difficult to assess their value either as general methods or in particular usages except against an appreciation of their nature. We shall return to this later in considering "simulation methods".

As well as constructing files from individual records, and scanning files to construct tabulations and statistical summaries, the computer can also assist in the construction of the records themselves. One way of doing this is through a direct link with a data-acquisition system such as an ADC device or a typewriter tele-terminal, but in a statistical context we are concerned more particularly with the construction of large records from smaller—the method subsumed under the heading of "record linkage". This is achieved by comparing pairs of records in the same file or in different files to determine "matches" and "non-matches" in terms of labels such as surnames, dates of birth, mothers' maiden names, or index numbers (Acheson, 1967, 1968).

Record linkage operations carried out between different files may be used to link obstetric records with those of later school performance, hospital discharges with notifications of death to the Medical Officer of Health, registration of cancer diagnosis with the Registrar General's file of Death Certificates, infant risk-registers with lists of children in schools for the physically and mentally handicapped, and maternity records with files of drug prescriptions. There are usually problems of different record-formats and incompatible recording media, and high rates of error in hand-prepared records. There may be non-standardized identity labels and a massive data-preparation task to be undertaken, together with difficult logical syntax analysis problems to identify "near miss" identity matches. However, with suitable investment time and ingenuity, massive linkage operations of these kinds have been undertaken that would have been quite impossible without a computer.

Record linkages within single files are usually less massive operations. They can be very simple indeed, and a set of laboratory reports, stored in daily sequence, can be re-sorted into order according to the patients' registration numbers so that all records of each patient are in juxtaposition. Secondary sorting in order of dates will arrange each patient's reports in correct order. Sorting procedures are well worked out in programming terms, and for most machines they are supplied by the manufacturer. Their efficiency depends upon the configuration, notably the number of magnetic tape decks if sorting is done on tapes, and the provision or non-provision of random-access devices such as discs or drums, which make sorting a relatively rapid procedure. Linkage *between* files is also carried out in this way, the files being merged and interleaved after they have both been sorted, or they may be mixed first and sorted later.

In applications where retrieval of a linked set is required within a response time too short for a sorting operation, the problem is more difficult. It is met in the maintenance and analysis of "live" files in hospital laboratory systems, where time-sequenced records are required at intervals in order to calculate the accuracy and performance of the laboratory itself, and where patient-sequenced records are required at short notice for clinical purposes. One of the two purposes must be met by a lengthy search, the file held in duplicate in two different orders, or a complex cross-reference system maintained at each addition of a new item.

In other situations complexity arises because the linkage system is branched rather than consisting of simple pairs and chains. This problem is met in genetic studies where each person's record contains the identity of his mother and father. Matings are then recognized by the parental declarations, sibship pairs by common parentage. By extension the whole complex of relationships can be discovered and either printed out, recorded permanently in augmented internal records, or simply pursued step by step on each occasion that it becomes necessary to identify a particular relationship. Thus it is possible to seek and identify all cousin-cousin pairs, or all uncle-niece pairs, or granddaughter-paternal-grandfather pairs. Pair-studies are not limited to genetic analyses and have been used also to examine immunization sequences in rhesus haemolytic disease (Knox, 1964) and the effects upon intelligence of position in family. Some analyses of these kinds can involve the systematic matching of enormous numbers of pairs of records. Hundreds of computing hours may be used.

Record-pairing and record-chaining for individual patients also enables us to derive observations which could not have been made in either record alone. Notably this refers to clinical *events*, which may be defined as changes of clinical *states*. Some events are observed directly and recorded as events, but others are inferred because a change of specified degree has occurred between two records. The recognition of events in this way is a crucial step in the evaluation of progress of patients with chronic disease, the effectiveness of treatment, the detection of deviations from baseline assessments, and secondarily for the measurement of attack rates of diseases in large populations. These problems are met in therapeutic trials, in monitoring morbidity in populations, and in the development and evaluation of large-scale disease-control measures in populations, notably screening services.

Epidemiology

Epidemiological research in recent years has relied more and more on the statistical contingency method, tabulating one variable against another in order to find out what tends to go with what: smoking and cancer, radiation and leukaemia, pre-natal medication and malformation, analgesics and chronic nephritis, lack of exercise and coronary disease, atmospheric pollution and chronic bronchitis, asbestos dust exposure and mesothelioma, fluoride deficiency in water supplies and dental decay. The technical computing aspects of these approaches are statistical and have already been discussed.

However, other classes of epidemiological research are also concerned with the distribution of disease in space and time, although no longer exclusively preoccupied with infective processes. Time-based analyses depend for their interpretation on the detection of trends, cycles, or non-cyclical clusters. These features can be demonstrated with large numbers of events, either by a graphical or tabular display of material across a time-base; the technical problems are again those of statistical tabulations and tests. Paradoxically, smaller numbers of events occurring at low intensity make more serious technical demands and require more difficult logical decision-networks. This is particularly so when decision-making must be made currently and urgently (is this the beginning of an epidemic?) rather than at leisure and on completion of all the available data.

The demonstration of trends can depend upon linear regression calculations, various accumulating and differencing calculations, and upon different forms of graphical display, all standardized and corrected if necessary for changing population-size and age-structure. These methods are not absolutely dependent upon a computer, but it is very convenient if it is necessary to scan a moderate or large number of conditions in such a way (e.g. in Cancer Registry work), or if a smaller group of conditions is to be reassessed at regular intervals (e.g. congenital malformations). Cohort analysis presentations are also amenable to computer programming, and "survival studies" (e.g. between treatments) can be facilitated by automatic comparison of observed survivals and survivals expected on the basis of age/sex life-tables.

Cyclical variations may be tackled using Fourier techniques, which make no initial assumptions about the number of cycle components, nor about their phase registration, but a simpler approach is adequate for most epidemiological studies. Sets of dates can be converted to tabular or graphical presentations of distributions by season, phase of moon or day of week, or directly correlated with environmental factors such as temperature, humidity or rainfall. A range of positive and negative lag intervals can also be tested here. Tests of significance for tabulated results may also be computed if desired. If a suitable test does not exist, then *ad hoc* "Monte Carlo" methods may be devised. Monte-Carlo methods will be discussed under the heading of "simulation" techniques.

Irregular clustering of events is also susceptible to computer analysis using any of a number of available statistical methods; auto-correlation techniques and 'runs tests' examine for likeness of length of adjacent intervals, and a simple presentation in graphical form may be sufficient in many cases to indicate an aberration from an earlier pattern.

Spatial concentrations of events, corrected for population density, may be presented in tables, or as print-outs of maps with density shadings. For tests of distributions too finely variegated to use existing tabulations of population distribution it is possible to specify both the physical geographical features of the map and the disease events in terms of map references, and to derive from this a plot of distributions of nearest-proximities between different disease-groups and different map features. A set of distributions can be compared and aberrant patterns identified.

Finally, we must mention those epidemiological studies which must use the contingency time and space method in various combinations. Computer methods have been applied to the study of clusters jointly in space and time. When a disease produces a small cluster in one place at one time and in another place at another, the pattern in time over the area taken as a whole need not be remarkable. Yet the detailed pattern, if it can be demonstrated, may be of crucial importance to understanding the nature of the disease. Several methods of tackling this problem have been suggested. The simplest is a method which examines every possible pair of events in a series, calculating for each pair both the distance and time apart, and tests for a correlation between time and distance (Knox, 1964; Meighan and Knox, 1965) over the whole series of pairs. The arithmetic and manipulation of the permutations are considerable tasks. Other methods, such as testing for various lag-times between hypothetical contacts and various radii of effectiveness surrounding disease locations, are even more demanding on computer time, especially if a range of options is tested. The statistical significance of findings displayed by these techniques has also been a problem to which Monte-Carlo techniques have been applied.

Display techniques

Almost any experienced computer user will confirm that the most tangible benefits of automation come from its simplest applications. This has been enshrined in the declaration of the KISS principle (Keep It Stupid and Simple). One of the things the computer can do stupidly, simply and well is to display information (Healy, 1968). Humans on the other hand are very quick and accurate in performing a wide range of cognitive tasks related to patterns—the recognition of misspelt and variously spelt names, of faces, of inversion errors in numbers and dates. They not only mis-file records but trace them quickly when they are mis-filed. The onset of an epidemic, an urban-rural patchiness on a map distribution, a systematic gradient of prevalence across a geographical area, overlaid chromosomes in photographs, a combination of two abnormalities in one X-ray, a number-preference artefact in a set of laboratory investigations, a shifting mean duration of stay in a medical unit—all these are recognized quickly in a way which is not well understood and certainly not easy to program. The obvious conclusion is that we should use humans to perform the cognitive acts and the machines to display the results.

A continuous oscilloscope display of cardio-respiratory data of patients in intensive care units, displayed within sight of a supervisor, may be a quicker and more sensitive way of detecting changes—certainly of identifying them—than attempting to program the syntax of the wide range of possible changes in a computer program.

The displays more characteristically associated with preparation of data in a computer are those produced on a line printer or on automatic typewriters. The incremental graph plotter has not yet been used widely for these purposes in medicine: it is expensive in machine time and a fair graphical representation can be achieved on a printer. Developed techniques can produce histograms, frequency polygons and maps on an ordinary printer. The Cathode ray oscilloscope is another method of producing graphical displays, though many CR tubes are designed or programmed only for the display of character-information. The light pen is a device for indicating positions and features on the face of an oscilloscope so that selections can be made on the basis of a complex pattern-display, or so that alteration of the display can be achieved. It follows the principle of using a human being to perform the difficult-to-program cognitive acts of an iterative process. The light pen can also be used for manipulating character information, as can various touch wire devices applied to the face of the tube.

For the time being, however, the use of a light pen in the construction and modification of graphical displays must be regarded as a highly specialized device and, as yet, has not found many applications in medicine.

Simulation Methods

Pattern recognition

The general pragmatic rule that it is often better to display data in a recognizable pattern than it is to classify it is not always applicable. There are many circumstances where automatic classification would be useful if it were reliable, and where the technical problem of defining pattern recognition criteria seems surmountable.

One approach is to use some kind of formal analysis in a series of cases where the "true" classification is known on grounds other than those of the data being inspected. An example was a discriminant analysis carried out on amniotic fluid spectograms in rhesus-immunized women in order to find a reliable method of predicting intra-uterine death (Knox, Fairweather and Walker, 1965). This analysis suggested what intuitive analyses had failed to reveal, namely that almost all the predictive information of the spectograms was held in the optical density determinations at two specific wavelengths, and that if these were known consideration of the rest of the spectogram was at best futile and at worst confusing.

The alternative to a formal approach is to try to mimic a human being carrying out his cognitive process, and to write down in program form the steps (he thinks) he takes. We can call this the cybernetic approach, and it is at least as instructive in helping us understand how humans think they work as it is in defining the syntax of the pattern being investigated. The cybernetic approach is the one most frequently applied to the analysis of electrocardiograms. The cardiographer, guided by his knowledge of the physiological mechanisms of the normal and abnormal ECG, declares first how he recognizes single complexes, how he recognizes the parts within the complex, notes the shape and duration of the segments, and their variation between complexes, leads and patients. He describes the more frequent and obvious abnormalities and later the less frequent and less obvious. The programmer writes it all down (Pipberger, 1965).

It is some measure of the self-deception of a process such as this that a powerful computer will take much longer than a human cardiographer to analyse a trace, and as long to recognize a normal as an abnormal recording. There is also the unfortunate corollary that the best of programmers will produce a result less efficient than the cardiographer himself and cannot improve on his best performance. Indeed, we must expect that the translated method will be a good deal worse. Of course it will be more consistent, and it may be better than the cardiographer when not at his best or short of time, and it may be better than other cardiographers.

Another well-known application of the cybernetic method to pattern recognition is in the field of karyotype analyses of cell cultures halted in metaphase (Rutovitz, 1968; Butler, Butler and Stroud, 1964-8). Human analysts face the laborious task of selecting cells, photographing them, printing, cutting out chromosomes on the print, and arranging them in "best" pairs. At a crude level they are interested in counting the chromosomes and separating the artefacts, but at finer levels in recognizing corresponding pairs, in sequencing the pairs, and in recognizing small deletions within chromosomes and translocations of materials between them. In family studies they are interested in following the transmission of individual chromosomes from parent to child, the chromosomes being recognized by small individual variations of outline and staining reactions. Implicit in all this is the recognition of a "good" cell, of staining artefacts, of overlaid chromosomes and of single chromosomes with twists, bends and crossed arms. But if humans can do it, can their behaviour not be mimicked?

Ledley and Riddle (1965) describe a syntactic analysis of chromosome pictures in terms of a "bug" which they program to pass systematically across the picture. The photographed cell has first been scanned by a photoelectric device and converted to an array of spots of graded density (0 to 7) within the computer core. The bug scans the raster until it meets a non-zero spot, when its behaviour changes. It feels its way around the opacity, registering lengths of straight line, of convex curve and concave curve until it reaches its starting-point. The sequence of elementary features is processed by seeing whether it corresponds with a complex combinatorial syntactical definition of a "chromosome" and as soon as a chromosome has been recognized and its characteristics tabulated, its image is deleted and the bug resumes its raster search. Nobody believes that a human cytologist analyses a chromosome like this, but it is still properly regarded as a cybernetic method in that it represents the way in which it might be done if a fretwork pattern were to be analysed with a fingertip—or by a bug.

One of the problems of the cybernetic approach in situations such as this is that there is no guarantee, beyond an intuitive feel for the subject, that the method will be valid for all the situations it may meet, or that statistical conclusions based on many analyses are not biased by some artefact. In pragmatic terms the syntax of the pattern may be defined adequately for nine out of ten occasions, yet be beaten unexpectedly on the tenth.

An example of this was encountered in an analysis of geographical proximities where it was important to determine not only how far a disease occurrence was from a line upon the map, but also, since the line was a closed boundary, whether the point was inside or outside the area. The "bug" method was employed, the boundary of the area being traversed in segments in a clockwise fashion and the disease reference classified as "on the left" or "on the right" at the point of closest approach. Problems were met at vertices and overcome, but it was found then that the syntax could still be beaten in various indented boundary forms. In the end the problem was solved in quite a different manner through the use of Jordan's theorem. This method recognizes the fundamental mathematical difficulty of defining "inside" and "outside", and the relative ease of defining "same side" and "other side". A point (the origin of the map references for example) is *declared* to be outside, and joined by a line to the test point; boundary crossings are detected with respect to each section of the boundary and counted. An even number of crossings signifies same side (outside) and an odd number signifies other side (inside). Thus an analytical method was adopted because a cybernetic one was seen to be unreliable and difficult to program, and even if it ha not been seen to be unreliable we would in general have more faith in a method with some claim to a logical proof of correctness than in one without.

Incidentally, this example raises the intriguing problem of how humans distinguish inside from outside so accurately and so well, but this is outside the scope of this discussion.

Medical diagnosis may also be seen as a problem in pattern recognition. The possibility of its automatic accomplishment is one of the most persistent images of computer usage in medicine, yet on analysis one of the more remote. The complexity of the process of intuitive diagnosis in a general situation is far greater than the problem of recognizing a limited range of electro-cardiographic or chromosomal classifications and requires that we introduce the consideration of *prior probabilities* of different diagnoses being correct (Card, 1969; Lusted, 1965; Anderson and Boyle, 1968).

Briefly, this means that a particular diagnosis of a disease, an ECG or of a karyotype, once made, carries a risk that it is wrong, and this in turn depends in part upon the risk that it would be wrong if the diagnosis were purely a guess. This depends on the relative frequencies of the alternative diagnoses in the circumstances. As everyone knows, we improve our diagnostic odds if we diagnose common conditions commonly.

Several methods of *differential* diagnosis have been developed using computers, based often upon statistical rather than cybernetic methods, and they distinguish reasonably well between a relatively narrow range of alternatives presenting in some specific circumstances such as the investigation of goitre or of cyanotic heart disease, or in a dyspepsia or hypertension clinic. It should be clear from what has been said in relation to prior probabilities that the results of analyses in one place do not necessarily apply in another. A notable illustration of this difficulty (quite apart from computer applications) is the attempted application of diagnostic methods developed in hospital contexts as population screening procedures; they may be satisfactory in hospital where the yield of true positives is high, but in a context where the yield is very low indeed they may be heavily outnumbered by a substantial yield of false results.

But for general diagnosis the range of alternatives is so wide, their relative frequencies so variable and so unstable in time (and in any case not usually known), the complexity of the branching logic such, that any hope of approaching the efficiency of intuitive methods seems far away. In addition, we must remember that diagnosis is a dynamic classification more or less frequently revised to meet a sequence of decision requirements and its minutiae often judiciously abandoned. The relatively static, limited-range, frequency-measured sets of alternatives amenable to formal differential-diagnosis methods are rather uncommon.

The recognition of new diagnostic categories, as opposed to the classification of patients in existing categories, is a different matter, and we shall return to this under the heading "Numerical Taxonomy".

Dynamic Models

Physiological and patho-physiological models

Biological systems tend to be complicated, and although it may be possible to isolate and investigate individual subsystems, the understanding of the whole may depend on a more or less arbitrary synthesis. Thus, for example, the activities of individual enzymes may be investigated rigorously in specialized experimental environments, but the sum of the separate investigations may not necessarily serve as a rigorous determination of their activities when they are interacting in a more complex and changing environment. Complexities of this kind occur in hormone-based, neurologically-based and nucleic-acid-based information transmission systems, as well as in the energy transformation chains and cycles mediated through enzymes, and of course in combinations of systems of different kinds.

The construction of complex hypotheses always suffers from the difficulty that so many options are open that it is difficult to envisage them all and often impossible to test rigorously the adequacy of all those that might be formulated as alternatives. Computer modelling of complex constructions offers a means of elucidating the consequence.

An example of an information transmission model described by Moe (1965) concerns the understanding of atrial fibrillation. A formalized concept of myocardium consists of a region of parallel fibres, packed so that in cross-section they appear as a lattice of hexagons. Each fibre, except for those at the edges, has six neighbour contacts. The model depends upon statements which can be varied on different runs, of triggering rules and excitability levels, refractory periods, and longitudinal and transverse transmission rates, and a stated degree of intrinsic variation for each of these is permitted. The overall geometry of the myocardial model may also be varied by the introduction of cavities and of lines of transmission-block, and with each variation the model can be run and its behaviour monitored and recorded. The conditions for "physiological" and "pathological" modes of activity were thus delineated and hypotheses of the mechanism of action and control progressively developed.

Neurophysiological transmission models demand a conceptual neuronal network with connections somewhat more complex than the nearest neighbour-stimulation hypothesis of the myocardial syncytium and the comparison of model-produced and *real world* results is experimentally more difficult. Nevertheless, attempts have been made both to model neuronal discharge patterns in the mass to produce model "EEG" patterns and to simulate unit-discharge patterns on a micro-scale for purposes of developing hypotheses appropriate to unit-activity measurements in experimental animals. Farley (1965) and Adey (1965) describe studies of this kind.

Enzyme energy-transformation systems have been studied extensively using computer models. The activities of enzymes are dependent on their intrinsic characteristics, local substrate concentrations, and diffusion rates of the substrates and temperature (also a local diffusion problem), but for single enzymes an adequate expression of function can often be made in algebraic terms and time-based graphical representations. Even complex systems with many enzymes can be expressed in this way provided that "steady state" models are proposed. However, it is more difficult to evaluate the adequacy of an algebraic model of activity as a suitable explanation of an adaptive system and to say with confidence how it would respond in all its parts to transient disturbances in one of its parts, or in its environment. At molecular levels the effect of random processes (Brownian movement, thermal noise) are quite difficult to allow for in algebraic terms, particularly with respect to the less frequent random contingencies which must occasionally occur in a "chemical vat". Garfinkle (1965) has discussed these problems in detail and describes the application of computer models to them.

A combined/energy/diffusion/information system model is described by Campbell and Matthews (1968) in a study of respiratory function control. In this context carbon dioxide is treated as a "hormone", the concentration of which increases respiratory activity, and also as a diffusable chemical whose concentration is affected by respiratory activity. It is easy enough to understand this as a simple feedback system capable of existing in a steady state, but less easy to predict the consequences of sudden changes in the rate of production of carbon dioxide and the behaviour of a complex of transient diffusion gradients across body compartments such as muscles, blood and brain. What are the limits within which the system is stable and within which the rate of return to stability is physiologically adequate? Does it oscillate? Campbell and Matthew's model envisages an eight-compartment system, and they succeed in developing the parameters which adequately describe experiments upon human volunteers with carbon-11-labelled carbon dioxide.

Current studies of these kinds abound and it is clear that a very wide range of physiological mechanisms is susceptible to such examination, including embryogenesis, structure-function relationships and homeostatic systems of all kinds (see also Berman, 1965).

Population models

The chemical sequences, energy flows, transportation patterns and control systems of individual living organisms have analogies on the population scale in the behavioural interactions between organisms, the dynamics of population growth and function, and changing patterns of births, deaths, health and sickness. Mankind as well as individual men can be seen as a combined energy-, transport- and information-system. Scientific enquiry within the field thus delineated is largely subsumed under the headings of demography, economics, engineering, sociology, and anthropology and is only in part to be seen as a direct concern of medical researchers, but the parts which are their concern present the same complexities of synthesis and testing, and therefore amenability to model methods, as those within individual organisms.

We begin here with principles rather than achievements, because despite the clear validity of computer studies in this field the method has not yet been very widely exploited.

Monte Carlo statistical methods were mentioned earlier and can be seen as a population modelling technique, but a very simple one in concept: a model of the process of sampling from the population rather than a process within the population. For example, suppose we find in a series of disease events that there were several pairs and triplets of cases which combined close proximities on the map with a short interval of time between their onsets; how are we to know the likelihood that our sampling procedure alone (choice of area and time) is capable of producing such a result? Suppose also that we cannot find or devise an algebraic test of significance. We can enter the dates and places to the computer, scramble them so that the dates are attached to the places at random, and count again the number of pairs and triplets meeting the proximity description. We can repeat the scrambling and counting process a thousand times and measure the proportion of occasions on which a coincidence as great as our observation occurs. Such a method was used by Pike (David and Barton, 1966) on a set of leukaemia data originally assembled by Knox (1964). Results of Monte Carlo tests may themselves suggest simpler algebraic methods which, while unproven mathematically, serve as empirical approximations.

Direct modelling of infective processes has been used as an aid to understanding observed patterns of epidemic behaviour (Kendall, 1965; Bailey, 1967). Modelling methods based upon algebraic analysis have been used for many years, and at least one large study from pre-computer days used large colonies of mice as "model systems", but the computer has opened new possibilities. First, of course, it permits the evaluation of the more complex classical algebraic relationships, but in addition it permits evaluation of "stochastic" processes. Just as an adequate model of the molecular dynamics of an enzyme system must take account of, and perhaps even depend upon, the random processes of thermal agitation and Brownian movement, so must a realistic model of an epidemic take account of indeterminate factors such as contacts with susceptibles, occurring nevertheless with determinate probabilities. Program-models taking such elements into account, usually on the basis of a random number generating subroutine, are called stochastic models, in contrast with models which do not use random processes, which are called deterministic models. A stochastic epidemic model may be run many times to build a picture of how it is *likely* to, rather than how it *must* behave (Garland, 1964).

Apart from the intuitive acceptability of a stochastic as opposed to a deterministic process, the validity of stochastic models has been confirmed to some extent by their apparent ability to explain the indefinite recurrence of major epidemics such as measles. Deterministic models do not appear able to do this and the wave-forms become progressively spread out and damped in amplitude. The effects of control policies such as isolation and immunization rates can be examined in model situations so developed. On the whole, however, any success of stochastic epidemic studies has been in confirming intuitive conclusions rather than producing new ones.

One major problem is the spatial element of real epidemics and the irregular spatial clustering of populations, and it has been difficult even with a large computer to reconcile the formalization of models capable of manipulation with the complexity of real situations. However, some attempts have been made in this direction, and Pike, Williams and Wright (1967) constructed a model of contagious spread for Burkitt's lymphoma which seems adequately to account for time and space observations which are very difficult to explain in any other way.

Studies of population genetics may use computer models. The situation is analogous with the studies of contagious epidemic models in that many problems of gene-flow, selection, and balance can be expressed in algebraic terms. On the other hand, stochastic models including gene-extinction probability problems at low frequencies in small populations, are rather more difficult to handle purely in algebra and may prove intractable when combined with complex selection situations.

Even where algebraic methods exist, their validity and efficiency can be tested by applying them to the results of running computer models (Ken-Ichi, 1965; Kirkman, 1966). A complex chromosomal linkage problem was recently approached in this way (Fraser and Mayo, 1968).

Service development and management models

The development and management of medical services requires a picture, that is a model, of how those services operate, how they could operate, and how the different alternatives would influence the health of the population they serve. Model manipulations are at least implicit in every policy decision about the deployment of medical resources, and they are often highly complex models, the operation of which depends on a large number of variables not easily amenable to algebraic formulation. This characteristic, accompanied by a need to predict future patterns, makes computer model applications particularly appropriate. They provide for the first time a realistic way of making the foundations of policy explicit, and enable alternative policies to be tested in some degree before they are actually applied, without having to wait for years for an unsatisfactory result before re-planning.

One study of this kind was concerned with rhesus haemolytic disease and the evaluation of the appropriate services. First, there was the problem of determining to what extent the incidence might vary in response to population changes in birth-rank distribution and to what extent it must be attributed to causes other than this, including proposed prophylactic procedures. Secondly, there was the problem of how best to deploy the limited resources to produce a maximal effect, in particular to determine the probable response to treating women having first babies only, or having demonstrable foetal transfusions, or both. There was also the estimate to be made of the degree to which available methods could be regarded as having solved the problem, or whether further major research and development was necessary. The answer to this question was in the affirmative (Knox and Walker, 1968).

Another example amenable to computer model procedures—although not yet implemented—concerns predictions about medical manpower availability and requirements in the face of a range of contingencies concerning the number of medical schools, their throughputs, patterns and timings of specific postgraduate trainings, immigration and emigration rates, proportion of female students and the patterns of work disabilities resulting from marriage, relative salary and promotion prospects in different parts of the world, and the possibility of restriction upon emigration of Indian and Pakistani doctors (Morrison, 1968).

Complex relationships such as these in the scientific study of evolving medical services, multiple interacting determinants of health and disease, and optimized deployment of resources, all rely on a multiplicity of "in-put" premises whose values and limits must be examined until a plausible combination is found which adequately explains the available observations. Preferably, we must find some observations which were not taken into account in deriving the model or its premises, on which we can test the model after it has been developed: in the haemolytic disease study the birth rank distribution of cases in the population was accurately predicted by the model. We may find, of course, that we can mimic the observations from more than one set of input premises, and that the model is not a unique explanation. Our investigation may then suggest additional critical observations or experiments which could distinguish between alternatives.

Results of this kind have for example emerged from studies of the natural history of carcinoma *in situ* of the cervix uteri, where a wide range of natural history patterns is capable of explaining existing prevalence observations made upon populations, so that the observations themselves do not specify the natural history. Studies of this disease have not so far been treated by computer simulation, but again it illustrates the scope for such usage. It should be mentioned that "natural history" is in itself a model. It is not a quantity or distribution that can be calculated directly from observations in the same way as a mean or standard deviation. It is an entity that must be constructed first and tested later to see what results derive from it and how far they conform with observations.

The management of existing medical services should be seen not only as a matter for professional managers and administrators but as a matter for everyone engaged in providing the services and for those engaged in their study. Indeed, the difference between a good and a bad medical service— we take it that adequate diagnosis and choice of treatment can generally be taken for granted—is the difference between the efficient and less than efficient routing of patients through the various facilities required and the organization of those facilities to receive the patients. This is partly a question of overall load and overall investment, but is also very largely a question of organization, and we enter the world of the systems designer. The equivalent here of the algebraic equation is the flow diagram, a diagrammatic layout of the facilities, linked by routes, divided by branches, governed by rules. A flow diagram is a model (Harris, 1968).

This kind of model may be used for describing the appointment/surgery/ visiting routine of a general practice partnership; the place of the local authority services in maternity arrangements; the relationship between general practitioners and the hospitals and between outpatient and inpatient departments; the transfer of patients between wards and their transport to and from service departments; the design of a laboratory request system, a specimen transport system, a reporting system or a discharge procedure; the staff structure; ordering and re-stocking procedures. Indeed, the whole function of a complex service can be expressed in this way (Weir, Fowler and Dingwall Fordyce, 1968).

Used as a statement of existing services, the flow chart often has a very limited value and may reveal only the egocentric viewpoint of its draughtsman. But used as a planning device, in system design and engineering as opposed to systems analysis, it imposes and requires a harder discipline. A wide range of alternative systems can be envisaged for almost any new or re-designed service, and their formulation and evaluation can reasonably be seen as a scientific activity. Moreover, some of them are so complex, containing complicated feedback systems and facilities with inconstant capacities subject to stochastic demands, and with rigorous requirements for fail-safe contingency plans, that computer simulation models are the only practical way to examine them.

A particularly intriguing example of computer simulation methods is the mimicking of computer systems themselves. These methods are used extensively by computer manufacturers in specifying configurations of equipment for customers, as well as being used increasingly by customers in developing tender documents and contractual arrangements. For example, a hospital group installing a computer data-handling system utilizing real-time video-display terminals in conversational mode with the central processor and its files must satisfy itself that the equipment chosen will handle the traffic, and if it will not, what the bottle-necks will be. The use of the computer for this purpose has several advantages. First, it enables many alternatives of equipment to be examined. Secondly, it enables a check to be made on the adequacy of different equipments for different estimates and limits of load at different parts of the system, at different times of day and at different stages of development. Thirdly, because a computer simulation system demands statements of the parameters it requires; it defines the things that must be measured in order to state requirements, even if a computer simulation technique is not in fact employed.

Evaluation of computers and other data handling systems in a medical service requires a simulation study wider than that of the configuration itself. There is little to be gained in efficiency through the elimination of data-handling bottle-necks, if there are overriding limits of efficiency outside the data handling system. One suspects that proper evaluation of such situations may often produce results of this kind.

For example, simulation studies of hospital units are in progress in which a complex set of rules is built up for the conduct of model operations in which each item of service and each action depends upon the completion of others, each is subject to capricious delays and also to the constraints that certain kinds of operation cannot be carried out simultaneously or within a short time of each other, and that there are limits to the number of procedures any patient can have in a given time. One type of operation is the transmission of such data as requests and reports whose timing and delay distributions may be entered to the simulation system, and comparison may be in terms of patient stay and patient costs between efficient and less efficient data-handling timings. Thus the limits of the likely benefits can be assessed at least and alternative methods of approaching these limits through data-handling automation can be compared. Also the effects of alternative investment of resources into buildings, secretarial staff, telephone calls (or even doctors) can be evaluated.

Another aspect of service evaluation assisted or enabled by computers is in costing. Doctors tend to take a naïve view of service-costing with its implied life-costing, or even regard it as improper. However, lack of criteria for determing the deployment of limited resources has resulted in decisions being taken elsewhere: the doctors' own views are taken about as seriously as doctors themselves regard a women's magazine slimming diet that mentions neither quantities nor calories, or an estate agent's specification that ignores the existence of square feet. It is important to appreciate that computing methods, and simulation methods in particular, place within the hands of those interested the means of making explicit cost-evaluations of any changes they propose.

The notion of the model permits us to distinguish between a "cost" and "costing". A "cost" may be regarded as a naïve concept fostered in the minds of shoppers by shopkeepers, and associated with the (false) notion that goods and services have absolute cash values that have only to be discovered and displayed. A "costing" may be regarded as something more appropriate to service evaluation, the results depending upon which of a number of methods of costing is adopted, the choice depending upon the purpose. Thus a method suitable for one context may not be suitable to another. Within a given context a costing may be regarded as adequate rather than accurate, and the criterion applied to any costing is its usefulness rather than its correctness. This is the test of a model.

For example, we may find that the costing of a service within a hospital budget is not the same as one appropriate to a wider context. An automatic same-day computer-implemented notification to general practitioners of their patient's discharge or death is a pure cost (postage stamps) against the hospital budget, but gives an entirely different result in a wider context where a proper costing is made of the work-time and work-efficiency of the general practitioner and of the benefit to the patient.

The acceptance of a costing as a model procedure permits us logically to offer different models appropriate to different frames of reference, and to choose the model according to the efficiency of service which follows from its adoption, rather than to choose the form of service on the basis of a single cost, as if the cost were absolute. Budgets may still have to be balanced, but a search can be made for a budgeting system which gives the best overall value for a range of applications, and which meets the requirements of the health care system which it is supposed to service, rather than allowing the budgetary system itself to determine the system.

Research into costing and evaluation techniques for the health services is one of the crucial areas of work on which efficiency depends, and the computer is a necessary tool for their investigation and development.

Numerical taxonomy

We have mentioned numerical taxonomy before. It is an automatic pro-
gram-expressed method of classifying heterogeneous material in the sense
that a new system of classification is derived from the data themselves,
rather than in the sense that the items of data are classified according to a
pre-existing system. In analogy it consists of the differentiation of the disease
typhoid from the disease typhus, rather than the diagnosis of either. There
are several methods of conducting such analyses, and all methods have been
shown to be sub-sets of a general method in which the user has to express
the "intensity" of the grouping which his derived taxonomy must show
(Lance and Williams, 1966, 1967). In effect, the user of such a system can
have a wide variety of results depending on the purpose for which he requires
them. Once more we recognize the appropriate criterion of useful or not useful
rather than right or wrong, and again we recognize that we are dealing with a
modelling technique. This point has been made explicitly by several workers
engaged in numerical taxonomic analyses (Baron and Frazer, 1968). From
this point of view we may deprecate studies purporting to detect new syndromes without at the same time showing that this achieves something useful
in terms of understanding or decision-making. Some studies have shown that
automatic analysis may successfully mimic the intuitive diagnostic groupings
of human classifiers, and these results are of interest. If they suggest additional
groupings that human intuition has not declared, then they certainly bear
examination. Numerical taxonomy is an elaborate method of displaying
information for human interpretation. Multiple regression techniques can
also be regarded in this light.

A corollary is that we need not limit numerical taxonomic examinations
to the biological classification purposes for which they were designed.
Indeed, as with other population simulation methods, the major applications
may turn out to be elsewhere, particularly in the area of service management.
Vigorous applications of numerical taxonomic techniques are currently
under way to discover the main reasons for variations in duration of hospital
stay and to investigate other crude and not so crude indices of service
efficiency.

SERVICE USES

General Considerations

Few of the service applications of computers can yet be regarded as proven.
By service uses we mean established applications carried out regularly day
by day or week by week on the basis of a relatively unchanging program and
data system. It is of course difficult to draw a line between developing and
developed usages, but for the purposes of this chapter applications still in

the process of rapid development and recurrent appraisal have been considered as scientific rather than service uses.

This point of view must also be made explicit that a service usage has not been regarded here as proven just because it has been shown to be possible. Indeed, as we stated earlier, a computer can do anything with data that logically can be done, and except where a logical impasse is encountered (possibly for example in the logic of open-ended diagnosis) we can assume that with adequate time, investment and ingenuity all problems can be solved. The question is not so much "Can we do them?" but "*Should* we?" In making these decisions we are not entitled to justify our conclusions simply by comparing the way things *were* (or were not) done with how they are now done or how it is intended they should be done, but upon the basis of comparing alternative ways of proceeding. Therefore it is always necessary to state the special benefits a computer seems likely to provide.

There are two main kinds of benefit, one relating to the quality of the service and the other to improvements in the cost of providing it. Cost-savings themselves can be of two kinds, the saving of recurrent cost already incurred, and the avoidance of cost that would otherwise arise. The subject of costing has already been discussed and its importance as a research and development field declared, but it is also necessary to say that within the frame of reference of current *budgeting* systems it is seldom that cash savings can be demonstrated. When they are, it is often with respect to some special application rather than to the system as a whole. In many health service units such as hospitals any increase in efficiency is likely to be reflected in an increased throughput, and therefore costs are *higher* than were previously budgeted. Exceptions apart, health service computer uses are not to be justified in terms of budget savings, and the problem is often to justify extra expenditure. This returns us to the problem of measuring non-budgetary benefits in terms of an improved quality of service. The non-cash benefits are of three kinds: saving of time in handling patient-data; saving of error in handling patient-data; capturing and displaying statistical and service management data. In view of the large expenditure of money and effort involved this may appear pedestrian, but it is recommended as a realistic and comprehensive statement of what can be hoped for. It might be added that time-saving is itself of two kinds—work time and real time. Work time is saved if doctors, technicians or other personnel are relieved of work such as that involved in retrieving records or the graphic display of results, or more usually if work that would otherwise be impossible is undertaken, such as quality control or optimization of radiotherapy dosage (Farr and Newell, 1968; Whitehead, Becker and Peters, 1968). Real time (clock time) is saved when a report is delivered at 3 p.m. instead of 6 p.m., though any benefit will depend on the making of a decision based upon the report between these times. Errors saved are also of more than one kind, including quantitative errors detected by routine statistical quality control of laboratory reporting, identification errors on requests and reports, obsolescence errors arising from delays, and errors of omission, such as "flagging" omitted investigations in antenatal clinics, or non-attendance of patients at follow-up clinics. Once more the benefits to the patient depend on other things, notably the nature of the error and its consequences, and on the cost and reliability of alternative means of correcting the errors. Indeed, the cost of erroneous records can often be translated into nothing worse than a waste of staff time, such as the expenditure by the telephonist of three minutes rather than ten seconds to make a connection, or by the records officer of ten minutes rather than one minute to find a folder. Criteria of computer benefits *per se* can be declared only in terms of data manipulation, and benefits to the patient depend entirely on the context of this improvement.

Patient Management Applications

Registration discharge systems

There are in existence several computer systems for registering patients with a service, storing their identities for retrieval, and recording discharge from the service or transfer between its parts. In some cases this may constitute the entire task, but usually the registration system serves also as a Master Index to which is attached one or more additional facilities or files, such as those used for the billing of hospital patients, registrations of immunization-status, listing of infants at risk of handicap or in need of supervision, calling cervical cytology patients for follow-up, diagnostic indexing, or as a key for linking together files of related material held in different places of the same data system or in different data systems.

Typical of the best of these are the hospital systems at Karolinska Hospital, Stockholm, Boston Children's Hospital, Boston, Mass., Queen Elizabeth Hospital, Birmingham, Monmouth Hospital, Longbranch, New Jersey, and the local health immunization project pioneered in West Sussex (Cross, Droar and Roberts, 1968; Dale and Roberts, 1968a; Hall *et al.*, 1967); Fahey, 1969).

Variously, such systems use paper tapes, cards, optical marks and real time terminal inputs, and they may operate in batch-mode or on a one-at-a-time basis for input and output. They have a common need for very large file storage devices (preferably of direct access type) and the common predominant operations are "putting" and "taking" records. Their main common internal technical problems and external system problems are those of identifying and locating records and people. They are more or less massive in scale and in the main replace the work of clerks rather than of doctors and nurses, but they are operationally effective and some of them at least are cost-comparable with alternative methods of achieving so efficient a service.

The Birmingham system registers patients as they attend either for admission to hospital or on their first attendance at an antenatal clinic, and standard document-preparation equipment is used simultaneously to label paper records, and to punch an admission card. The equipment also produces a small pack of punch cards carrying abbreviated identities in the first 28 columns but leaving the remainder of the card available to one of several additional purposes, notably for recording laboratory requests or carrying out the discharge procedure. Daily processing at the computer checks new identities for validity and initiates correcting procedures. At the same time it establishes the patient on a magnetic disc model of the hospital. Daily ward-lists are provided and sent to the wards for verification (they were previously handwritten at midnight) and to the administrative office, while transfer of patients from ward to ward is notified centrally with a card. Daily listings of patients' states, alphabetically by ward, are also prepared for checking and transferred to the telephone room in order to answer relatives' enquiries. Bed occupancy statements are prepared daily for the administrative office, operations and diagnoses entered and listed, and hospital activity analysis statistics prepared. Antenatal clinic lists are prepared in advance, and advance booking states for the Maternity Hospital computed, thyroid follow-up listings prepared and despatched, diagnostic indices printed, and diagnostic and other listings prepared on request. Files are available for scientific investigation of patients, to study the operation of different parts of the service or the geographical distribution of patients serviced by different specialities. The cards are used by doctors as request forms. The patient's identity having been previously recorded on the card, the request is written on it. The cards are used first to generate laboratory work sheets. When the results are available the patient's identity on the report is generated automatically from the card to continuous stationery through an automatic typewriter; when the result is added to the report it is punched simultaneously into the card. The card then forms the basis of daily quality control analyses of laboratory results and periodic statements of laboratory work. The computer stores different laboratory results in separate disc-files, linked through cross-indexing to the disc-Master-File, and the Master File-link is the basis of a chain-linking operation within each laboratory sub-file, between successive records belonging to the same patient. Whenever a patient has many investigations, a cumulative report is put together by the computer and sent to the ward to replace previous separate reports or any previous cumulative layouts. On discharge the whole of the patient's record is consolidated into a single location and transferred from the discs to the magnetic tape, from which it can be recovered on re-admission, or as required. Laboratory archive tapes are also kept. All this results in a great reduction in the very large error rates associated with handwritten data systems, and a concurrent saving in staff time (Dale and Roberts,

1968b). A more advanced laboratory system under development transfers specimen identities and laboratory results directly from equipment to patient files, removing yet another of the hand-operated and therefore error-prone links.

The Birmingham example is described here at some length largely because it is the one most familiar to the author but also because it demonstrates that a not-over-ambitious batch-mode system can carry out a wide range of simple and necessary tasks effectively and accurately and at a *saving* of staff time and effort. Too often the image of computer applications is that they make work rather than save it, and unfortunately this is sometimes true.

Scheduling

The use of computers to arrange the scheduling of patients through health care systems appears superficially to be one of their most promising applications. Budgetary costs might be inflated by increased efficiency of patient routine, but one might reasonably expect a significantly improved usage of capital investment and a decreased unit-of-care-cost. From the patient's point of view there would also be advantages. He might be admitted from a waiting list earlier, or if not earlier his admission might be more appropriate to the availability of the facilities he needs, and he might be investigated, treated and discharged more expeditiously. It might be sufficient to demonstrate the saving of one day from each two-week admission in order to justify a very large hospital installation on these grounds alone.

In the long run this may prove to be the case, but in the short term there are problems. This is because many scheduling problems are either so simple ("the back of an envelope type of problem") that they do not justify automation, or so difficult that they must still be considered far from service-ready. Small waiting lists can be maintained very effectively with a diary, and larger ones, which require a more sophisticated card index (perhaps even punch cards) and the services of a secretary, may not yet justify the use of the computer for their maintenance even when one is available. Some computer applications in fact mimic the diary in that the clerk enquires and has displayed upon a terminal the booking status of "slots" in each clinic (e.g. as in Boston Children's Hospital) and she can enter new bookings to vacant times. This has advantages in a busy booking department where many clerks require access to the same diary from separated places. However, for many other situations a reorganization of the booking system to a central point might prove quicker and easier. Airline booking systems are an example of highly developed schedules where the use of a computer is necessitated by the large flow of data traffic and the impossibility of centralization. Larger systems may also use machine logic to *select* a booking or a set of alternatives, based on requirements signalled in advance. This is a much more difficult field technically, and one which must still be regarded as experi-

Q

mental in the medical field on the basis of benefit for cost in relation to alternative methods.

None of the diary approaches is necessarily registration-based. The booking entries and displays can consist of any string of symbols, the interpretation of which is a matter for the operator of the terminal or the reader of the printed list. Therefore it is true, and is observed in practice, that simple scheduling systems such as waiting lists can exist and be developed alongside registration-based file operations, yet not interact. Nevertheless, the accomplishment of the *automated* scheduling of a sequence of investigations and treatments is a major potential source of saving, especially in a hospital, and this must depend upon integration of this kind. These problems cannot be separated from the scheduling of work items within all the departments concerned, and the adaptation of the management structure and work pattern of the hospital or service to the new situation. The programming, data transport and human problems are very large indeed, and there are at present no comprehensive automatic hospital scheduling systems that appear capable of early implementation. This is a far greater problem technically than an airline scheduling system (of say 150 man-years work) in a very fluid situation which will itself not remain unresponsive to any data handling system that is installed.

The simpler scheduling systems will of course continue to grow, but they will probably develop most effectively on the basis of displayed lists interpreted and manipulated by clerks, and optimized intuitively rather than through machine logic. In many respects the problem is analogous with the statistical conundrum known as the "Traveller's Walk"—the problem of finding the shortest route round a number of points on the map. In practice, an experienced traveller will do this very quickly and efficiently compared with the best program method.

Clinical data operations

The use of computers to handle clinical data, particularly histories and medical examinations, is almost entirely unproven, and the results of some experiments have been disappointing. Moreover, many of the applications which have been envisaged require real-time terminals attached in some numbers to a time-sharing processor, and the pace of transactions at each terminal is so slow in computer terms and the equipment used at such low intensity that the transactions carried out on such a system are particularly expensive. It is quite unlikely that such applications will ever be justified in terms of the "electronic notebook" concept alone, or on grounds of legibility or paper-saving or compactness of storage, or even—since this can be achieved in other ways—in terms of the systematic and standardized character of the information so compiled.

The proper evaluation of clinical data handling techniques on computers must be in terms of those processing operations carried out on the data entered, and in terms of the transport of data. Medical records are of two main kinds—observational and executive. Both may need to be processed and moved about quickly, so that they can be delivered gratuitously or made available on demand in many different places. In system terms the computer is competing with the letter and telephone rather than with the clinical notes. Observational records (e.g. clinical details) may be required by the biochemist to evaluate a biochemical profile and decide on further investigation, by the anaesthetist or by the physicist. It should be noted that there are problems of confidentiality and authorization which need to be resolved, and it makes little sense to use this expensive equipment to make information widely available and then to limit access—as has in fact been recommended—to the person responsible for entering the data. There are also some legal problems, notably with respect to the deletion of information. It may not be possible to delete anything, but only to amend it, because it must always be possible to show at a later date that action taken was justified on the basis of the information as it existed at the time it was taken.

Executive data such as prescriptions and orders involve fewer problems with respect to confidentiality because they are addressed to whom they concern and because transport is their essence. Again, however, their justification depends upon inability to find a cheaper method of their effective delivery. There is another legal problem here of establishing responsibility, and one way is to produce hard copy (a print-out) at the site of entry, which is signed by the person responsible and held as evidence of authorization.

There are three main approaches to the entry of clinical data to a computer.

The first requires completion of a schedule. This is a questionnaire form in which either patient or doctor ticks boxes or rings numbers for later transfer to punch card or paper tape, makes pen marks on the form for reading through an on-line optical mark senser, or graphite marks on a puch card coded in parallel with the questionnaire form, for automatic punching on a graphite mark-sense machine. The "Porta Punch" system enables him to perforate the card directly. The questionnaire can be of the "straight through" type, or it may be branched, the respondent being instructed to skip or enter particular sections depending on the answer he has just supplied. This approach can be used for compiling self-taken histories and the forms may be supplied in several languages. Questionnaires of this type tend to be bulky, and some patients have difficulty in following the instructions.

The second approach uses cards with questions printed upon them and the patient is asked to sort them into yes/no boxes. Codes are punched into them so that the machine can recognize which question is which. Technically this limits questions to those of the yes/no type, which in turn means that more questions must be asked and it is more difficult to control branches.

The third approach uses on-line terminals and the patient sits at a typewriter which presents the questions to him and invites responses by pressing particular keys. The program decides the branches but the patient may occupy the terminal (and it him) for an hour or so. Oscilloscope terminals can display the questions more rapidly than the typewriter and also more complex patterns of alternatives; this permits fewer steps. At this level the terminal begins to become a practical proposition for use by the doctor; he can cope with the high information contents of complex displays thus permitting a system with a relatively small number of steps. High resolution displays with light pen or touch wire selection (on the face of the CR tube) may eventually establish methods of work which would be impracticable with a typewriter keyboard. Another approach to providing good resolution is the "keymat" keyboard which has a matrix of buttons overlaid by a coded plastic mat, one for each particular type of transaction. The mat in use, and therefore the transaction type, is recognized physically by the device.

The resistance to terminal usage by patients may not be as great as has been feared; indeed, there is some evidence that patients are less embarrassed by a machine than by a doctor and offer more reliable data. But for nurses and doctors the main question is the time taken by a transaction in comparison with the use of pen and paper, or whether there are advantages in other terms that would justify extra time taken. It seems unlikely for transactions such as making prescriptions, which may depend on perhaps six levels of conversational response between doctor and machine, that a response of more than one to two seconds, or a considerable walking distance to the nearest terminal, will be acceptable. The success or failure of each of these approaches will depend on the design of flexible terminals, their acquisition in quantity, good response times and high resolution, together with alternative fail-safe procedures, all at reasonable costs (Baruch, 1965; Collen, et al. 1965).

Quite a different set of problems is posed by automated methods of acquiring physical data directly from the patient. The justification here is in terms of acquisition and processing rather than in terms of transport. In the developmental stages at least they do not rely on large-scale integrated systems, and many experimental approaches have been possible with small to medium-size machines.

Some data from ECG records, spirometry and other respiratory function tests, and cardiac catheterization data, have been entered directly through a real-time input system, converted to coded data inside the computer, or reprinted in graphical form with parameters calculated. Both these and other applications, such as sequential dye dilution data in the study of circulatory dynamics have also been digitized off-line and processed at a later stage. Some on-line applications have been conceived as continuous monitoring operations rather than definitive clinical investigations, especially in intensive care units. Here the primary function is the remote display of continuous clinical data, any processing being limited to the detection of critical warning signals. This, and similar monitoring of laboratory equipment, is the only medical application truly analogous with that referred to in industry as process control. Analogue devices or small specialised digital devices may prove more suitable to this kind of work than large time-sharing systems, although general purpose machines may be invaluable in their development.

Service Management

Lists and tables

Many administrative tasks require references to updated lists, tedious to produce by hand yet readily produced by machines. With a computer they can be held on magnetic media and referred to through a terminal, but there are many situations where the computer-printed list is as good or better. These uses comprise telephone directories arranged by name and department, daily listing of patients in hospitals and other units, lists of medical, nursing, clerical and technical staff on the payroll, on duty and in different stages of training, examination results and training records, sessional lists, and committee memberships. All these lists need to be re-compiled more or less frequently. Lists related to patient care were discussed earlier, but one other kind should be mentioned, that relating to a transfer of a responsibility from one service to another. This occurs in the notification of infectious disease, the transfer of responsibility from Maternity Hospitals to Local Authorities, or in the case of handicapped children from Health Authorities to Education Departments.

All such lists depend on the existence of "live" regularly updated files kept either on a magnetic medium or in a computer readable form. Simple but effective systems can be based on office-kept punch-card files. The cards can be "interpreted"—i.e the characters are printed along the tops of the cards, and they can serve to some extent as a day-by-day office file. The listings can be performed at intervals with a "borrowed" computer.

Accounts

Salaries, wages, insurance, superannuation, accounts, billing, invoicing, inventories, departmental stock control, mileage claims, capitation fees, are increasingly serviced with computers. Usually this amounts to the programming of existing part-mechanized systems, and there are few major conceptual problems but a surprising amount of difficult detail. Attempts are being made to devise generalized systems applicable to all health service personnel such as those in NHS hospitals, but the complexity of the system has so far defeated them and the methods are still fragmentary. Not all branches of the Health Service use computers and even large and eminently amenable systems such as the maintenance of general practitioner lists and the calculation of remuneration are largely performed by hand. There is little doubt that this picture will change, and as general practitioners themselves begin to use computers to calculate what they should have been paid, the Executive Councils will also have to do so if only to defend themselves.

Simple accounting procedures require only batch computer processes and they can often be contracted out. Indeed, the maintenance of programs and their adaptation to new wage or salary agreements may make centralization of service desirable even when a local computer is available. More complex accounting systems, particularly those integrated with service data in such a way as to permit automatic running financial audits of different units within a service, will require that the accounting is done on the local system or at least that the data are transferable to it. However, there are truly formidable technical, methodological and managerial problems to be overcome before this is likely to be achieved.

Service statistics

A range of service statistics about hospitals, general practitioner services and local authority services are usually collected and tabulated in a more or less effective way. The work is tedious, error-prone and often badly done as well as irrelevant to any conceivable managerial purpose. The computer can remove the tedium and eliminate the errors. It can also multiply the irrelevance. It is also capable of providing any results that are relevant at a time when they are still useful and it permits experimentation with new and better methods of presentation.

Fortunately, improved presentations are being developed, and Hospital Activity Analysis (HAA) methods at least constitute a departure from frankly token measurements. However, all the hospital audit systems currently in use have the fundamental difficulty that the true output of the hospital is not measured. We may show that the range of hospital stay for a particular treatment is very wide and that curtailment of the longer admissions should be possible, but we cannot say what the results of longer and shorter admissions would be, or even what a short-term comparison would reveal if costs to services outside the hospital, and to the patient and community, were computed. For this we must first declare the task which the hospital could be said to have undertaken with respect to each patient, and to devise criteria of success or failure according to each type of task. Developments of such methods are in progress both in this country and in the United States, and may lead to a realistic routine computer-based audit of the performance of services.

Ad hoc management studies

Present techniques of routine service monitoring are so primitive that we must for some time look to *ad hoc* studies as the chief source of effective management statistics. A major purpose of computers used in management must therefore be the provision of a service for such studies. In part, this amounts to the provision of a scientific service of program testing facilities and programming assistance and machine time, but various kinds of generalized study systems can also be supplied. Although they have been little used so far in medical applications, network analysis techniques have been developed in industrial environments and provide ways of laying out complex sequential and parallel/sequential operations, i.e. those involved in the building/staffing/equipping/systems-design/and stage-by-stage opening of developments such as new hospital complexes. Critical decision points are detected and signalled and consequences of different decisions or lack of decision specified. Generalized simulation systems and languages have also been developed for industrial use, and it is possible that these can be adapted to the medical scene and supplied as a service.

A notable example of a general basis for *ad hoc* research in service management is the Oxford Record Linkage Study which provides the techniques and facilities for linking together files of records from different services. Thus admission to hospital for treatment of fractured neck of femur has been studied by linking the hospital files with the files of death certificates, and this has produced realistic statements of the results of the treatment provided. Maternity service statistics have been assembled for the first time on a total service basis rather than in terms of unrelated parts. Such applications are beginning to find uses in the assessment of long-term hazards of particular occupations, and through linking hospital and other diagnostic indexes to population registers, such as those based in birth notifications, to the evaluation of developing population services. Examples are the detection and control of phenylketonuria, of congenital dislocation of the hip, of deafness in childhood and of other handicap risks.

Whilst presentations of this kind may often be appropriate to the management of existing divisions of the Health Service, it is also possible to present data in relation to a service which perhaps ought to exist but does not. For example, there is no "Maternity Service" under the National Health Service, nor a unified management of the needs of handicapped children, nor a geriatric service, nor a screening service. Imaginative presentation of data permits evaluation of these service functions and where defects are demonstrable it may help to call into being the organisations necessary to deal with them.

Policy design

Finally, the computer must have some impact on the larger issues of health care policy formulation. This is subsumed very largely under "research" and in the study of models of different ways of developing resources. However, the requirement of computer methods that the premises of an operation should be explicit and unambiguous must make uncomfortable any juxtaposition of those policy formulations based on declared premises and available evidence, and those which are not.

Appropriately enough, policies for the development of computers within the Health Services are shaping up to provide an example of a confrontation of this kind.

GENERAL BIBLIOGRAPHY AND SOURCES

BAILEY, N. T. J. (1967). *The Mathematical Approach to Biology and Medicine*. London: Wiley.

BRITISH MEDICAL ASSOCIATION (1969). Computers in Medicine in Planning Report No. 3. London.

BRITISH COMPUTER SOCIETY (1969). Medical Computing Progress and Problems. Proceedings of Conference.

ENSLEIN, K. (ed.) (1961–1966). *Data Acquisition and Processing in Biology and Medicine*, Volumes 1 to 5. Oxford: Pergamon.

GURLAND, J. (ed.) (1964). *Stochastic Models in Medicine and Biology*. Wisconsin: Madison.

HOLLINGDALE, S. H. (1965). *Electric Computers*. Pelican.

LEDLEY, R. S. (1965). *Use of Computers in Biology and Medicine*. New York: McGraw-Hill.

McCRACKEN, D. D. (1962). *A Guide to Algol Programming*. New York: Wiley.

McCRACKEN, D. D. (1963). *A Guide to Cobol Programming*. New York: Wiley.

McCRACKEN, D. D. (1965). *A Guide to FORTRAN IV Programming*. New York: Wiley.

McLACHLAN, G. & SHEGOG, R. F. A. (1968). *Computers in the Service of Medicine*, Volumes I and II. London: O.U.P.

MEDICAL RESEARCH COUNCIL (1965). *Mathematics and Computer Science in Biology and Medicine*. London: H.M.S.O.

SPICER, C. C. (1968). Computing in medicine. *Brit. med. Bull.*, **24**, 3.

STACEY, R. W. & WAXMAN, B. D. (ed.) (1965). *Computers in Biomedical Research*, Volumes I and II. New York: Academic Press.

STIBITZ, G. R. (1966). *Mathematics in Medicine and the Life Science*. Chicago: Year Book Medical Publishers.

REFERENCES

ACHESON, E. D. (ed.) (1967). *Medical Record Linkage*. London: O.U.P.

ACHESON, E. D. (ed.) (1968). *Record Linkage in Medicine*. Edinburgh: Livingstone.

ADEY, W. R. (1965). Computer analysis in neurophysiolology. In STACEY & WAXMAN, Vol. I, p. 223. New York: Academic Press.

ANDERSON, J. A. & BOYLE, J. A. (1968). Computer diagnosis: statistical aspects. *Brit. med. Bull.*, **24**, 230.

BARON, D. N. & FRASER, PATRICIA M. (1968). Medical applications of taxonomic methods. *Brit. med. Bull.*, **24**, 236.

BARUCH, J. J. (1965). Hospital automation via computer time-sharing. In STACEY & WAXMAN, Vol. II, p. 291. New York: Academic Press.

BERMAN, M. (1965). Compartmental analyses in kinetics. In STACEY & WAXMAN, Vol. II, p. 173. New York: Academic Press.

BUTLER, J. W., BUTLER, M. K. & STROUD, AGNES (1964, 1966, 1968). Automatic classification of chromosomes. In ENSLEIN, Vol. 3, p. 261; Vol. 4, p. 47; Vol. 5, p. 21. Oxford: Pergamon.

CAMPBELL, E. J. M. & MATTHEWS, C. M. E. (1968). The use of computers to simulate the physiology of respiration. *Brit. med. Bull.*, **3**, 249.

CARD, W. I. (1969). The diagnostic process. In *Medical Computing Progress and Problems*. Published by British Computer Society.

COLLEN, M. F., RUBIN, L. & DAVIS, L. (1965). Computers in multiphasic screening. In STACEY & WAXMAN, Vol. I, p. 339. New York: Academic Press.

CROSS, K. W., DROAR, J. & ROBERTS, J. L. (1968). Electronic processing of hospital records. In MCLACHLAN & SHEGOG, Vol. I, p. 23. London: O.U.P.

DALE, J. W. & ROBERTS, J. L. (1968a). The identification of patients and their records in a hospital using electronic data processing equipment. In MCLACHLAN & SHEGOG, Vol. I, p. 41. London: O.U.P.

DALE, J. W. & ROBERTS, J. L. (1968b). Errors in a hospital record system. In MCLACHLAN & SHEGOG, Vol. II, p. 63. London: O.U.P.

DAVID, F. N. & BARTON, D. E. (1966). Two space-time interaction tests for epidemiology. *Brit. J. prev. soc. Med.*, **20**, 44.

FAHEY, J. J. (1969). A hospital information system. In *Medical Computing Progress and Problems*. Published by the British Computer Society.

FARLEY, B. G. (1965). A neural network model and the slow potentials of electrophysiology. In STACEY & WAXMAN, Vol. I, p. 265. New York: Academic Press.

FARR, R. F. & NEWELL, J. A. (1968). Radiotherapy treatment planning. In MCLACHLAN & SHEGOG, Vol. I., p. 135. London: O.U.P.

FRASER, F. R. & MAYO, O. (1968). A comparison of the two-generation and three-generation methods of estimating linkage values in the X-chromosome in man with special reference to the loci determining the Xg groups and glucose-6-phosphate dehydrogenase deficiency. *Amer. J. hum. Genet.*, **20**, 535.

GARFINKEL, D. (1965). Simulation of biochemical systems. In STACEY & WAXMAN, Vol. I, p. 111. New York: Academic Press.

GARFINKEL, D. (1965). Simulation of ecological systems. In STACEY & WAXMAN, Vol. II, p. 205. New York: Academic press.

HALL, P., MELLNER, CH. & DANIELSSON, T. (1967). A data processing system for medical information. *J. Meth. med. Res. Inf. Doc.*, **6**, No. 1.

HARRIS, F. T. C. (1968). Systems analysis and hospitals. In MCLACHLAN & SHEGOG, Vol. II, p. 33. London: O.U.P.

HEALY, M. J. R. (1968). The disciplining of medical data. *Brit. med. Bull.*, **24**, 210.

KENDALL, D. G. (1965). Mathematical models of spread of infection. In *M.R.C.*, p. 213.

KEN-ICHI, KOJIMA (1965). The evolutionary dynamics of two gene systems. In STACEY & WAXMAN, Vol. I, p. 197. New York: Academic Press.

KIRKMAN, H. N. (1966). Properties of X-linked alleles during selection. *Amer. J. hum. Genet.*, **18**, 424.

KNOX, E. G. (1964). Epidemiology of childhood leukaemia in Northumberland and Durham. *Brit. J. prev. soc. Med.*, **18**, 17.

KNOX, E. G. (1968). Obstetric determinants of rhesus sensitization. *Lancet*, **1**, 433–7.

KNOX, E. G., FAIRWEATHER, D. V. I. & WALKER, W. (1965). Spectrophotometric measurements on liquor amnii in relation to the severity of haemolytic disease of the newborn. *Clin. Sci.*, **28**, 147.

KNOX, E. G. & WALKER, W. (1968). A working population model of haemolytic disease of the newborn. *Arch. dis. Childh.*, **43**, 562.

LANCE, G. N. & WILLIAMS, W. T. (1966). A general theory of classification sorting strategies. I. *Computer Journal*, **9**, 373.

LANCE, G. N. & WILLIAMS, W. T. (1967). A general theory of classification sorting strategies. II. *Computer Journal*, **10**, 271.

LEDLEY, R. S. & RIDDLE, F. F. (1965). Automatic analysis of chromosome karyograms. In *M.R.C.*, p. 189.

LUSTED, L. B. (1965). Computer techniques in medical diagnosis. In STACEY & WAXMAN, Vol. I, p. 319. New York: Academic Press.

MEIGHAN, S. S. & KNOX, E. G. (1965). Leukaemia in childhood. *Cancer*, **18**, 811.

MOE, G. K. (1965). Computer simulation of atrial fibrillation In STACEY & WAXMAN, Vol. II, p. 217. New York: Academic Press.

MORRISON, S. L. (1968). Medical manpower in National Health Service. In *Problems and Progress in Medical Care*, 3rd series, ed. G. McLachlan, for Nuffield Provincial Hospitals Trust. London.

PIKE, M. C., WILLIAMS, E. H. & WRIGHT, BARBARA (1967). Burkitt's tumour in the West Nile district of Uganda 1961–5. *Brit. med. J.*, **2**, 395.

PIPBERGER, H. V. (1965). Computer analysis of electrocardiograms. In STACEY & WAXMAN, Vol. I, p. 377. New York: Academic Press.

RUTOVITZ, D. (1968). Automatic chromosome analysis. *Brit. med. Bull.*, **24**, 260.

WEIR, R. D., FOWLER, G. B. & DINGWALL FORDYCE, I. (1968). Prediction and simulation of surgical admissions. In MCLACHLAN & SHEGOG, Vol. II, p. 141. London: O.U.P.

WHITEHEAD, T. P., BECKER, J. F. & PETERS, MARGARET (1968). Data processing in a clinical biochemistry laboratory. In MCLACHLAN & SHEGOG, Vol. I, p. 113. London: O.U.P.

14 The Medical Management of Affective Disorder and Schizophrenia

W. A. LISHMAN

AFFECTIVE DISORDER. DRUG TREATMENT. SCHIZOPHRENIA. PHYSICAL TREATMENTS

IN the present review of the clinical management of certain psychiatric disorders, pharmacological treatment will be described in detail, since this is the area in which the non-psychiatric physician will most often find himself involved. It is also the area that has witnessed some of the most dramatic changes in psychiatric practice over the past two decades and has helped to break down some of the barriers which have tended to separate psychological and physical medicine. In psychopharmacology it should not be forgotten that both the phenothiazines and the antidepressant drugs made their debut on the psychiatric scene after the observation of their effects, or that of their precursors, in patients under treatment for physical disorders and nowadays the psychiatrist is obliged to keep more closely in touch with the total field of medicine, if only to avoid doing physical harm with the drugs at his command. Conversely, it is easy to see how quickly the non-psychiatrist has learned to include psychotropic drugs in his therapeutic repertoire, when previously a diagnosis of "merely functional" was usually a gloomy foreboding that very little indeed could be done by way of treatment. The patient with an entrenched somatic neurosis or severe personality disorder remains as ever a formidable management problem, but in the generality of patients with "functional" complaints there is sufficiently often a basis in anxiety or depression to make the prescription of psychotropic drugs worth serious and careful consideration.

For psychiatry itself, the advent of useful drugs has done much in addition to adding another point of therapeutic attack. It has helped to shift the whole emphasis of treatment away from prolonged in-patient stay in mental hospitals, and has brought more realistic contact with patients in the community and in out-patient clinics. At least in theory treatment can be started in earlier and milder stages of mental disorder. Patients can more readily continue treatment in a general hospital setting where their initial referral may have led them, or when conjoint management of both physical and psychological aspects of an illness is required. But perhaps the greatest long-term benefit of all is that the psychiatrist has been drawn into an acute awareness of the need to evaluate treatment of all kinds. Authoritative statements no longer suffice, and controlled trials have come to be employed in psychiatry in many fields apart from that of psychopharmacology.

Treatment in psychiatry, as in other branches of medicine, cannot be fully considered in isolation from matters of diagnosis and aetiology. Equally pharmacological treatment can be properly discussed only along with other aspects of management. Thus, while the accent in the present review will be placed on psychopharmacology, broader aspects of psychiatric practice will also need to be considered.

AFFECTIVE DISORDER

Problems of Diagnosis and Classification

The present possibilities for pharmacological treatment of depression have thrown into prominence the old controversies over the classification of affective disorders, and indeed of separating them from "normal" changes of mood. Depression is a normal affect in that it is universally experienced from time to time in any psychologically healthy human being. It can be experienced equally certainly with abnormal intensity or frequency in such a way that it disrupts healthy functioning, and can then be seen to warrant medical intervention. In the presence of accompanying somatic symptoms, such as sleep and appetite disturbance or motor retardation, or of the more florid psychological symptoms which accompany severe depression, it is easy to view the condition as an illness. Indeed, affective disorder is often accompanied by objectively measurable disturbances in body physiology— alterations in amine metabolism, electrolyte distribution, and adrenal cortex activity (see review by Coppen, 1967). But people coming before doctors for treatment of depression as a symptom vary enormously in the intensity of the affective change, and in the physical and psychological symptoms which are found along with it. It may sometimes be correspondingly difficult to decide how far the individual case should properly be regarded as unwell rather than showing an expected and understandable response to antecedent circumstances.

Many attempts have been made to classify depression according to descriptive epithets, some aetiological and some descriptive of the presenting clinical picture. Critical studies have often shown that these have oversimplified the problem. For example, classification into *reactive* and *endogenous* groups, based on assessment of provocative factors and of genetic predisposition, is often found to be unsatisfactory. Provocation towards depression is a highly individual matter, depending much on the personal meaning of events and circumstances surrounding them. The idea has gained ground of continuity along a spectrum, with extreme cases illustrating classical reactive and endogenous states, but the great majority showing graded admixtures of provocative factors and innate susceptibility. Subdivisions based on the presenting mental state, for example into apathetic and agitated depressions, remain useful as clinical shorthand terms. The more complex classifications into psychotic, neurotic and involutional depressions run into considerable difficulties, and here the most recent and sophisticated studies have failed to reach agreement (compare Kiloh and Garside, 1963, with McConaghy *et al.*, 1967, and Kendell, 1968). Much of the evidence suggests that the clinical pictures produced by psychotic and neurotic depressions, also the so-called involutional depressions, merge gradually into one another, with only the extreme examples upholding the classical descriptions formerly found in psychiatric texts. These problems of classification have of course an important bearing on any attempts to recommend specific treatment procedures for different types of depressive illness, and on the comparability of drug trials which are carried out on samples from different populations of depressed patients.

Hill (1968) has reviewed the confusing picture that has resulted from these various approaches to the taxonomy of depression. He suggests that a more satisfactory subdivision of depressive disorders may come eventually, not from symptom inventories or analysis of antecedent circumstances but by objective measurement of the various admixtures of physiological arousal and physiological inhibition from which much of the symptomatology derives and which may underly the individual stamp given to the overall clinical picture. This approach has much to recommend it in seeking a solution to the problems of classification posed by the so-called anxiety states. These have sometimes been considered to represent a clinical entity quite separate from depressive disorders, sometimes simply as minor variants of agitated depression. Present opinion on the matter remains divided, and the whole subject has recently been well reviewed by Woolfson (1968). This group of disorders is perhaps especially relevant to the work of the general physician, in that somatic symptoms are often pronounced and may serve as the prime focus for the anxiety, thereby leading the patient to the general medical clinic.

Manic and hypomanic phases of affective disorder are relatively rare, and in addition are much less likely to come the way of the non-psychiatric physician. Accordingly, they will receive only very brief consideration here.

Atypical Presentation of Affective Disorder

A second problem highlighted by modern possiblities for treatment is that of the atypical presentation of affective disorder. Not all depressed patients complain of altered mood as the presenting symptom. Somatic complaints may be to the forefront, and even when the mood change is recognized by the patient it may be considered to be the result rather than the cause of the physical symptomatology. Such somatic symptoms commonly include fatigue, a general feeling of malaise, abdominal discomfort and indigestion, constipation, pains in the limbs and neck, headache, and abnormal body sensations, as well as the very common anorexia and insomnia. Specific enquiry for confirmatory signs of depression should be carefully made whenever the patient appears unduly concerned about such bodily symptoms, or when they affect a number of body systems together. Partially masked depression will be discovered only when it is among the specific conditions for which the patient is examined, and only after it has been diagnosed can the most effective treatment be instituted.

The association of atypical facial pain with depressive disorders has been well demonstrated by Lascelles (1966). Here, as with other somatic presentations, melancholia, self-recrimination and retardation may sometimes be relatively slight, and anergia with hypochondriacal preoccupation may dominate the picture. Another picture, commonly seen, is that of the acute onset of florid somatic symptoms in a setting of intense anxiety. Awareness of the action of the heart, fluttering in the abdomen, bizarre paraesthesiae, visual disturbances, and dyspnoea leading to hyperventilation tetany, may all be seen in varying combinations. Such attacks may be recurrent and without obvious precipitation (Walker, 1959). Profound anxiety dominates the picture rather than depression of affect, yet response to antidepressant medication is again found to be good. In late middle and old age, affective disorder may sometimes mimic dementia, especially when failing memory is accompanied by carelessness of habits and decrepitude due to loss of weight. Post (1966) has shown that one in six of his elderly depressives ran the risk of being misclassified in this way when too great reliance was placed on assessment of intellectual function alone, yet response to antidepressant treatment and follow up showed very satisfactory results.

In the above examples, affective disorder, though partially masked, can usually be seen to be present with the discerning eye or with hindsight. Response to antidepressant treatment is generally reasonably satisfactory. A more difficult therapeutic problem is posed by patients in whom depression might have been expected but has not occurred—patients Hill (1968) describes as producing "first-line neurotic defensive postures" in place of true affective disorder. Such reactions may include delinquent or acting-out behaviour in the adolescent; excessive eating, drinking or sexual behaviour; hypochondriasis; hysterical or obsessional symptoms. Here, antidepressant treatment is usually of little help and a more comprehensive approach to the total situation is usually necessary.

In addition to these risks of erroneous diagnosis the general physician must be alert to the affective disorder which may aggravate some physical diseases—asthma, peptic ulcer, migraine, Parkinson's disease—and which may participate in a vicious circle of increasing disability; likewise the depression which hinders convalescence from surgical operations or disabling physical disease, and which may act as a bar to rehabilitation after head injury or cerebrovascular accidents. Depression is well recognized after influenza, infectious mononucleosis, pneumonia and hepatitis, and may be induced by drugs such as rauwolfia alkaloids, alpha methyl dopa, guanethidine, steroids, and sulphonamides.

General Principles of Management

While the problems of classifying affective disorder have failed to reach a satisfactory resolution, they have given important leads to the correct approach in the management of individual cases. We know that some patients will present with a classical picture of recurrent endogenous swings of mood, divorced from discernible precipitating factors, and often with ample evidence of genetic loading. Here the first emphasis in treatment will be placed on physical measures, drugs or ECT, together with efforts to help the patient over the disruptions in his life produced by the disorder. We know that in other patients depression will be a self-limiting episode, in response to clearly defined stresses which commonly embody threats to self-esteem or some form of loss. A very substantial number of such patients will prove on enquiry to be particularly vulnerable to such events, some perhaps even to have sought out life patterns and personal relationships which predispose to their occurrence. Thus neurotic patterns of behaviour may sometimes be found here, and psychotherapy needed for the proper resolution of the psychological conflicts contributing to the present illness or predisposing to recurrence. Extreme examples may prove to suffer from fundamental personality disturbance, the so-called "depressive personality", and some may be very resistant to treatment of any sort in the long run. But between extremes we should be prepared to meet gradations along a continuum, requiring treatment from both physical and psychological points of view.

The availability of effective antidepressant drugs, while helping enormously in management, should not be allowed to lead to short-cuts in clinical appraisal. In some ways they call for special care over certain management decisions, such as whether the patient should be treated in or out of hospital. This must depend principally on the severity of the depressive illness, viewed in conjunction with the support and supervision which the patient may expect to receive if he remains at home. The possibility of out-patient treatment means that the assessment of suicidal risk must be undertaken with particular care. It should not be shirked for fear of causing embarrassment, and the patient who harbours suicidal ideas is often relieved when the subject is broached in a tactful way. Hospital admission may be indicated in order to remove the patient from precipitating circumstances or from an environment which militates against improvement. On the other hand, pronounced inadequacy or dependency of personality may mean that admission to hospital will ultimately delay recovery and lead too readily to long periods of harmful institutionalization.

This is not the place to discuss psychotherapeutic techniques, nor to consider in detail the value of social help for patient and relatives. But it must be emphasized that while the remainder of the section will deal with physical methods of treatment, therapeutic efforts cannot be allowed to rest here in the great majority of patients. That many patients stand to benefit from antidepressant drugs alone is shown by the success that can be gained from the treatment of depression by busy general practitioners, though even here the doctor-patient relationship and the total understanding of the physician are often more significant therapeutic factors than is explicitly recognized. Nevertheless, a great number even of mild cases of depression still come before the psychiatrist, often after drug treatment alone has given a temporary benefit, and often because the complexities of what seemed a straightforward problem have now become overt.

Drug Treatment in Depression

Controlled trials have shown beyond doubt that several drugs possess a true antidepressant action. They are not merely euphoriants, and have in fact little effect on mood in the non-depressed person. In depressive illness they not only relieve the abnormal mood state, but typically bring about progressive improvement in the whole range of physical and psychological disturbances which accompany depression.

Observer bias and observer enthusiasm have been shown to operate powerfully in the assessment of psychotropic drugs of all kinds, and anti-depressive medication is no exception. Impressionistic statements about the value of newly introduced antidepressants, or about competing claims, are notoriously unreliable, and fully controlled trials should be quoted in evidence for any serious claims. Unfortunately, depressive disorders are a heterogeneous collection of clinical states classified variously by different workers, and therefore even strictly controlled trials have not surprisingly sometimes led to incompatible results. Furthermore, the exigencies of clinical practice sometimes require a careful trial of less well-proved agents when the theoretically optimal drug has failed to produce benefit.

Theoretical background to antidepressant drug action

Recent work seeks to equate depletion of certain brain monoamines, particularly free noradrenaline and 5-hydroxytryptamine, with depressive disorder. This theory originally leant heavily on the use of reserpine sedation in animals as a pharmacological model for human depression, although recently rather more direct evidence has accumulated from studies of the metabolism of 5-hydroxytryptamine and its precursors in man. This chapter in neurochemistry has recently been reviewed by Gibbons (1968). The first class of pharmacological agents found to be of real value in the treatment of depression, the monoamine oxidase inhibitors, act on the enzymes which normally metabolize monoamines released from the deeply bound intra-cellular pool. Under their influence the level of free monoamines in the brain is made to rise. The second group of antidepressant drugs, the tricyclic compounds, are without effect on intracellular monoamines, but inhibit the re-uptake of the free noradrenaline which is released at nerve endings by presynaptic stimulation. Thus both types of antidepressants have possible modes of action in line with the "biogenic amine" hypothesis of depression, in that both have the property of increasing readily available noradrenaline and perhaps other monoamines at receptor sites in the brain (Pare, 1968). How far such a theoretical model for their pharmacological action will be upheld by further work remains to be seen. Unfortunately it has not proved possible to draw any satisfactory parallel between therapeutic potency and potency in inhibiting monoamine oxidase among the various monoamine oxidase inhibitor antidepressants; nor is the clinical response clearly tied to presently available indices for assessing these neurochemical changes in man.

Monoamine oxidase inhibitor drugs

Iproniazid (Marsilid), introduced for the treatment of tuberculosis, was found to produce euphoria and overactivity in some patients. This led to its use in psychiatric patients, initially with outstanding claims for its effectiveness in the treatment of depression. Though itself falling into disfavour, iproniazid paved the way for study of other monoamine oxidase inhibitors, several of which have found wide therapeutic application. These are listed in Table 14.1, which also shows the dosage range usually recommended.

In controlled trials, this group of drugs has generally been found to be less potent than the tricyclic antidepressants described below. However, as they were introduced before the tricyclics they have gained a firm foothold and are still frequently prescribed. Several careful trials have failed to show any benefit whatever, compared to placebo treatment, while others have revealed definite antidepressant action where the more potent members are concerned. In general, it may be stated that their proven value lies mainly in the less severe depressive disorders, trials on out-patients being much more liable to yield positive results than trials on in-patients (Bennett, 1967). Current opinion favours tranylcypromine, iproniazid and phenelzine as most efficacious, but relative merits are far from clearly established.

The idea has gained ground that this group of antidepressants is of particular value for depressive disorders which are accompanied by much neurotic, particularly phobic symptomatology, for those characterized by anergia rather than retardation, and when there is difficulty in getting to sleep rather than early morning waking, i.e. for depressive disorders commonly labelled "neurotic" or "reactive" (West and Dally, 1959). This suggestion has not been very fully tested, and may mean little more than that the monoamine oxidase inhibitors, being weak antidepressants, are most easily shown to be efficacious when the depressive disorder is mild.

TABLE 14.1

Monoamine Oxidase Inhibitor Antidepressants

Name	Usual daily dose (mg)
Non-hydrazine Derivatives	
Tranylcypromine (Parnate)	10–30
Hydrazine Derivatives	
Iproniazid (Marsilid)	50–150
Phenelzine (Nardil)	30–75
Mebanzine (Actomol)	10–30
Isocarboxazid (Marplan)	10–60
Nialamide (Niamid)	100–300

Pare *et al.* (1962, 1965) have put forward the interesting suggestion that there may be two biochemically distinct types of depression founded on genetic constitution, one of which responds better to monoamine oxidase inhibitors and the other to tricyclic antidepressants. They have indicated that in individual patients with recurrent depressive episodes, drugs of one class are likely to give consistently better results than the other, while the same preferential drug response in first degree relations is very frequently seen.

Tranylcypromine (Parnate) has some pharmacological actions which differ from the remainder of the group. It possesses amphetamine-like effects in addition to ability to inhibit monoamine oxidase, and is correspondingly said to have a stimulating effect in anergic depressions. A tablet incorporating tranylcypromine 10 mg with trifluoperazine 1 mg (Parstelin) has been advocated for conditions where depression and anxiety coexist. Controlled trials have confirmed the antidepressant action of tranylcypromine, which appears to act rather more quickly than the remainder of the group considered below. However, an increased tendency to produce hypertensive crises has caused its popularity to decline.

Iproniazid (Marsilid), the first monoamine oxidase inhibitor to be introduced is also generally regarded as one of the most powerful antidepressants in this group. Unfortunately it also shows the greatest incidence of side-effects, particularly toxic liver damage, and on this account has been withdrawn from sale in the U.S.A. In Britain it is still very occasionally prescribed for refractory depressions. Like the other hydrazine derivatives its clinical effect may be delayed, usually commencing only after one to three weeks.

Phenelzine (Nardil) is perhaps the most widely used monomine oxidase inhibitor, despite inconsistent results from clinical trials. While some trials have shown definite benefit in less severe depressions, others have yielded equivocal results. In the large M.R.C. trial which compared ETC, imipramine and phenelzine in the treatment of in-patient depressives, phenelzine was found to be no more effective than placebo (M.R.C., 1965). Used in conjunction with chlordiazepoxide (Librium), it is still widely promulgated as useful treatment in neurotic depressive states with coexistent phobic or anxiety symptoms.

Mebanzine (Actomol), more recently introduced, is regarded as roughly equivalent in potency and usefulness to phenelzine.

Isocarboxalid (Marplan) and *Nialamide (Niamid)* have in general given poor results in strictly controlled trials.

Unwanted effects of monoamine oxidase inhibitors

Quite apart from lessened confidence in their clinical efficacy, the side-effects of this group of drugs have led to a decline in their popularity.

Autonomic effects include hypotension, blurred vision, dryness of the mouth, constipation and delay with micturition. These may be troublesome initially, but tend to improve with continued exposure to the drug. Impotence and delay in ejaculation are fairly common, and the latter has led to the therapeutic use of these drugs in some cases of premature ejaculation. In the presence of prostatic enlargement or glaucoma the drugs are contraindicated. Ankle oedema, of uncertain pathogenesis, may occasionally be very troublesome.

Drowsiness is common early in treatment, except with tranylcypromine, which may produce insomnia. Hepatocellular jaundice has been reported with most members of the hydrazine group, but not with tranylcypromine. This complication is relatively rare, but is associated with a disturbingly high fatality rate. Iproniazid has been particularly associated with liver damage and may also induce peripheral neuropathy.

Interaction with other drugs is a special hazard, and it is now usual for patients taking any monoamine oxidase inhibitor to carry a warning card. Many drugs used in emergency procedures may be potentiated to a serious degree—morphine, pethidine, ether, phenothiazines, cocaine, procaine, and barbiturates. Ganglion-blocking hypotensive agents are potentiated, whereas the effect of guanethidine is antagonized. The control of diabetes may be upset by intensification of the action of insulin. States of drug-induced delirium and excitation may occasionally occur with monoamine oxidase inhibitors alone, but more particularly if they are given along with rauwolfia alkaloids, tricyclic antidepressants, anti-parkinsonian agents, or alpha methyl dopa. As might be expected, sympathomimetic amines are very considerably potentiated and must be strictly avoided. Hypertensive crises producing a clinical picture similar to phaeochromocytoma, and sometimes resulting in death from intracranial haemorrhage, have been reported after the administration of adrenaline, noradrenaline, amphetamine, ephedrine, or phenylephrine.

Hypertensive crises with severe headache are also produced after the ingestion of certain foodstuffs. Cheese is the best known and most studied example, but Marmite, Bovril, broad beans, beer, wines, cream, yeast extracts, chicken livers and game have also been incriminated. Blackwell et al. (1967) have reviewed the mechanisms underlying these phenomena, which appear to depend on the content of tyramine and other substances in the foodstuffs involved. The reactions may be extremely dangerous, but are to some extent idiosyncratic, some patients apparently continuing to eat all foods with impunity. Tranylcypromine is the most liable of all the drugs in the group to provoke hypertensive crises. The treatment of an acute episode is the intravenous injection of phentolamine (Rogitine) 5 mg.

The tricyclic antidepressants

Imipramine (Tofranil), the first of this group to be used, was found to have antidepressant properties while investigations were being made into the tranquillizing properties of various phenothiazine derivatives. The tricyclic antidepressants have now come to be recognized as the most reliable antidepressant drugs available, and numerous strictly controlled trials have confirmed their value. Imipramine and amitriptyline (Tryptizol), still the most firmly established members of this group, have been followed by the synthesis of a number of further derivatives, many of which also appear to be efficacious. These are listed in Table 14.2, along with indications that some members of the group have sedative or stimulating properties which accompany their antidepressant action. These additional effects are commonly transient and liable to individual variation.

The better attested members of the group have been clearly shown to have a more marked antidepressant action than the monoamine oxidase inhibitors. They have proved valuable in the treatment of hospitalized depressed patients, even those showing marked evidence of biological disturbance such as insomnia and psychomotor retardation. Patients with psychotic phenomena such as delusions and hallucinations may also respond. Thus, except in the most extreme cases they are well worth a trial before commencing ECT, since they can be given repeatedly in recurrent attacks and over more prolonged periods of time without detriment to the patient. Nevertheless, ECT still remains the most effective treatment for severe depressive illnesses; both the M.R.C. (1965) trial and Bennett's (1967) survey of therapeutic trials establish the efficacy of imipramine but also the superiority of ECT in relieving depressive symptoms among patients ill enough to be in hospital.

TABLE 14.2

Tricyclic Antidepressants

Name	Usual daily dose (mg)	Sedating or stimulating
Imipramine (Tofranil)	75–150	—
Desipramine (Pertofran)	75–150	Stimulating
Trimipramine (Surmontil)	75–150	Sedating
Iprindole (Prondol)	45–90	—
Opipranol (Insidon)	100–150	Sedating
Amitriptyline (Tryptizol)	75–150	Sedating
Protriptyline (Concordin)	15–60	Stimulating
Nortriptyline (Aventyl, Allegron)	30–75	—

With all the tricyclic drugs it is essential to explain the drug régime carefully to the patient. This should begin with half or less of the expected therapeutic dose for the first four days, increased gradually over several days to the full amount. In this way tolerance will be acquired to the less serious side-effects and the patient encouraged to persevere. Elderly patients are often extremely sensitive to small doses and should generally be started very cautiously on less than the normal starting dose; for this purpose 10-mg tablets of imipramine and of amitriptyline are available. The patient should be told not to expect any improvement until he has been on the optimum dose for 10–14 days. Continued improvement can then be expected for three or four weeks more, and in some cases pronounced extra benefit may result from a further small increase of dose beyond the usual level indicated in the table.

Imipramine (Tofranil) remains one of the most fully investigated and well-proved antidepressants available. Reviewing the available literature, Shepherd et al. (1968) note that improvement rates of between 60 and 80 per cent have in general been reported. In restless or anxious patients imipramine may aggravate tension and is therefore often prescribed along with chlordiazepoxide (Librium) or diazepam (Valium). Results are better in "endogenous" than "reactive" depressions but a demonstrable effect is present in both. Kiloh et al. (1962) have attempted to delineate the factors associated with good outcome among out-patients treated with imipramine; these include age over 40, a subjective experience of mood change qualitatively different from "normal" depression, weight loss of over seven pounds, early waking, an insidious onset, and a duration of less than one year.

Certain atypical depressive illnesses, including patients with primary complaints of pain and other somatic symptomatology, have been found to respond. Imipramine has found a useful place in the treatment of depressive components in general medical disorders. Kaplan *et al.* (1961) were able to demonstrate convincingly that it reduced the incidence of asthmatic attacks in one patient and the requirements of insulin in another. It was found to be beneficial in cases of neurodermatitis, rheumatoid arthritis, ulcerative colitis, functional amenorrhoea, and narcolepsy, while others have reported its value in psoriasis, cardiovascular disease, myalgia, vasomotor rhinitis and gastro-intestinal disorders. Imipramine has been widely reported to be of value in Parkinson's disease, certainly by relieving depression but possibly also by virtue of its anticholinergic effects (Strang, 1965).

It is not clearly established whether imipramine and other antidepressant drugs do more than merely suppress the manifestations of the depressive illness until a natural remission occurs. Certainly, many patients are seen who relapse if treatment is withdrawn too quickly. Investigation of the problem is difficult, but an M.R.C. trial of the value of maintenance therapy is now under way. Present practice usually advises cautious and gradual withdrawal of the drug only after some three to four months of optimal health, though in many patients it should probably be continued much longer depending on the severity of the illness, the previous history, and the environmental problems which remain to be faced.

Desipramine (Pertofran) was introduced in the hope of producing more rapid action than imipramine, since desipramine represents a stage in the body's metabolism of the latter. There is, however, little evidence that in practice it is superior to imipramine.

Trimipramine (Surmontil), introduced more recently, is said to compare favourably with imipramine and to have the advantage of being less prone to cause orthostatic hypotension. It is apparently less liable to aggravate tension and to have sedative properties.

Iprindole (Prondol) awaits full clinical assessment, but preliminary reports suggest a very low incidence of autonomic side effects. It may therefore find a special place in the treatment of patients with coexistent physical disease where such side effects would be dangerous.

Opipranol (Insidon) is mid-way in chemical structure between imipramine and chlorpromazine, and is said to combine the antidepressant action of the one with the tranquillizing effect of the other. It does not, however, emerge as a powerful antidepressant.

Amitriptyline (Tryptizol) is the only drug for which an antidepressant effect equivalent to that of imipramine has been widely established. It's main difference appears to lie in more powerful sedative properties which have led to its adoption as the treatment of choice in depressive illnesses accompanied by much tension or anxiety. Hordern *et al.* (1963, 1964), in a large controlled trial, showed that amitriptyline was superior to imipramine in depressed female in-patients, especially those in the older age-groups. This result has been confirmed by others. Shepherd Lader and Rodnight (1968) conclude that imipramine may be more efficacious for the "retarded male patient" and amitriptyline for the "agitated female patient".

Recently a preparation combining amitriptyline 25 mg with perphenazine 2 mg (Tryptafen) has been reported to show particularly effective anti-depressant properties (Browne, 1969).

Protriptyline (Concordin) and *nortriptyline (Aventyl, Allegron)* are more recently introduced tricyclic compounds which, although not yet fully evaluated, are gaining wide acceptance. Both are more potent pharmaco-logically (though not necessarily more effective clinically) than amitriptyline in that a smaller dosage is required. Protriptyline has stimulant properties which are claimed to be of value when anergia and apathy are prominent.

Unwanted effects of the tricyclic antidepressants

Some autonomic effects are almost universal in the early stages of treat-ment, and the patient deserves to be warned against them—dryness of the mouth, blurring of vision, tachycardia and constipation. Postural hypotension and increased sweating may also be troublesome. Difficulty with micturition may proceed to retention of urine in patients with prostatic enlargment, and paralytic ileus may also constitute a definite therapeutic risk. Tricyclic antidepressants are contra-indicated in glaucoma. They block the antihyper-tensive effects of guanethidine and similar adrenergic blocking agents (Mitchell *et al.*, 1967). Impotence is frequently reported, and loss of libido sometimes occurs in the female.

Drowsiness is common in the early stages of treatment with amitriptyline and may be extreme. The problem may sometimes be overcome by restarting at a very low dose indeed (10 mg per day) and increasing very gradually, but even then treatment may have to be abandoned. Fine tremor of the hands is occasionally a troublesome side-effect, more rarely muscular twitching and ataxia. Numbness and tingling in the limbs have sometimes been reported with tricyclic antidepressants, and very occasionally peripheral neuropathy. Toxic confusional states may occur including nocturnal hallucinatory episodes. Other psychiatric side-effects include the precipitation of hypo-mania (a risk with any effective antidepressant treatment) or the reactivation of latent schizophrenic symptoms.

Epileptic fits may be induced or increased in susceptible patients, and in known epileptics it is wise to increase anticonvulsant medication. Rare

allergic effects include skin reactions, mild cholestatic jaundice and agranulocytosis. Teratogenic effects have not been demonstrated in man or in animals,
but nevertheless administration during the first trimester of pregnancy should
only be considered if there are compelling reasons.

Some concern is now felt about the cardiac effects of the tricyclic antidepressants. A variety of ECG changes have been reported, including flattening or inversion of T waves, depressed ST segments and left axis deviation.
These may make their first appearance or be aggravated by exertion. Careful
studies (Schou, 1962) involving serial ECGs have confirmed the causative
relationship between the drugs and the ECG changes which, however, always
returned to the pre-treatment reading within a week or two of stopping the
drug. Thus, in spite of some reassuring reports that patients with established
heart disease can be treated with impunity with tricyclic antidepressants,
it is generally recommended that they should not be prescribed in the presence
of cardiac failure, known ischaemic heart disease, or recent myocardial
infarction.

Combined antidepressant drug treatment

Monoamine oxidase inhibitors given in conjunction with tricyclic antidepressants have been reported to produce severe reactions, including toxic
psychoses with acute excitement, and excessive central sympathetic stimulation with muscle twitching, convulsions, hyperpyrexia and even death
(Bowen, 1964; Lockett and Milner, 1965). Though such reactions are rare
it is generally recommended that 10–14 days should elapse between stopping
monoamine oxidase inhibitors and starting tricyclic antidepressants. A
change in the reverse direction can be allowed with a gap of only two
or three days owing to the more rapid clearance of the effects of tricyclic
drugs.

Nevertheless, the risk is said to have been overstated provided that imipramine and tranylcypromine are avoided, and combined treatment has
been advocated for the treatment of very refractory depressions. Amitriptyline combined with either phenelzine or isocarboxazid, for example, is
reported to have been employed in a great number of patients without ill
effect (Gander, 1967). Sargant et al. (1966) have used combined drug treatment, with in addition ECT and continuous narcosis, for patients with very
refractory tension states.

The claims of combined drug treatment are, of course, extremely hard to
evaluate in the absence of controlled trials, and in view of the considerable
difficulties encountered in reaching firm decisions about the rival merits of
drugs used even singly. It would certainly seem wise to embark on such
treatment only very cautiously indeed, and as something of a last resort
prior to leucotomy.

Drugs used in the Treatment of Anxiety Symptoms

Considerable strides have been made in treating specific anxiety symptoms, especially circumscribed phobias, by a variety of desensitization techniques derived from behaviourist psychological theory, but this is not the place to discuss such specialized psychiatric procedures. The problem of treating diffuse pervasive anxiety remains, and presents itself in the general medical clinic as well as to the psychiatrist. In all such cases it is necessary first to be scrupulous in searching for evidence of truly depressive symptomatology which may be masked in the presence of florid anxiety symptoms which command the patient's first attention. Symptomatic relief of anxiety in such cases can bring only temporary benefit until the underlying depressive illness is treated. Fortunately, the drugs described below can without exception be given with antidepressants or indeed with ECT, so that in cases of doubt it is often wise to prescribe both classes of drug together.

Barbiturates remain extremely useful for the treatment of acute severe anxiety, and for controlling the tension and restlessness of agitated depression. Many patients with chronic anxiety symptoms report more relief from small doses of amylobarbitone (60–100 mg t.d.s.) than from the newer anxiety-relieving drugs, though here much care must be taken to guard against an increase of dose and eventual addiction. It is probably for this reason, along with the risk of suicidal overdose, that barbiturates are not used more extensively as the treatment of choice for anxiety symptoms. An early controlled trial (Raymond et al., 1957) showed the superiority of barbiturates over benactyzine, meprobamate, rauwolfia, chlorpromazine and placebo. More recent trials comparing amylobarbitone with chlordiazepoxide have failed to demonstrate conclusively that the latter is more effective (Shepherd et al., 1968).

Meprobamate (*Equanil, Miltown*), a derivative of the muscle relaxant mephenesin, has enjoyed a vogue in the treatment of anxiety, usually in large doses of 800–1600 mg daily. However, controlled trials have in general thrown doubt on its effectiveness, and it has rapidly yielded in recent years to the more effective compounds described below. Untoward effects include drowsiness, a variety of anaphylactoid reactions and, more rarely, blood dyscrasias. Both addiction and successful suicide have been reported with meprobamate.

The benzodiazepines, including *chlordiazepoxide* (*Librium*), *diazepam* (*Valium*) and *oxazepam* (*Serenid-D*) have come to be the drugs of choice in the treatment of anxiety and tension. All have been demonstrated in adequate controlled trials to be effective therapeutic agents. Chlordiazepoxide is given in doses of 10–20 mg t.d.s., diazepan 5–10 mg t.d.s., oxazepam 15–30 mg t.d.s. An effect is usually noticeable from the start of treatment, but since the drugs are cumulative, regular medication is required. Effectiveness tends to diminish with prolonged use, but nevertheless this group of drugs appears often to remain of substantial benefit in chronic tension states. These drugs have no antidepressant effect, but are frequently given along with antidepressants, especially those which do not themselves have a sedative effect. Diazepam (and to a less extent chlordiazepoxide) also shows marked anticonvulsant properties, and is used in the treatment of status epilepticus. It is also a muscle relaxant, which makes it of considerable potential value in the treatment of tension headaches and the somatic manifestations of heightened muscle tone which may accompany anxiety. Perhaps an outstanding reason contributing to the popularity of these drugs is that successful suicide from overdosage is excessively rare, if indeed it has occurred at all.

The most common side-effect is drowsiness, which may usually be circumvented by increasing the dose gradually from a small beginning. Diazepam is more prone to produce this effect than chlordiazepoxide and may in addition produce ataxia. A common side-effect much resented by women patients is excessive gain in weight. As with barbiturates, confusion may be caused in the elderly. Lapses of attention while driving may lead to accidents and are probably commoner than is generally realized (Murray, 1961). Physical and psychological dependence have been reported, but when viewed against the enormous extent of prescribing this does not appear to be a substantial problem. Withdrawal after administration in high dosage may result in epileptic fits. Hypersensitivity reactions in the form of rashes may occur but do not appear to be frequent.

Other anxiety relieving drugs, including *methyl pentynol (Oblivon)*, *benactyzine (Suavitil)* and *hydroxyzine (Atarax)*, continue to be used in treatment of mild anxiety, but their clinical effectiveness is greatly overshadowed by the benzodiazepines. The Phenothiazines, at one time widely tried in the treatment of neurotic tension and anxiety, have not proved their value in this sphere (Merry *et al.*, 1957; Raymond *et al.*, 1957). However, in crises of anxiety and excitement in severe agitated depression their tranquillizing effect may be very beneficial, and their potentiating effect on barbiturates is exploited as an integral part of treatment by continuous narcosis.

Another drug in which psychiatrists have recently shown an interest is *propanolol (Inderal)*. This adrenergic beta-receptor blocking agent was shown to control the sinus tachycardia seen in anxiety states as well as in thyrotoxicosis (Turner *et al.*, 1965). Following this, Granville-Grossman and Turner (1966) carried out a double blind trial of propanolol, 20 mg q.d.s. in patients with anxiety symptoms, and found that it controlled a wide range of disturbances mediated by the autonomic nervous system. Coincident with this there was improvement in subjective anxiety, suggesting that control of somatic symptoms had a favourable effect on the mental state. Frohlich *et al.* (1966) reported two patients in whom they postulated primary sensitivity of beta-receptor mechanisms to circulating adrenergic substances, and who benefited from propanolol with a reduction of anxiety. These observations should perhaps warn us against too readily diagnosing a primary emotional disorder in anxious patients with prominent tachycardia and other autonomic disturbances. Further work clearly needs to be done, and it remains to be shown that propanolol counteracts anxiety *via* beta-adrenergic blockade and not merely by virtue of central sedative effects.

DRUGS USED IN THE TREATMENT OF MANIA

The standard treatment for mania or hypomania continues to be chlorpromazine (Largactil), beginning with 50 mg t.d.s. and increasing the dose rapidly over several days until overactivity and excitement are controlled. Most patients respond satisfactorily, though very large doses of 1500 mg per day or more are sometimes necessary. In the early stages of treatment, intramuscular chlorpromazine to obtain a more rapid effect, and with due care barbiturates (e.g. sodium amytal 100–200 mg t.d.s.) may be given coincidentally so that the two drugs may potentiate one another. It is usually necessary to prescribe anti-parkinsonian medication along with chlorpromazine to prevent extrapyramidal side-effects, as will be described more fully in the section on schizophrenia. There is no firm evidence that chlorpromazine shortens the course of the hypomanic illness or in any way does more than damp down the outward manifestations of the disorder. A cautious trial of withdrawal after the symptoms have been fully controlled for three weeks or more is the only certain way of determining when treatment should cease.

Haloperidol (Serenace) is now increasingly used in the treatment of mania and hypomania. This drug is considered more fully in the section on schizophrenia. It is a useful alternative in patients who tolerate chlorpromazine poorly, and some patients respond well to haloperidol after chlorpromazine in large dosage has failed to alleviate hypomanic symptoms. Nevertheless, the higher incidence of side-effects prevents haloperidol from being the drug of first choice.

The Use of Lithium in Affective Disorders

A great deal of interest centres on the use of lithium salts in affective disorders, particularly because claims have recently been made that they have a prophylactic effect in preventing recurrences of both manic and depressive episodes in manic-depressive disorder.

Lithium has been used in the treatment of mania and hypomania since 1949 when Cade reported a beneficial effect. However, problems of toxicity prevented lithium from achieving widespread popularity in this disorder, and the subsequent introduction of phenothiazine drugs tended greatly to displace it. Two carefully controlled trials (Schou *et al.*, 1954; Maggs,

1963) have nevertheless firmly established the effectiveness of lithium in mania and hypomania, and with increased confidence resulting from laboratory control of serum levels this form of treatment is now used extensively. It is generally used only when other drug treatments have failed, though in some centres it has been advocated as the treatment of choice. A careful comparison of the relative merits of these various treatments for mania is awaited. Improvement with lithium sets in gradually after the sixth day when adequate blood levels have been reached, and the disorder may in favourable cases be brought under control within a further week.

There is no convincing evidence that lithium has any therapeutic effect in an attack of depressive illness. But interest centres here around the claim that maintenance treatment with lithium over long periods of time can diminish the frequency of episodes of affective disorder in patients who suffer recurring attacks. Baarstrup (1964) initially reported a small group of such patients treated with encouraging results, and Baarstrup and Schou (1967) later reported on 88 patients observed over six and a half years and treated for periods varying from one to five years. In the latter group the pre-treatment average frequency of relapse had been at eight-month intervals, whilst that in the group under treatment was 60–85 months. Treatment was found to be equally effective in preventing attacks both in patients who experienced manic and depressive episodes and in patients who had suffered recurrent depression only. The patients were also said to be more stable in mood between relapses. On discontinuing lithium episodes of affective disorder occurred with the same frequency as before. The authors' claim that "lithium is the first drug for which a clear-cut prophylactic action against one of the major psychoses has been demonstrated" is very important if fully substantiated.

This effect appears at first sight to obtain some theoretical backing from what is known of electrolyte balance in affective disorder, in that lithium reduces the residual body sodium which is known to be raised in mania and to a less extent in depression (Coppen et al., 1966). More recent studies, however, show that the true position is complex and uncertain (Coppen and Shaw, 1967). The therapeutic claim has been criticized by Blackwell and Shepherd (1968), who dissect in detail many aspects of the methodology of the study by Basstrup and Schou which might have led to spurious results.

Dosage and side-effects. Lithium is usually given as the carbonate in 250-mg tablets. In the treatment of acute mania, it is wise to start with 250 mg t.d.s., then increase gradually with frequent checks to ensure that the serum level does not exceed 2 mEq/litre. Up to 2000 mg per day may be required in the initial stages for the control of acute symptoms, though the dosage required to ensure an adequate blood level appears to fall with improvement in the mental state. Maintenance therapy usually requires between 500 and 1000 mg per day in order to maintain serum levels between

0·6 and 1·5 mEq/litre. Serum estimations should be performed at least twice a week in the initial stages and once a month throughout maintenance therapy. *Treatment should be initiated in hospital.* Fluctuations in the daily intake of sodium chloride affect the serum levels, and patients should be instructed to keep up an adequate intake of salt. It is recommended that treatment be withheld for 24 hours once a week, to diminish the risk of a cumulative effect leading to dangerously high blood levels. Recently a controlled release preparation of lithium carbonate has been produced (Priadel) which needs to be taken only once daily during maintenance therapy.

Common side-effects include fine hand tremor and transient drowsiness. More severe effects, which must never be ignored, are diarrhoea, nausea and vomiting, anorexia, thirst, polyuria, ataxia, coarse limb tremor and muscular twitching. Serious signs which indicate a developing encephalopathy include nystagmus, dysarthria and epileptic fits. Several reports of fatalities have occurred, mostly due to neurological complications. Renal damage may also occur, but is said to be reversible in the early stages. A teratogenic effect found in animals has not as yet been reported in human subjects, but lithium salts should not be given to pregnant patients. There have been recent reports of non-toxic goitre in patients treated for long periods with lithium (Schou *et al.*, 1968).

Nevertheless, most patients can take lithium over prolonged periods with safety, provided that subjects with renal disease, cardiac disease or any other clinical condition liable to cause disturbance of sodium balance are excluded, and provided that serum levels in excess of 2 mEq/litre are avoided.

Electroconvulsive Therapy

Electroconvulsive therapy, introduced by Cerletti and Bini in 1938, remains the most effective treatment for severe depressive illnesses. Its therapeutic value has been amply demonstrated and is in no way impaired by the present-day practice of administering the shock under full anaesthesia together with muscle-relaxant drugs. The effectiveness of the procedure depends not on the intensity of current flowing through the brain but on the incidence and duration of the epileptic dysrhythmia engendered within it (Cronholm and Ottoson, 1960). By contrast, the troublesome side-effect of memory disturbance depends on the strength of shock given; therefore the aim of each treatment must be to achieve an epileptic fit with the minimum possible shock. Six to eight treatments given at intervals of three or four days generally suffice, though if continuing improvement is occurring, courses may sometimes be further extended very cautiously. Three-quarters of straightforward depressive illnesses treated in hospital may be expected to respond.

The advent of antidepressant drugs has brought renewed attention to the special indications for ECT, and several studies have sought to compare its effectiveness with that of the drugs themselves. Hobson, in 1953, had already outlined some of the chief factors in depressive illness which indicated a good outcome with ECT—sudden onset, duration of less than one year, good preservation of insight, self-reproach, pronounced retardation and obsessional personality traits. Bad prognostic factors included neurotic disturbances, hypochondriasis, emotional liability, an hysterical attitude to the illness, and an ill-adjusted previous personality. This supported the widely held belief that the so-called "neurotic" depressions fared less well with ECT than did "endogenous" depressions. More recently, Carney et al. (1965), in a study of 129 in-patients, were able to confirm that the presence or absence of features considered to discriminate between neurotic and endogenous depression had a marked effect on ECT response. They were further able to delineate ten features which could be weighted for prediction of outcome of treatment at six months: a favourable outcome was indicated by weight loss exceeding seven pounds (+3), pyknic body build (+3), early waking (+2), somatic delusions (+2), and paranoid delusions or gross ideas of reference (+1), whereas poor outcome was indicated by hysterical features or attitudes (−3), hypochondriasis (−3), worsening of depression in the evenings (−3), anxiety (−2), and self-pity (−1).

With regard to the relative merits of ECT and antidepressant drugs, the great majority of studies agree in finding that ECT remains the most powerful and the most rapidly effective treatment. In the M.R.C. (1965) multicentred trial on 250 in-patients, which compared ECT, imipramine, phenelzine and placebo, ECT caused the most rapid improvement and induced the most marked amelioration of individual symptoms. The results with ECT were particularly outstanding in the group of patients with the most severe illnesses. Imipramine, however, compared favourably with ECT in the less severely ill group (bearing in mind that all patients were ill enough to require hospitalization) whereas phenelzine proved no better than placebo. The short-term results at four weeks after commencing treatment were upheld at six months. An unexpected finding was that imipramine was especially effective in men and ECT especially effective in women. Several smaller studies have confirmed these main findings—that ECT is very definitely superior to monoamine oxidase inhibitor drugs, and generally superior to tricyclic antidepressants also. Against this must be set the practical problems of administering the treatment, the small but definite risk accompanying it, the anaesthetic hazard in the physically ill, and the limitations imposed on repeated or long-continued treatment by virtue of amnesic defects. Moreover, while out-patient ECT is widely prescribed in many centres, this has obvious limitations. Certainly the antidepressant drugs offer a certain advantage over ECT when long-standing personality and environmental problems need to be tackled over a considerable period of time, during which sustained relief of depressive symptoms must also be maintained.

Two recent developments of ECT deserve attention—the full evaluation of unilateral ECT and the elaboration of convulsive treatments based on the inhalation of hexafluorodiethyl ether (Indoklon).

The first studies of unilateral ECT applied to the non-dominant hemisphere suggested that this was equally effective in relieving depression and less inclined to disturb memory than the conventional bilateral treatment (Lancaster *et al.*, 1958; Cannicott, 1962). This has been confirmed by several recent careful studies (Zinkin and Birtchnell, 1968; Valentine *et al.*, 1968), the latter also showing that pulse currents produce less disturbance than sinusoidal currents. In Levy's (1968) study, however, the advantages of unilateral ECT were far from clear, despite excellent experimental design. Three studies have compared bilateral ECT with unilateral ECT administered to either hemisphere of the brain (Zamora and Kaebling, 1965; Gottlieb and Wilson, 1965; Halliday *et al.*, 1968). ECT given to the non-dominant hemisphere was shown to produce less disturbance of verbal memory than either dominant hemisphere or bilateral ECT. This indicates that the benefit is due not merely to a generalized reduction of current flow through the brain, but depends on the different neuronal circuits traversed by the current. In Halliday's study non-verbal learning was selectively impaired by ECT to the non-dominant hemisphere, but even here this was less persistent as time went by than in the group receiving bilateral ECT. These important experimental studies are therefore accumulating in favour of adopting unilateral non-dominant ECT as the treatment of choice in helping to minimize the most troublesome side effects of the procedure.

In several centres, trials are now being conducted into the relative merits of ECT and of convulsions induced by inhalation of hexafluorodiethyl ether (Indoklon). Some reports (Rose and Watson, 1967) have suggested that post-ictal confusion is reduced. In a recent study by Gander *et al.* (1967) Indoklon was found to be a satisfactory method of inducing therapeutic convulsions, but was attended by more side-effects and proved rather cumbersome in practice. It is therefore not possible at this stage to judge whether this form of treatment will find a firm place in therapeutics.

Leucotomy

The more restricted forms of leucotomy evolved in recent years have a place in the management of severe and long-standing affective disorders when other treatments have failed. Undesirable effects on personality are not inevitable for a therapeutic effect, but still occur in a small proportion of patients, and along with post-operative epilepsy still constitute a definite risk. Thus leucotomy can be recommended only with caution. A sound premorbid personality without sociopathic traits remains an important criterion if untoward sequelae are to be avoided. Obsessional traits in the personality are generally regarded as increasing the likelihood of a good therapeutic outcome.

Intractable states of tension from whatever cause are a principal indication for leucotomy. Kelly *et al.* (1966) have reported its value in patients with long-standing anxiety symptoms including panic attacks, and have demonstrated the immediate benefit on pathological anxiety mechanisms by objective physiological measures. Chronic depressive illness can also respond to leucotomy; Sykes and Tredgold (1964) reported that restricted orbital undercutting helped a high proportion of patients with chronic depressive illnesses resistant to other forms of treatment, and furthermore could bring a halt to frequently recurring attacks. Post *et al.* (1968), in a careful evaluation of the results of bimedial leucotomy, confirmed the benefits to be seen in depressive illness; amongst a variety of psychiatric conditions depression, especially in the elderly, showed the best response. Knight (1965, 1969) has evolved a technique for implanting radio-active Yttrium Y.90 into the substantia innominata of the frontal lobes under radio-active control. The critical brain areas lie immediately beneath the striatum and overlie the posterior orbital cortex of areas 13 and 14. This operation is claimed to be virtually without risk, and to be applicable to patients of advanced years and in poor physical condition. The procedure has again been reported to be particularly effective in chronic depression.

REFERENCES

BAARSTRUP, P. C. (1964). The use of Lithium in manic-depressive psychosis. *Comprehens. Psychiat.*, **5**, 396.

BAARSTRUP, P. C. & SCHOU, M. (1967). Lithium as a prophylactic agent. *Arch. gen. Psychiat.*, **16**, 162.

BENNETT, I. F. (1967). Is there a superior antidepressant? In *Antidepressant Drugs.* ed. S. Garattini and M. N. G. Dukes. Excerpta Medica Foundation.

BLACKWELL, B., PRICE, J. & TAYLOR, D. (1967). Hypertensive interactions between monoamine oxidase inhibitors and foodstuffs. *Brit. J. Psychiat.*, **113**, 349.

BLACKWELL, B. & SHEPHERD, M. (1968). Prophylactic lithium: another therapeutic myth? *Lancet*, **1**, 968.

BOWEN, L. W. (1964). Fatal hyperpyrexia with antidepressant drugs. *Brit. med. J.*, **2**, 1465.

BROWNE, M. W. (1969). A comparison of two drug treatments in depressive illness. *Brit. J. Psychiat.*, **115**, 693.

CADE, J. F. J. (1949). Lithium salts in the treatment of psychotic excitement. *Med. J. Aust.*, **36**, 349.

CANNICOTT, S. M. (1962). Unilateral electroconvulsive therapy. *Postgrad. med. J.*, **38**, 451.

CARNEY, M. W. P., ROTH, M. & GARSIDE, R. F. (1965). The diagnosis of depressive syndromes and the prediction of E.C.T. response. *Brit. J. Psychiat.*, **111**, 659.

CERLETTI, U. & BINI, L. (1938). Electroshock. *Boll. Acad. med. Roma*, **64**, 36.

COPPEN, A. (1967). The biochemistry of affective disorders. *Brit. J. Psychiat.*, **113**, 1237.

COPPEN, A., SHAW, D. M., MALLESON, A. & COSTAIN, R. (1966). Mineral metabolism in mania. *Brit. med. J.*, **1**, 71.

COPPEN, A. & SHAW, D. M. (1967). The distribution of electrolytes and water in patients after taking lithium carbonate. *Lancet*, 2, 805.

CRONHOLM, B. & OTTOSON, J. O. (1960). Experimental studies of the therapeutic action of electroconvulsive therapy in endogenous depression. *Acta. psychiat. scand., Suppl.*, 145, 69.

FROHLICH, E. D., DUNSTAN, H. P. & PAGE, I. H. (1966). Hyperdynamic beta-adrenergic circulatory state. *Arch. intern. Med.*, 117, 614.

GANDER, D. R. (1967). The clinical value of monoamine oxidase inhibitors and tricyclic antidepressants in combination. In *Antidepressant Drugs*. ed. S. Garattini and M. N. G. Dukes. Excerpta Medica Foundation.

GANDER, D. R., BENNETT, P. J. & KELLY, D. H. W. (1967). Hexafluorodiethyl ether (Indoklon) convulsive therapy: a pilot study. *Brit. J. Psychiat.*, 113, 1413.

GIBBONS, J. L. (1968). Biochemistry of depressive illness. In *Recent Development in Affective Disorders*. ed. A. Coppen and A. Walker. *Brit. J. Psychiat.*, special publication No. 2. Ashford, Kent: Headley Brothers.

GOTTLIEB, G. & WILSON, I. (1965). Cerebral dominance: temporary disruption of verbal memory by unilateral electroconvulsive shock treatment. *J. comp. physiol. Psychol.*, 60, 368.

GRANVILLE-GROSSMAN, K. L. & TURNER, P. G. (1966). The effect of propanolol on anxiety. *Lancet*, 1, 788.

HALLIDAY, A. M., DAVISON, K., BROWNE, M. W. & KREEGER, L. C. (1968). A comparison of the effects on depression and memory of bilateral E.C.T. and unilateral E.C.T. to the dominant and non-dominant hemispheres. *Brit. J. Psychiat.*, 114, 997.

HILL, D. (1968). Depression: disease, reaction, or posture? *Amer. J. Psychiat.*, 125, 445.

HOBSON, R. F. (1953). prognostic factors in electroconvulsive therapy. *J. Neurol. Neurosurg. Psychiat.*, 16, 275.

HORDERN, A., BURT, C. G., GORDON, W. F. & HOLT, N. F. (1964). Amitriptyline in depressive states: six month treatment results. *Brit. J. Psychiat.*, 110, 641.

HORDERN, A., HOLT, N. F., BURT, C. G. & GORDON, W. F. (1963). Amitriptyline in depressive states: Phenomenology and prognostic considerations. *Brit. J. Psychiat.*, 109, 815.

KAPLAN, S. M., KRAVETZ, R. S. & ROSS, W. D. (1961). The effects of imipramine on the depressive components of medical disorders. *Proc. 3rd Wld Congr. Psychiat.*, 2, 1362.

KELLY, D. H. W., WALTER, C. J. S. & SARGANT, W. (1966). Modified leucotomy assessed by forearm blood flow and other measurements. *Brit. J. Psychiat.*, 112, 871.

KENDELL, R. E. (1968). The problem of classification. In *Recent Developments in Affective Disorders*. ed. A. Coppen and A. Walk. *Brit. J. Psychiat.*, special publication No. 2. Ashford, Kent: Headley Brothers.

KILOH, L. G., BALL, J. R. B. & GARSIDE, R. F. (1962). Prognostic factors in treatment of depressive states with imipramine. *Brit. med. J.*, 1, 1225.

KILOH, L. G. & GARSIDE, R. F. (1963). The independence of neurotic depression and endogenous depression. *Brit. J., Psychiat.*, 109, 451.

KNIGHT, G. C. (1965). Stereotactic tractotomy in the surgical treatment of mental illness. *J. Neurol. Neurosurg. Psychiat.*, 28, 304.

KNIGHT, G. C. (1969). Bifrontal stereotactic tractotomy: an atraumatic operation of value in the treatment of intractable psychoneurosis. *Brit. J. Psychiat.*, 115, 257.

R

LANCASTER, N. P., STEINERT, R. R. & FROST, I. (1958). Unilateral electroconvulsive therapy. *J. ment. Sci.*, **104**, 221.

LASCELLES, R. G. (1966). Atypical facial pain and depression. *Brit. J. Psychiat.*, **112**, 651.

LEVY, R. (1968). The clinical evaluation of unilateral electroconvulsive therapy. *Brit. J. Psychiat.*, **114**, 459.

LOCKETT, M. F. & MILNER, G. (1965). Combining the antidepressant drugs. *Brit. med. J.*, **1**, 921.

McCONAGHY, N., JOFFE, A. D. & MURPHY, B. (1967). The independence of neurotic and endogenous depression. *Brit. J. Psychiat.*, **113**, 479.

MAGGS, R. (1963). Treatment of manic illness with lithium carbonate. *Brit. J. Psychiat.*, **109**, 56.

MEDICAL RESEARCH COUNCIL (1965). Clinical trial of the treatment of depressive illness. Report by Clinical Psychiatry Committee. *Brit. med. J.*, **1**, 881.

MERRY, J., PARGITER, R. A. & MUNRO, H. (1957). Chlorpromazine and chronic neurotic tension. *Amer. J. Physchiat.*, **113**, 988.

MITCHELL, J. R., ARIAS, L. & OATES, J. A. (1967). Antagonism of the antihypertensive action of guanethidine sulfate by desipramine hydrochloride. *J. Amer. med. Ass.*, **202**, 973.

MURRAY, N. (1961). Covert effects of chlordiazepoxide therapy. *J. Neuropsychiat.*, **3**, 168.

PARE, C. M. B. (1965). Some clinical aspects of antidepressant drugs. In *Scientific Basis of Drug Therapy*. ed. J. Marks and C. M. B. Pare. London: Pergamon Press.

PARE, C. M. B. (1968). Recent advances in the treatment of depression. In *Recent Developments in Affective Disorders*. ed. A. Coppen and A. Walk. *Brit. J. Psychiat.*, special publication No. 2. Ashford, Kent: Headley Brothers.

PARE, C. M. B., REES, L. & SAINSBURY, M. J. (1962). Differentiation of two genetically specific types of depression by response to antidepressant drugs. *Lancet*, **2**, 1340.

POST, F. (1966). Somatic and psychic factors in the treatment of elderly psychiatric patients. *J. psychosom. Res.*, **10**, 13.

POST, F., REES, W. L. & SCHURR, P. H. (1968). An evaluation of bimedial leucotomy. *Brit. J. Psychiat.*, **114**, 1223.

RAYMOND, M. J., LUCAS, C. J., BEESLEY, M. L., O'CONNELL, B. A. & FRASER ROBERTS, J. A. (1957). A trial of five tranquillising drugs in psychoneurosis. *Brit. med. J.*, **2**, 63.

ROSE, L. & WATSON, A. (1967). Flurothyl—a new inhalant convulsant agent. *Anaesthesia*, **22**, 425.

SARGANT, W., WALTER, C. J. S. & WRIGHT, N. (1966). New treatment of some chronic tension states. *Brit. med. J.*, **1**, 322.

SCHOU, M. (1962). Electrocardiographic changes during treatment with lithium and with drugs of the imipramine type. *Acta psychiat. scand.*, **38**, 331.

SCHOU, M., AMDISEN, A., JENSEN, S. E. & OLSEN, T. (1968). Occurrence of goitre during lithium treatment. *Brit. med. J.*, **3**, 710.

SCHOU, M., JUEL-NIELSON, N., STROMGREN, E. & VOLDBY, H. (1954). The treatment of manic psychoses by the administration of lithium salts. *J. Neurol. Neurosurg. Psychiat.*, **17**, 250.

SHEPHERD, M., LADER, M. & RODNIGHT, R. (1968). *Clinical Psychopharmacology*. London: English Universities Press.

STRANG, R. R. (1965). Imipramine in treatment of Parkinsonism: a double-blind placebo study. *Brit. med. J.*, **2**, 33.

SYKES, M. K. & TREDGOLD, R. F. (1964). Restricted orbital undercutting. A study of its effects on 350 patients over the ten years 1951-60. *Brit. J. Psychiat.*, **110**, 609.

TURNER, P. G., GRANVILLE-GROSSMAN, K. L. & SMART, J. V. (1965). Effect of adrenergic receptor blockade on the tachycardia of thyrotoxicosis and anxiety states. *Lancet*, **2**, 1316.

VALENTINE, M., KEDDIE, K. M. G. & DUNNE, D. (1968). A comparison of techniques in electroconvulsive therapy. *Brit. J. Psychiat.*, **114**, 989.

WALKER, L. (1959). The prognosis for affective illness with overt anxiety. *J. Neurol. Neurosurg. Psychiat.*, **22**, 338.

WEST, E. D. & DALLY, P. J. (1959). Effects of iproniazid in depressive syndromes. *Brit. med. J.*, **1**, 1491.

WOOLFSON, G. (1968). Recent advances in the anxiety states. In *Recent Developments in Affective Disorders*. ed. A. Coppen and A. Walk. *Brit. J. Psychiat.*, special publication No. 2. Ashford, Kent: Headley Brothers.

ZAMORA, E. N. & KAEBLING, R. (1965). Memory and electroconvulsive therapy. *Amer. J. Psychiat.*, **122**, 546.

ZINKIN, S. & BIRTCHNELL, J. (1968). Unilateral electroconvulsive therapy: its effects on memory and its therapeutic efficacy. *Brit. J. Psychiat.*, **114**, 973.

SCHIZOPHRENIA

In the last 20 years the medical management of schizophrenia has changed in many important respects, one of which is the almost universal use of phenothiazine drugs. That phenothiazines have come to form the mainstay of treatment in this disorder was shown by a questionnaire issued to senior psychiatrists in England by Willis and Bannister (1965); 96 per cent of those who replied used phenothiazines, with or without ECT and other drugs, in the management of schizophrenic patients. Indeed, a study of diagnosis-treatment relationships in psychiatry showed the highest concordance of all for this particular clinical practice (Bannister *et al.*, 1964).

This therapeutic enthusiasm rests on a firm foundation of careful clinical observation described below, but one must guard against assuming too readily that drugs alone have been responsible for recent progress in the management of schizophrenia. It has been variously claimed that in psychiatry the phenothiazines have "heralded the clinical revolution that has transformed treatment and medical attitudes" (Sargant and Slater, 1963), and that they are "responsible for the essential progress of psychiatry during the past decade" (Haase and Janssen, 1965). These statements represent only part of the truth, and fail to take into account other complex aspects of the transition which has been occurring in the treatment of the mentally ill. In an admirable survey, Hoenig (1967) traces the developments in the management of schizophrenia both before and after the introduction of phenothiazine drugs. Important changes in legislation and in mental hospital practice set in well before the advent of phenothiazine drugs in the 1950s. The dangers of institutionalization and the importance of planned rehabilitation were already receiving attention, and statistics bearing on the efficacy of mental hospital treatment have indicated that considerable improvement began before the introduction of psychiatric drugs (Odegaard, 1964). Certainly these social and administrative developments, and the further growth of open door policies and community care have been helped to reach fruition by the use of drugs, but the latter should not be viewed in isolation or given exclusive credit for the achievements of the past 15 years. Wing and Brown (1961) have shown that the clinical state of chronic schizophrenics in different mental hospitals relates more closely to the social environment within each hospital than to differences in the drug dosages employed. Thus it seems that two factors—improvement in social policy and application of effective drugs—have developed hand in hand, and probably each has helped to realize the potentialities of the other.

General Management of Schizophrenia

Our diagnostic criteria for schizophrenia are by no means clear-cut; in fact it seems likely that more than one disease entity is subsumed under this title. For this reason it is often preferable to talk of schizophrenic illnesses rather than of schizophrenia generally. Some schizophrenic illnesses are symptomatic in the sense that they are clearly related to a precipitating or predisposing cause, such as amphetamine abuse or temporal lobe epilepsy, though in most cases no such factors can be discovered. Certainly the clinical pictures produced by schizophrenia are very diverse, and the amount of disruption of normal functioning occasioned by the disease may vary greatly from one individual to another. Among this diversity, however, certain cases are regarded by common consent as representing true or "nuclear" schizophrenia, whereas others represent atypical or transitional forms of illness. The present review of management will concentrate on the former group alone; it is, however, important to remember that much is written on groups of cases selected by less stringent criteria, and that schizophrenia is more readily diagnosed by practitioners in the U.S.A. than in the U.K.

As a general statement, it may be said that all patients newly suspected of suffering from a schizophrenic illness should be admitted to hospital for an initial spell, if only for careful observation which will help to clarify what is often a difficult diagnostic problem. Moreover, physical treatments for the disease should be pursued thoroughly from the earliest possible moment after the diagnosis is made, and are best instituted in an in-patient setting.

Treatment in hospital is a relatively short-lived phase in almost all cases of recent onset. In the majority, the more prominent symptoms of the initial attack are brought under control, and as soon as possible the patient is thereafter encouraged to resume his place in society and at work. Those who respond less completely need careful assessment of the particular problems which remain, so that an early start can be made with rehabilitation either within the hospital or in specialized rehabilitation units. The aim is the same, to attempt very strenuously to avoid prolonged hospitalization with the attendant risks to which the schizophrenic patient is particularly vulnerable, such as restriction of activities and interests, and withdrawal from involvement and communication with those around him.

Except where recovery is complete, discharge from hospital is merely the beginning of long-term supervision which aims at helping the patient to cope with the handicaps engendered by the illness. The success of early discharge depends on the quality of care which can be provided thereafter. Community care has evolved to a high degree in many centres, with close out-patient medical supervision and comprehensive social support for the patient and his family. Of prime importance are the maintenance of appropriate medication, the securing of suitable employment, dealing with family and interpersonal problems, and prompt attention to any emergencies which arise including the need for re-admission to hospital. While some patients even with established chronic schizophrenia remain self-supporting, others need special facilities such as day hospitals, hostels, occupation centres, sheltered workshops and social clubs.

Medical management in the out-patient clinic needs above all else close attention to medication and to means of ensuring that it is taken regularly. but much may also be done by way of supportive psychotherapy. Every effort must be made to help the patient to improve his social contacts and to maintain relationships within the family and elsewhere, to develop interests, and to formulate realistic plans for his future. Much can be done by sympathetic discussion to help the patient gain better insight into abnormal experiences and paranoid delusions, or at least to persuade him to keep them to himself during more florid phases of the disease. All this, of course, represents attempts to assist in the healing and encapsulation of symptoms rather than their exploration in depth; any attempts at analytic or "uncovering" psychotherapy are contra-indicated and are generally agreed to be more likely to precipitate relapse.

In spite of modern developments in out-patient care, some patients need long-term, even permanent, hospital care when their difficulties are viewed realistically. It is often claimed that the proportion of such cases is likely over the years to become very small. Among present long-stay patients, however, schizophrenia clearly remains a chronic and severe disease. It is important to remember that schizophrenic patients in 1967 still occupied 60,000, or one sixth, of all hospital beds in England and Wales (Bennett, 1967). Catterson et al. (1963) found that in a hospital with a tradition of active treatment and well-developed rehabilitation services only 13 per cent of such patients appeared likely to be able to hold down stable jobs and be discharged from hospital in the near future. In hospital, however, the policies of long-term care have evolved in important directions which seek to minimize the harmful effects of former regimes, and leave the patient more ready to benefit from future remissions should these occur. Techniques of social stimulation and occupation to the limits imposed by the illness have been shown to halt deterioration. The aim is to provide an environment that approximates as closely as possible to everyday life, to maintain links with the world outside, to give attention to individual needs, and to awaken in the patient a sense of responsibility towards his own achievements and progress.

The Phenothiazine Drugs

Chlorpromazine, synthesized in 1950, found its first clinical applications in anaesthesia (Laborit and Hugenard, 1951). Here, amongst other valuable properties, it was found to produce a state of calm relaxation and apparent indifference to distracting stimuli when used as a premedication, yet without producing the degree of somnolence seen with other sedative agents. This unique tranquillizing effect was soon found useful in conjunction with other drugs for producing prolonged narcosis in patients with a variety of mental illnesses (Deschamps and Cadoret, 1953). But something much more significant was revealed by Delay et al. (1952); these workers showed that chlorpromazine could control violent psychotic excitement, without producing confusion or persistent somnolence, in patients suffering from mania and schizophrenia. Thereafter reports multiplied from mental hospitals all over the world, confirming that the drug could effectively calm excitement, aggression and overactivity in emotionally disturbed hospitalized patients. Chlorpromazine proved greatly superior to existing chemical remedies— barbiturates, paraldehyde and bromide—which commonly controlled excitement only at the expense of profound torpor and sleepiness. Elkes and Elkes (1954) were able to show in a fully controlled study that a true pharmacological action lay behind these enthusiastic reports. The rauwolfia alkaloids, introduced at about the same time, were soon ousted by the phenothiazines on account of their tendency to produce depression and their relative slowness to take effect. Only the butyrophenones, considered further below, have been able in recent years to compete where clinical effectiveness is concerned, yet even now phenothiazines remain almost universally the drugs of first choice.

The phenothiazines have come to be one of the most frequently prescribed drugs in medicine. In psychiatry their principal use is in the management of schizophrenia in all of its forms. They are also employed in mania and hypomania in which a high proportion of patients respond from the outset and come rapidly under control. They are valuable in combating agitation and tension in severe depressive illnesses (though without antidepressive effect) and in reducing restless disturbed behaviour among patients with dementia (Baker, 1955). Organic confusional states from a variety of toxic and infective causes have been shown to benefit, including post-operative and puerperal psychotic states. Chlorpromazine has been held to account for the decreased mortality of *delirium tremens* (Coirault *et al.*, 1956).

Before discussing the use of phenothiazine drugs in schizophrenia in detail, chlorpromazine and its more recent derivatives will be briefly described along with their pharmacological actions. Table 14.3 shows the principal

TABLE 14.3

Phenothiazine Drugs used in Schizophrenia

Name	Usual daily dose (mg)
Aliphatic Radical at R_2	
Promazine (Sparine)	75–1000
Chlorpromazine (Largactil)	150–600
Triflupromazine (Vesprin)	20–150
Piperidine Ring at R_2	
Mepazine (Pacatal)	25–100
Thioridazine (Melleril)	100–500
Piperazine Ring at R_2	
Prochlorperazine (Stemetil)	15–100
Thioproperazine (Majeptil)	30–60
Thiopropazate (Dartalan)	15–30
Perphenazine (Fentazin)	6–24
Trifluoperazine (Stelazine)	15–30
Fluphenazine (Moditen)	2·5–15

phenothiazine drugs currently in use. All share the common structure shown at the bottom of the table and vary in the radicals attached to C_2 and N. Substitution at these points may profoundly alter their pharmacological properties, including therapeutic potency milligram for milligram, and perhaps also their efficacy in psychiatric disorders. Substitution of Cl for H at R_1 increases potency (i.e. promazine→chlorpromazine) and this is still further increased by the substitution of a CF_3 radical (triflupromazine). The replacement of the aliphatic side chain at R_2 by a piperidine ring or by a piperazine ring provides a further series of compounds. The piperazine compounds show enormously increased potency, milligram for milligram, but also an equivalently increased liability to produce extrapyramidal side-effects. In the table the compounds are arranged very approximately in order of increasing potency as the table is descended.

Chlorpromazine may be taken as representative of the group. Its pharmacological range is wide, including antiadrenaline, antiacetylcholine and antiserotonin actions. Its own antihistaminic properties are weak, but those of other phenothiazines (e.g. promezathine) are strong. It potentiates a large number of analgesic, hypnotic and anaesthetic agents. In the central nervous system there is little direct action on the cortex, and the principal actions which can be demonstrated are on the hypothalamus and brain stem. The effect on brain-stem mechanisms is particularly interesting in that the drug has little effect on the arousal response to direct stimulation of the reticular formation (whether measured behaviourally or by EEG), but markedly raises the threshold for arousal by incoming stimuli along the ascending sensory pathways. (Bradley, 1963). This dissociation of action is not seen with barbiturates, which raise the thresholds for both direct and indirect arousal. Thus we have a neurophysiological paradigm for the unique clinical tranquillizing effect of the drugs in which an excessive response to stimuli is abolished without a marked general lowering of alertness. Behaviourally, chlorpromazine can be shown to increase sociability in cats, to abolish sham rage in the decorticate cat, and to tame rhesus monkeys. In man, of course, the outstanding behavioural effect is sedation without impairment of consciousness; a large initial dose may produce transient impairment of cognitive function and psychomotor control, but with continued administration this effect soon recedes (Kornetsky et al., 1959). This parallels the clinical observation of some initial drowsiness which passes in spite of a steadily increasing dose.

Phenothiazine drugs in schizophrenia

The usefulness of phenothiazines in acute schizophrenia is beyond doubt. They quieten overactive and aggressive behaviour, and in addition cause a wide range of other schizophrenic symptoms to recede. The more florid the clinical picture the more obvious the therapeutic effect. Several comprehensive controlled studies have been carried out. The N.I.M.H. (1964) multi-hospital trial involved 344 acute schizophrenics and compared phenothiazines with placebo: 95 per cent of the patients showed improvement with phenothiazines (50 per cent with placebo), and in 75 per cent this was judged marked to moderate in degree (23 per cent with placebo). After six weeks, 45 per cent of drug-treated patients were symptom-free, or very nearly so. Specific areas of improvement included thought disturbance, delusions, auditory hallucinations, ideas of persecution, social withdrawal and loss of self-care, in addition to diminution of anxiety and agitation. Noting this range and scope of effect, together with the rapidity and completeness of recovery in many cases, some have been tempted to postulate a true "antischizophrenic" action for phenothiazine drugs. This conception, however, lacks pathological, biochemical or epidemiological support. It is not easy to discount the influence of hospital environment and social aftercare in contributing to the completeness of recovery which may be seen in favourable cases; and since we know so little about the ways in which schizophrenic symptoms may depend one upon another, it would seem premature to suggest that any fundamental "psychotic process" is affected directly by the action of the drugs.

In chronic schizophrenia the evidence is less impressive, though substantial benefits are still found to occur. Phenothiazines remain invaluable for tiding patients over acute recurrences of symptoms, and in the established chronic disease they very often control aggressiveness, overactivity and tension. Hallucinatory experiences and the intensity of delusions are substantially reduced in a great number of cases, though less success is found with the so-called negative symptoms such as withdrawal, inertia and underactivity. Post (1966) has reported substantial success with phenothiazines in obtaining marked improvement and even full remission in the chronic paranoid illnesses of later life. With very high dosage, sustained remission has been claimed in up to 40 per cent of chronic schizophrenics (Rosati, 1964), though in general the more rigorous the therapeutic trial the less enthusiastic the claims put forward (Heilizer, 1960). Reports continue to be made, particularly in the chronic apathetic states which may supervene after many years of illness, that no benefit whatever can be demonstrated (Letemendia and Harris, 1967). It seems in general that the longer the duration of unremitting illness, the less decisive are drugs and the more prominent are social and environmental factors in determining the degree of symptom relief and social adjustment which can be obtained (Cawley, 1967).

The question of maintenance therapy and the effect on long-range functioning of schizophrenic patients has not yet been fully worked out. This is perhaps not surprising in view of the wide range of clinical pictures and natural histories which may be seen in schizophrenic illnesses. Several studies have indicated that relapse and rehospitalization are significantly reduced by long-term phenothiazine medication, and that long-term social adjustment is improved (Gross et al., 1961; Katz and Cole, 1962; Pasamanick et al., 1964). Englehardt et al. (1964), however, suggest that relapse is merely delayed rather than prevented, so that the final outcome may not be significantly altered. Certainly, several recent papers have suggested that among hospitalized chronic schizophrenics maintenance therapy may sometimes be continued unnecessarily and even to the long-term detriment of the patient (Prien et al., 1969).

Differences between different phenothiazines

A great number of different phenothiazines are in use in schizophrenia, as indicated in Table 14.3, and the literature contains bewildering claims about their relative merits. Improvements over chlorpromazine have been sought in terms of diminished side-effects and greater efficacy in certain types of schizophrenic illness.

Chlorpromazine (*Largactil*) remains the drug of choice for the great majority of cases and has only rarely been shown in strictly controlled trials to be surpassed by new derivatives. It has the great advantage of being first in the field, and therefore still the most tried and trusted phenothiazine drug. It is usually given in a starting dose of 50 mg t.d.s., increased over several days to 200 mg t.d.s. The dose may be increased further when necessary; relatively enormous dosages of up to 3000 mg per day have sometimes been advocated, but it is doubtful whether increases above 1000 mg per day confer any additional benefit. The dose should be adjusted to the level which controls symptoms or to within the limits imposed by extrapyramidal side-effects. The necessary dose appears to depend on individual susceptibility rather than on type or severity of illness. For maintenance therapy, 50–100 mg t.d.s. is the dose usually prescribed. Anti-parkinsonian medication (benzhexol 2–5 mg t.d.s. or orphenadrine 50–100 mg t.d.s.) is usually given concurrently to minimize extrapyramidal effects. A liquid preparation of chlorpromazine is available for patients resistant to swallowing tablets, and an intramuscular injection (100 mg) may be given for rapid control of acute disturbance.

Thioridazine (*Melleril*) has found especially wide application in the treatment of elderly patients. There is a considerably diminished tendency to cause extrapyramidal disturbances or photosensitivity, and allergic side effects are also said to occur more rarely.

Trifluoperazine (*Stelazine*) is the best tried member of the piperazine group of phenothiazines. Like the other piperazine derivatives it is very much more potent milligram for milligram than chlorpromazine, and the liability to cause extrapyramidal disturbances is correspondingly increased. The usual dose is 5–10 mg t.d.s. The advantage claimed for trifluoperazine, and for piperazine compounds in general, is that they have a lessened tendency to sedate, and indeed arouse and activate the patient. For this reason they are often recommended as the drugs of choice for apathetic and underactive patients, and occasional careful studies have appeared to confirm that this is so (Gwynne *et al.*, 1962). Superiority over chlorpromazine has also been claimed in paranoid schizophrenia, especially of late onset. Nevertheless, several extensive and rigorous studies have failed to demonstrate significant qualitative differences between piperazine compounds and chlorpromazine, or between the various members of the piperazine group themselves, when properly tested one against the other according to a flexible dosage schedule (Casey *et al.*, 1960; Adelson and Epstein, 1962; N.I.M.H., 1964). This does not mean, of course, that individual susceptibility may not still vary, and it remains possible that with better methods of evaluation certain differences in clinical effect may yet become firmly established. In the meantime, clinical practice justifies the trial of different phenothiazines in the patient who responds poorly to the initial therapeutic endeavour.

Fluphenazine hydrochloride (Moditen) is one of the most recent and powerful phenothiazines to be introduced. It is given orally in the very small dose of 2·5–15 mg once daily only. The special value of this drug is its availability in forms for intramuscular injection which provide slow release and sustained blood levels for a very considerable period of time. *Fluphenazine enanthate (Moditen enanthate)* is given as 25 mg (1 ml) by deep intramuscular injection every 10–14 days, or the newer preparation *fluphenazine decanoate (Modecate)* in the same dose at intervals of approximately four weeks. The timing of injections can be adjusted to individual needs. These powerful preparations should be given initially only in hospital, starting with a trial dose of half the normal amount and preferably only after oral fluphenazine has been shown to be well tolerated and effective. Extrapyramidal side-effects may be troublesome in the first few days after injection, but are generally controlled by oral anti-parkinsonian medication. They are said to be considerably less common with Modecate, and here routine use of anti-parkinsonian medication is said to be unnecessary. In elderly female patients the risk is greater, and half the normal dose is recommended. Experience to date has indicated that these preparations are safe. Hypotensive episodes occasionally occur, and may prove a risk in patients undergoing surgery. In such an event noradrenaline should be given as the vasopressor agent; adrenaline should not be used since phenothiazine derivatives have been found to reverse its action causing further lowering of blood pressure.

These intramuscular preparations are of special value for maintenance therapy in relapsing schizophrenic patients who, through lack of insight or of motivation fail to persist with oral medication. They are, of course, less useful in the treatment of acute schizophrenia where a more flexible dosage régime is needed.

The other phenothiazines listed in Table 14.3 will not be considered individually. All are used in the treatment of schizophrenia and their value has been established. It is generally agreed that *promazine (Sparine)* and *mepazine (Pacatol)* are inferior to the others in controlling psychotic symptoms. Some (e.g. prochlorperazine) have achieved widespread use in other medical disorders such as migraine and Menière's disease.

Overall outcome of treatment

It is extremely hard to obtain firm information about changes in prognosis which may have followed the use of phenothiazine drugs. Conflicting information is derived from different studies which deal with different samples of schizophrenic patients. As explained earlier, it is also hard to disentangle the effect of drugs from the effect of other changes in management which have proceeded concurrently.

The subject is reviewed in detail by Hoenig (1967). The general pattern of change appears to be clear—time spent in hospital has decreased and discharge rates have risen appropriately. Some studies show that readmission rates have also risen in compensatory fashion, whereas others show more encouragingly that these too have fallen since the introduction of phenothiazine drugs. Much must depend on the facilities which exist for comprehensive aftercare and supervision on discharge.

The overall results that can be expected from present-day treatment are illustrated by the four-year follow-up survey conducted by Hoenig and Hamilton (1966). This covered the entire intake of schizophrenic patients incepted for the first time from a given area in the north of England: 14 per cent of these patients were never in hospital, 21 per cent for less than two months, and a further 35 per cent for less than one year. Only 5 per cent were hospitalized for more than two years. Twenty-six per cent were symptom free for at least three years during the survey period, and only 46 per cent for less than two years. One-third were in employment for at least three of the four years, whereas almost one-third were unemployed throughout. At the end of the four-year period, 27 per cent remained more or less symptom free, 27 per cent were much improved, 16 per cent were not improved at all, 10 per cent had died, and in the remainder information could not be obtained.

It seems doubtful whether the use of drugs has in any way altered the factors known to be associated with good or bad prognosis (Cawley, 1967). Factors indicating a relatively good prognosis include an acute onset, physical precipitants (e.g. infection, childbirth, trauma), good previous personality, cyclothymic personality, pyknic build, higher intelligence, and higher social class. Catatonic schizophrenia carries a better prognosis than hebephrenic forms of illness, and illnesses beginning in later adult life generally run a more favourable course than those which start in adolescence. Atypical forms of illness, including those varieties designated as schizophreniform, pseudo-neurotic, reactive psychosis, periodic psychosis, or schizo-affective psychosis fare better than classical presentations of "nuclear" schizophrenia. Certain symptoms, such as clouding of consciousness, good preservation of affect, or the admixture of manic-depressive symptoms are generally held to indicate an improved prognosis.

Unwanted effects of phenothiazine drugs

Despite their many pharmacological actions, the phenothiazines are remarkably safe drugs. Successful suicide does not appear to have been recorded despite overdoses of up to 20 g of chlorpromazine (Hollister, 1961) and they appear also to be safe during pregnancy (Kris, 1962). Habituation and addiction are virtually unknown.

The most common unwanted effect is drowsiness, which usually passes with continued use and is less often seen with the piperazine derivatives. A variety of autonomic side-effects are common, especially in the early stages of treatment—hypotension, tachycardia, dryness of mouth, blurred vision, nasal congestion and constipation. The latter may very occasionally progress to paralytic ileus. Urinary retention may sometimes occur and the drugs are contra-indicated in the presence of prostatic hypertrophy. Impotence and inhibition of ejaculation may be pronounced, and thioridazine has been advocated in the treatment of premature ejaculation. Phenothiazines are strictly contraindicated in the presence of glaucoma.

Weight gain is common, and more rarely there are hormonal changes including feminization in men and menstrual irregularity and lactation in women.

Hypersensitivity effects with chlorpromazine include jaundice, blood dyscrasias and skin complications. Jaundice, which occurs in approximately 0·5 per cent of cases, is usually benign and resolves rapidly on withdrawal of the drug. It is of the acute intrahepatic cholestatic type, and if it is to occur it occurs during the early weeks of treatment. It is not related to the dose employed, and there is no evidence of subclinical hepatocellular damage even after very prolonged administration among the patients who do not develop jaundice (Cohen and Archer, 1955). Among blood dyscrasias a variety of disturbances of white blood corpuscle formation, thrombocytopaenia, and pancytopaenia have been reported, but only rarely. A variety of skin rashes may occur. The commonest skin complication is photosensitivity, and patients on chlorpromazine should be advised to avoid exposure to the sun.

Non-specific electrocardiographic abnormalities may occur, including flattening of T-waves and widening of QRS complexes (Graupner and Murphree, 1964). Whilst specific cardiotoxicity has not been proved, phenothiazines should generally be avoided in patients with severe cardiac deficiency. Recently they have been incriminated in contributing to sudden unexplained death in a very small minority of patients (Hollister and Kosek, 1965); intramyocardial lesions have been found at post-mortem, and acute ventricular fibrillation has been suggested as the mechanism of death.

Long continued phenothiazine medication has come under more critical review in recent years on a number of counts, chiefly the severe buccal dyskinesias which will be considered below. In addition, stellate lens opacities have been reported (Barsa et al., 1965) often in conjunction with progressive skin pigmentation. Disturbances of melanin metabolism occur in schizophrenia and appear to be aggravated by long continued phenothiazine medication. Nicholson et al. (1966) have reported that pigment deposition is increased in many organs of the body in addition to the skin, and that the distribution closely follows that of phenothiazine metabolites.

Extrapyramidal effects of phenothiazine drugs

The effects of phenothiazines on the extrapyramidal nervous system deserve a section on their own. These are usually regarded as their chief disadvantage in therapy, though some have maintained that they represent the key to their action in psychotic illness. It is certainly a striking observation that almost all drugs of value in schizophrenia, often very diverse in pharmacological structure, should also have in common a capacity to disturb extrapyramidal function.

Three main syndromes occur. *The Parkinsonian syndrome* is the most common. The signs are similar to if not identical with those of naturally occurring Parkinson's disease, i.e. slowing of movement, muscular rigidity, and the typical gait, posture and facial expression. Tremor may accompany the changes in tone or occur in isolation. The onset is usually in the first weeks of treatment and is closely related to the dose employed. Individual susceptibility varies greatly but increases with age. Mirianthopoulos *et al.* (1962) have shown a threefold increase in the incidence of naturally occurring Parkinson's disease among the relatives of patients who develop this complication on phenothiazines, which may therefore be related to a genetic factor. Anti-parkinsonian drugs are usually very effective in delaying the complication or in causing the symptoms to recede.

Dystonic syndromes are relatively rare. They are more common in the young, and if they are to occur they set in abruptly within the first few days of treatment or even after a single large dose. They are very much more common with the powerfully acting piperazine drugs. A variety of syndromes are seen, all with spasmodic or sustained tonic contraction of muscle groups —torticollis, retrocollis, trismus, deviation of the head and eyes, oculogyric crises, opisthotonus, or torsion of the trunk and limbs. In severe cases protrusion of the tongue and stridorous breathing may embarrass respiration. Fortunately, the condition responds rapidly to anti-parkinsonian drugs, which should be given intravenously in an emergency (biperiden lactate (Akineton) 2–5 mg, or procyclidine hydrochloride (Kemadrin) 10 mg). The clinical picture may give rise to confusion, especially in casualty departments, when it is not known that phenothiazines have been recently prescribed, and is quite often misdiagnosed as dystonia musculorum, tetanus or hysteria.

Dyskinetic syndromes include akathisia (inability to sit still) and takathisia (constant shuffling of the feet). They usually respond to anti-parkinsonian medication but are sometimes difficult to control completely. Recently, attention has been focused on a more serious syndrome of "facio-bucco-linguo-masticatory dyskinesia", which has been reported in up to 5 per cent of female patients treated over long periods of time with phenothiazines (Hunter *et al.*, 1964). Onset may occur only after many years of treatment, and sometimes while on régimes previously well tolerated. The clinical picture is of continuous grimacing, blinking, munching, sucking movements, with protrusions of the tongue, bulging of the cheeks, and writhing movements of the jaw. When accompanied by dyskinetic movements of the limbs it may suggest Huntington's chorea, and many cases were probably formerly ascribed to schizophrenic mannerisms. It is most commonly seen amongst patients with evidence of brain damage, or in those who have had leucotomy or ECT in addition to phenothiazines (Faurbye et al., 1964). Some cases respond to stopping the drugs, but others appear to persist indefinitely (Uhrbrand and Faurbye, 1960; Schmidt and Jarcho, 1966).

The precise mechanisms underlying these various extrapyramidal effects remain unknown. It has often been suggested that there is a causal relationship between the elicitation of extrapyramidal effects and a therapeutic response in schizophrenia (Haase and Janssen, 1965). Some clinicians have therefore recommended massive intermittent doses of phenothiazines with the aim of producing short-lived episodes of severe extrapyramidal disturbance (Denham and Carrick, 1960, 1961). There is much, however, which argues against a causal association. Many carefully controlled trials have failed to reveal differences in therapeutic effect between one phenothiazine and another while at the same time showing marked differences in their liability to cause extrapyramidal disturbances. Thioridazine in particular is considerably less likely than most phenothiazines to produce extrapyramidal effects yet remains effective in schizophrenia. Nor is there good evidence that therapeutic effect is diminished when phenothiazines are given in such a way, and with such anti-parkinsonian cover, that extrapyramidal signs are not allowed to occur.

Other Drugs used in Schizophrenia

While the phenothiazines continue to hold pride of place in the drug treatment of schizophrenia, several other preparations have recently been introduced and some enthusiastic claims made for them. Some of these other "major tranquillizers" are pharmacologically quite distinct from the phenothiazines, but nevertheless almost all share the ability to induce extrapyramidal side effects along with their tranquillizing properties.

Two situations appear to warrant a trial of these alternative drugs—failure of phenothiazines adequately to control acute symptoms in the individual patient (sometimes by virtue of sensitivity to side-effects), or the need for a drug which will activate the withdrawn chronic schizophrenic and enable him to participate in rehabilitation. It is in the latter group of patients that the newer drugs are most often claimed to be superior to phenothiazines. Adequate proof of their efficacy is not often available to date, but may yet be obtained with continuing clinical experience.

The butyrophenones, haloperidol (Serenace) and *trifluperidol (Triperidol)* are probably the best known of the non-phenothiazine drugs. Chemically, they are substituted pethidine derivatives. These pharmacologically powerful agents are given in very small dosage, haloperidol 3–15 mg per day and tri-fluperidol 1–5 mg per day. In acute schizophrenia, they are said to be at least equivalent to chlorpromazine in ability to control florid psychotic symptoms and overactivity, and possibly take effect somewhat more quickly (Pratt et al., 1964). In chronic schizophrenia it has been claimed that they are superior in activating withdrawn inert patients, and that they sometimes abolish hallucinations and paranoid delusions when other treatments have failed (Gallant et al., 1963; Okasha and Tewfik, 1964; Clark et al., 1968). Extrapyramidal disturbances, particularly dystonic spasms of head and neck, are very common and may be very severe, but respond to anti-parkinsonian medication. Somnolence and drowsiness are less likely to occur than with chlorpromazine, which may partly account for the claimed superiority in inert chronic schizophrenics. Disturbance of ocular accommodation is common, but experience to date suggests that other side-effects are rare and that the drugs may be tried with relative safety.

Oxypertine is an indole derivative with a piperazine side-chain. Opinions vary regarding its ability to control acute schizophrenic symptoms, though in high dosage it has been claimed to have an effect comparable to phenothiazines. In lower dosage (40–120 mg per day) it has been reported to have an activating effect, and valuable mood-elevating properties in chronic schizophrenics. The evidence is by no means unanimous to date and the place of oxypertine in therapeutics has yet to be fully established (Skarbek and Jacobsen, 1965; Hunt, 1967; Skarbek and Hill, 1967). Extrapyramidal side-effects occur but appear to be mild.

Certain *thiaxanthene derivatives* have been reported to show a clinical effect and field of action similar to the phenothiazines. These include *chlorprothixene* (*Taractan*) 30–150 mg per day, and *thiothixene* (*Navane*) 10–50 mg per day (Petersen and Nielsen, 1964; Browne, 1968). Again a stimulating effect in chronic schizophrenics has been claimed. A lower incidence of side-effects, including extrapyramidal disturbances, is said to occur.

Benzoquinoline derivatives including *tetrabenzene* (*Nitoman*) and *benzquinamide* (*Quantril*) are synthetic reserpine-like compounds which share the disadvantage of reserpine in sometimes inducing depression. They have been used in schizophrenia with some success (Lingjaerde, 1963; Bishop et al., 1963), but have not achieved popularity.

Other substances for which claims have been made include *ascorbic acid* in high dosage (Milner, 1963) *nicotinic acid,* and *penicillamine.* The situation regarding nicotinic acid and nicotinamide adenine dinucleotide has been the subject of controversy (Hoffer, 1963; Kilne et al., 1967; Hoffer and Osmond, 1968). The claim that such substances can help in schizophrenia and avert relapses still awaits confirmation. D-penicillamine in conjunction with a low copper diet has been tried in a very small controlled study with interesting preliminary results (Nicholson et al., 1966). This was undertaken in view of the evidence of increased melanogenesis in some schizophrenic patients.

OTHER PHYSICAL TREATMENTS IN SCHIZOPHRENIA

Electro-convulsive therapy is still widely employed in the treatment of schizophrenia, especially in acute and florid phases of the disease. Its judicious use may help symptoms to recede when drugs alone have failed. It is widely believed on the basis of clinical experience that phenothiazine drugs and ECT used together are sometimes more effective than either used alone, though adequate proof of this has yet to be demonstrated. The combination certainly appears to be safe and to benefit individual patients (Gonzalez and Imahara, 1964). ECT remains the most effective treatment for catatonic stupor, and may profoundly benefit withdrawn and anergic patients in whom an element of depression coexists. Its routine use over prolonged periods of time in established chronic schizophrenia has however fallen into disrepute.

Insulin coma therapy, introduced by Sakel in 1935, was for some 25 years regarded as the treatment of choice for schizophrenic illnesses of recent onset. It has now virtually disappeared from the therapeutic scene. This has been largely due to the introduction of effective drugs, together with the demonstration under carefully controlled conditions that induction of comas by barbiturates was of equal therapeutic value (Ackner and Oldham, 1957, 1962). Thus it now appears that the benefits produced by insulin coma therapy were due not to insulin as a specific therapeutic agent but to non-specific aspects of the coma régime, including improvement in weight, physical health and well-being, together with the increased attention and enthusiasm of the nursing staff which involved the patient in a beneficial kind of group situation. Nevertheless, when all other treatments have failed and the patient remains severely disturbed, some still regard insulin coma treatment as worth a trial (Sargant, 1965). *Modified insulin therapy*, as opposed to insulin coma therapy is still occasionally employed as a means of stimulating appetite and producing a gain in weight in debilitated patients.

Modified prefrontal leucotomy continues to be employed on a small scale in carefully selected patients, though the former enthusiasm for such procedures in schizophrenia has declined markedly, and more than their use in other psychiatric illnesses. However, leucotomy still finds application in some paranoid syndromes resistant to other treatments, and in schizophrenic patients who display marked and intractable tension (Pippard, 1962; Sykes and Tredgold, 1964; Sargant, 1965).

REFERENCES

ACKNER, B., HARRIS, A. & OLDHAM, A. J. (1957). Insulin treatment of schizophrenia. A controlled study. *Lancet*, **1**, 607.

ACKNER, B. & OLDHAM, A. J. (1962). Insulin treatment of schizophrenia. *Lancet*, **1**, 504.

ADELSON, D. & EPSTEIN, L. J. (1962). A study of phenothiazines with female and male chronically ill schizophrenic patients. *J. nerv. ment. Dis.*, **134**, 543.

BAKER, A. A. (1955). Observations on the effect of Largactil in psychiatric illness. *J. ment. Sci.*, **101**, 175.

BANNISTER, D., SALMON, P. & LEIBERMAN, D. M. (1964). Diagnosis—treatment relationships in psychiatry—a statistical analysis. *Brit. J. Psychiat.*, **110**, 726.

BARSA, J. A., NEWTON, J. C. & SAUNDERS, J. C. (1965). Lenticular and corneal opacities during phenothiazine therapy. *J. Amer. med. Ass.*, **193**, 10.

BENNETT, D. (1967). The management of schizophrenia. *Hospital Medicine*, **1**, 589.

BISHOP, M. P., GALLANT, D. M. & STEELE, C. A. (1963). A controlled evaluation of benzquinamide: behavioural toxicity with high dose levels in schizophrenics. *Curr. ther. Res.*, **5**, 238.

BRADLEY, P. B. (1963). Phenothiazine Derivatives. In *Physiological Pharmacology*, Vol. I, ed. W. S. Root and F. G. Hofmann. New York: Academic Press.

BROWNE, M. W. (1968). Experiences with thiothixene. *Brit. J. Psychiat.*, **114**, 123.

CASEY, J. F., LASKY, J. J., KLETT, C. J. & HOLLISTER, L. E. (1960). Treatment of schizophrenic reactions with phenothiazine derivatives. *Amer. J. Psychiat.*, **117**, 97.

CATTERSON, A. G., BENNETT, D. H. & FREUDENBERG, R. K. (1963). A survey of long-stay schizophrenic patients. *Brit. J. Psychiat.*, **109**, 750.

CAWLEY, R. H. (1967). The present status of physical methods of treatment in schizophrenia. In *Recent Developments in Schizophrenia*. ed. A. Coppen and A. Walk. *Brit. J. Psychiat.*, special publication No. 1. Ashford, Kent: Headley Brothers.

CLARK, M. L., HUBER, W. K., KYRIAKOPOULOS, A. A., RAY, T. S., COLMORE, J. & RAMSEY, H. R. (1968). Evaluation of trifluperidol in chronic schizophrenia. *Psychopharmacologia*, **12**, 193.

COHEN, I. M. & ARCHER, J. D. (1955). Liver function and hepatic complications in patients receiving chlorpromazine. *J. Amer. med. Ass.*, **159**, 99.

COIRAULT, R., LABORIT, H., MISSENARD, R., JOLIVET, B., HAINAULT, J. & WEBER, B. (1956). Le Delirium Tremens. *Encépale*, **45**, 762.

DELAY, J., DENIKER, P. & HARL, J. M. (1952). Utilisation en thérapeutique psychia-triaqe d'une phenothiazine d'action centrale élective. *Ann. med.-psychol.*, **110**, 112.

DENHAM, J. & CARRICK, D. J. E. L. (1960). Therapeutic importance of extra-pyramidal phenomena evoked by a new phenothiazine. *Amer. J. Psychiat.*, **116**, 927.

DENHAM, J. & CARRICK, D. J. E. L. (1961). Therapeutic value of thioproperazine and the importance of the associated neurological disturbances. *J. ment. Sci.*, **107**, 326.

DESCHAMPS, A. & CADORET, M. (1953). Cures de sommeil prolonge. *Pressé méd.*, **61(i)**, 878.

ELKES, J. & ELKES, C. (1954). Effect of chlorpromazine on the behaviour of chroni-cally overactive psychotic patients. *Brit. med. J.*, **2**, 560.

ENGLEHARDT, D. M., FREEDMAN, N., ROSEN, B., MANN, D. & MARGOLIS, R. (1964). Phenothiazines in prevention of psychiatric hospitalisation. *Arch gen. Psychiat.*, **11**, 162.

FAURBYE, A., RASCH, P. J., PETERSEN, P. B., BRANDBORG, G. & PAKKENBERG, H. (1964). Neurological symptoms in pharmacotherapy of psychosis. *Acta psychiat. scand.*, **40**, 10.

GALLANT, D. M., BISHOP, M. P., TIMMONS, E. & STEELE, C. A. (1963). Trifluperidol: a butyrophenone derivative. *Amer. J. Psychiat.*, **120**, 485.

GONZALEZ, J. R. & IMAHARA, J. K. (1964). Electroshock therapy with the phenothiazines and reserpine. *Amer. J. Psychiat.*, **121**, 253.

GRAUPNER, K. I. & MURPHREE, O. D. (1964). Electrocardiographic changes associated with the use of thioridazine. *J. Neuropsychiat.*, **5**, 344.

GROSS, M., MITCHMAN, I. L., REEVES, W. P., LAWRENCE, J. L. & NEWELL, P. C. (1961). Discontinuation of treatment with ataractic drugs. *Recent Adv. biol. Psychiat.*, **3**, 44.

GWYNNE, P. H., HUNDZIAK, M., KAVTSCHITSCH, J., LEFTON, M. & PASAMANICK, B. (1962). Efficacy of trifluoperazine on withdrawal in chronic schizophrenia. *J. nerv. ment. Dis.*, **134**, 451.

HAASE, H-J. & JANSSEN, P. A. J. (1965). In *The Action of Neuroleptic Drugs— A Psychiatric Neurologic and Pharmacological Investigation.* Amsterdam: North Holland Publishing Company.

HEILIZER, F. (1960). A critical review of some published experiments with chlorpromazine in schizophrenic, neurotic and normal humans. *J. chron. Dis.*, **11**, 102.

HOENIG, J. (1967). The prognosis of schizophrenia. In *Recent Developments in Schizophrenia.* ed. A. Coppen and A. Walk. *Brit. J. Psychiat.*, special publication No. 1. Ashford, Kent: Headley Brothers.

HOENIG, J. & HAMILTON, M. W. (1966). The schizophrenic patient under new management. *Compr. Psychiat.*, **7**, 81.

HOFFER, A. (1963). Nicotinic acid: an adjunct in the treatment of schizophrenia. *Amer. J. Psychiat.*, **120**, 171.

HOFFER, A. & OSMOND, H. (1968). Nicotinamide adenine dinucleotide in the treatment of chronic schizophrenic patients. *Brit. J. Psychiat.*, **114**, 915.

HOLLISTER, L. E. (1961). Current concepts in therapy. Complications from psychotherapeutic drugs. I. *New Engl. J. Med.*, **264**, 291.

HOLLISTER, L. E. & KOSEK, J. C. (1965). Sudden death during treatment with phenothiazine derivatives. *J. Amer. med. Ass.*, **192**, 1035.

HUNT, P. V. (1967). A comparison of the effects of oxypertine and trifluoperazine in withdrawn schizophrenics. *Brit. J. Psychiat.*, **113**, 1419.

HUNTER, R., EARL, J. C. & THORNICROFT, S. (1964). An apparently irreversible syndrome of abnormal movements following phenothiazine medication. *Proc. roy. soc. Med.*, **57**, 758.

KATZ, M. M. & COLE, J. O. (1962). Research on drugs and community care. *Arch. gen. Psychiat.*, **7**, 345.

KLINE, N. S., BARCLAY, G. L., COLE, J. O., ESSER, A. H., LEHMANN, H. & WITTENBORN, J. R. (1967). Controlled evaluation of nicotinamide adenine dinucleotide in the treatment of chronic schizophrenic patients. *Brit. J., Psychiat.*, **113**, 731.

KORNETSKY, C., PETTIT, M., WYNNE, R. & EVARTS, E. V. (1959). A comparison of the psychological effects of acute and chronic administration of chlorpromazine and secobarbital (quinalbarbitone) in schizophrenic patients. *J. ment. Sci.*, **105**, 190.

KRIS, E. B. (1962). Children born to mothers maintained on pharmacotherapy during pregnancy and postpartum. *Recent Adv. biol. Psychiat.*, **4**, 180.

LABORIT, H. & HUGENARD, P. (1951). L'Hibernation artificielle par moyens pharmacodynamiques et physiques. *Presse méd.*, **59(ii)**, 1329.

LETEMENDIA, F. J. J. & HARRIS, A. D. (1967). Chlorpromazine and the untreated chronic schizophrenic: a long-term trial. *Brit. J. Psychiat.*, **113**, 950.

LINGJAERDE, O. (1963). Tetrabenzene (nitoman) in the treatment of psychoses. *Acta. psychiat. scand., Suppl.*, **170**.

MILNER, G. (1963). Ascorbic acid in chronic psychiatric patients—a controlled trial. *Brit. J. Psychiat.*, **109**, 294.

MIRIANTHOPOULOS N. C., KURLAND, A. A. & KURLAND, L. T. (1962). Hereditary predisposition in drug-induced Parkinsonism. *Arch. Neurol. (Chic.)*, **6**, 6.

N.I.M.H. PSYCHOPHARMACOLOGY SERVICE CENTRE COLLABORATIVE STUDY GROUP (1964). Phenothiazine treatment in acute schizophrenia. *Arch. gen. Psychiat.*, **10**, 246.

NICHOLSON, G. A., GREINER, A. C., McFARLANE, W. J. G. & BAKER, R. A. (1966). Effect of penicillamine on schizophrenic patients. *Lancet*, **1**, 344.

ODEGAARD, O. (1964). Pattern of discharge from Norwegian psychiatric hospitals before and after the introduction of the psychotropic drugs. *Amer. J. Psychiat.*, **120**, 772.

OKASHA, A. & TEWFIK, G. I. (1964). Haloperidol: a controlled clinical trial in chronic disturbed psychotic patients. *Brit. J. Psychiat.*, **110**, 56.

PASAMANICK, B., SCARPITTI, F. R., LEFTON, M., DINITZ, S., WERNERT, J. J. & McPHEETERS, H. (1964). Home versus hospital care for schizophrenics. *J. Amer. med. Ass.*, **187**, 177.

PETERSEN, P. V. & NIELSEN, I. M. (1964). Thiaxanthene derivatives. In *Psychopharmacological Agents*, Vol. I. ed. M. Gordon. New York: Academic Press.

PIPPARD, J. (1962). Leucotomy in Britain today. *J. ment. Sci.*, **108**, 249.

POST, F. (1966). *Persistent Persecutory States of the Elderly*. Oxford: Pergamon Press.

PRATT, J. P., BISHOP, M. P. & GALLANT, D. M. (1964). Trifluperidol and haloperidol in the treatment of acute schizophrenia. *Amer. J. Psychiat.*, **121**, 592.

PRIEN, R. F., COLE, J. O. & BELKIN, N. F. (1969). Relapse in chronic schizophrenics following abrupt withdrawal of transquillising medication. *Brit. J. Psychiat.*, **115**, 679.

ROSATI, D. (1964). Prolonged high dosage ataractic medication in chronic schizophrenics. *Brit. J. Psychiat.*, **110**, 61.

SARGANT, W. (1965). Use of physical methods. *Brit. med. J.*, **1**, 648.

SARGANT, W. & SLATER, E. (1963). *An introduction to Physical Methods of Treatment in Psychiatry*. Edinburgh: Livingstone.

SCHMIDT, W. R. & JARCHO, L. W. (1966). Persistent dyskinesias following phenothiazine therapy. *Arch. Neurol. (Chic.)*, **14**, 369.

SKARBEK, A. & HILL, G. B. (1967). An extended trial of oxypertine in five selected cases of chronic schizophrenia. *Brit. J. Psychiat.*, **113**, 1107.

SKARBEK, A. & JACOBSEN, M. (1965). Oxypertine: a review of clinical experience. *Brit. J. Psychiat.*, **111**, 1173.

SYKES, M. K. & TREDGOLD, R. F. (1964). Restricted orbital undercutting. A study of its effects on 350 patients over the ten years 1951–60. *Brit. J. Psychiat.*, **110**, 609.

UHRBRAND, L. & FAURBYE, A. (1960). Reversible and irreversible dyskinesia after treatment with perphenazine, chlorpromazine, reserpine and electroconvulsive therapy. *Psychopharmacologia*, **1**, 408.

WILLIS, J. H. & BANNISTER, D. (1965). The diagnosis and treatment of schizo-phrenia. A questionnaire study of psychiatric opinion. *Brit. J. Psychiat.*, **111**, 1165.

WING, J. K. & BROWN, G. W. (1961). Social treatment of chronic schizophrenia: a comparative survey of three mental hospitals. *J. ment. Sci.*, **107**, 847.

15 Alcoholism

M. M. GLATT

ALCOHOL DEPENDENCE, STUDENT EDUCATION. PREVALENCE, AETIOLOGY. THE "ALCOHOLISMS". PHYSICAL COMPLICATIONS. TREATMENT. CONCLUSION.

ALCOHOLISM was briefly alluded to in a short chapter in the second edition of this volume in 1952.

It began with the statements: "The treatment of alcoholics is fraught with disappointment as anyone who has treated such patients is aware. They are a very serious challenge indeed and any method which offers hope is worth consideration." This was followed by a description of three therapeutic approaches: conditioned reflex treatment, antabuse, and Alcoholics anonymous (A.A.). Of these three methods at least the latter two are still among the most widely used the world over. Similarly, the two sentences quoted remain essentially true today.

However, in the intervening two decades there has been a definite change in attitudes towards the problem of alcoholism, probably as a consequence of the work in the scientific field of E. M. Jellinek—who in the early 1950s was Consultant on Alcoholism to the World Health Organization—as well as of the success of A.A. The latter—a fellowship of recovering and recovered alcoholics—was often able to help alcoholics who had proved resistant to all other therapeutic approaches. By proudly admitting their alcoholism A.A. members have provided many thousands of visual demonstrations that alcoholics can in fact recover. Their approach has had a great influence on medical and psychiatric thinking and treatment methods. What may be even more important, the success of A.A. has contributed greatly towards improving the public image of the alcoholic. It is now widely recognized by professional workers in this field that the outlook in the case of many alcoholics is much better than previously thought. A summary of several published follow-up reports shows that out of unselected samples about two-thirds can improve considerably. There is of course no such person as "the" alcoholic: among a large unselected sample of alcoholics one finds many different personality types and various types of alcoholism. Factors such as underlying personality and social stability are among the most important factors in prognosis. Alcoholics of good personality, emotionally not too unstable or too immature, and of good social stability (domestic, marital, occupational, residential) can be expected to do fairly well: the emotionally unstable and highly immature, "psychopaths", and those with poor social stability have a worse prognosis.

Whatever therapeutic methods are used, a proportion of patients will go on drinking and relapsing, so that results will often be disappointing. In fact, alcoholism has to be regarded as essentially a relapsing disorder, and the members of the therapeutic team have to view a relapse as a challenge to try again, and not to throw up their arms because of a feeling of personal failure or affront. Moreover, one has to accept that some alcoholics will fail whatever is tried. On the other hand, just as alcoholism is a family disease, and the alcoholic's family are closely affected, so his improvement and recovery may bring about remarkable improvement also in the emotional state of health of his close relatives. In some alcoholics one has to be satisfied with a more modest, limited goal, but here again it matters to his family a great deal if the alcoholic, instead of being on a more or less perpetual "bender", is now having no more than two to three short-lived bouts a year, and in the meantime is a good husband, father and breadwinner. Thus treatment of alcoholics, whilst often fraught with disappointments, often also brings rich rewards. However, as in the past, in aspects of treatment, as well as in research and lay and professional education, alcoholism still presents a great challenge.

Unfortunately, the medical profession has been slow to accept this challenge. In general, doctors and alcoholics have kept out of each other's way—although this has been slowly changing in recent years. Alcoholism has also social, economic, legal and ethical aspects, but it is—or should be—to a large extent a medical problem. On the whole, doctors in their student days have learned little about the essential earlier phases of alcoholism. Thus many come to identify alcoholism with its complications, such as liver cirrhosis and psychoses, and think of the diagnosis only when such secondary disorders have made their appearance. Fortunately, these complications are rare and late. Thus, liver cirrhosis as a complication of alcoholism, whilst greatly varying from country to country, has been estimated to occur in no more than 8 per cent of chronic alcoholics (Haggard and Jellinek, 1950) and alcoholic psychoses in not more than 10 per cent (WHO, 1952). Other physical and definite mental complications, such as Korsakoff's and Wernicke's Syndrome and dementia, are likewise comparatively rare. In 1959 Jellinek, stating that in the 1940s the relative incidence of alcoholic complications had changed in North America but not in Europe, published the following Table, relating to North America, showing the "Relative Incidence of Alcoholic

Complications (among Alcoholics with Complications) Prior to 1942 and Currently (in Per Cent)":

TABLE 15.1

Complication	I Prior to 1942	II Current
1. Polyneuropathy	30	5
2. Cirrhosis of the liver	9	14
3. Alcoholic encephalopathies	15	20
4. Gastritis	40	61
5. Other alcoholic complications	6	0
Totals	100	100

DEVELOPMENTAL PROCESS OF ALCOHOL DEPENDENCE

Diagnosis should be made early in the alcoholic's drinking career, long before the onset of complications. This is often extremely difficult because the practising alcoholic, unable to give up drinking, hides behind a long list of rationalizations, projections and outright denials. Often the diagnosis cannot be made without calling in the assistance of somebody who knows the drinker's habits intimately, such as his wife. Another difficulty is that the early symptoms of alcoholism are largely subjective. Jellinek (1952), on the basis of replies to an extensive questionnaire obtained from over 2000 male American A.A. members, drew up a chart of the development of alcohol "addiction". He divided the chart into four phases, each with a number of symptoms. Not every alcoholic has all the symptoms, and not all occur in the same order. Moreover, the fact that A.A. members are not necessarily a representative group of alcoholics—by and large they come, especially in this country, more from the middle class than from the working class, and in wine-drinking countries different alcoholic drinking patterns may prevail—limits its usefulness. On the other hand, as investigations at Warlingham Park Hospital have shown, Jellinek's description also applies to the English middle-class alcoholic (Glatt, 1961a). The four phases are named by Jellinek as the "pre-alcoholic", prodromal, crucial, and chronic phases respectively—the whole process taking, on the average 10 to 20 years in men, and considerably less in women. Most important from the early diagnostic aspect are the symptoms of the prodromal phase, listed by Jellinek as: alcoholic amnesias, surreptitious drinking, preoccupation with alcohol, "gulping" drink, guilt feelings about drinking behaviour, and avoidance of reference to alcohol. To these symptoms could be added another, i.e. repeated alcohol-impaired driving in basically non-psychopathic individuals (Glatt, 1964). If people who otherwise would never dream of falling foul of the Law repeatedly drive in an alcohol-impaired state, despite their knowledge of the risks involved, this may denote a certain degree of dependence on alcohol. Among male patients at Warlingham Park Hospital, alcohol-impaired driving started at an average of 27 years, alcohol amnesias (described as introducing the "prodromal phase" at an average age of 30, "loss of control" (initiating the third, "crucial" phase) at 34·4 and alcoholic benders (starting the "chronic" phase) at 35 years.

THE NEED FOR EDUCATION OF MEDICAL STUDENTS

Medical students are taught little about the early stages of alcoholism, and this may contribute greatly to the unfortunate fact that in this as well as in most other countries alcoholism is diagnosed late, if at all. Moreover, alcoholics often do not tell their doctors about their drinking habits, though they often complain of stomach upsets, headaches, fatigue, etc. Thus, it is little wonder that general practitioners are so often unaware of the presence of alcoholics in their practices. This is well illustrated by the findings of an enquiry carried out by Parr (1957) into the number of alcoholics known to family doctors in England and Wales. He chose as his definition of "alcoholics" the one proposed by the World Health Organization (1952) which, despite its limitations, is still the one most widely used:

> "Alcoholics are those excessive drinkers whose dependence upon alcohol has attained such a degree that it shows a noticeable mental disturbance or an interference with their bodily and mental health, their inter-personal relations, and their smooth social and economic functioning: or who show the prodromal signs of such developments. They therefore require treatment."

One may wonder how many general practitioners had heard at that time of alcoholic "prodromal" symptoms. The figure arrived at of alcoholics known to family doctors was about 35,000—and it is interesting to note that doctors with small lists knew proportionately more alcoholics than those with larger lists. Whilst nobody knows for certain even the approximate number of alcoholics in this country, most experienced observers are inclined to accept an older WHO estimate (1951) of about 350,000. This would mean that the average practitioner fails to diagnose nine out of ten alcoholics in his practice! Alcoholism is generally regarded as a progressive illness and early diagnosis is therefore highly important. It leads to much suffering and misery and a not inconsiderable mortality from such causes as intercurrent infections associated with lack of nutrition and lowered resistance; liver damage; suicides; and accidents caused by overdosage, on the road, at work, and also at home. An American Insurance Company (1968) found that among 847 fatal home accidents, in 15 per cent of the men and 20 per cent of the women such deaths were associated with drinking. Per Sundby (1967) found in a study of Norwegian male alcoholics an "extra loss of lives" of 113 per cent of the Norwegian expectation or 69 per cent of the Oslo expectation. "Extra deaths" occurred mainly from respiratory tract tuberculosis, cancer of the larynx and upper digestive organs, accidents, apoplexy, suicide, other cancers, and coronary heart disease. Special instruction of medical and other professional students about alcoholism is therefore vital, but it is rarely practised. Not only would it give future doctors a more balanced picture of alcoholism but it would help them to accept alcoholism as an illness worthy of and often benefiting by medical help. Once doctors have shown that they regard alcoholism as a genuine illness the general public will follow suit, and the stigma still attached to such a diagnosis will gradually fade away. These sufferers will come forward at an earlier stage, and their families will no longer have to be so careful to hide the "skeleton in their cupboard".

PREVALENCE OF ALCOHOLISM

Reference has been made to doubts about the prevalence of alcoholism in this country. *Indirect indices* are often employed, such as prosecutions or convictions for drunkenness, admissions to hospitals, or deaths from cirrhosis of the liver. All these are highly unreliable. For example, drunkenness is obviously not synonymous with alcoholism, although English alcoholics very often get drunk, in contrast to wine-drinking French alcoholics. But many drunks are obviously not alcoholics: only public drunkenness is an offence and most policemen turn a blind eye to drunks. Hospital admissions for "alcoholism" and "alcoholic psychoses" may reflect to some extent not the changes in the incidence of alcoholism but the inclination of practitioners to diagnose the condition, and of hospitals to admit them. As to liver cirrhosis, in this country as compared with France for example, only a small proportion of cases of cirrhosis are alcoholic in origin. Many alcoholics suffer from a reversible fatty liver which clears up with abstinence and a balanced diet and never develop cirrhosis. Nor are doctors keen to mention cirrhosis on the death certificate. However, of the indirect indices, the WHO (1951) regarded the connection between alcoholism and liver cirrhosis as the least unsatisfactory one.

On the assumption of a relation between mortality rates from cirrhosis and the number of alcoholics alive, and using a complicated formula (Jellinek's formula), Jellinek (1951) arrived at a "probably reliable" estimate of 86,000 "chronic" alcoholics in England and Wales. The term "chronic alcoholism" is unfortunately used in a very different sense by various observers. Jellinek employed the term to indicate those alcoholics who as a consequence of their excessive drinking have developed definite mental or physical complications. Such alcoholics form only a minority compared to those who do not develop such complications. In the U.S.A. the proportion of alcoholics with complications among all alcoholics was then one in four: according to later estimates by Jellinek (1959) it had decreased to less than one in five. Multiplying the figure of 86,000 by four, Jellinek arrived at an approximate estimate of 350,000 alcoholics in England and Wales. Jellinek himself regarded this estimate as no more than a rough guess, but in the absence of other more reliable estimates it has since formed the basis of most statements on the prevalence of alcoholism in this country.

Another interesting point regarding the findings obtained from the use of the indirect indices is the general "upward" trend shown. Thus, drunkenness convictions, though still much lower than for example at the turn of the century (200,000 in 1900), have gradually risen despite certain ups and downs from their all-time post-war low of 20,000 to 79,000 in 1968; admission for "alcoholism" to psychiatric hospitals and psychiatric units in England and Wales from 464 in 1952 to 5836 in 1967; death rates from liver cirrhosis (4000 in 1900) from 816 in 1948 to 1350 in 1967.

Whilst an upward trend in one indirect index might have little significance, the matter may be different if all these various indices seem to point in the same direction. The impression of an increase in alcoholism in recent years is in line with one's findings of a rising referral of alcoholic patients, at a time when little attention is given to alcoholics in contrast to the headline-stealing and news-making addicts to other drugs. Another important point to bear in mind is the rising rates of drunkenness convictions among the young and of alcoholism among relatively young age groups of 20–30 (Glatt and Hills, 1968; Hassal, 1968).

However, it is clear that the only reliable method is *field surveys*. Two such surveys have been undertaken in this country in recent years. The first was carried out under the auspices of the Steering Group on Alcoholism set up by the Rowntree Social Service Trust (Prys Williams and Glatt, 1966). It aimed at discovering which of the two previously mentioned estimates—the WHO (350,000) or the G.P. enquiry (35,000)—was more likely to come nearer the truth. To this end, and with the active co-operation of the local Medical Officers of Health, health visitors and probation officers in five selected English towns attempted to determine the number of alcoholics among their clientele. In looking for agencies other than medical practitioners suitable to act as recorders of the incidence of alcoholism, essential requirements were that such an agency should have access of right and routine to all households, and the adequacy of access should enable the observer to determine whether a person was an alcoholic in the sense of the WHO definition, quoted above. Such requirements are of course difficult or impossible to fulfil through any single agency, and Probation Officers and health visitors were thought the two most suitable agencies, provided care was taken to avoid double counting as far as possible. The study was carried out between 1960 and 1963. The Probation Officers' enquiry arrive at an estimate of 11·4 alcoholics per 1000 families, indicating for England and Wales a total of just over 10,000 alcoholics in those segments of the population particularly likely to become the Probation Officers' responsibility. The Health Visitors enquiry showed an average incidence of 2/5 per 1000 families, or rather over 1/1000 individuals—a figure slightly lower than that obtained in the G.P. investigation of 1957 (1·1/1000).

The type of alcoholic coming to the notice of Probation Officers is as a rule unlikely to be adequately observed by family doctors. For that reason the enquiry concluded that, used in combination, adequate representative samples of doctors with smaller lists and of Probation Officers might serve quite well as recorders of the trend of advanced well-established alcoholism. The number of such alcoholics in England and Wales, estimated on the basis of this enquiry, was thought to be of the order of at least 70,000—a figure that compared well with Jellinek's (1951) estimate of 86,000 "chronic alcoholics".

The ideal field survey would be one designed to approach all agencies in a given area likely to come in contact with alcoholics. This was the aim of a more recent survey of the number of alcoholics in an English county (Cambridgeshire) carried out by Moss and Beresford Davies (1967). Sources consulted were hospital records, general practitioners, the Police, Probation Service, hostels, Marriage Guidance, A.A., Samaritans, etc. The incidence was found to be 62/10,000 of the population among males aged 15 and over: among females, 14/10,000. The total figure for alcoholics in England and Wales would thus amount to 136,000, but the authors state that in their view "the incidence in Cambridgeshire is lower than that in many other parts of England and Wales". Other important findings of this excellent study were that in fact more than 40 per cent of the total number in the survey were so much affected by alcoholism that they consulted their doctors either for the alcoholism *per se* (25 per cent) or for a physical or psychiatric condition attributable to it: 10·2 per cent of alcoholics found in the survey attempted suicide at some time during the study period—women significantly more often, i.e. 24 per cent of the women as against 6·8 per cent of the men, the incidence of achieved suicide being 1·7 per cent, an incidence lower than that obtained by some other studies (Kessel and Grossman, 1961; Sainsbury, 1955).

Alcoholism affected the work of more than half the males in the survey (absenteeism, loss of job, etc.), and the authors quote a WHO estimate that the cost of alcoholism to British industry amounts to £30 million a year. The "most telling effects" were found in the disruption of family life; 70 per cent of the wives and 58 per cent of the husbands of alcoholics complained of their alcoholic spouse's behaviour, a finding at variance with the general impression that wives of alcoholics bear the alcoholic's behaviour better than husbands of alcoholic women. The health of approximately one-third of the wives was adversely affected because of the husbands' drinking, usually by the development of reactive depression or psychosomatic disorder. In over 25 per cent the children were adversely affected. The community was affected by the drinking behaviour of nearly two-thirds of the male alcoholics and over half of the females (social problems, including aggressive behaviour). All these findings are of course well known to students of alcoholism, but this study gives the actual proportions found in a field survey. It bears out the fact that alcoholics closely involve many others by their drinking behaviour; the total number of alcoholics would have to be multiplied by three or four to include those closely affected by the condition. Alcoholism is thus an important public health problem.

The Cambridgeshire survey showed the proportion of male to female alcoholics as 4/1, the G.P. enquiry in 1957, 2·2/1. These findings of a relatively high proportion of female alcoholics are borne out by clinical impressions in this country. It is interesting that this ratio is apparently lower than anywhere else in the world, although everywhere in the past few years the proportion of female alcoholics has risen. Women alcoholics tend to be secret drinkers and more difficult to diagnose. As a result of the slowly diminishing stigma they now show greater readiness to come forward for treatment, but most observers feel that there is an actual increase in the number of female alcoholics.

AETIOLOGY

The fact that throughout history, and all over the world, male alcoholics have always outnumbered their female counterparts illustrates the influence of environmental factors on the aetiology of alcoholism. Because of the greater taboo of society on heavy female drinking, only women with more than their fair share of personality problems or external stresses will expose themselves to this taboo by heavy drinking, whereas in the case of men, heavy drinking is often encouraged, so that even relatively normal personalities can become excessive drinkers.

While the aetiology of alcoholism is as yet not clear, three interesting factors are generally held to be of importance: personality make-up, environmental (e.g. cultural and traditional influences), and the pharmacological role of alcohol as a potentially dependence-producing drug itself—or, in a rough analogy with infectious diseases, host, environment and agent. The important role of the mental make-up is generally accepted. As regards the role of the physical make-up it is probably fair to say that most observers feel that so far no definite evidence has been put forth, which does not exclude the possibility. The possible role of genetic factors in the causation of alcoholism is under active investigation in a number of countries. Thus, Mardones (1968) quotes three examples where in his view genetic influences have been demonstrated:

1. The genetic origin of individual fluctuations in alcohol preference of rats (preferring alcohol solutions to water), such fluctuations probably being related to the normal "physiological appetency" for alcohol.

2. The discovery by Chilean workers (Cruz-Coke and Varela, 1966) of a significant correlation between colour-blindness (an X-linked trait), liver cirrhosis and alcoholism.

3. The existence of an atypical alcohol dehydrogenase six times more active than the typical one (von Wartburg and Schenker, 1968).

Although alcoholism is limited to man, it has been shown that in most animal species, as in man, ethyl alcohol is converted over acetaldehyde and acetyl coenzyme A to carbon dioxide and water; nearly 90 per cent of the ethanol is oxidized in the liver by the enzyme alcohol dehydrogenase (ADH). Investigations showed a heterogeneity of human ADH in two respects: in 5–20 per cent of individuals an atypical variant enzyme occurs with a higher catalytic activity than the normal human liver alcohol dehydrogenase. Moreover, isoenzymes of ADH were found in tissues of various species in varying proportions. This important work continues.

Other studies relating to the possible importance of inheritance in the genesis of alcoholism include that by Camps and Dodd (1967), who found a higher incidence among alcoholics of individuals not secreting in their saliva ABH blood group substances than among the random (norm 1) population; and Finnish twin studies showing an influence of inheritance in practices such as normal and heavy drinking, abstinence and loss of control among the young (Partanen et al., 1966), but no such influence in other aspects. However, in general these investigators refrained from drawing far-reaching conclusions from their findings; and some 25 years ago Roe (1952) found no evidence of hereditary influence on the development of alcoholism in an American study on the adult adjustment of foster children of alcoholic parentage. Thus, the question of a genetically determined predisposition to alcoholism remains open.

THE "ALCOHOLISMS"

Since there is no such person as the alcoholic and since different types of alcoholism prevail in various countries, Jellinek (1960) prefers to talk of the "alcoholisms" rather than of alcoholism, which he regards as a fairly broad genus with a large number of species. He enumerated five common species which he called by letters of the Greek alphabet.

"**Alpha alcoholism**" is a purely psychological dependence or reliance on the effect of alcohol to relieve bodily or emotional pain. It is symptomatic of some underlying pathological condition. This species may last for many years without any signs of progression, or it may gradually progress to "gamma alcoholism".

"**Beta alcoholism**" may result from certain cultural drinking patterns which in conjunction with poor nutritional habits may lead to nutritional deficiency diseases and such alcoholic complications as polyneuropathy and cirrhosis of the liver, even in the absence of physical or psychological dependence.

"**Gamma alcoholism**" and "**Delta alcoholism**". In Jellinek's view, these two species constitute diseases in the pharmacological sense. Gamma alcoholism predominates in Anglo-Saxon countries, and is characterized by increased tissue tolerance to alcohol, adaptive cell metabolism, withdrawal symptoms, craving or physical dependence, and loss of control. Delta alcoholism predominates in wine drinking countries and shows the same features with the difference that there is inability to abstain in place of loss of control. In Delta alcoholism the drinker tops up intermittently throughout the day without necessarily getting drunk but he is unable to go "on the wagon" without developing withdrawal symptoms. In Gamma alcoholism, on the other hand, the drinker may often end up drunk, yet he sometimes manages to stay completely sober for days, weeks or months.

"**Epsilon alcoholism**" is periodic alcoholism, formerly often called dipsomania. While it sometimes appears to be a disease *per se* it may also be symptomatic of a number of underlying conditions.

"**Loss of control**"—possibly more suitable terms suggested are "loss of freedom" (Stewart, 1956) or "loss of choice"—does not mean that this type of drinker gets drunk whenever he starts drinking. Rather it means that once he has started to drink on a given occasion he can never be certain of being able to stop drinking when he wants to. The rule is therefore not that the first drink is "fatal" but that it *may be* "fatal". The "loss of control" phenomenon explains the main rule which the alcoholic will have to follow for the rest of his life; that is, at least at the present state of knowledge, *no alcohol in any shape or form.*

THE PHYSICAL COMPLICATIONS OF CHRONIC ALCOHOLISM

Complications affecting the alimentary and the nervous system are especially prevalent. Certain aspects of the problem of liver disease in alcoholism were discussed in the second edition (pp. 74–82) of this book, including:

> *Liver function tests* (prior to the advent of the transaminase tests). In a battery of such tests some are often pathological just after the alcoholic has finished an acute bout, but may revert to normal soon after a short period of abstinence and balanced nutrition.
>
> *Liver biopsy.* Leevy and Hove (1967) described this as the only means of recognizing cirrhosis in its early phases: "This represents an optimum time for diagnosis since the lesion may become arrested with appropriate therapy. Unfortunately the disease often is first evident with the appearance of manifestations of liver failure or portal hypertension, such as bleeding oesophageal varices, ascites, or hepatic coma. Once these clinical features appear, prognosis is guarded, despite control of alcoholism." The histologic features of alcoholic fatty liver and alcoholic cirrhosis are well described and depicted in Shorter's *Liver Biopsy* (1961). Fatty liver is by far the most common hepatic abnormality seen in hospitalized alcoholics (Leevy and Hove, 1967).
>
> *The relation of nutrition to liver disease.* In the 1952 edition this chapter contained the statement "Alcohol itself is probably devoid of toxic effects on liver cells", a view which is no longer generally held. Thus Leevy and Hove state: "Prospective studies indicate that both alcohol and dietary deficiency contribute to the fatty liver, hepatic necrosis, iron overload, and cirrhosis seen in the alcoholic. . . . The amount of alcohol consumed and the nutritional state both influence its oxidation and toxicity." Lieber (1967) carried out investigations indicating that the alcoholic fatty liver was not simply a consequence of a lack of available calories but resulted from alcohol *per se*, of which the capacity for producing a fatty liver was found to be greater than that of fat itself. Rubin and Lieber (1968) concluded from studies in alcoholics and non-alcoholic volunteers that alcohol can damage the liver of alcoholics and non-alcoholics, independently of nutritional factors, within two days, and in their view the amounts of alcoholic drink consumed by many social drinkers are injurious even if they do not get drunk.

Other points of interest in this connection are the development of hepatoma in a high proportion of alcoholics with severe cirrhosis who survive for long periods (Leevy and Hove, 1967): the relatively better prognosis in alcoholic cirrhosis than in the cryptogenic form (*Lancet*, 1960; *Brit. med. J.*, 1968); and the description of a new syndrome by Zieve (1958) in chronic alcoholism, consisting of transient hyperlipaemia, jaundice and haemolytic anaemia, with an alcoholic fatty liver and cirrhosis.

Alcohol and the blood. Folate deficiency (Sullivan and Herbert, 1964; *Lancet*, 1969) following dietary restriction, with megaloblastic erythropoiesis and macrocytic anaemia, is probably one of the most important factors responsible for the chronic alcoholic's anaemia; other factors involved may be gastro-intestinal dysfunction with poor iron absorption, and liver disease. The diet of chronic alcoholics often contains less than the minimum oral folate requirements of 50 μg daily. Alcohol can suppress the response of bone-marrow haemopoiesis to such minimum amounts of dietary folic acid, but there is a response when larger doses of folic acid are given such as are present in an ordinary hospital diet, or when alcohol intake ceases. This may explain the finding that the anaemia of a chronic alcoholic usually improves rapidly on hospital admission and alcohol withdrawal.

Excessive alcohol intake can cause suppression of formation of red cells, granulocytes, and platelets. MacLeod and Michaels (1969) have found thrombocytopenia a common complication of excessive alcohol ingestion. This may cause an abnormal tendency to bruise and may add yet another hazard to the alcoholic who is already accident-prone, frequently exposed to trauma, subject to head injury with subdural haematoma, liable to bleed from peptic ulceration or oesophageal varices, and a frequent candidate for emergency operations.

As regards the *neurological complications* of chronic alcoholism, Victor and Adams (1961) conclude that delirium tremens, alcoholic epilepsy, and acute auditory hallucinosis are causally related to habituation to and withdrawal of alcohol and are not of nutritional origin; whereas Wernicke's disease, alcoholic Korsakoff's pyschosis, polyneuropathy and the neurological manifestations of pellagra are clearly nutritional in origin; in a third group, alcoholic cerebellar degeneration, central pontine myelinolysis and Marchiafava-Bignami disease pathogenesis and the role of nutritional factors remain uncertain. The prognosis of alcoholic neuropathy is regarded as good. According to Hornabrook (1961), almost all patients recover on a regimen of parenteral vitamins, a good diet and bed rest, the moderately severe cases in six to eight weeks, the more severe after a somewhat longer period.

Certain other conditions sometimes associated with protracted alcoholism and discussed in the recent literature includ *Renal cortical necrosis* (Bull et al., 1957) and *Cancer of the pharynx, larynx, mouth and possibly oesophagus*, stated to be commoner in alcoholics than in other people (*Brit. med. J.*, 1957; Wynder and Boss, 1957; Kennaway, 1957).

Alcoholic cardiomyopathy. Brigden (1957) studied 50 cases of "non-coronary"cardiomyopathy, 13 of whom had histories of severe alcoholism without beri-beri. Of these, seven had drunk beer only, the rest spirits; among the spirit drinkers symptoms appeared earlier and were more severe. All presented with dyspnoea on exertion, as did 10 of 20 patients suffering from alcoholic cardiomyopathy observed by Evans (1959). Evans considers that alcoholic cardiomyopathy is commoner than generally assumed because the features are usually attributed to ischaemic heart disease, but diagnosis can

S

be made by certain characteristic ECG changes, the commonest being the "dimple T wave". Early diagnosis is essential because at an early stage abstinence is said to lead to complete recovery, continued drinking to intractable heart failure.

Thus, in many of the conditions described stress is laid on early diagnosis and the possibility of recovery on alcohol withdrawal and proper nutrition. As a rule one sees a remarkably rapid improvement in an alcoholic's general physical state under such conditions. It is surprising that in very long-standing chronic drunkenness offenders—despite their prolonged neglect of food and of all rules of personal hygiene—the state of general health is not too bad. This has been ascribed by some of these people themselves to their repeated spells of imprisonment when their staple diet—alcohol, often including surgical spirit—is replaced by ordinary food.

TREATMENT

The question of "normal" drinking in "loss of control" alcoholism

Interest in the question of the need for lifelong abstinence in alcoholism has been revived since, according to a number of recent reports, several alcoholics managed to resume "normal" drinking (Davies, 1962; Kendell, 1965). On the other hand, the great majority of experts the world over who have treated large numbers of alcoholics state that they have hardly ever encountered such patients. The few alcoholics reported to have achieved "normal" drinking (and of course every therapist knows alcoholics who have been trying it for years only to end up drunk) were often individuals whose life situation had altered a great deal, as by a change of job or marriage, who were no longer under the same stress, or who had changed their type of drink. In our own experience there has been the occasional alcohol "addict" who managed moderate drinking for a short-term period under special circumstances and taking special precautions (Glatt, 1967), such as drinking only whilst in a contented or cheerful frame of mind; sticking to beer or wine only and taking at most two to three drinks on one occasion; sipping slowly rather than "gulping"; drinking in company and with meals only. In virtually all such patients, however, such efforts were short-lived and soon led to uncontrolled drinking once again. One might also question whether such techniques of cautious "nibbling", with one's eyes glued to the clock or on the company can be called normal drinking. At any rate, exceptional successes cannot alter the rule that alcoholics have to learn to accept and adjust to a life of total abstinence. There is a consolation in that once alcoholics have managed to get over their first three to six months of sobriety the going becomes progressively easier, since the great majority of first relapses happen during the first six months after treatment and more rarely afterwards (De Morsier and Feldman, 1950; Glatt, 1961b).

The physical abstinence syndrome in "Gamma alcoholism" and the treatment of the acute phases of alcoholism

Only during the past 15 years has the existence of a dangerous physical abstinence syndrome following sudden cessation or rapid decrease of alcohol intake in very heavy drinkers been generally accepted. This has been largely due to the experimental work of Isbell *et al.* (1955) with ex-morphine addicts: of six patients who drank average daily amounts of 346 to 489 c.c. of absolute alcohol for 48 to 87 days, all but one developed symptoms such as convulsions, hallucinations or delirium tremens on abrupt alcohol withdrawal. Nevertheless, sudden withdrawal is still the method commonly adopted in the treatment of alcoholics although one must watch for the appearance of fits or delirium tremens in very heavy drinkers, and try to prevent them by anticonvulsants and tranquillizers. Dehydration, salt depletion and malnutrition may require liberal administration of fluids, salt and vitamins parenterally or orally. Tranquillizers such as the phenothiazines and benzodiazepines are usually needed to calm the tense, anxious, agitated and restless patients. Because of the risk of psychological and physical dependence, meprobamate is best avoided in alcoholics. Occasional cases of such dependence have also been described after prolonged administration of high doses of benzodiazepines (Hollister *et al.*, 1961; Kryspin-Exner, 1966a) but they do not seem to have occurred in this country, possibly because of the smaller dosages employed and shorter duration of administration.

A sedative-hypnotic frequently employed in recent years during the alcohol withdrawal period, and in particular delirium tremens, is chlormethiazole ("Heminevrin") (Frisch, 1966) which is derived from the thiazole fraction of the B_1 molecule. Many workers in Sweden and Germany regard it as the best method of preventing and treating delirium tremens (Lundquist, 1966). In severe states therapy may begin with the intravenous injection of the 0·8 per cent solution or with infusion, the most severe cases sometimes requiring up to 500–1000 ml over six to twelve hours. In this country, where delirium tremens seems milder than in some foreign countries, oral administration is usually adequate, the approximate dosage being 2 g (4 tablets) to start with, followed by about 1 g, every two to four hours until adequate sedation is obtained (e.g. up to 8–10 g on the first day). Over the following days the dose is gradually reduced. Like other sedatives, chlormethiazole carries a risk of psychological and rarely physical dependence, and administration should therefore not continue, as a rule, beyond six days. In delirium tremens a longer period may be necessary, but there is some evidence that the type of alcoholic more likely to develop this condition (Kryspin-Exner, 1966b; Lundquist, 1966) is less prone to abuse other drugs. Chlormethiazole was shown in a controlled trial to be significantly more effective during the alcohol withdrawal period than a placebo (Glatt *et al.*, 1965). Because of its anticonvulsant action it may diminish the risk of withdrawal convulsions as well as of delirum tremens, but it is probably wise to add some such anticonvulsant as phenytoin during the alcohol withdrawal phase. Reported side-effects such as transient fall of blood pressure and slight respiratory depression are rare and usually mild.

Insomnia during the withdrawal period often necessitates the administration of hypnotics. In alcoholics they should be used sparingly and discontinued as soon as possible since many alcoholics tend to abuse and become dependent on them. Because of this risk barbiturates and oral paraldehyde are best avoided in alcoholics, as well as such stimulating drugs as amphetamines and phenmetrazine. On the whole this danger seems rather less with non-barbiturate hypnotics. Cases of psychological and physical dependence have been described with drugs such as glutethimide and methaqualone but not yet with the more recently introduced nitrazepam (Mogadon).

In view of the prevalence of barbiturate abuse among alcoholics one should always enquire directly whether the patient has taken barbiturates, because of the risks of barbiturate-withdrawal convulsions and delirium tremens. Where alcoholics have also taken barbiturates these must of course be tapered off, and never withdrawn abruptly.

In this country delirium tremens is usually a manifestation of withdrawal, but in countries such as Sweden it seems often to be precipitated by other factors (Lundquist, 1961) such as infection, head injury and poor nutrition.

Long-term treatment of alcoholism

Detoxication and sobering-up are no more than first-aid measures in alcoholics which must always be followed up by long-term measures aimed at assisting the alcoholic to reach a state of contented sobriety. To withdraw therapy after the sobering-up phase does no more than to render the alcoholic fit to resume drinking again. Quite different approaches, including psychological, physical and social methods have achieved success in the hands of various therapists. The common denominator may lie either in the breakdown of the original attitudes of the alcoholic himself so that he may be able to adopt other, more constructive attitudes in their place (Williams, 1956), or in the approach by the therapist who accepts the alcoholic as a sick man instead of adopting a moralistic, judging, and condemning attitude. The therapists' basic attitude is probably more decisive than the technique he chooses. There have been heated arguments as to whether psychotherapy or behaviouristic techniques are more successful in alcoholics. It would seem more realistic, however, instead of adopting from the beginning a rigid, partisan "Freud *or* Pavlov" approach, to assess the factors of aetiological importance in the given patient and then to select the method or combination of methods best suited to his individual needs. At any rate, in as complex a condition as alcoholism, with its multifactorial aetiology, it seems highly unlikely that one and the same treatment is the best for each and every patient.

The three different types of approaches employed today are:

Physical methods

By and large, conditioned reflex treatments (apomorphine, emetine, and the recently revived electrical methods) seem less popular today, whereas alcohol sensitizing and deterrent drugs such as disulfiram (Antabuse) and citrated calcium carbimide (Abstem) are widely used all over the world. Abstem was described by Canadian investigators (Ferguson et al., 1956; Armstrong, 1957) and is on the whole somewhat milder than Antabuse: sensitization to alcohol starts and fades away more rapidly with CCC than with disulfiram, the alcohol reaction and the side-effects are milder: the deterrent effects are therefore less strong and the "protection" afforded less long with the newer drug compared to the older disulfiram. Whether Antabuse or Abstem are preferred may depend largely on an assessment of the individual patient's personality (Glatt, 1959a). The minimum maintenance dosage should be chosen, usually in the range of half an Antabuse tablet (i.e. 0·25 g) at night (because of its sedative effect) or one Abstem tablet (50 mg) in the morning. In general, a preliminary Antabuse or Abstem alcohol test is no longer recommended, but alcoholics who are likely to gamble on getting away with drinking on top of these drugs, such as psychopaths, are probably best excluded. On such a small antabuse maintenance dose the occasional serious toxic effects like psychotic episodes and peripheral neuropathy should be very rare.

It is often alleged that these forms of treatment are useless because so many alcoholics find it easier to forget to take the Antabuse and Abstem tablets than to give up drink. However, no treatment can succeed with alcoholics unless it is possible to enlist their co-operation and motivation. Merely to give Antabuse as the main method of treatment is useless, but like other physical treatments, it can be very helpful as an adjunct to the psycho-social approach. In practice, these drugs will often be found helpful after the patient has been informed about their purpose and his co-operation enlisted. And although these tablets are not claimed to reduce craving one may often find in practice that the knowledge that for the next few days alcohol is definitely "out", effectively reduces the conflict within the alcoholic—"shall I or shan't I drink?"—and thus indirectly the desire.

From time to time new drugs are introduced with the claim that they may be very helpful in the treatment of alcoholism, but no others have stood the test of time. Recently metronidazole (Taylor, 1964), a drug used in trichomoniasis, has been claimed to possess disulfiram-like properties, to diminish alcohol withdrawal symptoms, and to decrease craving for alcohol, thus possibly facilitating social drinking by alcoholics. A double-blind controlled trial (Gelder and Edwards, 1967) in which the drug, in a dosage of 400 mg t.d.s., and a placebo were given to alcohol addicts, showed no evidence of an Antabuse-like effect or of a therapeutic effect on alcoholics, though it made alcoholic drink less pleasant. Two Italian observers (Bonfiglio and Donadio, 1967) who treated 60 male alcohol addicts concluded that the drug was active in a high percentage of patients provided it was administered for a prolonged period in a daily dosage of 750 mg for a month, followed after an alcohol test by a maintenance dose of 250 mg per day. Hungarian observers (Kardos and Szabados, 1967) noted that the drug led to a much milder alcoholic reaction than disulfiram, and that it contributed "to aborting dependence on alcohol". Thus, the place and value of metronidazole in alcoholism therapy is not yet clear.

Another drug frequently reported in recent years as of value in alcoholism is LSD. No definite answer as to its value as an adjunct to the therapy of alcoholism can as yet be given. However, a careful review of the relevant literature and a controlled trial were recently reported from the Addiction Research Foundation in Ontario (Smart *et al.*, 1967). It was concluded that "... the results as a whole fail to indicate that the LSD experience as described here is an effective adjunct to the clinical treatment of alcoholism . . .", and that "earlier reports that LSD was an effective adjunct to therapy for alcoholism may have resulted from lack of adequate controls in the evaluation of its utility".

The physical treatments employed in alcoholism are not without danger, especially the aversion methods. Doctors who use them should have familiarized themselves with the techniques and the risks. A full physical examination, ECG and certain laboratory investigations must precede the employment of such physical methods.

Tranquillizers and thymoleptics are sometimes used in the long-term management of alcoholics, for purposes such as helping the "dry" alcoholic over periods of anxiety, tension, or depression, and encouraging him to keep in regular touch with the therapist. Undue dependence of an alcoholic on any drug should however be avoided. It is often difficult to decide ". . .when there is so much anxiety present as to hinder the patient's peace of mind and progress and require alleviation by drugs, or whether it may be sufficiently bearable so that, when tolerated, it may act as a spur to arouse and to develop the patient's own adaptive potentialities" (Glatt, 1959b).

Not much will be said here about psychotherapy and the role of A.A. Psychoanalysis has not proved to be of value in alcoholics, nor is deep psychotherapy required in most alcoholics. However, brief electric psychotherapeutic techniques and in particular group-psychotherapy have often proved useful in helping such patients to gain insight into their problems and personality difficulties, so that they learn to cope with inner tensions and environmental stresses in a more mature and less destructive manner than by seeking refuge and oblivion in alcohol or drugs.

Alcoholics Anonymous, the fellowship of recovered alcoholics, has proved of enormous value to many alcoholics. They are now established in every part of the British Isles, and doctors would be well advised to work in close co-operation with them, in particular in the aftercare phase, which is so vital in determining the success or failure of any method of treatment in alcoholism. One word of caution: A.A. has created its own image of the alcoholic from its early experiences with the American Gamma-type of alcoholism. When recommending other types of alcoholics to attend A.A. Meetings, the therapist should therefore inform such a patient about the difference between this and the average English pattern of alcoholism.

Alcoholic units. Memoranda recommending the establishment of Regional Alcoholic Units were sent by the Ministry of Health Boards in 1962 and 1968. The first alcoholic unit in this country was established at Warlingham Park Hospital in 1952 (Glatt, 1955). There are at present 13 units in England and Wales, and units have also been established in Scotland and Ireland. It has been suggested that the concept of such an Alcoholic Unit should also include out-patient clinics and special half-way houses apart from in-patient wards (Glatt, 1965). The work in such units is based on the principles of living in a therapeutic community and on group-therapy, collaboration with A.A., and the use of physical methods as adjuncts. Some units are very selective in their admission policies, others less so. Some admit alcoholics with marked physical complications, others do not. In general, alcoholics with definite mental and physical disorders are admitted to psychiatric and general hospitals respectively. However, certain units abroad specialize in the treatment of alcoholic diseases. The centre in West Berlin, for example, admits patients with liver cirrhosis, peptic ulcer (a history of duodenal ulcer and partial gastrectomy is very common in alcoholics) and pancreatitis (Schmidt, 1968).

CONCLUSION

As clearly evident from the brief but yet fairly comprehensive recent WHO report on "Services for the Prevention and Treatment of Dependence on Alcohol and Other Drugs" (1967), much progress has been made during the past two decades; a great deal more remains to be done in the fields of treatment, education, research and prophylaxis. Doctors should be in the forefront in the task of preventing and fighting alcoholism, but they need to be better equipped by adequate education in this field during their student days. This important task can no longer be left to the postgraduate private enterprise of a few individuals.

REFERENCES

ARMSTRONG, J. D. (1957). The protective drugs in the treatment of alcoholism. *Canad. Ass. J.*, **77**, 228.

BONFIGLIO, G. & DONADIO, G. (1967). Results of the clinical testing of a new drug "Metronidazole" in the treatment of chronic alcoholism. *Brit. J. Addict.*, **62**, 249.

BRIGDEN, W. (1957). Uncommon myocardial diseases. *Lancet*, **2**, 1179, 1243.

British Medical Journal (Any Questions) (1957). Cancer in chronic alcoholics. **1**, 1195.

British Medical Journal (L. A.) (1968). Slow progress in cirrhosis. **1**, 445.

BULL, G. M., JOEKES, A. M. & LOWE, K. G. (1957). Acute renal failure due to poisons and drugs. *Lancet*, **1**, 134.

CAMPS, F. E. & DODD, B. E. (1967). Increase in the incidence of non-secretors of ABH blood group substances among alcoholic patients. *Brit. med. J.*, **1**, 30.

CRUZ-COKE, R. & VARELA, A. (1966). Inheritance of alcoholism. *Lancet*, **2**, 1282.

DALEY, R. & MILLER, H. (eds) (1952). *Progress in Clinical Medicine*, 2nd edition, pp. 74–82, 367-370. London: Churchill.

DAVIES, D. L. (1962). The problem of normal drinking in recovered alcohol addicts. *Quart. J. Stud. Alcohol*, **23**, 94.

DE MORSIER, G. & FELDMAN, H. (1950). Biological treatments of chronic alcoholism by apomorphine. *Brit. J. Addict.*, **47**, 50.

Drinking involved in home accidents, company finds (1968). *Illinois med. J.*, **133**, 423, 543.

EVANS, W. (1959). The electrocardiogram of alcoholic cardiomyopathy. *Brit. Heart J.*, **21**, 445.

FERGUSON, J. K. W., ARMSTRONG, J. D., KERR, H. T. & BELL, R. G. (1956). A new drug for alcoholism treatment. *Canad. med. Ass. J.*, **74**, 793.

FRISCH, E. P. (1966). Chlormethiazole. (Proceed. of a sympos.). Copenhagen: Munksgaard.

GELDER, M. G. & EDWARDS, G. (1967). Metronidazole in the treatment of alcohol addiction: a controlled trial 13th Internat. Institut. Prev. Trtmt. Alcoholism. Internat. Col. Alcohol. Alcoholism. *Zagreb*, p. 14.1.

GLATT, M. M. (1955). Treatment centre for alcoholics in a mental hospital. *Lancet*, **1**, 1318.

GLATT, M. M. (1959a). Disulfiram and citrated calcium carbimide in the treatment of alcoholism. *J. ment. Sci.*, **105**, 476.

GLATT, M. M. (1959b). The use and abuse of tranquillizers in alcoholics. *Brit. J. Addict.*, **55**, 111.

GLATT, M. M. (1961a). Drinking habits of English (middle-class) alcoholics. *Acta psychiat. scand.*, **371**, 88.

GLATT, M. M. (1961b). Treatment results in an English mental hospital alcoholic unit. *Acta psychiat. scand.*, **37**, 143.

GLATT, M. M. (1964). Alcoholism in "impaired" and drunken driving. *Lancet*, **1**, 161.

GLATT, M. M. (1965). Alcoholism in Britain. In *New Aspects of the Mental Health Services*. ed. H. Freeman and J. Farndale, p. 115. Oxford: Pergamon Press.

GLATT, M. M. (1967). The question of moderate drinking despite "loss of control". *Brit. J. Addict.*, **62**, 267.

GLATT, M. M., GEORGE, H. R. & FRISCH, E. P. (1965). Controlled trial of chlormethiazole in treatment of the alcoholic withdrawal phase. *Brit. med. J.*, **2**, 401.

GLATT, M. M. & HILLS, D. R. (1968). Alcohol abuse and alcoholism in the young. *Brit. J. Addict.*, **63**, 183.

HAGGARD, H. W. & JELLINEK, E. M. (1950). *Alcohol Explored*, p. 190. New York: Doubleday.

HASSALL, C. (1968). A controlled study of the characteristics of young male alcoholics. *Brit. J. Addict.*, **61**, 193.

HOLLISTER, L. E., MOTZENBECKER, F. P. & DESAN, R. O. (1961). Withdrawal reactions from chlordiazepoxide (Librium). *Psychopharmacologia (Berl.)*, **2**, 63.

HORNABROOK, R. W. (1961). Alcoholic neuropathy. *Amer. J. clin. Nutr.*, **9**, 398.

ISBELL, H., FRASER, H. F., WIKLER, A., BELLEVILLE, R. E. & EISENMAN, A. J. (1955). An experimental study of the aetiology of "rum fits" and delirium tremens. *Quart. J. Stud. Alcohol.*, **16**, 38.

JELLINEK, E. M. (1951). Jellinek estimation formula. *World Hlth Org. techn. Rep. Ser.*, **42**, 20, 21. Geneva.

JELLINEK, E. M. (1952). The phases of alcohol addiction. *Ibid.*, **48**, 26.

JELLINEK, E. M. (1959). Estimating the prevalence of alcoholism. *Quart. J. Stud. Alcohol.*, **20**, 261.

JELLINEK, E. M. (1960). *The Disease Concept of Alcoholism*, pp. 35, 41, 82, 111, 145, 152. New Haven, Conn.: Hillhouse Press.

KARDOS, G. & SZABADOS, P. (1967). Trials with drug therapy in the treatment of chronic alcoholism. II. Metronidazole-alcohol reaction. *Ideggyog. Szle.*, **20**, 362 (in Hungarian). (English abstract: *Quart. J. Stud. Alcohol.*, 1969, **30**, 793.)

KENDELL, R. E. (1965). Normal drinking by former alcohol addicts. *Quart. J. Stud. Alcohol.*, **26**, 247.

KENNAWAY, SIR E. (1957). Some questions on cancer of the lung, larynx, and urinary tract. *Brit. med., J.*, **1**, 299.

KESSEL, N. & GROSSMAN, G. (1961). Suicide in alcoholics. *Brit. med. J.*, **2**, 1671.

KRYSPIN-EXNER, K. (1966a). Missbrauch von Benzodiazepinderivaten bei Alkoholranken. *Brit. J. Addict.*, **61**, 283.

KRYSPIN-EXNER, K. (1966b). In *Chlormethiazole*. ed. E.P. Frisch, p. 205. Copenhagen: Munksgaard.

Lancet (Annot.) (1960). Alcoholic cardiomyopathy. **1**, 536.

Lancet (Annot.) (1960). Alcoholic versus non-alcoholic cirrhosis. **1**, 814.

Lancet (L. A.) (1969). Alcohol and the blood. **2**, 675.

LEEVY, C. M. & HOVE, W. (1967). Pathogenesis and sequelae of liver disease in alcoholic man. In *Biochemical Factors in Alcoholism*. ed. R. P. Maickel, p. 151. Oxford: Pergamon Press.

LIEBER, C. S. (1967). Alcoholic fatty liver, hyperlipemia and hyperuricemia. In *Biochemical Factors in Alcoholism*. ed. R. P. Maickel, p. 167. Oxford: Pergamon Press.

LUNQUIST, G. (1961). Delirium tremens. *Acta psychiat. scand.*, **36**, 443.

LUNQUIST, G. (1966). In *Chlormethiazole*. ed. E. P. Frisch, 113 p. 209. Copenhagen: Munksgaard.

MacLEOD, E. C. & MICHAELS, L. (1969). Alcohol and the blood. *Lancet*, **2**, 1198.

MARDONES, J. (1968). 28th Internat. Congr. Alcohol and alcoholism. Washington, D.C.

MOSS, M. C. & DAVIES, E. BERESFORD (1967). *A Survey of Alcoholism in an English County (Geigy)*. Cambridge: C.U.P.

PARR, D. C. (1957). Alcoholism in general practice. *Brit. J. Addict.*, **54**, 25.

PARTANEN, J., BRUUN, K. & MARKKANEN, T. (1966). *Inheritance of Drinking Behaviour*. Helsinki: Finnish Foundation for Alcohol Studies.

PRYS WILLIAMS, G. & GLATT, M. M. (1966). The incidence of long-standing alcoholism in England and Wales. *Brit. J. Addict.*, **61**, 257.

ROE, A. (1952). Children of alcoholic parents raised in foster homes. In *Alcohol, Science and Society*. ed. Newhaven, Conn. *Quart. J. Stud. Alcohol.*, p. 115.

RUBIN, E. & LIEBER, C. S. (1968). *Studies of the Effect of Time, Dose and Diet on Alcoholic Liver Injury in Alcoholics and Non-alcoholic Volunteers*. 28th Internat. Congr. Alcohol and Alcoholism. Washington, D.C.

SAINSBURY, P. (1955). *Suicide in London*. Maudsley Monograph Ser. 1. London.

SCHMIDT, L. (1968). *Development of a Psychosomatic Centre for Treatment and Research in Alcoholism in West Berlin*. 28th Internat. Congr. Alcohol and Alcoholism. Washington, D.C.

SHORTER, R. G. (1961). *Liver Biopsy*, pp. 20–22, 31, 32. Figs. 37–40, 64. Oxford: Pergamon Press.

SMART, R. G., STORM, T., BAKER, E. F. W. & SOLURSH, L. (1967). *LSD in the Treatment of Alcoholism*, p. 89. Toronto: Univ. of Toronto Press.

STEERING GROUP ON ALCOHOLICS (J. Rowntree Social Service Trust) (1965). *Chronic Alcoholics*. ed. G. Prys Williams. London.

STEWART, D. A. (1956). *Preface to Empathy*. New York: Philosophical Library.

SULLIVAN, L. W. & HERBERT, V. (1964). Suppression of hemopoiesis by ethanol. *J. clin. Invest.*, **43**, 2048.

SUNDBY, PER (1967). *Alcoholism and Mortality*, p. 172. Oslo: Universitetsforlaget.

TAYLOR, J. A. (1964). Metronidazole—a new agent for combined somatic and psychic therapy of alcoholics. *Bull. Los Angeles neurol. Soc.*, **29**, 158.

VON WARTBURG, J. P. (1967). In *Biochemical Factors in Alcoholism*. ed. R. P. Maickel, p. 3. Oxford: Pergamon Press.

VON WARTBURG & SCHENKER, T. M. (1968). *Metabolism of Ethanol*. 28th Internat. Congr. Alcohol and Alcoholism. Washington, D.C.

VICTOR, M. & ADAMS, D. R. (1961). On the aetiology of the alcoholic neurologic diseases. *Amer. J. clin. Nutrit.*, **9**, 379.

WILLIAMS, L. (1956). *Alcoholism*, p. 39. Edinburgh: Livingstone.

WORLD HEALTH ORGANIZATION (1951). Alcoholism Subcommittee. *Wld Hlth. Org. techn. Rep. Ser.*, **42**, 20, 21. Geneva.

WORLD HEALTH ORGANIZATION (1952). Alcoholism Subcommittee. *Ibid.*, **48**, 16, 37. Geneva.

WORLD HEALTH ORGANIZATION (1954). Expert Committee on Alcohol. *Ibid.*, **84**, 10. Geneva.

WORLD HEALTH ORGANIZATION (1967). Services for the Prevention and Treatment of Dependence on Alcohol and other Drugs. *Ibid.*, **363**, Geneva.

WYNDER, E. L. & BOSS, I. D. (1957). Aetiological factors in mouth cancer. *Brit. med. J.*, **1**, 1137.

ZIEVE, L. (1958). Jaundice, hyperlipemia and hemolytic anaemia: a heretofore unrecognised syndrome associated with alcoholic fatty liver and cirrhosis. *Ann. intern. Med.*, **48**, 471.

16 Drug Addiction

P. H. CONNELL

LEGAL DEFINITION. DRUG DEPENDENCE AND ABUSE: EVALU-
ATION AND CRITERIA FOR CONTROL. THE GROWTH OF DRUG
DEPENDENCE IN THE UNITED KINGDOM. DRUG DEPENDENCE
IN OTHER COUNTRIES. THE PERSONALITY OF THE DRUG-DEPEN-
DENT INDIVIDUAL. DRUG DEPENDENCE AND CRIME. THE RISK
OF DRUG DEPENDENCE. THE DIAGNOSIS OF DRUG DEPENDENCE.
TREATMENT OF DRUG DEPENDENCE. WITHDRAWAL IN HOSPITAL
REHABILITATION. GOALS OF REHABILITATION. METHODS OF
REHABILITATION. SPECIAL METHODS. THE PHOENIX HOUSE
PROGRAMME. CRIMINAL COMMITMENT PROGRAMMES. RESULTS
OF TREATMENT. DRUG DEPENDENCE AND DOCTORS. THE
PHILOSOPHY OF SOME DRUG PRESCRIBING. THE PRESENT AND
THE FUTURE.

THE subject of drug addiction and habituation has long been a confusing
one in that definitions of the terms addiction and habituation have varied.
If one goes back to the original World Health Organization's report (WHO,
1950) one reads the following:

> Drug addiction is a state of periodic or chronic addiction detrimental
> to the individual and to society, produced by the repeated consumption
> of a drug (natural or synthetic). Its characteristics include
>
> 1. an overpowering desire or need (compulsion) to continue taking
>   the drug and to obtain it by any means;
> 2. a tendency to increase the dose;
> 3. psychic (or psychological) and sometimes a physical dependence on
>   the effects of the drug;
> 4. a detrimental effect on the individual and on society.

It will be seen that in (3) above the emphasis was on psychic or psychological aspects. Some years later, however, the World Health Organization
(WHO, 1957) Expert Committee thought again and changed point (3) of

their original definition so that the word *sometimes* became *generally* a physical dependence.

The Interdepartmental Committee (1961), in this country under the Chairmanship of Lord Brain, came out firmly in favour of the old classical definition of addiction as follows:

> Drug addiction is a state of periodic or chronic intoxication produced by the repeated consumption of a drug (natural or synthetic). Its characteristics include
>
> 1. an overpowering desire or need (compulsion) to continue taking the drug and to obtain it by any means;
> 2. a tendency to increase the dose, though some patients may remain indefinitely on a stationary dose;
> 3. a psychological and physical dependence on the effects of the drug;
> 4. the appearance of a characteristic abstinence syndrome in a subject from whom the drug is withdrawn;
> 5. an effect detrimental to the individual and to society.

This was distinguished from drug habituation which was defined as follows—Drug habituation (habit) is a condition resulting from the repeated consumption of a drug. Its characteristics include

> 1. a desire (but not a compulsion) to continue taking the drug for the sense of improved well being which it engendered;
> 2. little or no tendency to increase the dose;
> 3. some degree of psychological dependence on the effect of the drug but absence of physical dependence and hence of an abstinence syndrome;
> 4. detrimental effects, if any, primarily on the individual.

The Thirteenth Report of the World Health Organization (1964), however, re-examined the whole question of addiction, habituation and dependence and came out strongly in favour of using the word dependence and then to define the type of dependence according to the drug used. The definition used was similar to previous definitions but went into details about the specific effects of the drug. For instance, amphetamine type of dependence was defined as follows:

> A state arising from repeated administration of amphetamine or an agent with amphetamine like effects on a periodic or continuous basis. Its characteristics include
>
> 1. a desire or need to continue taking the drug;
> 2. consumption of increasing amounts to obtain greater excitatory or euphoric effects or to combat more effectively depression and fatigue, accompanied in some measure by the development of tolerance;

3. a psychic dependence on the effects of the drug related to a subjective and individual appreciation of the drug's effects; and
4. general absence of physical dependence so that there is no characteristic abstinence syndrome when the drug is discontinued.

Barbiturate dependence was defined as follows:

A state arising from the repeated administration of a barbiturate, or an agent with barbiturate-like effect, on a continuous basis, generally in amounts exceeding therapeutic dose levels. Its characteristics include:

1. a strong desire or need to continue taking the drug; the need can be satisfied by the drug taken initially or by another with barbiturate-like properties;
2. a tendency to increase the dose, partly owing to the development of tolerance;
3. a psychic dependence on the effects of the drug related to subjective and individual appreciation of those effects; and
4. a physical dependence on the effects of the drug requiring its presence for maintenance of homeostasis and resulting in a definite, characteristic, and self-limited abstinence syndrome when the drug is withdrawn.

Heroin dependence was defined as follows:

A state arising from repeated administration of morphine, or an agent with morphine-like effects, on a periodic or continuous basis. Its characteristics include:

1. an overpowering desire or need to continue taking the drug and to obtain it by any means; the need can be satisfied by the drug taken initially or by another with morphine-like properties;
2. a tendency to increase the dose owing to the development of tolerance;
3. a psychic dependence on the effects of the drug related to a subjective and individual appreciation of those effects; and
4. a physical dependence on the effects of the drug requiring its presence for maintenance of homeostasis and resulting in a definite, characteristic and self-limited abstinence syndrome when the drug is withdrawn.

The older rigid definitions of addiction which required an abstinence syndrome were unhelpful in that

(a) they did not take into account the dangers of drugs like amphetamines which have since been shown to produce severe dependence and a hazard to public health;
(b) they tended to confer the title "habituation" on such drugs as amphetamines which had the result of lulling doctors into a false sense of

security in their prescribing so that they were prescribed freely and thus many instances of amphetamine dependence were produced:

(c) the borderline between drugs which do not produce overt physical dependence syndromes and those which do is a blurred one in that some drugs may produce physical dependence in some instances but not in all instances, and certain physical symptoms which are not very distressing to the patient hardly have the quality of the abstinence syndrome which is present with drugs such as morphine.

The attempt of the World Health Organization to deal with this whole subject in terms of "dependence" is to be applauded but in general conversation we are short of a word which can replace "addict" in that it seems wrong to talk about a drug dependant in the same way as we talk about a drug addict.

Furthermore, the general term "dependence" is only satisfactory if the medical profession regard this as equivalent in severity and importance to the term "addiction". Otherwise, the word "dependence" would lead to a watering down of anxiety towards all drugs producing dependence.

Finally, the whole situation is confused further in that the classical withdrawal syndromes are now thought to contain a considerable psychological element and last year a report of "dependence on a placebo" (Vinar, 1969) relates a case history in which a middle-aged schizophrenic woman became dependent on a placebo which was presented as "a new major tranquillizer without any side-effects" which relieved her anxiety and tiredness and which in time she increased to 25 tablets a day and on withdrawal from them she was reported to have an abstinence syndrome with physical symptoms. Honigfeld (1964) reported the substitution of saline injections for morphine in addicts, without withdrawal symptoms appearing until the saline injections were stopped.

Legal Definition

The Dangerous Drugs Act, 1967, defined in its regulations an addict as follows:

... a person shall be regarded as addicted to a drug only if, as a result of repeated administration, he has become so dependent upon the drug that he has an overpowering desire for the administration of it to be continued.

In these regulations "drug" means any substance for the time being specified in Part I of the Schedule to the Dangerous Drugs Act, 1965, and the regulations (Dangerous Drugs (Notification of Addicts) Regulations, 1968).

Drug Dependence and Abuse: Evaluation and Criteria for Control

The WHO Expert Committee on Drug Dependence (1969) in its Sixteenth Report attempted to go into the question of evaluation and criteria for control. It adopted the following definitions for use in the present context:

Drug. Any substance that, when taken into the living organism, may modify one or more of its functions.

Drug Abuse. Persistent or sporadic excessive drug use inconsistent with or unrelated to acceptable medical practice.

Drug Dependence. A state, psychic, and sometimes also physical, resulting from the interaction between a living organism and a drug, characterized by behavioural and other responses that always include a compulsion to take the drug on a continuous or periodic basis in order to experience its psychic effects, and sometimes to avoid the discomfort of its absence. Tolerance may or may not be present. A person may be dependent on more than one drug.

Physical Dependence Capacity (P.D.C.). The ability of a drug to act as a substitute for another upon which an organism has been made physically dependent, i.e. to suppress abstinence phenomenon which would otherwise develop after abrupt withdrawal of the original dependence-producing drug.

Drug Control. National law or international agreement governing and restricting production, movement and use of a drug to medical and scientific needs in the interests of public health and for the prevention of drug abuse.

Methods of evaluation of the dependence liability included evidence concerning the presence and degree of psychic dependence drawn mainly from case histories, subjective statements and general observations, but it was suggested that more reliable evidence may be obtained from a controlled, double-blind quantitative procedure for the measurement of subjective effects and behavioural responses. Studies of patients with illness requiring continued medication with or without persistent pain, those with terminal illness, especially of a painful character, and persons who are already drug dependent and who have been incarcerated for law violation were referred to. The use of adjective check lists or some form of questionnaire to assess subjective reactions was referred to, particularly the work of the Addiction Research Center (U.S.A.), which had developed the Addiction Research Center Inventory (A.R.C.I.) which consists of 550 questions or items answerable by "Yes" or "No" (Haertzen *et al.*, 1963).

Studies in several centres employing electroencephalographic techniques in order to assess dependence liability were reported in the WHO Sixteenth Report as were studies relating to the effect of dependence-producing drugs on central nervous system transmitter systems. Studies depending on technical arrangements which give an animal the opportunity to self-administer a drug such as the bar press method developed by Seevers and his co-workers were particularly helpful in suggesting dependence-producing liability of drugs but still not conclusive evidence of the possibility of man developing psychic dependence on a new agent (Deneau *et al.*, 1964).

Physical dependence

Methods are available for the study of drug dependence of morphine and barbiturate type in animals and in man (Halbach and Eddy, 1963; WHO, 1964).

Criteria for determining the need for drug control

In a consideration of the criteria for determining the need for control, the Sixteenth Report of the WHO (1969) suggests that there are two main conditions, at least one of which must exist for a drug to be considered in need of control:

1. The drug is known to be abused other than sporadically or in a local area and the effects of its abuse extend beyond the drug taker; in addition, its mode of spread involves communication between existing and potential drug takers, and illicit traffic in it is developing.
2. It is planned to use the drug in medicine and experimental data show that there is a significant psychic or physical dependence liability; the drug is commercially available or may become so.

If neither of these conditions is fulfilled, there is no need for an agent to come under consideration for control.

Drugs already in Use

Where a drug is already in use the World Health Organization (1969) suggested that the decision on the need for control must be based upon evaluation of the risk; this may lead to a recommendation for control at the national or international level, depending upon the interpretation of "local area", seriousness of adverse effects, degree of communicability, and the extent of illicit traffic.

At a practical level, mobile emergency teams trained in many disciplines, such as sociology, psychology, epidemiology, psychiatry, etc., would have an important part to play in assessing the relevant facts, the epidemic risk, and the possible methods of spread.

In the following account of other aspects of drug addiction and drug dependence no individual who is dependent upon a therapeutic dose of a drug, who does not attempt to obtain it by any means, and who does not escalate the size of the dose will be considered as being included under the heading of drug dependence or addiction. Thus, the tired housewife who takes two Drinamyl a day year after year and keeps to this dose will not be included in the general consideration of amphetamine dependence.

The Growth of Drug Dependence in the United Kingdom

The history of the development of drug dependence in the United Kingdom has recently been clarified by a paper on the growth of heroin addiction (Spear, 1969). The annual figures for heroin addicts known to the Home Office had remained remarkably constant for many years up to 1959 when the total number of known heroin addicts was 68. In 1960, however, the figure had risen to 94 and the situation rapidly worsened following this. However, after the war there was a considerable increase in cannabis use, particularly amongst the coloured seamen of the East End and the clubs frequented by Negro theatrical performers and others in the West End of London. By 1950 it was clear that the traffic in cannabis was now of much greater importance in the United Kingdom than the traffic in opium and the figures of the total numbers of persons prosecuted for offences involving cannabis had risen steadily. Although the use of this drug continued to be linked mainly with the coloured populations the year 1950 saw the first evidence that, unlike opium, cannabis was a drug which was being used by our own indigenous population. Spear (1969) describes the activities of a hospital employee whom he names "Mark" who was sentenced to a term of imprisonment in April 1951 and who had broken into a hospital dispensary and taken considerable quantities of heroin, morphine and cocaine. The removal of "Mark" from the scene resulted in the appearance of a number of new heroin addicts and it was considered that some 63 individuals were connected either directly or indirectly with the activities of "Mark"! Spear notes that the evidence from events themselves and the testimony of those involved in them suggested that until "Mark" appeared on the scene there was little or no heroin circulating in the West End of London but that his appearance coincided with the scarcity of cannabis with the result that many persons may have changed from cannabis smoking to the use of heroin and cocaine.

The situation in relation to drug addiction was explored by the Brain Committee which was convened in 1958, and their first report (Interdepartmental Committee, 1961) noted that the problem was small, static and that no special measures needed to be taken. It emphasized, among other points, that the problem was a medical one rather than a form of criminal behaviour; that satisfactory treatment was only possible in suitable institutions but that compulsory committal was undesirable; that the problem was too small to warrant the establishment of specialist institutions exclusive to the treatment of drug addiction; that a system of registration of addicts would not be desirable or helpful—and that further statutory powers to control new analgesic drugs were not needed at present. It also noted that the situation regarding drugs affecting the central nervous system which are potentially habit-forming required watching but that no further statutory control was required.

However, this Committee was reconvened in July 1964 because of an increase in the problem (see Fig. 16.1).

ADDICTS INDEXED BY THE HOME
OFFICE

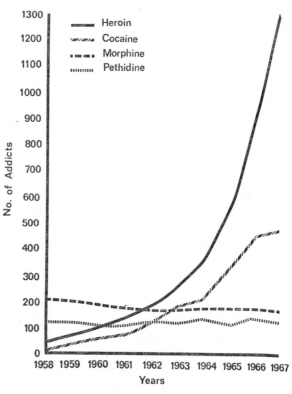

FIG. 16.1

It will be seen that in July 1964 there was a clear increase in heroin and cocaine addiction and the problem was achieving rapid increase which, if unchecked, would lead to very serious proportions.

The findings of the second report (Interdepartmental Report, 1965) noted that a small number of doctors (not more than six) who prescribed these drugs very freely were responsible for the availability of heroin and cocaine.

Paragraph 11 states:

". . . from the evidence before us we have been led to the conclusion that the major source of supply has been the activity of a very few doctors who have prescribed excessively for addicts. Thus we were informed that in 1962 one doctor alone prescribed almost 600,000 tablets of heroin (i.e. 6 kilograms) for addicts. The same doctor, on one occasion, prescribed 900 tablets of heroin (9 grams) to one addict and, three days later, prescribed for the same patient another 600 tablets (i.e. 6 grams) "to replace pills lost in an accident". Further prescriptions of 720 (i.e. 7·2 grams) and 840 (i.e. 8·4 grams) tablets followed later to the same patient. Two doctors each issued a single prescription for 1000 tablets (i.e. 10 grams). These are only the more startling examples. We heard of other instances of prescriptions for considerable, if less spectacular, quantities of dangerous drugs over a long period of time. Supplies on such a scale can easily provide the surplus that will attract new recruits to the ranks of the addicts."

The sweeping recommendations of the Brain Committee were made not only because of the rapid increase of abuse of these drugs but because it was quite clear that informal methods of controlling doctors who were prescribing dangerous drugs freely were ineffective. The Second Report also stresses the Committee's anxiety about the use by young people of amphetamines, amphetamine barbiturate mixtures and other drugs, and recommended that a Standing Advisory Committee be set up to keep a close watch on developments.

The march of events in relation to the increase of drug taking appears to have been the development of a sociocultural pattern of behaviour springing up in the adolescent population (Connell, 1964, 1965a, b, 1966, 1970) which involved young people staying out at weekends, going to the Soho area of London and taking amphetamines or amphetamine barbiturate mixtures to keep awake. Some of these, probably a small proportion, became dependent on the drug and some found their way to psychiatric clinics. The presence of a fringe group of small numbers of prostitutes, transvestites, homosexuals and heroin and cocaine users was noted (Sharpley, 1964; Connell, 1964, 1968) in the same coffee bars and clubs and this might be one factor explaining why the attitude to drug taking in this young population changed from that of regarding taking hard drugs as "mad" or "nutty", "stupid" and "taboo", to a more accepting attitude towards involvement with hard drugs and intravenous use of drugs. As time went on there was a spread from the West End to outlying districts of London and to other towns, particularly the coastal resorts in the south of England. Spread throughout the country did not take place at the same rate. Studies of heroin use in a new town (Alarcon and Rathod, 1968) and in a provincial town (Kosviner *et al.*, 1968) showed that the population using this drug were different in many respects.

The mode of spread of heroin abuse in Crawley has been described (Alarcon, 1969). The chain of transmission from one subject to another, relating to 58 young people, is described. It is interesting that they do not

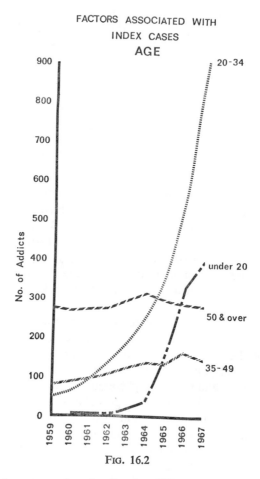

FACTORS ASSOCIATED WITH
INDEX CASES
AGE

Fɪɢ. 16.2

appear to have been turned on by "pushers" from London and other towns but by local boys who had acquired the habit whilst visiting or living in another town. These then spread the habit amongst their peers. In all cases between the initiators and the initiated there had been long-standing or current links of common school and neighbourhood, or common haunts of amusement. Heroin users from nearby towns who visited Crawley and accompanied Crawley boys on trips to London and seaside resorts also provided further mutual inter-reactions.

The age distribution up to and including 1967 is shown by Fig. 16.2 which demonstrates that it was the younger population which was becoming involved and drawing attention to the fact that since 1963 there has been a large increase in the younger individuals under 20 taking heroin.

The age and sex distribution in 1966 heroin cases is shown by Fig. 16.3 and the preponderance of males has continued since.

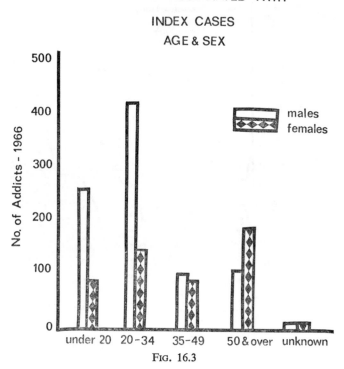

FACTORS ASSOCIATED WITH

INDEX CASES

AGE & SEX

Fig. 16.3

The convictions for offences against the drug laws including the Drugs (Prevention of Misuse) Act, 1964, is shown on a log scale by Fig. 16.4 and demonstrates the very serious increase in convictions for offences against cannabis, manufactured drugs, and drugs such as amphetamines.

Drug Dependence in Other Countries

The problem of heroin addiction has for many years been of major concern in the United States of America and Puerto Rico. Estimates as to the numbers of heroin addicts in the United States vary, some authorities suggesting that there are 50,000 in New York alone, whilst others suggest that there are 100,000 in that city. Heroin is a banned drug not used in clinical practice so that supplies are only available from illicit sources. Bags of "junk" are sold and contain varying amounts of heroin adulterated with lactose, caffeine, or other substances. Few American addicts are now taking more than 1 grain to $1\frac{1}{2}$ grains of heroin a day. Opium and morphine abuse have been the concern in Singapore and Hong Kong for many years.

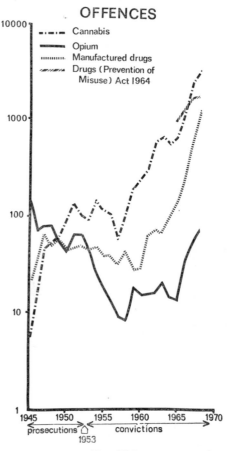

FIG. 16.4

In 1956 Professor Massaki submitted a report to the World Health Organization Expert Committee on Drugs liable to produce Addiction (WHO, 1957) noting that there was widespread abuse of amphetamines and that in the city of Kurume about 1·1 per cent of the whole population and about 5 per cent of the 16 to 25-year-old population were amphetamine addicts. In May and June 1954, 10,148 persons were taken into custody because of offences against the Awakening Drug Control law (amphetamines were known as Wake-amines). Of these, 52 per cent were found to be addicts.

The total number of misusers of amphetamines in Japan in June 1954 was estimated at between 500,000 and 600,000, of whom half were considered to be addicts. Out of 60 murder cases in Japan during May and June 1954, 30 convicted murderers had some connection with amphetamine misuse.

This problem appears to have sprung up after the war when there were considerable supplies of amphetamines, mainly methamphetamine, and the common route was to take the drug intravenously. Illegal manufacture of this drug developed and considerable changes in the laws relating to amphetamines were required. A recent paper (Nagahama, 1968) notes that at the peak there were one million amphetamine addicts, and now with a combination of stricter laws to ban the drug and their precursors, more severe penalties, setting up of treatment facilities in mental hospitals to which addicts could be admitted against their will, and the creation of general headquarters for campaign against amphetamine abuse as well as local campaigns had produced the beneficial disappearance of this problem. This approach would appear to be a truly comprehensive one and represents an immense investment of money, personnel, hospital facilities and so on. Details are not given in this short chapter and there is no follow-up of amphetamine-dependent individuals, or any comment as to whether they have, for instance, turned to barbiturates. More recently, however, a serious problem of glue and other vapour sniffing has beset Japan and estimates suggest that there may be 30,000 young people misusing these substances. Deaths occur since plastic bags are placed over the head in which to sniff the vapour, and if unconsciousness develops suffocation by the bag can occur.

In Sweden a serious problem has sprung up relating to the misuse of phenmetrazine (Preludin). This has been used by young people intravenously and there may well be as many as 10,000 such persons in Stockholm alone. The characteristics of this problem have been described (Goldberg, 1968). Even in Czechoslovakia there has been a problem with phenmetrazine (Vondracek et al., 1968).

More recently there has been a small epidemic of diethylpropion abuse in Sweden (Allmark and Rylander, 1968). It is important in considering experiences of different countries to recognize that it is unwise to extrapolate the experiences of one country to another. For instance, methods of treatment of heroin addiction appropriate in the United States of America are not necessarily appropriate elsewhere because of the differences in individual groups, differing sociocultural pressures in the realms of law enforcement, punishments etc., which vary widely from those existing, for instance, in Great Britain. Furthermore, even the two major programmes (Methadone Maintenance, Drug Free Hostels) are still only dealing with a small proportion of the heroin addicts the majority of whom have to continue to obtain heroin illicitly and to obtain the money to maintain their 'habit'.

The Personality of the Drug-dependent Individual

Many attempts have been made to search for and define the personality of the addict, but with disappointing results. These attempts have largely included statements based upon subjective assessments and uncontrolled clinical interviews. Attempts have, however, been made to define typologies on the basis of standard tests. Osnos and Laskowitz (1966) considered the following characteristics to be of importance:

1. Inadequate control of impulses.
2. Avoidance of stress and tensions.
3. An intense desire for immediate and effortless gratifications.
4. A disturbed relationship to authority manifest by either total resistance or submission to external direction.
5. Persistent exploitive behaviour.

Other authors stress in psychoanalytical terms the addict's relationship with his mother, and a weak and immature ego which becomes, in the face of tension or depression, threatened by disintegration. Astin (1959) factor analysed the responses of 250 male addicts on the Minnesota Multiphasic Personality Inventory and found that persons with identical scores on one scale could present very different clinical pictures. Other studies using the Wechsler IQ tests, educational tests and the Rorschach gave the general impression of the addict as an individual who displays immature, labile emotional reactions and has a low frustration tolerance. Difficulties seem to be repressed and withdrawal into fantasy seems a characteristic response.

Chein et al. (1964) note that "as far as psychiatric classification goes there is no single type or syndrome of maladjustment specific to the adolescent opiate addict". In a comprehensive study of personality in terms of ego pathology these authors claim to be able to predict factors in the addict's family background which would be conducive to such psychopathology. Particular traits considered typical included unresponsiveness, flattened affect, frustration, intolerance, lack of realistic orientation, lack of purpose, deficiency in healthy self-regard, inability to form close warm relationships, problems of identity and in particular of sexual identity, general inadequacy and so on. These authors also put forward a typology which is as yet untested.

A recent and perhaps more promising approach to the problem of typologies is that of Brotman et al. (1965). This approach is predominately sociological and the concept of "life-style adaptation" was chosen in an attempt to relate the behaviour of the addicts to social and cultural context within which that behaviour must take place and be responsive. The life-style was "the degree of an addict's involvement in conventional and in criminal areas of life". It was found possible to classify patients pre-hospitalization life-style as being one of four main types.

Suffice it to say that in this very difficult area there are very few definitive statements which can be made at the present time. Perhaps one can fairly say that those who become dependent on drugs are likely to be suffering from personality disorders, and that some of these will be akin to psychopathic states. There seems to be no direct correlation between drug addiction and intelligence, and extrapolation of findings from one culture to another is hazardous.

Finally, it is probably wise to say that it should not be assumed that all drug addicts show signs of personality disorder before they become addicted to drugs. This is particularly relevant when one is considering the young adolescent population who are at a period of adjustment which can sometimes be regarded as "normal maladjustment" and who have not yet developed their clear personality structure and identity. In this group one must accept that the risks of becoming dependent on drugs are much higher than at any other time of life, since anxieties, sensitivities, mood swings, depression and stresses and strains are operating at a considerable intensity on individuals who have not yet learned adequately to deal with them and are at risk of adopting drug use as a panacea for these problems.

Drug Dependence and Crime

Criminal activities as a means of obtaining money for drugs are well known. Removing those drug-seeking crimes from consideration, the position is not so clear, as Chein *et al.* (1964) have noted. A study of remand home amphetamine users in London by Scott and Willcox (1965), who compared them with control groups who had been shown not to be taking amphetamines (they had negative urines for amphetamines) and also with a control group of young persons admitted to the remand home in 1949 before drug taking became prevalent, failed to demonstrate any correlations between the drug taking and frequency and types of crime, family and social backgrounds, ethnic groups and many other factors. These authors also state, "While amphetamine can be a drug of addiction, in the great majority even of this very selected sample which may be assumed to include the most serious problems of delinquency, the taking of amphetamine appears to be incidental to delinquency, probably having similar roots in opportunity and predisposition. No more definite conclusion will be possible until the drug-taking habits of non-delinquent adolescents are known, and this will be a matter of great difficulty."

Nevertheless, it is noted in Sweden (Goldberg, 1968) that the delinquent population there tend to go for drugs, and this may be a manifestation of their delinquency rather than a cause.

It seems unlikely that drug abuse will be involved in the production of criminal activities except in the following situations:

(*a*) Criminal activities which are directly associated with the need to obtain the drug to maintain equilibrium. This includes not only offences but also such activities as breaking into pharmacies, etc.

(*b*) Offences involving the effect of a drug in allowing a trait of character to manifest itself because of the effects of the drug either on dis-inhibiting this trait or on encouraging directly the manifestation of the trait. This, of course, is well known in the case of alcohol, but recent experience with intravenous Methedrine abuse has suggested that aggressive activity is facilitated by the use of this drug in this way.

(*c*) Criminal activities consequent upon the effects of the drug on menta-tion. This would include activities based upon the development of delusions or hallucinations caused by the drug (such as amphetamine psychosis) in which the individual may firmly believe that he is being chased by the police; that his friends are really enemies and are about to attack him and do him harm.

(*d*) Offences directly related to other aspects of the drugs effect such as diminished neuromuscular skill, incoordination, ataxia, etc. This would therefore include traffic accidents and the like.

It is likely that the same criteria in relation to "responsibility" and "intent" will apply in due course, and after the courts have established case law to such drugs as amphetamines, LSD and others as now apply to alcohol. In this respect a case of murder committed under the influence of LSD was dealt with by the Court and the accused was found guilty of manslaughter. This verdict was upheld on appeal (*The Times*, 1969).

The Risk of Drug Dependence

In the section on personality, reference has already been made to the fact that drug addicts tend to have personality disorders of varying types including those sometimes labelled psychopathic disorders. Reference has also been made to the particular vulnerability of the adolescent in relation to developing drug dependence when introduced to drugs at a period of life development which is usually accompanied by anxieties, depressions, challenges, stresses; the facing of which, and the solution of which, contribute to the production of the adult personality pattern.

Those at risk, therefore, of developing drug dependence are likely to be those disturbed or maladjusted children who usually show exaggerated problems of adolescence if their disturbance is not dealt with before then, and would number, according to different surveys, between 5 to 10 per cent of our child population or more. There has, however, been no study of the incidence of drug dependence in adolescence for a number of reasons which will be clear in the discussion of the diagnosis of this problem. The development of a cyclothymic personality which begins to show itself in adolescence is particularly relevant here. Might it be, for instance, that an adolescent developing this form of normal personality might find that the use of drugs relieves the short-lived depressive swings and thus may become dependent on it for such relief? Might some adults also become dependent on this basis?

Examination of adolescent drug users shows amongst the reasons they give for taking the drug a high incidence of social factors such as relief of sensitivity, anxiety in mixing, difficulties in communication and so on.

Certain professions are, of course, at risk in terms of drug dependence. Before the sociocultural pressures of the early 1960s towards drug taking in the younger population it was mainly the professional classes which were involved in drug taking, including doctors, nurses, pharmacists, and others in related activities.

The statement, often made by those who wish to justify the use of certain drugs, that normal people never become dependent upon drugs is, in this writer's opinion, untrue. Normal people may well be at risk in terms of drug dependence when under excessively severe stresses or strains and it should not be forgotten that everyone has his breaking-point. The use of psychoactive drugs in such periods often by prescription from family doctors or others can lead to severe problems of addiction in some instances. In a series of 42 cases manifesting amphetamine psychosis (Connell, 1958) a small number had shown no evidence of instability as measured by the usual criteria of work record, personal relationships and so on when they were prescribed or given amphetamine.

The Diagnosis of Drug Dependence

The difficulty of determining the presence of drug taking, either by sporadic or continuous use, is not generally known. When the intravenous route is used it is relatively easy because of the presence of injection marks in the antecubital fossa or elsewhere. It is also relatively easy to diagnose the use of drugs such as morphine and heroin because of the presence of constricted pupils—an effect of the drugs to which tolerance does not develop. In the case of amphetamines taken orally it may be impossible to tell whether or not the patient is taking the drug. Dilated pupils, raised blood pressure, tachycardia and mild tremor are common in individuals who are seen by a doctor and by those who suffer from anxiety states who are not taking amphetamines. Even persons with long experience of amphetamine addiction using refined techniques of interview may be hood-winked. It is vital to accept the fact that although in every other way the patient may be of unimpeachable honesty he is very unlikely to tell the truth about his drug taking, either in terms of size and frequency of the dose used, or in terms of denying drug taking altogether, or in terms of only mentioning one drug when he is in fact taking several. An essential part, therefore, of the diagnostic process is the determination of the presence of drugs in biological fluids—especially urine—by special methods such as thin layer chromatography and gas liquid chromatography. However, it must not be assumed that one positive result indicates drug dependence. Only serial positives are likely to indicate continuous use and it must be noted that some professed heroin addicts who attended the new special clinics were found, by the use of such serial assessments, to be sporadic and not continuous users and an occasional case was found not to be using it at all. If problems of drug abuse continue to spread it will be necessary to develop laboratory services in order to make use of these objective methods of assessing drug use. Even so, the results are only qualitative and it is not yet possible to extrapolate from either blood levels or urine levels the actual dose of drug taken, but assessment of dose level taken by the addict must remain, at the moment, on the basis of a clinical empirical judgment. When large doses are claimed it is best to assess the reliability of the statement made by the patient by admission to hospital, or by attendance as a day patient and observation for the development of withdrawal symptoms or to observe the effect of taking the claimed dose.

Treatment of Drug Dependence

Treatment of drug dependence can be split up into various phases (Connell, 1966) where the following phases in relation to amphetamine-dependence were defined:

1. Treatment of the withdrawal phase.
2. Treatment of the early abstinence phase.
3. Long-term treatment and/or rehabilitation.

Treatment, of course, cannot take place unless the individual attends for treatment, so that prior to treatment there will need to be referral to an out-patient clinic or centre where the assessment of the intial problems and the optimum methods of treatment as indicated at the time can be formulated. Since the individual is still taking the drug at that period it needs to be borne in mind that evaluations at this time may be inaccurate in that the effects of the drug may be producing a picture difference from the underlying picture which has led to the problem of drug dependence.

Out-patient treatment will be mainly directed towards encouraging patients to accept withdrawal from the drug and to come to terms with the possibility of a life without it. In those cases, particularly of heroin dependence, now that heroin can only be prescribed to addicts in special clinics, an out-patient period during which a maintenance policy is adopted can be envisaged. In this writer's experience withdrawal from drugs on an out-patient basis is only possible in those rare instances where motivation for cure is very high. The vast majority of individuals require to come into hospital which involves removal from stresses and strains which may be contributing to the continuation of drug use, and will require to come to terms with the fact that withdrawal from the drug is only the first stage in treatment.

Once the drug is withdrawn, the early abstinence phase commences and it is not widely enough appreciated that during this phase even though the patient is no longer on the drug the general physiological reactions and psychological reactions may not be normal and may indeed not return to normal for some time.

It is important, therefore, to encourage patients to stay for longer rather than shorter periods in order that they can be as normal as possible before discharge and also to allow of a more penetrating and accurate assessment on which more realistic plans for treatment and rehabilitation can be based.

Rehabilitation will include the complex process of helping to re-establish the ex-drug-dependent person in the community. This requires close liaison between medical and many other social agencies whether they be attached to law-enforcement facilities, voluntary bodies or other social services. It is now generally recognized that whatever the system of medical treatment, inadequate rehabilitation provision is likely to vitiate the earlier efforts of patients, doctors and other staff.

Withdrawal in Hospital

Heroin and other opiates

The most widely used method of withdrawal in hospitals is that of replacing heroin or another opiate directly with methadone, and once withdrawal symptoms are controlled to reduce methadone by 10 mg every 24 hours so that withdrawal is effected in 7–14 days. Wikler (1967) and Blachly (1966) used this method and give the following methadone equivalents:

$$1 \text{ mg methadone} = \begin{array}{l} 3 \text{ mg morphine sulphate} \\ 1 \text{ mg heroin} \\ 20 \text{ mg pethidine} \\ 30 \text{ mg codeine.} \end{array}$$

Blachly (1966) describes abstinence signs in sequential appearance in time after the last dose of narcotics in patients with well-established intravenous use and suggests five grades (0–4). He advises 10 mg methadone given orally when grade 2 signs are present—in other words, when there is an increase of grade 1 signs (yawning, perspiration, lachrymation, rhinorrhea, "yen" sleep) and the development of gooseflesh (pilo-erection), mydriasis, tremors (muscle twitches), hot and cold flushes, aching bones and muscles and anorexia. Should the patient vomit, 10 mg methadone is given parenterally and 20 mg repeated in 12 hours. If debilitating illness is present, a slower withdrawal regime is recommended, withdrawing 5 mg each 24 hours.

Blachly warns that should the patient show severe restlessness, anxiety and insomnia, in the absence of the autonomic symptoms characteristic of opiate abstinence, he may well be dependent on barbiturates as well. In such a case the appropriate barbiturate-withdrawal regime must be instituted. Insomnia is a common and almost universal complaint after the second or third day of withdrawal and Blachly recommends that pentobarbitone 100–200 mg is given at night to combat this. Extra fruit juices and hot soaks in a bath are given if there are muscular cramps. Wikler (1967) also using a methadone withdrawal regime or subcutaneous morphine as a system of rapid withdrawal, emphasizes the need for a slower regime in cases of debilitating disease, active pulmonary tuberculosis or cardiac insufficiency. He advocates the use of codeine in the final stages of withdrawal and the use of aspirin 10 grains (600 mg) if there are aches and pains. Barbiturates 100–200 mg are given at night for insomnia.

Since the average dose of heroin taken by addicts in the United States of America is only of the order of 60 mg (1 grain) it is necessary, in the United Kingdom, to take into account the much higher doses used by some addicts. Bewley (1968) suggests that methadone up to a total of 100 mg in 24 hours or more might be required and the withdrawal takes place over a period of 14 days. He quotes one patient who was said to be taking 1080 mg of heroin daily which was withdrawn by the use of this method in 14 days. Before following the routine of Blachly, the regime Bewley uses in the high dosage cases is modified initially by the use of heroin itself in reducing quantities for the first three days. During this time it is replaced by increasing quantities of methadone, and on the fourth day the methadone withdrawal regime is instituted.

Other methods of withdrawal have been employed using electroconvulsive therapy (Thigpen et al., 1955), diphenoxylate hydrochloride (Lomotil) (Goodman, 1968) and prolonged sleep therapy (Schlomer, 1955; Owens, 1968). Withdrawal under methadone cover remains, however, the most widely used method, whether or not it be supplemented by the use of barbiturates or tranquillizers.

Pethidine. Withdrawal from pethidine should be treated differently from withdrawal of other opiates since substitution of methadone or morphine may lead to excessive sedation. Wikler (1967) suggests that a patient who is dependent on a high dose-level may develop withdrawal fits which may be followed by extreme restlessness, profuse sweating and isolated muscle twitches. The accustomed dose of pethidine may lead to the cycle being repeated. A withdrawal regime using pethidine by intramuscular injection in diminishing doses given three hourly for the first week is therefore suggested.

Barbiturates. The withdrawal regime for chronic barbiturate addicts which is widely used has also been fully worked out at Lexington (Fraser et al., 1953, 1954; Isbell et al., 1950. Blachy (1964) chooses pentobarbitone

(Nembutal) for withdrawal because it has a moderate duration of action and because most addicts use it, or quinalbarbitone (Seconal). He advises against the use of phenobarbitone since its long action prevents flexible manipulation of doses. Gradual withdrawal is necessary, according to these workers, in order to prevent the occurrence of barbiturate withdrawal fits and barbiturate withdrawal psychosis, a psychosis very similar to delirium tremens. Blachly modifies his regime for three groups of patients: those who have normal tolerance, those who are highly tolerant and those with debilitating illness (Blachly, 1964).

James (1962) prefers to withdraw the barbiturate over the space of a few days and control withdrawal symptoms with chlorpromazine or chlordiazepoxide (Librium). He gives phenytoin for the first three weeks before tailing it off. Essig and Carter (1962) found, however, that diphenylhydantoin and selected anticonvulsants were ineffective in suppressing the general depressant withdrawal syndrome in dogs and concluded that they were probably without value in man.

Although gradual withdrawal is the method used nearly everywhere, Wulff (1959) advocates abrupt withdrawal and gives neither hypnotics nor sedatives. However, with the first sign of withdrawal psychosis or the development of more than one fit phenobarbitone is given immediately. A dose of 0·2 g at least three times a day is recommended and this dose is maintained until psychotic symptoms have disappeared, when there is a gradual reduction over ten days in the dose. The rationale of Wulff's approach is partly based on the belief that gradual withdrawal strengthens the patient's belief that he cannot exist without barbiturates so that he resists final withdrawal—and partly because he found that none of his nine cases dependent on long-acting barbiturates developed delirium or seizures. He therefore hypothesizes that intoxicating the patient first with short-acting barbiturate is an added risk which might produce the very withdrawal symptoms the treatment is designed to prevent. This hypothesis remains to be confirmed by further work.

Non-barbiturate hypnotics. Essig (1964) drew attention to the fact that there did not appear to be any controlled trials in man to determine the best method of withdrawal from drugs such as meprobamate, glutethimide, chlordiazepoxide, etc., and suggested that the principles of barbiturate withdrawal were applicable. He noted that convulsions and delirium had been reported on withdrawal in patients dependent on these drugs.

Amphetamines. Abrupt withdrawal of amphetamines has been advocated (Connell, 1958a, 1964). There are no physical withdrawal symptoms which produce physical distress, but sleepiness and depression are a feature of the withdrawal phase. The depression may be severe and associated with definite risk of suicide, thus requiring hospitalization for withdrawal. Amphetamine psychosis, which is a psychosis often indistinguishable from paranoid schizophrenia (Connell, 1958), usually passes within the first day though occasionally it can continue for up to a week. Phenothiazines are useful in combating the severe restlessness and overactivity as well as for controlling fear attendant on paranoid delusions and hallucinations, and the aggression which may be produced by these phenomena. The addition of ammonium chloride to facilitate the excretion of amphetamines in the urine has been advocated (Connell, 1966) and is based upon the findings of Beckett *et al.* (1965).

The post-withdrawal phase. As previously mentioned, it is not generally recognized that even though a patient may have been withdrawn from his drug of dependence his body physiology and psychology may not return to normal for some time. This is particularly so for the opiates. Furthermore, the post-withdrawal phase is often referred to by the patient as normality since the patient considers that "cure" is merely to be withdrawn from the drug. It is important that the patient is warned that being withdrawn from the drug is only one phase of treatment and that it may be some time before it would be advisable to leave hospital after such withdrawal. During the post-withdrawal phase a full examination of the factors which have led to drug dependence must be made and this may well take several weeks. It is only at this time when the patient is no longer under the direct effects of a drug that a truer picture of the total situation, both personal and environmental, can be made. In this phase it may be that an underlying depression is revealed and that this will require treatment by the usual methods. Occasionally it will be found that other forms of psychiatric disorder are present such as anxiety states, obsessive-compulsive states, or even schizophrenia. In the majority of cases, however, the problems which emerge are related to personality development and adjustment of personal relationships and relationships with society and societal controls.

REHABILITATION

It is frequently said that without adequate rehabilitation and all the various services this word implies, previous treatment in hospital or by other methods is likely to be of no avail.

The recent report on Rehabilitation of the Advisory Committee on Drug Dependence in the United Kingdom (1968a) notes "the aims of rehabilitation must be to re-educate the individual to live without drugs and to assume or resume a normal social life". In the recommendations this report states "rehabilitation begins with the first contact with the addict".

This very broad concept of rehabilitation is perhaps too wide since it merely draws attention to the fact that subsequent care may be dependent upon the quality and quantity of data obtained during the first contact with the patient. This assumption can be easily accepted.

Goals of Rehabilitation

Although the ideal goal—namely to withdraw a person from drugs and rehabilitate him so that he is no longer needing to take drugs and is socially adjusted—is certainly one which should be aimed at, it is being increasingly realized that the goal of rehabilitation must be tempered to the particular weaknesses and problems of the addict. In other words, a more limited goal, which is now being aimed at in the United States and other countries, is the maintenance of a heroin addict on methadone with the hope that by the proper use of this drug by mouth the individual will be able to resume his life in the community, will become gainfully employed and socially stable. In the United Kingdom a goal is to maintain heroin addicts on heroin in order to guard against the possibility that heroin addicts who are determined to take heroin would create a black-market criminally-organized supply or the adverse social phenomena which come with it.

A definition of the appropriate goals in any individual case would depend upon the characteristics of the personality of the patient, the reasons why he has embarked upon drug taking, his basic potential and skills, his family background and possibilities of rehabilitation within the family circle and, above all, his motivation. It is a very difficult and probably impossible task to rehabilitate an addict who wishes to continue to take drugs, who has every resolve to start to use them as soon as he is discharged from hospital or prison, and who is quite prepared to obtain them by any means. In this instance, perhaps, one should look at the goals in terms of the needs of society rather than the individual wishes of the addict, and in this case, therefore, the question of compulsory controls to be placed on the addict is relevant. Again it must not be forgotten that there would be no drug addiction if drugs of addiction were not available, and that included in the ideal goal might also be the goal of cutting down the availability of these drugs in society.

Methods of Rehabilitation

(a) General

General methods of rehabilitation will include industrial training, further education (carried out either whilst in hospital, penal institution or on discharge), social support at home, help with obtaining jobs, continuous social care and counselling and referrals to appropriate facilities for medical care for the patient or members of his family. Special attention requires to be paid to the need to refer emotional and nervous problems of children, marital problems between the addict and his partner, for help. These general methods are common to all groups who require social care but there is considerable resistance to including the drug addict, or the ex-drug addict, in the general facilities available for such social care and rehabilitation. The

T

fear of relapse and the fear of the "infectivity" of the addict are such that many services will refuse to help. Thus special facilities have, often to be created for addicts.

(b) Special methods

Methadone maintenance. Recognizing that many addicts are unable to keep free from drugs and some may be better on a drug such as methadone, which can be given once a day, rather than on heroin; methadone has been used in two ways in Canada and the U.S.A. The first way was to replace heroin with methadone either by in-patient transfer or by out-patient substitution from the outset using an equivalent dose or somewhat less dose. The second method was devised by Dole and he entitled it "narcotic blockade" (Dole and Nyswander, 1968).

The first method was described by Paulus (1966) in Vancouver, who noted that the patient "may be maintained on methadone until such time as he or she can either function without a narcotic or other factors warrant discontinuation of medication". ". . . prolonged methadone then provides a stepping stone to a more desirable way of life—less damaging to the addict and to the community." The study of Paulus (1966) showed that more patients on methadone maintenance could work, fewer had to sustain their habits by illegal means and consequently were less likely to be apprehended and convicted. Thus maintenance methadone meant less crime. Jaffe and Zaks (1968) have also shown encouraging results.

The second method—narcotic blockade—used a different principle. Dole (Dole and Nyswander, 1966) noted that psychiatric treatment had consistently failed as a treatment for chronic addiction to heroin. It seemed "reasonable to look for some medication to block the abnormal reactions of addicts to heroin and permit them to live as normal citizens in the community". He proposed certain criteria if the medication were to be of practical value.

1. It must eliminate the euphoric appeal of heroin and the abstinence syndrome that draws addicts back to drug use.
2. It must be sufficiently free from toxic or dysphoric effects for the patient to continue with treatment.
3. It must be orally effective, long-acting, medically safe and compatible with normal performance in work and at school and with responsible behaviour in society.

Patients were admitted to hospital and withdrawn from heroin. Gradually increasing doses of methadone were given until a level was reached at which the administration of heroin in the dose usually taken by the addict failed to produce euphoria. Doses of up to 120 mg a day or even more were sometimes necessary. This method, then, does not merely substitute equivalent or smaller doses of methadone but uses larger doses in an attempt to block the pleasurable actions of an intravenous dose of heroin should the addict be tempted to try this. A recent evaluation (Dole & Nyswander, 1968) noted that of 872 persons who were admitted to the programme between 1963 and 1968 inclusive, 59 per cent were working, 29 per cent although not working were socially acceptable, and only 12 per cent were failures. Reduction in criminality was demonstrated by a 90 per cent reduction in the rate of convictions. About 1000 patients were awaiting entry to the programme which had latterly been including a purely out-patient method of achieving the maintenance dose of methadone which would block the heroin effects. Other workers using this method have also achieved satisfactory results.

Narcotic antagonists. Cyclazocine, a synthetic analgesic related to nalorphine hydrochloride, antagonizes both the central and systemic effects of opiates and has a longer duration of action. Cyclazocine induction in hospital (Freedman *et al.*, 1967) has been employed and a narcotic challenge given in order to assess the suitable dose of cyclazocine. This was found to be of the order of 5 mg daily. Some side-effects were noted, including occasional hallucinations, and there were some withdrawal effects when cyclazocine was stopped. Results, though not at this stage as good as the methadone maintenance method, were encouraging. This drug is not yet available for use in the United Kingdom.

Self-help groups. Self-help groups have been developed mainly in the United States of America, the first of them being Synanon. The aim was to provide a drug-free community in which by a process of socialization and inter-reaction between addicts, personality changes could occur which would lead to permanent rejection of drug taking as a way of life. Holzinger (1965) reported on his experiences as a visiting psychologist for a week. He describes "Synanon sessions" which are held three times a week and were compulsory. Psycho-drama took place once a week, and high school educational and vocational and other help were provided where feasible. The Synanon sessions were devoted in the one and a half hours available, to verbal discussions which involved not only polite discussions but emotionally intense verbal exchanges in which individuals had roles "both as aggressors and aggrieved". The aim, said Holzinger (1965), would seem to be to find out the truth about oneself and to express hostilities and feelings without regard to the sensitivity of others. Physical aggression is not, however, permitted. Holzinger concludes that at Synanon there is a kind of tribal family which re-educates its members and because of the goal-directed life and the possibility of status advance—members have a purpose and develop an intense loyalty towards the Synanon movement. The Synanon sessions although appearing "unmerciful and even sadistic seem to constitute effective guidance and punishment adminstered by a basically loving 'family' ".

Other self-help groups have developed but the biggest programme is the Phoenix House Program in New York.

The Phoenix House Programme. This was based on the work of Dr Effram Ramirez in Puerto Rico, who came to New York to establish the programme. The theoretical assumptions defined by Ramirez (1968) include several concepts such as:

1. that drug addiction is a symptom of personality malformation and aberration;
2. that treatment specially designed to deal with characterological deviations must therefore be developed;
3. that the addict, unless psychotic, is responsible for the consequences of his behaviour;
4. that the role of the therapeutic personnel involved in the process is not the conventional one; and
5. that the treatment for the prevention of addiction cannot be accomplished merely through the rehabilitation of addicts.

There are more than 800 individuals now in Phoenix Houses which, in each house, accommodate about 80 addicts. The addict is required to be drug free before entering the Phoenix House, and this can be done either as an out-patient attending hospital or in an in-patient unit. When the drug has been withdrawn, transfer to the hostel is effected. Addicts in the hostels are required to be free from drugs and honest and non-violent. Group therapy takes place and there are two types of what is called "encounter". The basic one (Rosenthal, 1967) is the "floor encounter". This is specially for newcomers. "Emotional catharsis is the goal and the accuracy of psychological confrontation or interpretation is not important. It is a sort of training group where the newcomer can both loosen up and toughen up psychologically, learn that he can yell or be yelled at without anything happening to him or to anyone. There is no appointed leader. The more advanced encounter is the staff tutorial encounter. Here there is an appointed leader. He controls a group of experienced participants. He commands a powerful force. He can spearhead an attack and harness the energy, insight and experience of the group, bringing it into focus in turn on each participant. The impact is tremendous, participants are also instructed as to the process of the group and individual defences employed."

These self-help groups are highly organized and have built-in punitive systems. It is quite clear that anyone who stays the course, which may last a year or more, has to be highly motivated in order to submit to the training system. One feature of these groups is the use of ex-addicts in staffing, and the increasing employment of such ex-addicts in newly opened hostels which gives, of course, a kind of career for them or a career hope for addicts if they feel they wish to help in this area.

There are no follow-up studies of these addicts and there has been criticism of this lack. However, it would be true to say that if the 800 or so addicts at present living in Phoenix Houses lived at such houses for the rest of their lives one would have a group of drug-free individuals no longer causing depredations to society in terms of criminality, etc.

Criminal commitment programmes. These programmes, which operate in California and New York State, are an attempt to deal with the problem of heroin addiction under a "therapeutic" label. It is doubtful, however, if the addict regards them in any other way than he regards "prison", and if this is so it is unlikely that these programmes will be effective unless they include therapy and rehabilitation which are not available within the prison service. Kramer *et al.* (1968) has concluded "that commitment programmes for addicts can only be considered at this time an interim procedure between totally punitive and evolving non-punitive approaches to the issues of drug dependence, though perhaps they will persist as an alternative for those who are not helped by other programmes".

Behaviour therapy. The observations of behaviour of addicts and its relevance in terms of learning theory have been discussed (Wikler, 1961). Recently, an attempt has been made to create aversion to the syringe and the needle in the hope that this will prevent relapse by causing the addict to inject scoline (Thomson and Rathod, 1968). This method is in its infancy and its effect and practicability remain to be fully assessed. Other methods of desensitivation or deconditioning using electric shocks are soon to be explored.

It is too soon to assess how far these methods, which on theoretical grounds appear to offer hope, are practical and effective.

Leucotomy. Leucotomy is being used in a small number of cases of long-standing addiction and poor prognosis but its place in therapy is still obscure.

Results of Treatment

Follow-up studies of American addicts were reviewed (O'Donnell, 1965) and results are not encouraging. However, the studies lacked refinement and definite conclusions could not be drawn. A more recent study (Vaillant, 1966) of New York addicts who had been admitted to the Lexington Hospital found that compulsory after care of a group of these addicts produced a 67 per cent one year abstinence rate. This was a very encouraging reponse since in groups not subject to compulsory parole or aftercare, one year abstinence rates were of the order of 7–14 per cent. This group, however, was very different from our own United Kingdom addicts and extrapolation would be most unwise.

Furthermore, if one looks at the new methods described above relating to the use of methadone, cyclazocine and self-help groups, one must recognize that it would be most unwise to extrapolate from the American experience to that obtaining here. In the first instance, only a very small proportion of heroin addicts in the U.S.A. can obtain acceptance on any of these programmes. The alternative to these programmes is a life of hustling, crime and other activities which are essential if enough money is to be obtained to buy the heroin which is all provided by organized crime. To take the question of Phoenix House and look at the British scene, it must be stated that an attempt is being made in a hostel just opening in Lewisham (London) to put into practice some of the American Phoenix House experience. However, the regime is an authoritarian one with punitive aspects for non-conformity and it is somewhat doubtful whether the British populations of young addicts who can maintain themselves on National Assistance or on money from their parents and who can obtain heroin free on the Health Service, will find themselves able to submit to this kind of regime. Modifications of such an approach to suit the British population may have to be worked out.

Similarly, the use of methadone in this country which is being employed by some of the special treatment clinics is subject to different environmental factors in this country. It is an unfortunate fact that there are some general practitioners who, as in the case of heroin addiction, are prescribing methadone to addicts too liberally and we are now seeing an increasing number of young persons dependent on methadone who have never taken heroin. The special drug dependence clinic's use of methadone requires close evaluation since some of the methadone available in the black market comes from these clinics.

Further difficulties in assessing the results of treatment are presented by the fact that in this country the problem is a recent one and involves young persons, and in the United States by the fact that the problem is no longer limited to the deprived ghetto, Negro and Puerto Rican and Mexican populations. Increasing numbers of young persons from all social classes are now becoming involved in drug taking in America so that the population of addicts is changing. Thus comparison of success rates using different methods is unreliable unless the age and social background and other features of the addict are taken into account in making follow-up assessments.

The very weak and often absent motivation of the British addict is of particular concern and raises the question of whether or not compulsory powers should be taken to treat these people. To admit an individual who is dependent upon drugs to hospital against his will and against his wishes in so far as he still wants to remain on drugs, would seem to be putting the clock back because it is compulsorily detaining an individual in hospital when treatment is very unlikely to be of any avail.

Incarceration of mental patients in asylums in the old days was common, but all the developments of the past decade have been in terms of free access to hospital, voluntary treatment and avoiding compulsory detention except for those who, because of their illness, are so disturbed that they require hospitalization for treatment. In nearly all cases the compulsory element can be lifted within a short period of time. It would seem, therefore, a retrograde step to use compulsion in the case of an unwilling and unmotivated addict. Certainly such compulsion would require maximum security units which hospitals would be reluctant to run. Conversely, placement of addicts who are unmotivated in penal institutions has not been shown to be effective in the United States, but perhaps the detention is simply for the protection of society recognizing that because of crimes or for other reasons society cannot accept these people in its midst. The debate about the use of compulsory powers in this difficult area of drug dependence will continue and it may well be that special powers under the ambit of the Mental Health Act (1959) will be provided. If this were so, it is doubtful whether many addicts would be considered suitable to be dealt with under such powers.

Drug Dependence and Doctors

Doctors are in a particularly vulnerable position in relation to the field of drug dependence. This position has two limbs: (a) the responsibility of the doctor in avoiding producing drug dependence in his patients, and (b) the particular hazard to the individual doctor who can prescribe drugs for himself, in avoiding becoming dependent upon drugs.

In the latter context, before the development of drug taking in young people around 1960–63, the numbers of heroin addicts and addicts to other narcotic drugs was remarkably constant and included a considerable proportion of doctors and also patients who had been placed on these drugs legitimately and who had found themselves unable to give the drugs up after the resolution of their organic disorder. The numbers of the latter, the so-called therapeutic addicts, has remained remarkably constant also.

A study of 120 patients treated on account of drug addiction from 1949 to 1960 inclusive (Clarke, 1962 and 1965) noted that 65 belonged either to the medical or nursing professions. Findings on the latter were presented in detail. Fifteen were discarded because of inadequate follow-up data though there was no significant differences in many of the variables recorded such as age, sex, duration of addiction, etc.

The follow-up results of the 50 cases showed that 34 were male and 16 female, age at admission 24–64, with an average period of consumption of drugs four years prior to entering hospital.

Twenty-eight patients were addicted to drugs covered by the Dangerous Drugs Acts, 60 per cent were in general practice, 20 per cent in hospital practice and 20 per cent in the nursing profession. Morphine and pethidine were the commonest drugs used in this group whilst amphetamines and barbiturates were the commonest used in those addicted to drugs not covered by the Dangerous Drugs Act. A significantly higher proportion of the narcotic users commenced because of persistent physical pain whereas a higher proportion of the non-D.D.A. group regarded psychiatric illness as the cause of their addiction.

The follow-up was from 2 to 12 years and on assessment only four (14 per cent) had remained off drugs continuously since discharge, seven (25 per cent) had taken drugs continuously since discharge and 17 (61 per cent) had taken drugs at intervals since discharge. However, those addicted to non-D.D.A. drugs did rather better; 45·5 per cent remaining off drugs continuously since discharge; 45·5 per cent taking drugs at intervals and 9 per cent taking drugs continuously since discharge.

In terms of working capacity and employability, Clarke (1962) noted that of the 50 patients, 15 had successfully overcome their addiction and returned to their previous employment, but 13 other patients had remained apparently unemployable since discharge from hospital.

The problem of prescribing psycho-active drugs to patients is a difficult one. Prescribing habits differ very widely, and in 1958, 5·6 million prescriptions for amphetamines were issued. The Brain Committee (Interdepartmental Committee, 1961) noted this fact and also claimed that addiction to amphetamines was low.

The basic requirements relating to the responsibility of a doctor in prescribing psycho-active drugs have been stated (Connell, 1968). The responsibility includes proper security measures over drugs and prescriptions and requires that the drug is used sensibly for particular purposes and that full supervision of the patient is provided. Repeating prescriptions for these potent drugs *ad lib* without seeing the patient and continuing for years would seem to be irresponsible. Avoidance of prescribing drugs of this nature to unstable personalities would also seem to be important. These remarks do not apply only to family doctors but also to physicians and surgeons who, not keeping abreast of such problems as drug dependence, sometimes use psycho-active drugs in post-operative conditions or subsequent to severe medical illness in an unwise way.

Finally, doctors have a particular responsibility in relation to the Acts govening control of drugs.

The Dangerous Drugs Act, 1967, requires " . . . any medical practitioner who attends a person who he considers, or has *reasonable grounds to suspect*, is addicted (within the meaning of the regulations) to drugs of any description, to furnish, to such authority as may be specified by the regulations, such particulars with respect to that person as may be so specified".

This requirement for notification notes in the regulation "that a person shall be regarded as addicted to a drug only if as a result of repreated administration he has become so dependent upon the drug that he has an overpowering desire for the administration of it to be continued".

Drug in this context means "any substance for the time being specified in Part I of the Schedule to the Dangerous Drugs Act, 1965". Notification therefore is required from any doctor who attends a patient who is taking any of the large number of drugs covered and this includes not only heroin and cocaine but also a large number of other drugs such as dextromoramide, pethidine, methadone, etc. This fact is not widely enough known amongst medical practitioners who may well find themselves infringing the regulations. The other particular limb of the 1967 Act is the prohibition on a medical practitioner "from administering, supplying, and authorizing the administration and supply to persons so addicted, and from prescribing to such persons such drugs as may be so specified except under the authority and in accordance with the conditions of a licence issued by the Secretary of State in pursuance of the regulations". The regulations restrict this prohibition at the present time to the drugs heroin and cocaine but could be amended without another Act to include other drugs covered in Part I of the Schedule to the Dangerous Drugs Act, 1965.

The problem of dealing with the small number of irresponsible doctors who prescribe dangerous and psycho-active drugs irresponsibly still eludes a satisfactory solution. It is quite clear, however, that in the present socio-cultural climate in our young population an irresponsible doctor can, in a few months, create a serious epidemic of drug abuse by irresponsible prescribing. This was particularly evident when the epidemic of intravenous Methedrine taking developed at the end of 1967 and which came to a sudden stop in 1968 when, by the voluntary agreement of the medical profession, the pharmaceutical industry, and the Department of Health and Social Security, etc., preparations of Methedrine for parenteral use were withdrawn from retail distribution and only available for use within the hospital service.

The Philosophy of some Drug Prescribing

A recent review of the use of amphetamines (Connell, 1968) has suggested that the medical use of these drugs is now confined to a small number of conditions. The report of the British Medical Association Working Party on Amphetamines came to the same conclusion and in some countries amphetamines are banned. Opinions are hardening against the use of these drugs partly, therefore, on the basis that for specific clinical syndromes in which they have been used widely in the past there is little evidence to suggest that they are effective, but more importantly because of the anxieties about amphetamine dependence and in particular the danger to young people.

This raises a number of issues which could be regarded in a philosophical context. In the first instance, the data relating to the effectiveness of these drugs is provided by studies of specific clinical syndromes. Studies at depth of individuals taking the drug through legitimate medical channels in relation to what they themselves consider they need the drug for, and studies at depth into the proportion who are dependent on the drug, using the definition of the World Health Organization which requires a tendency to increase the dose, etc., are lacking.

The two main groups of amphetamine-dependent individuals have been defined and include the tired housewife or other adult under stress, and the adolescent (Connell, 1968). What is the position in relation to a woman of 46 with four children who, perhaps unwisely, was placed on Drinamyl because of mild depression and tiredness who finds that she cannot manage without her three tablets a day but who is able on this dose to be a reasonably effective housewife who can show reasonable affection for her children and her husband and who can cope? This is unlikely to be a placebo effect two years later, and experienced physicians and family doctors know only too well the difficulty of withdrawing such individuals from this drug. What is the position in relation to a tired executive who has a three-day period of intense committee meetings, etc., assuming that he does not have any depression or any other specific disorder which might, theoretically, be an indication for the use of amphetamine? If amphetamines were freely available, would a number of people use them for a short-term period to assist in the emergency in the same way as in war tired pilots and others who were given them to continue their important work? What is the risk of dependence in these people? It would seem that there is going to be a need to examine the philosophy of the use of such drugs under a much closer scrutiny than heretofore. This particular problem is related to, but not identical with, the problem raised by cannabis use which was the subject of a recent report (Advisory Committee on Drug Dependence, 1968).

The Present and the Future

The present situation in relation to drug dependence in this country is one of continuing concern. Although the special clinics set up to deal primarily with heroin and cocaine addiction have been operating for 18 months there have been certain disturbing developments. It would seem that the problem of heroin abuse has been contained and that the rationale on which the clinics were based (Connell, 1969) was realistic in terms of dealing with drugs, the use of which was denied to all except those with a special licence. The socio-cultural pressure to take drugs in the young population continues and patterns of use are now changing. Multiple drug use is becoming common and the use of methadone is increasing for the same reasons that the epidemic of heroin addiction occurred in the early 1960s. It seems likely that even if methadone were placed under the same restriction as heroin this would only give a breathing-space before a similar drug was prescribed irresponsibly. Furthermore, a disturbing feature has been the increasing use of barbiturates intravenously by young persons who cannot get the other drugs they want, with consequent production of abscesses and so on. LSD appears to be used at about the same level and rate as a year ago, but young persons are not appearing at the courts in anything like the numbers for offences involving possession of amphetamines as was the case a year ago. New potent drugs are likely to be discovered and become the subject of abuse.

The future would seem to lie between the production of flexible drug legislation which will allow of control of manufacture, distribution and use of drugs at the level which is necessary for the particular drug—flexible in so far as a drug can be placed under a control measure without the need for new legislation, and upon measures to limit the activities of over-prescribing doctors. The future would seem to rest also on the development of research at all levels from the molecular research of the basic scientist to the pharmacological, clinical, sociological, epidemiological and educational fields which may provide data on which to deal with this complex field which is only partly of medical concern.

Finally, a hope for the future may lie in the fact that adolescent culture patterns change and that perhaps in the not too distant future the growing population of young people will consider drug taking just as "square" as they now consider it "with it".

REFERENCES

ADVISORY COMMITTEE ON DRUG DEPENDENCE REPORT (1968a). *Rehabilitation.* London: H.M.S.O.

ADVISORY COMMITTEE ON DRUG DEPENDENCE REPORT (1968b). *Cannabis.* London: H.M.S.O.

ALARCON, R. DE & RATHOD, N. H. (1968). Prevalence and early detection of heroin abuse. *Brit. med. J.*, **1**, 549.

ALARCON, R. DE (1969). The spread of heroin abuse in a community. *Community Health*, **1**, 155.

ALLMARK, J. & RYLANDER, G. (1968). Annu en form av Narkomani. *Laekartidningen*, **65**, 1530.

ASTIN, A. (1959). A factor study of the MMPI psychopathic deviate scale. *J. Consult. Psycho.*, **23**, 550.

BECKETT, A. H., ROWLAND, M. & TURNER, P. (1965). Influence of urinary pH on excretion of Amphetamine. *Lancet*, **1**, 303.

BEWLEY, T. H. (1968). The diagnosis and management of heroin addiction. *Practitioner*, **200**, 215.

BLACHLY, P. H. (1964). Procedure for withdrawal of barbiturates. *Amer. J. Psychiat.*, **120**, 894.

BLACHLY, P. H. (1966). Management of the opiate abstinence syndrome. *Amer. J. Psychiat.*, **122**, 742.

BROTMAN, R., MEYER, A. S. & FREEDMAN, A. M. (1965). An approach to treating narcotics based on a community mental health diagnosis. *Compreh. Psychiat.*, **6**, 104.

CHEIN, I., GERARD, D. L., LEC, R. S. & ROSENFELD, E. (1964). *The Road to H. Narcotics, Delinquency and Social Policy.* London: Tavistock Publications.

CLARKE, J. A. (1962). The prognosis in drug addiction. *J. ment. Sci.*, **108**, 411.

CLARKE, J. A. (1965). Opiate Addiction. *Proc. Roy. Soc. Med.*, **58**, 412.

CONNELL, P. H. (1958). *Amphetamine Psychosis.* Maudsley Monograph No. 5. London: Oxford University Press.

CONNELL, P. H. (1964). Amphetamine misuse. *Brit. J. Addict.*, **60**, 9.

CONNELL, P. H. (1965a). *The Assessment and Treatment of Adolescent Drug taking with special reference to the amphetamines.* Proc. Leeds Symposium on Behaviour Disorders, 10. Dagenham, London: May & Baker.

CONNELL, P. H. (1965b). Adolescent drug taking.

CONNELL, P. H. (1968). The use and abuse of Amphetamines. *The Practitioner*, **200**, 234.

CONNELL, P. H. (1966). Clinical manifestations and treatment of Amphetamine type of dependence. *J. Amer. med. A.*, **196**, 718.

CONNELL, P. H. (1969). *Drug Dependence in Great Britain—A Challenge to the Practice of Medicine.* In Scientific Basis of Drug Dependence. ed. Hannah Steinberg. London: Churchill.

CONNELL, P. H. (1970). Clinical aspects of drug addiction. *J. Roy. Coll. Phycns.*, *London*, **4**, 254.

DANGEROUS DRUGS ACT (1965). London: H.M.S.O.

DANGEROUS DRUGS (NOTIFICATION OF ADDICTS) REGULATIONS (1968). London: H.M.S.O.

DENEAU, G. A., YANAGITA, T. & SEEVERS, M. H. (1964). Psychogenic dependence to a variety of drugs in the monkey. *Pharmacologist*, **6**, 182.

DOLE, V. P. & NYSWANDER, M.E. (1966). Rehabilitation of heroin addicts after blockade with Methadone. *New York J. Med.*, **66**, 2011.

DOLE, V. P. & NYSWANDER, M. E. (1968). The use of Methadone for narcotic blockade. *Br. J. Addict.*, **63**, 55.

ESSIG, C. F. & CARTER, W. W. (1962). Failure of Diphenylhydantoin in preventing barbiturate withdrawal convulsions in the dog. *Neurology, Minneap.*, **12**, 481.

ESSIG, C. F. (1964). Addiction to non-barbiturate sedative and tranquillizing drugs. *Clin. Pharmac. Ther.*, **5**, 334.

FRASER, H. F. & GRINDER, J. A. (1953). Treatment of drug addiction. *Amer. J. med.*, **14**, 571.

FRASER, H. F., ISBELL, H., EISENMAN, A. J., WIKLER, A. & PESCOS, F. (1954). Chronic barbiturate studies: further studies. *Arch. Internal Med.*, **94**, 34.

FREEDMAN, A. M., FINK, M., SHAROFF, R. & ZAKS, A. (1967). Cyclazocine and Methadone in narcotic addiction. *J. Amer. med. A.*, **202**, 191.

GOLDBERG, L. (1968a). Drug abuse in Sweden. *Bull. Narcot.*, **20**, No. 11.

GOLDBERG, L. (1968b). Drug abuse in Sweden. *Bull. Narcot.*, **20**, No. 29.

GOODMAN, A. L. (1968). Use of Diphenoxylate Hydrochloride in the withdrawal period of narcotic addiction. *J. Southern med. Ass.*, **61**, 313.

HAERTZEN, C. A., HILL, H. E. & BELLEVILLE, R. E. (1963). Development of the Addiction Research Center Inventory (ARCI)—Selection of items that are sensitive to the effects of various drugs. *Psychopharmacologia*, **4**, 155.

HALBACH, H. & EDDY, M. B. (1963). Tests for addiction (chronic intoxication) of morphine type. *Bull. Wld. Hlth. Org.*, **28**, 139.

HOLZINGER, R. (1965). Synanon through the eyes of a visiting psychologist. *Quart. J. Stud. Alcohol.*, **26**, 304.

HONIGFELD, G. (1964). Non-specific factors in treatment. *Dis. nerv. Syst.*, **25**, 145.

INTERDEPARTMENTAL COMMITTEE ON DRUG ADDICTION (The Brain Committee). First Report (1961). London: H.M.S.O. Second Report (1965). London: H.M.S.O.

ISBELL, H., ALTSCHUL, S., KORNETSKY, C. H., EISENMAN, A. J., FLANARY, N. G. & FRASER, H. F. (1950). Chronic barbiturate intoxication. An experimental study. *Archs. Neurol. Psychiat., London*, **64**, 1.

JAFFE, J. H. & ZAKS, M. (1968). *Experience with the use of Methadone.* Proc. First Nat. Conf. on Methadone Treatment, 23. New York: The Rockefeller University.

JAMES, I. P. (1962). The recognition and management of addiction and chronic intoxication with sedative drugs. *Med. J. Aust.*, **49**, 277.

KOSVINER, A., MITCHESON, M. C., MYERS, K., OGBORNE, A., STIMSON, G. V., ZACUNE, J. & EDWARDS, G. (1968). Heroin use in a provincial town. *Lancet*, **1**, 1189.

KRAMER, J. C., BASS, R. C. & BERECOCHEA, J. E. (1968). *Civil Commitment for Addicts: The California Program.* Proc. First Nat. Conf. on Methadone Treatment, 45. New York: The Rockefeller University.

NAGAHAMA, M. (1968). A review of drug abuse and counter measures in Japan since World War II. *Bull. Narcot.*, **20**, 19.

O'DONNELL, J. A. (1965). *The Relapse Rate in Narcotic Addiction: A Critique of Follow-up Studies.* Chap. Narcotics. ed. D. N. Wilmer and G. G. Kassebaum. 226. Univ. California Med. Extension Series. New York: McGraw-Hill.

OSNOS, R. & LASKOWITZ, D. (1966). A counselling center for drug addicts. *Bull. Narcot.*, **18**, No. 4, 31.

OWENS, J., NYMAN, M., HILL, E. D. & STEAD, P. (1968). Nursing the drug addict. *Nursing Times*, **64**, 584.

PAULUS, I. (1966). *A Comparative Study of Longterm and Shortterm withdrawal of Narcotic Addicts voluntarily seeking Comprehensive Treatment.* Vancouver, B.C., Canada: The Narcotic Addiction Foundation of British Columbia.

RAMIREZ, E. (1968). A new program to combat drug addiction in New York City. *Br. J. Addict.*, **63**, 89.

ROSENTHAL, M. S. (1967). *Phoenix Therapeutic Community: An overview.* New York City, N.Y.: Addiction Services Agency.

SCHLOMER, G. M. (1955). *Morphine Withdrawal in Addicts by the Method of Prolonged Sleep.* Chap. Management of Addictions. ed. E. Podolsky. New York: Philosophical Library Inc.

SCOTT, P. D. & WILLCOX, D. R. C. (1965). Delinquence and the Amphetamines. *Brit. J. Psychiat.*, **111**, 865.

SHARPLEY, A. (1964). *Evening Standard* (3–6 Feb., 1 May) London.

SPEAR, H. B. (1969). The growth of heroin addiction in the United Kingdom. *Br. J. Addict.*, **64**, 245.

THIGPEN, F. G., THIGPEN, C. H. & CLECKLEY, H. M. (1955). *Use of Electric-Convulsive Therapy in Morphine, Meperidine and related Alkaloid Addictions.* Chap. Management of Addictions. ed. E. Podolsky, New York: Philosophical Library Inc.

THOMSON, I. G. & RATHOD, N. H. (1968). Aversion therapy for heroin dependents. *Lancet*, **2**, 382.

TIMES, THE (1969). 30 July 1969.

VAILLANT, G. E. (1966). Some characteristics and determinants of abstinence. *Amer. J. Psychiat.*, **123**, 573.

VINAR, O. (1969). Dependence on a placebo: A case report. *Brit. J. Psychiat.*, **115**, 1189.

VONDRACEK, V., PROKUPEK, F., RISCHER, R. & AHRENBERGOVA, M. (1968). Recent patterns of addiction in Czechoslovakia. *Brit. J. Psychiat.*, **114**, 285.

WIKLER, A. (1961). On the nature of addiction and habituation. *Br. J. Addict.*, **57**, 73.

WIKLER, A. (1967). *Personality Disorders III: Sociopathic Type: The Addictions.* Chap. Comprehensive Textbook of Psychiatry. ed. A. M. Freedman and H. I. Kaplan. Baltimore: Williams & Wilkins.

WORLD HEALTH ORGANIZATION (1950). Report of Expert Committee on Addiction-producing Drugs. *Wld. Hlth Org. tech. Rep. Ser.*, **21**, 6.

WORLD HEALTH ORGANIZATION (1957). Report of Expert Committee on Addiction-producing Drugs. *Wld. Hlth. Org. tech. Rep. Ser.*, **116**.

WORLD HEALTH ORGANIZATION (1964). Report of Expert Committee on Addiction-producing Drugs. *Wld. Hlth. Org. tech. Rep. Ser.*, **273**, 13.

WORLD HEALTH ORGANIZATION (1969). Report of Expert Committee on Addiction-producing Drugs. *Wld. Hlth. Org. tech. Rep. Ser.*, **407**, 11.

WULFF, M. H. (1959). The Barbiturate Withdrawal Syndrome. *Electroenceph. clin. Neurophysiol.*, Suppl. 14. Copenhagen: Munksgaard.

17 Diseases of the Respiratory System

TREVOR STRETTON

CLINICAL ASSESSMENT. TESTING PULMONARY FUNCTION.
IMMUNOLOGICAL MECHANISMS IN RESPIRATORY DISEASE.
DIFFUSE AIRWAYS OBSTRUCTION. CHRONIC BRONCHITIS.
EMPHYSEMA. ASTHMA.

IN recent years the emphasis has been on the functional and immunological rather than the structural aspects of respiratory diseases. This is not to diminish the importance of morbid anatomical findings but simply reflects the growth in understanding of the other facets. Accordingly, the present review is selective and follows these recent trends.

Functionally, the lungs may be considered in two parts: the conducting airways, and the parenchyma or region of gaseous exchange between alveolar air and pulmonary capillary blood. Numerically, the most important group of patients with disturbed pulmonary function is that with disease predominantly affecting the conducting air passages and producing the syndrome of diffuse airways obstruction; this group will therefore be given special attention.

CLINICAL ASSESSMENT

The general approach to patients with respiratory disease is well described by Grant in Macleod's *Clinical Examination* (1967), though certain additional points in their clinical assessment deserve mention.

1. The problem of the nature and causation of breathlessness is one of considerable depth and has indeed been the subject of an entire symposium (Howell and Campbell, 1966). It should be recognized that in the intact subject information is continuously available to the central nervous system from a variety of sources regarding the performance and effectiveness of the act of breathing. Such information comes from the lung by the vagus nerve; from position receptors in the costo-vertebral joints and muscle spindles of the chest wall; from peripheral chemoreceptors which are monitoring arterial P_{O_2} and hydrogen ion concentration (and which are also influenced by arterial pressure); and from central chemoreceptive areas in the brain

stem. Integration of this information allows the rhythmic act of breathing to be adjusted so as to effect carbon dioxide elimination and oxygen uptake with a minimal expenditure of energy by the respiratory muscles. Diseases of the respiratory system most commonly produce breathlessness when the effort demanded of the respiratory muscles is increased, because either the airways are narrower (giving rise to an increased resistance) or the lungs or thorax are "stiffer" (less compliant). Alterations in the blood gases or pH appear to be of less importance and even marked disturbances in them apparently fail in some patients to have any effect on the sensation of breathlessness.

Sometimes the degree of a patient's breathlessness is disproportionate to the degree of his lung disease. This may be due to psychogenic factors. Burns and Howell (1969) have described their findings in 31 patients with chronic bronchitis who had disproportionately severe breathlessness of this type. Characteristically, these patients experienced a sudden onset of and rapid deterioration in their breathlessness rather than the insidious onset and gradual deterioration seen in most patients with chronic bronchitis. Marked fluctuation in the severity of symptoms, which might change within a few minutes, was common. Ninety per cent of their patients had attacks of breathlessness at rest; and exertional dyspnoea was not directly proportional to the severity of exercise. Nocturnal episodes of breathlessness were common, occurring in half of the patients. By contrast, waking at night with breathlessness was found by Burns and Howell in only a minority of a control group of chronic bronchitic subjects and those affected had the most severe degree of airways obstruction when tested objectively. It should be emphasized, however, that nocturnal attacks are common in asthmatic individuals and it is well known that left ventricular failure may present in this way. Patients with psychogenic breathlessness causing them to wake at night tended to do so earlier (around 1.30 a.m.) than those with organic causes (around 3 a.m.); although of interest this observation is unlikely to be of diagnostic significance in any given patient.

Many disproportionately breathless patients had symptoms related to acute or chronic hyperventilation. These include paraesthesiae of the extremities or around the mouth, muscle cramps or frank tetany, and disturbed consciousness (usually a feeling of faintness, though frank syncope might occur). Generalized sweating and palpitations were universal symptoms in these patients. Fatigue was described by almost all of them, and pain or discomfort in the chest was almost as common.

The psychological disturbances found in these patients by Burns and Howell were classified as depression in 52 per cent, anxiety in 22 per cent and a hysterical reaction in 26 per cent. The premorbid personality was noted to be obsessional in three-quarters of the depressed patients and all of the group with an anxiety reaction, whilst three-quarters of those classed as hysterical had previously revealed evidence of their psychoneurotic constitution. The most important single stress factor experienced during the three years before the development of the respiratory symptoms was bereavement. Other disturbances or sources of disharmony within the family unit were sometimes held responsible for the onset of breathlessness. In a few instances an iatrogenic factor was implicated: this might simply have amounted to injudicious handling of the patient by his medical adviser on a previous occasion.

On examination most of these patients are seen to be dyspnoeic, especially if observed during exercise; the ascent of a flight of stairs will often reveal distressing shortness of breath. Obvious attacks of hyperventilation are quite common and a disorder in the rhythm of breathing may be apparent. In particular, the patient may breathe for a period of time with the chest obviously held in a position of partial hyperinflation with accessory respiratory muscle activity. This disturbance in the normally orderly pattern of breathing may be readily demonstrated if a spirogram is recorded whilst the patient breathes from a closed-circuit spirometer (Fig. 17.1). At the same time it can be shown that airways obstruction due to coincidental chronic bronchitis is not excessively severe (Forced Expiratory Volume in 1 second greater than 1 litre). Indeed, there may be a normal or near normal vital capacity and F.E.V.$_1$. However, it may require firm persuasion and numerous attempts to secure a reliable reading of the patient's best efforts because their performance of spirometric tests such as the forced vital capacity manœuvre is often poor. Proof of hyperventilation is possible only by estimation of the arterial P_{CO_2}, when other causes of a low P_{CO_2}, such as a metabolic acidosis, should also be excluded.

With careful management and treatment of the underlying psychological disorder the outlook for the depressed patients and those with an anxiety reaction was found by Burns and Howell to be good. However, only a minority of the patients with a hysterical personality improved.

Patients with psychogenic breathlessness, although they may have associated (mild) diffuse airways obstruction, therefore present certain distinctive features and many of these may be recognized at the bedside.

2. During the examination of a patient in whom the history suggests the possibility of diffuse airways obstruction attention should be paid to the following:

(a) Is there evidence of hyperinflation of the lungs? It may be noted here that hyperinflation is not synonymous with the presence of emphysema and should not be interpreted as such; it is a natural consequence of severe expiratory obstruction. Signs of hyperinflation or lung distension include the well-known barrel-shaped chest with an increased anteroposterior diameter, use of the accessory inspiratory muscles, and loss

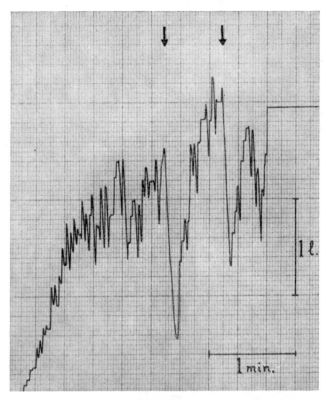

FIG. 17.1

Spirometric recording showing gross disorganization in the pattern of breathing found in a 40-year-old shipwright with mild chronic obstructive bronchitis who suddenly developed breathlessness, thoracic pains and attacks of light-headedness. Arrows indicate times at which he exhaled deeply on instruction; each time he again spontaneously overinflated his lungs. At his first visit to hospital he was found to have a respiratory alkalosis with a P_{CO_2} of 26 mm Hg; on a subsequent occasion the P_{CO_2} was 37 mm Hg. He had difficulty in performing a forced vital capacity and very variable results were obtained; the best results achieved (F.E.V.$_1$ 2·65 litres; vital capacity 4·5 litres) showed that the degree of airways obstruction was not severe. An anxiety state due to circumstances at home and work was found to be responsible for his psychogenic breathlessness.

of hepatic or cardiac dullness on percussion. Lesser known signs (Campbell, 1969) are best elicited with the patient breathing quietly whilst reclining at 45°. Since the sternum is elevated by the over-inflated lungs, less of the trachea is palpable above the sternal notch; normally, three to four finger-breadths of trachea can be palpated, and this may be reduced to zero in patients with severe airways obstruction. Also with each inspiratory effort the trachea tends to be pulled down further into the thorax and this may be detected by resting a fingertip on the most prominent point of the thyroid cartilage; in normal quiet breathing there is no inspiratory tug on the larynx. At the same time it should be noted whether there is inspiratory recession of the supraclavicular and suprasternal fossae.

Normal movement of the ribs may be lost as a result of the alteration in their position due to overdistension of the thorax. It may be recalled that normal rib movements can be resolved into a bucket-handle and a pump-handle action (Campbell, 1958). With the former the transverse diameter of the thorax is increased as the rib is rotated and its lateral extremity elevated about the vertebro-sternal axis. The pump-handle action increases the antero-posterior diameter of the chest as the downward-sloping rib is rotated upwards about the axis of the neck of the rib. In the overdistended thorax the bucket-handle action is lost as the ribs come to lie in a more horizontal position. This can be recognized by careful palpation of one of the upper ribs with the widely spread fingers, when an exaggeration of the pump-handle action may also be apparent. Palpation of the costal margin may reveal that this is pulled inwards during inspiration, probably by the flattened diaphragm, whereas in the normal thorax the action of the diaphragm tends to move the costal margin outwards.

(b) Is there auscultatory evidence of airways obstruction? Rhonchi may sometimes be best heard at the mouth or over the trachea rather than over the lungs. They may occasionally not be heard at all, but this must not be taken to deny the presence of airways obstruction: in the most severe grade there may be insufficient airflow through the narrowed air passages to generate a wheeze. The most useful and direct physical sign of airways obstruction is the demonstration of a prolongation in the forced expiratory time (Lal, Ferguson and Campbell, 1964). To accomplish this the patient is asked to take as deep a breath as possible, and after a momentary pause to blow the air out as fast and as far as he is able through the widely open mouth. The physician listens throughout this manoeuvre with the stethoscope placed over the patient's trachea and notes the time in seconds from the abrupt onset of expiratory airflow to its gradual cessation or until the subject is forced to take another breath. This is the forced expiratory time (F.E.T.) and corresponds approximately to the time taken to deliver a forced vital capacity (F.V.C.). The normal F.E.T. is less than four seconds. Airflow may persist for considerably longer than this in some normal older subjects (Leith and Mead, 1967), but the test is not invalidated as the rate of airflow is then so low as to be inaudible. In patients with airways obstruction the F.E.T. is prolonged to six seconds or more and is quite frequently found to be greater than ten seconds.

REFERENCES

BURNS, B. H. & HOWELL, J. B. L. (1969). Disproportionately severe breathlessness in chronic bronchitis. *Quart. J. Med.*, **38**, 277.

CAMPBELL, E. J. M. (1958). *The Respiratory Muscles and the Mechanics of Breathing.* London: Lloyd-Luke.

CAMPBELL, E. J. M. (1969). Physical signs of diffuse airways obstruction and lung distension. *Thorax*, **24**, 1.

GRANT, I. W. B. (1967). In *Clinical Examination*, p. 177. ed. J. Macleod. Edinburgh: Livingstone.

HOWELL, J. B. L. & CAMPBELL, E. J. M. (eds) (1966). *Breathlessness.* Oxford: Blackwell.

LAL, S., FERGUSON, A. D. & CAMPBELL, E. J. M. (1964). Forced expiratory time: a simple test for airways obstruction. *Brit. med., J.* **1**, 814.

LEITH, D. E. & MEAD, J. (1967). Mechanisms determining residual volume of the lungs in normal subjects. *J. appl. Physiol.*, **23**, 221.

TESTING PULMONARY FUNCTION

In most clinical situations it is possible to test pulmonary function adequately with relatively unsophisticated apparatus. For the analysis of pulmonary and thoracic mechanics a spirometer is required, preferably one which will give a permanent record of the spirogram.

When the vital capacity is recorded (several times to ensure repeatability) the observer should bear in mind factors which limit its magnitude. The limit of inspiration is reached when the inspiratory muscles, of which the diaphragm is the most effective, can no longer achieve an increase in thoracic volume; that is when the elastic recoil of the lungs and thorax is at its maximum. Therefore, the vital capacity will be reduced due to a limitation in the volume of air which can be drawn into the lungs when there is (a) impairment of inspiratory muscle power, as in neurological disorders; (b) a reduction in lung volume due to pulmonary resection; (c) reduced pulmonary distensibility (compliance) due to diffuse parenchymal disease; (d) occupation of intrathoracic space by, for instance, a large pleural effusion; (e) gross disease of the thoracic cage, such as a severe kyphoscoliosis.

As the lung volume diminishes during expiration the air-passages become narrower. This progressively impedes airflow until finally expiratory airflow ceases. Air—the residual volume—is still contained within the lungs at this time and cannot be expelled no matter what force is generated by the expiratory muscles (the most powerful of these being the abdominal muscles), suggesting that certain airways close at the end of deep expiration even in normal subjects.

It follows that diffuse obstruction of the airways by disease will impede expiration more than inspiration, and that the narrowed airways will tend to close during expiration at a higher lung volume than normally. In the presence of severe diffuse airways obstruction progressive overinflation of the lungs develops until ultimately the patient is breathing at a position close to the extreme upper end of his total lung capacity, giving rise to the physical signs previously described. The expiratory airflow obstruction is satisfactorily quantified by measurement of the forced expiratory volume in one second and the ratio of this to the forced vital capacity. The proportion of the F.E.V.$_1$ to the F.V.C. is customarily expressed as a percentage (F.E.V.%) and this is normally greater than about 70 per cent. In patients with severe airways obstruction the F.E.V.$_1$ is less than one litre and may be considerably lower, values of under 0·5 litre being found not infrequently. While the F.E.V.% in patients with airways obstruction is usually greatly reduced, the precise figure is of doubtful value when the degree of airways obstruction is very severe.

The expiratory peak flow rate may be measured as an alternative to the F.E.V.$_1$. This is conveniently done using the Wright peak flow meter (Wright and McKerrow, 1959) which has the great advantage of ease of portability. A patient may therefore measure his own expiratory peak flow rate (P.F.R.) and keep records, several times each day if necessary, of the behaviour of his airways obstruction and its response to treatment. Normal values in adults are from about 300 in females to 400 litres per minute and upwards in males. In extreme cases of airways obstruction patients may be barely able to deflect the needle at all.

When the presence of airways obstruction has been demonstrated by one of these methods the degree of responsiveness to a bronchodilator, usually isoprenaline, should be tested. The possible variability in the time course of a response to different drugs should be noted (Chamberlain, Muir and Kennedy, 1962) so that repeat observations of the F.E.V.$_1$ or P.F.R. may be made at an optimum time; in the case of isoprenaline, which acts rapidly, a five-minute pause after inhalation of the drug is appropriate. Long-term variations in the degree of airways obstruction may also be recorded and the response to drugs such as corticosteroids may be checked. In this way it can be decided whether the patient's airways obstruction is partially or completely reversible either spontaneously or as a result of treatment, or whether it is fixed.

By contrast to the patients who have an obstructive ventilatory defect those with a restrictive defect have no impediment to airflow. In them, spirometry shows simply a diminution in the vital capacity with a normal F.E.V.%, the F.E.V.$_1$ being reduced in proportion to the reduction of the vital capacity. Other clinical features will usually reveal whether a restrictive ventilatory defect is due to diffuse changes in the lung parenchyma leading to a reduction in the lung compliance, or to a large intrathoracic lesion which is encroaching on space available to the lungs, or to disease of the thoracic cage. Where a reduced vital capacity is secondary to neurological or muscular disease the ventilatory defect may be termed hypodynamic.

Scadding (1966) has suggested the use of the following classification of the various syndromes of disordered lung function:

1. *Ventilatory defects*
   (*a*) obstructive; the airways obstruction may be
       (i) reversible
       (ii) fixed
   (*b*) non-obstructive
       (i) restrictive
       (ii) hypodynamic.
2. *Defects of gas exchange.*

As already discussed, ventilatory defects can be separated into the different types by clinical observation, aided by spirometry; and a chest radiograph gives additional information about the state of the lungs, whether they are hyperinflated by airways obstruction or diffusely affected by some parenchymal disorder.

The recognition of defects in gas exchange, however, may require the use of equipment not universally available. Although reliable arterial P_{O_2} measurement cannot always be obtained it is usually possible to measure arterial pH and obtain the P_{CO_2} by the Astrup interpolation technique or to measure it directly with a CO_2 electrode; if not, a rebreathing method should be applied (Campbell and Howell, 1962). Knowledge of the P_{CO_2} and pH is essential to an understanding of problems in gas exchange. Precise knowledge of the state of arterial oxygenation is less important, even though hypoxia is the most common result of defects in gas exchange, some aspects of which will now be discussed.

Ventilation-perfusion inequality. For the efficient transfer of gas from alveoli to blood it is clearly essential to refresh the alveolar gas by ventilation at a rate appropriate for the rate of blood-flow through the pulmonary capillaries. If ventilation is excessive in relationship to the blood-flow through a lung unit, the P_{CO_2} in the alveoli and the capillary blood will fall and the P_{O_2} will rise. In the extreme situation where the ratio of ventilation to perfusion rises to infinity (i.e. alveoli that are ventilated but not perfused), the alveolar gas pressures will approximate to those in ambient room air which has been fully saturated with water vapour at body temperature. At the other extreme, if the ventilation-perfusion ratio falls to zero (i.e. non-ventilated alveoli which are still being perfused), the alveolar gas pressures would come to equal those in the venous blood flowing through the alveolar capillaries and unable to exchange gas; the P_{CO_2} would rise to the level found in mixed-venous blood, normally about 46 mm Hg, and the P_{O_2} would fall to mixed-venous blood levels, normally around 40 mm Hg. Such blood reaching the arterial system would lead to a modest elevation of arterial P_{CO_2} and an appreciable fall in arterial P_{O_2}.

Theoretically, all gradations of ventilation-perfusion ratio between these two extremes may exist in different parts of the lungs, though the overall ratio in normal lungs is approximately unity. In disease, the ventilation of different lung units will be disturbed if there is an alteration in their time-constants. The use of the term "time-constants" assumes that alveolar filling during inspiration follows an exponential curve (Fig. 17.2) so that

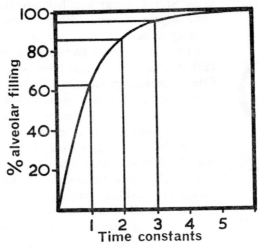

FIG. 17.2

Exponential curve of alveolar filling.

filling will be 63 per cent complete in 1 time-constant, 87 per cent complete in 2 time-constants and 95 per cent complete in 3 time-constants. The time-constant for a functioning lung unit (Fig. 17.3) may be calculated from the equation $T = R \times C$, where T is the time-constant in seconds, R is the resistance and C the compliance of the lung unit concerned. In the case of three lung units arranged in parallel as in Figure 17.4 it will be apparent that the normal unit in the centre will achieve a greater share of the alveolar ventilation than either the stiffer unit with reduced compliance on the left or the obstructed unit with a raised resistance on the right: the time-constant of the unit with low compliance will be shortened and filling will cease whilst the normal unit continues to fill; the obstructed unit will have a prolonged time-constant and it, too, will fail in a limited time to receive the one-third share of alveolar ventilation which each of the three units would get if their time constants were equal.

Disturbances of this kind account for the ventilatory component of alterations in regional ventilation-perfusion ratios due to lung disease. In the situation considered in Figure 17.4 the normal lung unit would be hyperventilated relative to the other units so that it would have a high ventilation-perfusion ratio, and the other two would have a low ventilation-perfusion ratio if the blood-flow to each unit remained equal. Readjustment of the blood-flow may occur, but it is less than perfect: vasoconstriction in vessels leading to the units with a low ventilation-perfusion ratio and a consequent fall in alveolar P_{O_2} will to some extent divert blood away from these units to those with a higher ventilation-perfusion ratio, but some degree of ventilation-perfusion inequality invariably remains.

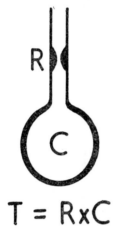

FIG. 17.3

Diagrammatic representation of a functioning lung unit consisting of an airway with resistance R and alveoli with compliance C. The time constant (T) of alveolar filling $= R \times C$.

There are two important consequences of widening of the ventilation-perfusion ratios present in the lungs. One is arterial hypoxaemia. This is due to the contribution of blood from regions with low ventilation-perfusion ratios, and cannot be compensated by increased ventilation in other regions since the P_{O_2} in these regions is already normal and blood flowing from them is fully saturated with oxygen. Any change in arterial P_{CO_2} due to regional ventilation-perfusion imbalance is unlikely to be marked; an increase due to regions with a low ventilation-perfusion ratio is itself not great and may be compensated by increased ventilation in other regions where the P_{CO_2} in alveoli and blood can be appropriately reduced.

The other consequences of ventilation-perfusion imbalance is the effective wastage of ventilation in regions where the ratio is high. The excess ventilation in these regions over and above that needed to arterialize the pulmonary capillary blood flowing through the region is, in effect, dead-space ventilation, and when added to the anatomical dead-space of the upper and lower conducting air passages it constitutes the physiological dead-space. The magnitude of the physiological dead-space, which is normally about 30 per cent of each breath in resting subjects, rises in disease, and patients with severe airways obstruction may have a physiological dead space which amounts to more than 60 per cent of their tidal volume.

A widening of the range of ventilation-perfusion ratios in the lungs constitutes the commonest indication for the administration of oxygen and is also seen in conditions other than lung disease. In shock, and especially after myocardial infarction, ventilation-perfusion inequality occurs for reasons which are not altogether clear. Pure oxygen is not necessary to overcome hypoxaemia due solely to ventilation-perfusion imbalance: 25–40 per cent oxygen is adequate since the aim is only to raise the P_{O_2} in badly ventilated alveoli sufficiently to saturate the blood flowing through them. On account of the shape of the oxygen dissociation curve of blood an alveolar P_{O_2} of 90 mm Hg will practically achieve this.

For those wishing to read a more comprehensive account of the ventilation-perfusion relationships within normal and diseased lungs the monograph by West (1965) is strongly recommended.

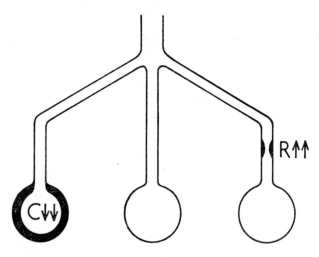

FIG. 17.4

A normal lung unit between two pathological units, the time constants of which are altered by a reduced distensibility (compliance), on the left, and an increased resistance, on the right.

Alveolar hypoventilation. This is characterized by a rise in arterial P_{CO_2} which in conscious healthy subjects is kept between 35 and 45 mm Hg, though it may rise a few mm Hg during sleep. Conversely, if alveolar hyperventilation occurs, the arterial P_{CO_2} will be reduced, since

$$Pa\ CO_2 \propto \frac{\text{metabolic production of } CO_2}{\text{alveolar ventilation}}$$

Alveolar ventilation and minute ventilation volume measured by collection of expired air are of course not synonymous, because of the effect of physiological dead-space. In patients with lung disease the minute ventilation volume may be normal or even increased, yet there can be serious alveolar hypoventilation. Inspection of a patient's breathing may therefore be totally misleading, and measurement of the arterial P_{CO_2} is the only means of establishing whether the level of overall alveolar ventilation is appropriate to the patient's metabolic rate. The qualification "overall" is necessary since within lungs in which there is overall hypoventilation there may still be regions of relative hyperventilation, but these are in effect overwhelmed by the hypoventilated regions.

With alveolar hypoventilation the P_{O_2} falls as the P_{CO_2} rises. If the respiratory exchange ratio (the rate of carbon dioxide elimination divided by the oxygen consumption) were unity then the fall in P_{O_2} would equal the rise in P_{CO_2}. But this is not so; the respiratory exchange ratio is usually about 0·8. This means that more oxygen is removed from the alveoli than carbon dioxide is liberated into them. For this reason the fall in alveolar P_{O_2} is greater than the rise in P_{CO_2}.

The alveolar P_{O_2} may be satisfactorily calculated from the modified alveolar air equation,

$$\text{Alveolar } P_{O_2} = \text{Inspired } P_{O_2} - \frac{P_{CO_2}}{R},$$

where P_{CO_2} is the arterial P_{CO_2} and R is the respiratory exchange ratio. Thus, in a normal subject breathing room air at sea level,

$$\text{Alveolar } P_{O_2} = 150 - \frac{40}{0·8} = 100 \text{ mm Hg.}$$

In a patient whose alveolar ventilation is halved so that his P_{CO_2} is doubled,

$$\text{Alveolar } P_{O_2} = 150 - \frac{80}{0·8} = 50 \text{ mm Hg.}$$

The arterial P_{O_2} of the patient will, however, probably be considerably lower than 50 mm Hg because of the additional effect of regional ventilation-perfusion inequality.

The commonest cause of alveolar hypoventilation is severe diffuse airways obstruction. Ineffective performance of the chest bellows also leads to alveolar hypoventilation, so this condition can be seen in certain non-obstructive ventilatory defects of either the restrictive or hypodynamic variety. The last may be due to lesions in the muscles, nerves, spinal cord or respiratory reticular formation; and the commonest of these seen in general medical wards is that due to serious drug overdosage leading to depression of the reticular formation. Hypoventilation also occurs in severe obesity and may rarely be found in otherwise normal individuals (Fishman, Goldring and Turino, 1966).

Carbon dioxide retention due to hypoventilation produces a respiratory acidosis, though the increase in hydrogen ion concentration (fall in pH) is minimized by the blood buffer systems; if the situation is chronic, the rise in hydrogen ion concentration is then compensated by renal tubular bicarbonate retention. In patients breathing room air a limit to the degree of elevation of the P_{CO_2} which they can sustain is set by the concomitant hypoxia (McNicol and Campbell, 1965). Thus, if the P_{CO_2} were to rise to about 100 mm Hg the alveolar P_{O_2} would be of the order of 25 mm Hg. Arterial P_{O_2} would be lower than this due to the effects of ventilation-perfusion inequality and would therefore be at a level which, if long sustained, is incompatible with life. For this reason such a high P_{CO_2} level is rarely found in patients with alveolar hypoventilation unless they have been breathing oxygen-enriched air. In practice, values greater than 80 mm Hg are uncommon (Refsum, 1963; McNicol and Campbell, 1965; Lal, 1965).

Alveolar hypoventilation is not in itself an indication for oxygen therapy. The aim should be to achieve an increase in the level of alveolar ventilation. Unfortunately this objective is often unattainable and oxygen is therefore usually administered. But this is done at the risk of inducing a further rise in P_{CO_2} by eliminating the hypoxaemic stimulus to breathing; hypoventilation is aggravated, the P_{CO_2} rises further, and carbon dioxide narcosis is liable to ensue. For this reason uncontrolled oxygen therapy must never be permitted in patients with a tendency to hypoventilation.

A reduction in the transfer factor (diffusing capacity) of the lungs. Patients with a restrictive ventilatory defect due to diffuse changes in the lung parenchyma characteristically have a low transfer factor. By the single-breath carbon monoxide method the transfer factor in normal adults is usually 18 ml/min/mm Hg or greater. The restrictive ventilatory defect is due to the low compliance of the stiff lungs. The reduction in the transfer factor is due to an effective loss of surface area available for diffusion of gas and not to a unique thickening of all alveolar-capillary membranes (Finley, Swenson and Comroe, 1962). The older usage of the term "alveolar-capillary block syndrome" is thus inappropriate though firmly established. Localized differences in the degree of thickening of alveolar walls, or interstitial fibrosis, accompanied by regional ventilation-blood flow inequality, therefore probably account for both the reduced transfer factor and hypoxaemia. In this syndrome there is often alveolar hyperventilation at rest; the reasons for this are not entirely clear though it is probably a neurogenic response rather than due to hypoxaemia (Lourenco et al., 1965).

A defect in gas transfer may also be demonstrated in emphysema. Here again it is the result of a reduction in the surface area of alveolar-capillary membrane available for diffusion, in part due to its destruction by the emphysema. A severe obstructive ventilatory defect is usual, though rare instances are encountered where this is not the case.

Respiratory failure. The presence of respiratory failure is implied by the presence of hypoxaemia in the absence of a right to left cardiovascular shunt, or by the presence of hypercapnia. Precise levels of arterial P_{O_2} and P_{CO_2} beyond which respiratory failure may be diagnosed are difficult to define, but for resting individuals living close to sea-level Campbell (1965) suggested the following values: P_{O_2} below 60 mm Hg and a P_{CO_2} above

49 mm Hg. Since hypercapnia is inevitably accompanied by hypoxia, Campbell suggested that respiratory failure could usefully be classified into ventilatory failure (P_{CO_2} high and P_{O_2} low) and hypoxaemic failure (P_{O_2} low with a normal or low P_{CO_2}).

From the foregoing discussion it is clear that ventilatory failure may result from ventilatory defects of obstructive, restrictive, or hypodynamic varieties. Hypoxaemic failure may antecede the onset of ventilatory failure in these conditions; thus asthmatic patients with obstructive ventilatory defects may be severely hypoxic yet continue to maintain an adequate alveolar ventilation (Tai and Read, 1967). The most characteristic examples of "pure" hypoxaemic respiratory failure are those patients with the "alveolar-capillary block syndrome" described earlier.

For a detailed consideration of the physiological, aetiological and therapeutic aspects of respiratory failure the reader is referred to Sykes, McNicol and Campbell (1969).

REFERENCES

CAMPBELL, E. J. M. (1965) Respiratory failure. *Brit. med. J.*, **1**, 1451.

CAMPBELL, E. J. M. & HOWELL, J. B. L. (1962). Rebreathing method for measurement of mixed venous P_{CO_2}. *Brit. med. J.* **2**, 630.

CHAMBERLAIN, D. A., MUIR, D. F. C. & KENNEDY, K. P. (1962). Atropine methonitrate and isoprenaline in bronchial asthma. *Lancet*, **2**, 1019.

FINLEY, T. N., SWENSON, E. W. & COMROE, J. H., Jr. (1962). The cause of arterial hypoxaemia at rest in patients with "alveolar capillary block syndrome". *J. clin. Invest.*, **41**, 618.

FISHMAN, A. P., GOLDRING, R. M. & TURINO, G. M. (1966). General alveolar hypoventilation: a syndrome of respiratory and cardiac failure in patients with normal lungs. *Quart. J. Med.*, **35**, 261.

LAL, S. (1965). Blood gases in respiratory failure: blood gases on admission to hospital and management. *Lancet*, **1**, 339.

LOURENCO, R. V., TURINO, G. M., DAVIDSON, L. A. G. & FISHMAN, A. P. (1965). The regulation of ventilation in diffuse pulmonary fibrosis. *Amer. J. Med.*, **38**, 199.

MCNICOL, M. W. & CAMPBELL, E. J. M. (1965). Severity of respiratory failure: arterial blood-gases in untreated patients. *Lancet*, **1**, 336.

REFSUM, H. E. (1963). Relationship between state of consciousness and arterial hypoxaemia and hypercapnia in patients with pulmonary insufficiency breathing air. *Clin. Sci.*, **25**, 361.

SCADDING, J. G. (1966). Patterns of respiratory insufficiency. *Lancet*, **1**, 701.

SYKES, M. K., MCNICOL, M. W. & CAMPBELL, E. J. M. (1969). *Respiratory Failure*. Oxford: Blackwell.

TAI, E. & READ, J. (1967). Blood gas tensions in bronchial asthma. *Lancet*, **1**, 644.

WEST, J. B. (1965). Ventilation/Blood Flow and Gas Exchange. Oxford: Blackwell.

WRIGHT, B. M. & MCKERROW, C. B. (1959). Maximum forced expiratory rate as a measure of ventilatory capacity. *Brit. med. J.*, **2**, 1041.

IMMUNOLOGICAL MECHANISMS IN RESPIRATORY DISEASE

Gell and Coombs (1963) classified immune or allergic reactions into four types, at least three of which may be implicated in respiratory tract disorders (Parish and Pepys, 1963).

Type I reactions occur when cells which have been passively sensitized by circulating antibodies are exposed to the appropriate antigen. Such exposure leads to the liberation of several pharmacologically active agents, notably histamine, 5-hydroxytryptamine, bradykinin, acetylcholine and a slow-reacting substance of anaphylaxis (SRS–A). Untoward effects of Type I responses are due to the release of these substances, which are held to be responsible for hay fever and extrinsic allergic asthma as well as for the classical anaphylactic reaction.

Atopic individuals are peculiarly liable to produce antibodies (reagins) which give rise to Type I reactions. The presence of reagins in serum was first demonstrated by the classic experiments of Prausnitz and Küstner in which the fish-allergy of the latter was transferred to Prausnitz's skin by intradermal injection of Küstner's serum. When a minute quantity of antigen is introduced into the skin of an atopic subject his skin reacts within minutes by a weal and flare reaction; this usually resolves within two hours. Attempts to demonstrate reagins by *in vitro* tests have mostly been unsuccessful or difficult to perform, but a new class of immunoglobulin (IgE) has been described which appears to represent reaginic antibody. The evidence relating IgE and reagin was reviewed in a leading article in the *Lancet* (1968). This class of globulin was first demonstrated by Ishizaka, Ishizaka and Hornbrook (1966) and Johansson, Bennich and Wide (1968). Raised levels of serum IgE have been found in patients with hay fever, extrinsic asthma and atopic eczema; it may be noted that the serum of normal subjects does contain some IgE (Johansson, 1967).

There is often a family history of allergy in atopic subjects who demonstrate their abnormality early in life; typically, infantile eczema is followed by hay fever and later by asthma. As well as producing positive skin reactions to the appropriate antigens the asthmatic patient will react to inhaled antigen by the development of airways obstruction—extrinsic asthma. The time course of this reaction is of the same order as the time course of the skin response. The atopic status of these patients varies from high, when multiple positive skin reactions occur to a wide variety of common antigens, to low, when only one or two positive reactions can be elicited.

Not all asthmatic patients have such direct evidence of antigen-antibody reactions. This is most likely to be the case where the asthma is of late onset. These patients, commonly middle-aged women, do not react vigorously on skin-testing to a variety of antigens as do the majority of atopic subjects, nor do they usually have a family history of allergic disease. Their serum does not contain abnormal levels of immunoglobulin IgE (Johansson, 1967). Nevertheless, immunological mechanisms may well be operative in the pathogenesis of their disease. This is suggested by the presence of eosinophils in their sputum (eosinophilic cellular infiltration of the bronchial mucosa is a characteristic of the Type I reaction of extrinsic asthma), the response to corticosteroid therapy, and the occurrence in some patients of circulating auto-antibodies (Hall, Turner-Warwick and Doniach, 1966). Patients of this type are usually classified as having "intrinsic asthma", though this is clearly an unsatisfactory term for it may simply reflect an inability to identify responsible allergens.

Type II antigen-antibody reactions are not at present implicated in human respiratory disease. In this type of reaction circulating antibody attaches to a cellular antigen or to a hapten attached to the cell, usually in the presence of complement, and cellular lysis results as in certain haemolytic anaemias.

Type III responses may occur in atopic or non-atopic subjects and ensuing disorders in the respiratory system may predominantly affect either the conducting airways or the gas-exchanging parts of the lungs. Allergic disorders of this class are mediated by circulating precipitating antibodies which may be demonstrated by *in vitro* tests. *In vivo* there is precipitation of the antigen by antibody and the resulting aggregates to which complement becomes fixed are ingested by neutrophils; these are then disrupted, resulting in the liberation of lysosomes which are responsible for the characteristic tissue damage with oedema, thrombosis and haemorrhage followed by cellular infiltration. When reactions of this type affect the lung parenchyma the syndrome of extrinsic allergic alveolitis is produced. Patchy infiltration of the alveolar walls occurs, with mononuclear and plasma cells predominating, polymorphonuclear cells being scanty; epithelioid cell granulomata with multinucleate giant cells may be present.

Skin tests with appropriate antigens in individuals with a Type III allergic disorder may give rise to a slowly developing diffuse oedematous swelling quite different from the weal and flare reaction mediated by reaginic antibody. The response takes several hours to develop and usually resolves in about twenty-four hours, being maximal at about seven or eight hours. Immunoglobulins of the IgA, IgG and IgM classes have been demonstrated, as well as complement both intra- and extracellularly at the site of this type of skin reaction (Pepys *et al.*, 1968).

Type III allergy may complicate Type I reactions in atopic asthmatic patients, as in the syndrome of allergic bronchopulmonary aspergillosis (Pepys *et al.*, 1959). The clinical aspects of the disorder are considered below. Skin tests with *Aspergillus fumigatus* antigen in this condition characteristically produce first an immediate Type I response followed by a later oedematous reaction; bronchial challenge with the antigen may produce an analogous effect with an immediate asthmatic response and a later more prolonged reaction after a delay of a few hours.

Precipitin-mediated reactions to inhaled organic antigen also occur at alveolar level, producing allergic alveolitis. The development of this kind of disorder probably requires repeated intensive exposure to an appropriate size of particle which can penetrate to the alveoli. Those who inhale the dust regularly tend to develop symptoms insidiously, while subjects exposed at intervals may present with episodic attacks of respiratory and systemic symptoms. The respiratory symptoms consist of cough, breathlessness and a sensation of tightness in the chest. Systemic symptoms include fever, malaise and sometimes loss of weight. On examination the most striking physical sign is the presence of crepitations on auscultation of the lungs. Physiologically there may be a restrictive ventilatory defect due to low lung compliance with a reduced transfer factor and arterial hypoxaemia, especially on exercise, due to widening of the range of ventilation-perfusion ratios within the lungs. Radiologically, a widespread micronodular infiltration is characteristic of early cases; and in the late stages pulmonary fibrosis may be apparent, together in some instances with the changes of honeycomb lung.

By contrast to the situation in Type I allergy where the variety of known antigens is immense, only a relatively small number of organic dusts have been shown to be capable of producing allergic alveolitis. Some of these are shown in Table 17.1, which is after Pepys (1968). It is reasonable to presume, however, that this list will continue to grow as more patients with the syndrome of acute or insidious alveolitis are recognized to have a disorder of extrinsic allergic origin.

Type IV, cell-mediated, delayed immune reactions are not associated with antibodies in the serum. The well-known tuberculin reaction is of this type. The skin response to injected allergen in this case is due to a local cellular aggregation producing the characteristic induration which is maximal at 48–72 hours.

In addition to these different types of immunological reaction to extrinsic agents the lungs may be involved in conditions in which there is evidence of *auto-allergy*. This subject has been reviewed by Burrell (1963) and by Turner-Warwick (1967). The role and exact significance of the antibodies in these conditions remains uncertain. Organ-specific autoantibodies may be produced as a purely secondary event due to the occurrence of non-specific tissue destruction, and it may be noted that anti-lung antibodies have been found in conditions as diverse as pulmonary tuberculosis and emphysema (Hennes *et al.*, 1961). The demonstration of organ-specific antibodies should therefore not be accepted as proof of a pathogenetic mechanism.

The lungs are not infrequently involved in the connective tissue disorders, especially rheumatoid disease, systemic sclerosis, polyarteritis nodosa and systemic lupus erythematosus, in all of which autoimmune processes have been implicated. Rheumatoid factor, anti-nuclear factor and complement-fixing autoantibodies which are not organ-specific may often be demonstrated in patients with these conditions. As with organ-specific antibodies their significance with regard to the presence or absence of pulmonary pathology remains obscure (Turner-Warwick, 1967). A high incidence of these various antibodies has also been shown in cases of fibrosing alveolitis (Turner-Warwick and Doniach, 1965; Turner-Warwick, 1967). Thus, in 109 patients with fibrosing alveolitis 31 per cent had circulating rheumatoid factor, 28·5 per cent had a positive antinuclear factor test (usually with negative rheumatoid factor) and 19 per cent had autoimmune complement-fixing antibodies in their serum. The majority of the last group also had either a raised titre of rheumatoid factor or positive antinuclear factor (Turner-Warwick, 1967). These findings suggest that fibrosing alveolitis may also fall into the category of connective-tissue disease.

TABLE 17.1

Extrinsic Allergic Alveolitis
(from Pepys, 1968)

Disease	Dust concerned	Precipitins against	Reference
Farmer's lung	mouldy hay	*Micropolyspora faeni Thermoactinomyces vulgaris*	Pepys and Jenkins, 1965
Bird fancier's lung	pigeon/budgerigar/hen droppings	antigens in bird droppings and serum proteins (avian)	Hargreave *et al.*, 1966
Pituitary snuff-taker's lung	pituitary powder (heterologous)	pituitary antigens/ serum proteins (beef or pig)	Mahon *et al.*, 1967
Bagassosis	mouldy, overheated sugar-cane bagasse	*T. vulgaris*	Salvaggio *et al.*, 1967
"New Guinea lung"	mouldy thatch dust	thatch from huts	Blackburn and Green, 1966
Maple-bark pneumonitis	mouldy maple bark	*Cryptostroma corticale*	Emanuel *et al*, 1966
Malt worker's lung	mouldy barley, malt dust	*Aspergillus fumigatus* and *clavatus*	Riddle *et al.*, 196?
Mushroom worker's lung	mushroom compost	*M. faeni* and *T. vulgaris*	Sakula, 1967
Suberosis	mouldy oak bark, cork dust	mouldy cork dust	Avila and Villar, 1968
Wheat weevil disease	infested wheat flour	grain weevil	Lunn and Hughes, 1967
Sequoiosis	mouldy redwood sawdust	*Graphium* and *Pullularia*	Cohen *et al.*, 1967

REFERENCES

AVILA, R. & VILLAR, T. G. (1968). Suberosis: respiratory disease in cork workers. *Lancet*, **1**, 620.

BLACKBURN, C. R. B. & GREEN, W. (1966). Precipitins against extracts of thatched roofs in the sera of New Guinea natives with chronic lung disease. *Lancet*, **2**, 1396.

BURRELL, R. G. (1963). Autoantibodies in pulmonary disease. *Amer. rev. Resp. Dis.* **87**, 389.

COHEN, H. I., MERIGAN, T. C., KOSEK, J. C. & ELDRIDGE, F. (1967). Sequoiosis: a granulomatous pneumonitis associated with redwood sawdust inhalation. *Amer. J. Med.*, **43**, 785.

EMANUEL, D. A., WENZEL, F. J. & LAWTON, B. R. (1966). Pneumonitis due to Cryptostroma corticale (Maple-Bark disease). *New Engl. J. Med.*, **274**, 1413.

GELL, P. G. M. & COOMBS, R. R. A. (eds) (1963). In *Clinical Aspects of Immunology*, p. 317. Oxford: Blackwell.

HALL, R., TURNER-WARWICK, M. & DONIACH, D. (1966). Autoantibodies in iodide goitre and asthma. *Clin. exp. Immunol.* **1**, 285.

HARGREAVE, F. E., PEPYS, J., LONGBOTTOM, J. L. & WRAITH, D. G. (1966). Bird breeder's (fancier's) lung. *Lancet*, **1**, 445.

HENNES, A. R., MOORE, M. V., CARPENTER, R. L. & HAMMARSTEN, J. F. (1961). Antibodies to human lung in patients with obstructive emphysema and pulmonar tuberculosis. *Amer. rev. Resp. Dis.* **83**, 354.

ISHIZAKA, K., ISHIZAKA T. & HORNBROOK, M. M. (1966). Physicochemical properties of reaginic antibody. V. Correlation of reaginic activity with Gamma E-Globulin antibody. *J. Immun.*, **97**, 840.

JOHANSSON, S. G. O. (1967). Raised levels of a new immunoglobulin class (Ig ND) in asthma. *Lancet*, **2**, 951.

JOHANSSON, S. G. O. BENNICH, H. & WIDE, L. (1968). A new class of immuno-globulin in human serum. *Immunology*, **14**, 265.

Lancet (1968). Reagin and IgE, **1**, 1131.

LUNN, J. A. & HUGHES, D. T. D. (1967). Pulmonary hypersensitivity to the grain weevil. *Brit. J. industr. Med.*, **24**, 158.

MAHON, W. E., SCOTT, D. J., ANSELL, G. MANSON, G. L. & FRASER, R. (1967). Hypersensitivity to pituitary snuff with miliary shadowing in the lungs. *Thorax*, **22**, 13.

PARISH, W. E. & PEPYS, J. (1963). In *Clinical Aspects of Immunology*, p. 390. Oxford: Blackwell.

PEPYS, J. (1968). Immunological mechanisms in allergic diseases of the lungs. *J. clin. Path.*, **21**, suppl. no. 2, 127.

PEPYS, J. & JENKINS, P. A. (1965). Precipitin (F.L.H.) test in farmer's lung. *Thorax*, **20**, 21.

PEPYS, J., RIDDELL, R. V., CITRON, K. M., CLAYTON, Y. M. & SHORT, E. I. (1959). Clinical and immunological significance of Aspergillus fumigatus in the sputum. *Amer. rev. Resp. Dis.* ,**80**, 167.

PEPYS, J., TURNER-WARWICK, M., DAWSON, P. L. & HINSON, K. F. W. (1968). Arthus (Type III) skin test reactions in man. Clinical and immunopathological features. In *Proc. VIth int. Congr. Allergology*. Quoted by Pepys J. (1968). *J. clin. Path.* **21**, suppl. no. 2, 127.

U

RIDDLE, H. F. V., CHANNELL, S., BLYTH, W., WEIR, D. M., LLOYD, M., AMOS, W. M. G. & GRANT, I. W. B. (1968). Allergic alveolitis in a malt worker. *Thorax*, **23**, 271.

SAKULA, A. (1967). Mushroom worker's lung. *Brit. med. J.*, **3**, 708.

SALVAGGIO, J. E., SEABURY, J. H., BUECHNER, H. A. & KUNDUR, V. G. (1967). Bagassosis: demonstration of precipitins against extracts of thermophilic actinomycetes in the sera of affected individuals. *J. Allergy*, **39**, 106

TURNER-WARWICK, M. (1967). Autoallergy and lung diseases. *J. Roy. coll. Phycns. Lond.*, **2**, 57.

TURNER-WARWICK, M. & DONIACH, D. (1965). Autoantibody studies in interstitial pulmonary fibrosis. *Brit. med. J.*, **1**, 886.

DIFFUSE AIRWAYS OBSTRUCTION

A characteristic feature in the history of most patients with diffuse airways obstruction is the wheezing breathlessness to which they are prone and which often limits their exercise tolerance. This is not a universal symptom, however; some with very severe obstruction do not experience wheezing. They may describe a sensation of "tightness" in the chest which must in turn be distinguished from angina of effort, in which breathlessness, though less obtrusive than pain, is often a significant feature (Phibbs, Holmes and Lowe, 1968). Epidemiological studies have also shown that some subjects may have diffuse airways obstruction without being aware of it (Fletcher *et al.*, 1959).

Bronchial irritability is often present in patients with diffuse bronchial disease. This is the tendency to develop acute symptoms such as cough, tightness in the chest or wheezing if they enter a smoky atmosphere or if they experience a sudden change in ambient temperature. Patients may not spontaneously report this tendency and it should therefore be specifically sought at the interview.

Mechanisms of airways obstruction. Elegant studies by Macklem and colleagues (Hogg, Macklem and Thurlbeck, 1968) have shown that in normal lungs the peripheral airways with a diameter of 2–3 mm or less contribute only a quarter of the total resistance to airflow. This is due to the dichotomous system of branching of the bronchial tree, in which the total cross-sectional area increases although the individual diameter of airways decreases as one progresses from the central to the smaller peripheral airways. In chronic obstructive lung disease it was shown that a considerable increase in the peripheral airways resistance could occur before this was sufficient to alter the total resistance of the tracheo-bronchial tree. The increased resistance of peripheral airways could therefore account for gross disturbance of ventilation distribution and hence gas exchange before conventional tests would detect an overall increase in resistance.

The usually quoted mechanisms of airways narrowing are bronchiolar muscle constriction, mucosal oedema, inflammatory stenosis, obstruction by secretions and, in emphysema, loss of radial traction applied to the bronchioles by surrounding lung tissue. Hogg *et al.* (1968) cast doubt on the last hypothesis. This presupposes that normally the small airways are tethered and supported by an outward pull due to the alveolar walls which extend radially like the spokes of a wheel from the outer wall of the airways. In emphysema the bronchioles would hypothetically lose this alveolar support because of the alveolar wall destruction, and would therefore collapse. In all cases of increased peripheral airways resistance Macklem and colleagues were able to show morphological lesions such as peribronchiolar cellular infiltration, bronchiolar stenosis and mucous plugging which could satisfactorily account for the obstruction.

In addition to the obstruction of the small airways, which was shown to be relatively fixed and affected both expiration and inspiration, Macklem, Fraser and Brown (1965) have shown that patients with chronic bronchitis or emphysema have a variable obstruction to larger airways and this is only present on expiration. Expiratory collapse of the larger airways may occur within the lung or in the main stem bronchi or trachea, and is probably due to intrinsic pathology of the bronchial wall.

Aetiological varieties. Chronic bronchitis, emphysema and asthma are the most important conditions associated with diffuse airways obstruction in adults. Occupational factors may be implicated and should be sought: examples are cotton dust which produces byssinosis in card-room workers; toluene or other volatile di-isocyanates used in the manufacture of poly-urethane materials (*Lancet*, 1966); proteolytic enzymes derived from *Bacillus subtilis* and utilized in the detergent industry (Flindt, 1969).

Circulatory disturbances may be accompanied by airways obstruction, as in left ventricular failure or acute pulmonary embolism. Although the airways obstruction is not usually very apparent it may occasionally be the dominant feature.

In children the most common cause is a lower respiratory tract infection of which the most serious variety is acute bronchiolitis (Gardner *et al.*, 1967). Asthma is also an important cause, though the other conditions seen in adults do not occur or are rare in children.

Chronic bronchitis. Stuart-Harris (1968) has reviewed this condition in all its aspects and in considerable detail. It is a condition in which there is hypersecretion of mucus in the absence of localized bronchial disease such as bronchiectasis. This gives rise to a productive cough and if this is present for most days during three months in two successive years or more a diagnosis of chronic bronchitis is tenable (M.R.C., 1965).

Patients with chronic bronchitis may be subdivided into those with simple bronchitis, where the sputum is mucoid, and infected, where the sputum is purulent. The discoloration of the sputum is then due to its cellular content and the dominant cell-type in bronchitis is the neutrophil polymorphonuclear leucocyte. Patients with simple chronic bronchitis do not necessarily have sterile sputum, but the presence of pus usually signifies a more active infection. The bacteria responsible for infection are *Haemophilus influenzae*, pneumococci and, less commonly, staphylococci or coliform organisms.

The third subdivision is chronic obstructive bronchitis. The defining characteristic of this group is the demonstration of an obstructive ventilatory defect. Either of the other two groups, the cases of simple chronic bronchitis or infected chronic bronchitis, may have airways obstruction. It is the development of narrowed airways which is responsible for converting them into respiratory cripples and ultimately killing them from respiratory failure with or without cor pulmonale.

The pathology of chronic bronchitis has been extensively studied by Reid and her co-workers. The essential features are hypertrophy of mucous glands in the bronchial walls and increase in numbers of goblet cells, which also appear in the smaller, more peripheral airways, where they are not normally found (Reid, 1954). The hypertrophy of bronchial mucosal glands has been expressed as a ratio of the thickness of the glandular layer divided by the thickness of the bronchial wall internal to the cartilage (Reid, 1960). In normal subjects the bronchial mucosal gland/wall ratio is less than 0·36 and in patients with chronic bronchitis it is greater than 0·4; there is said to be no overlap with the normal results. Changes of this type have been induced in experimental animals with irritants such as tobacco smoke and sulphur dioxide (Lamb and Reid, 1969).

The development and natural history of chronic bronchitis are still inadequately understood. Influences dating from childhood may play a more important part than generally recognized: Holland *et al.* (1969) showed that the area of residence and a previous history of lower respiratory tract infection all have a significant adverse effect on the peak expiratory flow rate of children between the ages of 5 and 16 living in Kent. Social class and family size also had an effect, though these did not reach the conventional 5 per cent level of statistical significance in all the subgroups they studied. In a different context the Newcastle Family Survey (Miller *et al.*, 1960) showed that 80 per cent of illness in the first five years of life was infective and 61 per cent of the infective illness was respiratory. In nearly one in every five instances the lower respiratory tract was involved. The different contributory factors such as social class, male sex, atmospheric pollution, have been reviewed by Court (1968). Unfortunately, little is known of the legacy which this high frequency of childhood lower respiratory tract infection has in adult life; nor is its potential role in the later development of chronic bronchitis known. However, McDonald *et al.* (1958) demonstrated the serious consequences of respiratory infections in young Royal Air Force recruits.

The role of infection in adults remains conjectural. It has long been held responsible both for the development and for the progressive deterioration of chronic bronchitis. And no clinician will seriously doubt the acute deterioration in a patient's condition induced by a lower respiratory tract infection. Evidence is accumulating, however (M.R.C., 1966; Fletcher, 1968), that such deterioration is usually transient and the patient usually recovers the ventilatory capacity he had before the infective episode. The organisms responsible for acute episodes of illness may be bacteria or viruses. The published data concerning the latter was reviewed by Grist (1968), who concluded that patients with chronic bronchitis were subject to infection with the same variety of viruses which attack the upper respiratory tracts of otherwise normal subjects; rhinoviruses and myxoviruses appear to be particularly important and in the bronchitic patient they can spread to involve the lower respiratory tract. However, not all episodes of acute deterioration in the condition of a patient with chronic bronchitis can be shown to be infective. For this reason the rather non-commital term "acute exacerbation" of chronic bronchitis has received general acceptance.

Cigarette smoking is now widely recognized to be a factor of major importance in the pathogenesis of chronic bronchitis (U.S. Department of Health, Education and Welfare, 1967). Lowe (1969) estimated that some three-quarters of the 32,000,000 working days and 30,000 lives lost in Britain in one year from bronchitis could be attributed to cigarette smoking. Urban atmospheric pollution is also an important contributory factor. By comparison with these two, occupational sources of inhaled pollution assume little significance (Lowe, 1969).

McDermott and Collins (1965) found that men with symptoms of chronic bronchitis had a greater increase in airways resistance after smoking a cigarette than did men without such symptoms. This suggested the possibility that increased bronchial reactivity might be related to the development of chronic bronchitis. Fletcher and his colleagues have confirmed the tendency to an increased bronchial reactivity to tobacco smoke in bronchitic subjects but were unable to relate this to a more rapid deterioration in ventilatory function than occurred in subjects whose response was normal (Fletcher, 1968). Robertson et al. (1969b) have shown that efficient filters can reduce this reaction to inhaled smoke and they have also shown that smoke from cigarettes made with cigar tobacco has the same effect as cigarette smoke when inhaled in the same way.

The rate of decline in the ventilatory capacity of patients with chronic bronchitis is a feature of great interest and practical importance. As ventilatory function judged by measurement of the F.E.V.$_1$ declines, the time comes in the course of the disease when ventilatory failure develops and the P$_{CO_2}$ rises. Further decline in the F.E.V.$_1$ due to an exacerbation of bronchitis is then liable to be associated with a brisk rise in P$_{CO_2}$, and the accompanying hypoxia may prove lethal. Regular records of a patient's F.E.V.$_1$ and P$_{CO_2}$ may permit anticipation of the time when this critical situation is likely to be encountered, though sudden unpredictable falls in

F.E.V.$_1$ can occur for no accountable reason (Howard, 1967; Howard and Astin, 1969). It should be noted that there is a steady decline in the F.E.V.$_1$ and vital capacity in normal subjects from the third decade onwards (Fig. 17.5). The rate of this decline is of the order of 30 ml/year (Cotes *et al.*, 1966) though a recent study of a Swedish urban male population aged 50 showed a significantly higher rate of almost 60 ml/year (Wilhelmsen, Orha and Tibblin, 1969).

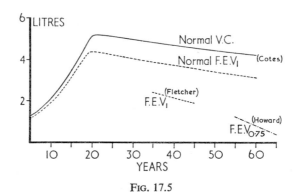

FIG. 17.5

Growth and decline of the vital capacity and F.E.V.$_1$ with age for a male subject (adult height approximately 69 in. (1·75 m); data from Cotes, 1968). Regression lines from data of Fletcher (1968) and Howard (1967) show average decline in F.E.V. in chronic obstructive bronchitis.

Patients with obstructive bronchitis have by definition a lower initial F.E.V.$_1$ and their rate of decline is greater than normal. Fletcher (1968) quoted a value of 51 ml/year for subjects with a mean F.E.V.$_1$ of below 2·25 litres; in an M.R.C. survey of the value of chemotherapy in early chronic bronchitis (1966) the average decline was 80 ml/year and this was un-influenced by chemotherapy. Howard (1967), studying a bronchitic population with a mean age older than in the other two groups, found that the F.E.V.$_{0·75}$ fell by 80 ml/year from a mean initial value of 1·2 litres.

No data are available to show how patients with chronic obstructive bronchitis reach their low level of F.E.V.$_1$ The periods of study of different groups of patients have all been for relatively few years and it is invalid to extrapolate retrospectively beyond these years. Yet if such a procedure were legitimate it could be seen from Figure 17.5 that the onset of airways obstruction either dated from many years earlier, possibly from childhood, or there had been a much more rapid rate of decline in F.E.V.$_1$ during previous years than that shown by the regression lines of Fletcher or Howard. Clinical experience suggests it is unlikely that there has often been a sudden decline from a near-normal value to the low values found in the majority of bronchitic patients attending hospital, whose rate of fall in F.E.V.$_1$ then averages 80 ml/year. This suggests that airways obstruction has probably been present and progressive for many years. The observations of Fletcher *et al.* (1959) that quite severe airways obstruction may be symptomless are in keeping with the latter hypothesis.

Emphysema. Up to ten years ago (Ciba Guest Symposium, 1959) little attempt was made by clinicians to separate emphysema from chronic bronchitis. Previously, the term "chronic bronchitis and emphysema" tended to be applied indiscriminately to most patients admitted to hospital in Britain with chronic diffuse airways obstruction. Such a diagnosis may be perfectly correct for there is considerable overlap between the two conditions. They may however occur quite independently, and for this reason strict diagnostic criteria are desirable. Those for chronic bronchitis have been given and depend essentially on the patient's history, with or without evidence of airways obstruction.

Emphysema can ultimately only be satisfactorily defined on morbid anatomical grounds as an "abnormal increase in the size of air spaces peripheral to the terminal bronchiole with destructive changes in their walls" (W.H.O., 1961).

Beyond the terminal bronchiole there are usually three orders of respiratory bronchiole with progressively larger numbers of alveoli in their walls as they proceed distally to the alveolar ducts from which the atria arise; several alveolar sacs arise from each atrium and their walls are made up of alveoli. The entire lung unit beyond the terminal bronchiole is the acinus or secondary lobule, and the alveolar duct with its distal connections constitutes the primary lobule.

In terms of functional derangement the varieties of emphysema of most importance are centrilobular and panlobular (panacinar). In the former the second and third order of respiratory bronchioles bear the brunt of the process, their walls being dilated, attenuated and disrupted. In the panacinar variety the process is more diffuse through the acinus, with dilatation of air sacs and alveolar ducts as well as respiratory bronchioles. It is the centrilobular variety of emphysema that is most often found in association with chronic bronchitis (Leopold and Gough, 1957).

Other varieties of so-called or true emphysema, such as compensatory, senile, focal and paraseptal are not of great functional significance. The term bullous emphysema implies the presence of emphysematous spaces which exceed 1 cm in diameter. If bullae enlarge to an extreme size they may act as intrathoracic space-occupying lesions.

Several studies in recent years (Fletcher *et al.*, 1963; Jones *et al.*, 1967) have shown that it is possible to identify typical cases of extensive panacinar emphysema (designated type A patients) from typical examples of chronic obstructive bronchitis (Type B) though intermediate cases with mixed features (type X) occur. A clinical spectrum of cases exists, ranging from those with pure emphysema through mixed cases to those who have bronchitis without any emphysema, and certain criteria enable the physician to diagnose them with greater precision than hitherto.

Severe emphysema (Type A disease) is diagnosed predominantly on radiological and physiological grounds. Chest X-rays show hyperinflation of the lungs with a flattened diaphragm, a long narrow mediastinum and, most importantly, marked attenuation of the pulmonary vessels as they radiate from the hila to the periphery (Fig. 17.6). Bullae may be seen, though not inflammatory opacities in the lung parenchyma. The lateral film shows an increased area of radiotranslucency behind the sternum and in front of the heart. Physiologically there is a severe irreversible obstructive ventilatory defect and the transfer factor is notably reduced. Despite these defects the patients tend to maintain alveolar ventilation until a very late stage, so that at rest the arterial P_{CO_2} is usually normal and hypoxaemia is insufficient to cause marked cyanosis; on exercise there is usually a rise in P_{CO_2} and a fall in P_{O_2} (Jones, 1966). Patients with these characteristics are often thin, elderly men with progressively severe dyspnoea in whom evidence of bronchitis is lacking or minimal. Chronic or recurrent congestive cardiac failure is unusual, possibly because of the tendency to maintain alveolar ventilation, though heart failure may complicate the inevitable terminal respiratory failure.

Patients with Type B disease have by definition chronic productive cough with an obstructive ventilatory defect and minimal or no evidence of emphysema. Patchy opacities in the lung parenchyma consistent with present or previous inflammatory disease are usual on the chest radiograph (Fig. 17.7). There tends to be a higher P_{CO_2} for the degree of airways obstruction and cyanosis is common. Chronic ventilatory failure is often found, and cor pulmonale occurs with recurrent episodes of congestive heart failure. By contrast with the Type A patients the transfer factor is relatively well preserved and may be normal. Type B patients do not typically lose weight and they are often of a mesomorphic build.

The reasons for the clinical and physiological differences between these polar groups, which correspond to the "pink puffers" and "blue bloaters" of Dornhorst (1955), remain unclear. Lane et al. (1968) have investigated the response to breathing carbon dioxide in certain of these patients. First they confirmed the general relationship between low levels of F.E.V.$_1$ and a rise in P_{CO_2}. They then showed how different subjects behaved within the general relationship: some maintained alveolar ventilation until the F.E.V.$_1$ fell to the order of 0·5 litre, when their P_{CO_2} rose abruptly to high levels; others had a high P_{CO_2} even at an F.E.V.$_1$ of 1·5 litres. Lane and Howell then studied the ventilatory response to breathing carbon dioxide in selected patients of each type. In studies of this kind the ventilatory response to carbon

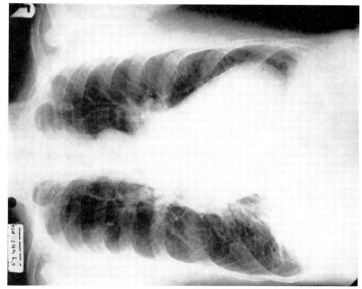

Fig. 17.7

The chest radiograph of a stocky, 45-year-old male with a long history of chronic bronchitis. The $F.E.V._{.1}$ was 0·7 and the vital capacity 2·75 litres; these rose only fractionally with bronchodilator drugs. His obstructive ventilatory defect was not accompanied by a reduction in the gas transfer factor (18 ml/min/mm Hg for carbon monoxide). There was mild chronic ventilatory failure (arterial P_{CO_2} 55 mm Hg, pH 7·36).

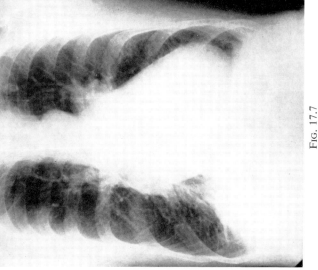

Fig. 17.6

Radiological appearances in a severely dyspnoeic, thin, 60-year-old male with emphysema. Physiological data showed a severe irreversible obstructive ventilatory defect ($F.E.V._{.1}$ 0·67; vital capacity 3·3 litres). His transfer factor (diffusing capacity) for carbon monoxide was severely reduced at 7 ml/min/mm Hg, consistent with extensive alveolar destruction. He was slightly hypoxic ($P_{O_2} = 60$ mm Hg) and the P_{CO_2} was at the extreme upper end of the normal range (48 mm Hg).

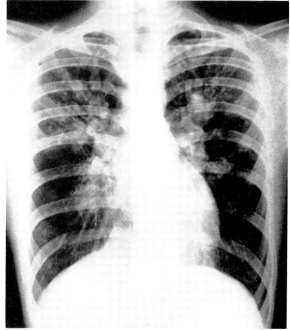

FIG. 17.8a

Chest radiograph of a 17-year-old atopic subject with severe
asthma associated with bronchopulmonary aspergillosis. With
corticosteroid therapy his asthma remitted and the radiological
opacities cleared.

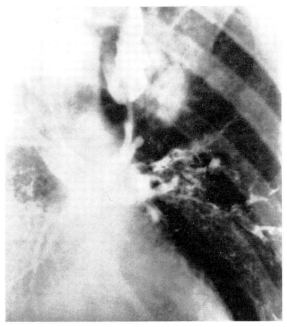

FIG. 17.8b

Detail of the bronchographic appearances from the left upper lobe
of the same subject as Fig 17.8a.

dioxide is not itself very meaningful because in the presence of severe airways obstruction it may be impossible to increase the total ventilation no matter what effort is made by the subject. Lane and Howell therefore measured the work rate of the inspiratory muscles whilst breathing carbon dioxide and used this as an index of carbon dioxide sensitivity. This was shown to be normal in patients who had a normal P_{CO_2} despite very low F.E.V.$_1$ levels (corresponding to the "pink puffers") and impaired in those with raised P_{CO_2} in the presence of lesser degrees of airways obstruction (the "blue and bloated" group). The results suggest the possibility that not only are there anatomical differences within the lungs of the two extreme varieties of patient but there may also be differences in their central respiratory control mechanisms.

In the aetiology of emphysema the same factors have been implicated as in chronic bronchitis, and emphysema has traditionally been thought of as a consequence of bronchitis. A more critical appraisal may be necessary in the future in view of the greater diagnostic precision which the recently defined criteria permit. One recently discovered abnormality which may be of aetiological importance in a few patients is a deficiency of the serum inhibitor of trypsin, alpha 1-antitrypsin (Eriksson, 1964; Tarkoff *et al.*, 1968). This glycoprotein is the main proteolytic-enzyme inhibitor in human serum and is a major component of the alpha 1-globulin band on electrophoresis of the serum proteins. Subjects who are homozygous for the defect have very low levels of alpha 1-antitrypsin, while heterozygous individuals have levels which are intermediate between those found in homozygotes and those found in normal serum. The possibility of this defect should be considered especially in patients who develop emphysema under the age of 40 and have a rapidly progressive course. Alpha 1-antitrypsin is able to inhibit proteolytic enzymes from leucocytes and may therefore limit their destructive capacity. Hypothetically, alpha 1-antitrypsin deficiency permits this destructive effect to go unchecked in the lungs, leading to the development of emphysema. Implicit in such a hypothesis is an association with infection or some other cause for leucocytic infiltration of the lungs so that the effects of alpha 1-antitrypsin deficiency may be manifest.

Asthma. Allergy of the Type I variety is a major cause of asthma. Some patients also develop Type III reactions. But not all asthmatics have demonstrable allergy, and for this reason the term is best avoided in a definition of asthma. This can be satisfactorily defined only in functional terms as diffuse airways obstruction that is variable in severity, usually over short periods of time; the variability may be spontaneous or the result of treatment.

Whether there is evidence of allergy or not, an asthmatic subject may have episodes triggered by events such as respiratory infection, exercise, or emotional disturbance. Exercise is sometimes the dominant or sole cause of asthmatic attacks (McNeill *et al.*, 1966) which may be attributable to the lactic acidosis of muscular work (Seaton *et al.*, 1969). Such observations indicate the need to consider the total environment, internal as well as external, of the asthmatic patient.

There is little difficulty about the diagnosis in many patients with asthma, especially in the younger age-groups. Their episodic attacks may be nocturnal as well as diurnal, may be predominant at some particular season (usually the summer months), and may be associated with symptoms of rhinitis, or with the fully developed eczema-hayfever-asthma syndrome of the atopic individual, leaving little doubt about the diagnosis.

Skin-tests with an appropriate range of allergens will reveal the atopic "status" of the individual. This may range from high, when positive reactions are obtained to a wide variety of substances, to low, when only one or two allergens give positive skin-tests. The choice of allergens is guided by the patient's history though the following are commonly used: house dust, dog hair, car fur, grass and other pollens, and moulds including *Aspergillus fumigatus*.

In recent years it has been recognized that house dust mites (Dermatophagoides species in particular) are the most important source of allergens in patients reacting to house dust (Voorhorst *et al.*, 1967). Material from these mites may therefore be usefully included in the range of allergens against which patients are tested. An alternative and clinically more relevant method of testing for hypersensitivity in asthmatic subjects is to observe changes in the F.E.V.$_1$ induced by inhalation of a nebulized aerosol of the allergen. Tests of bronchial hypersensitivity are unfortunately more cumbersome and time-consuming than skin-tests and are consequently less often used.

Diagnostic difficulties arise notably in two situations. One is the patient in whom a dominant symptom is the production of sputum, with or without recurrent infective episodes; such a patient is liable to masquerade as a case of chronic bronchitis. The other is the patient with little or no variation in the degree of his airways obstruction who runs the risk of being "written off" as a case of "irreversible obstructive lung disease" for which little can be done. In such cases repeated examination of the cellular content of samples of sputum should be made. An asthmatic patient has numerous eosinophils in the sputum whereas in other conditions the predominant leucocyte is the polymorphonuclear neutrophil. Also, the ventilatory response to different drugs, administered as aerosols, can be helpful in distinguishing the patient whose airways obstruction is essentially due to asthma.

Altounyan (1964) made detailed studies of the response to a variety of drugs in a large group of patients with diffuse airways obstruction. He divided them, broadly, into patients with "allergic" and "non-allergic" airways obstruction. The former group included cases of both extrinsic and intrinsic asthma, many of whom were difficult to distinguish on clinical grounds alone from patients with chronic bronchitis. Subsequently they were shown to respond to and require treatment with corticosteroids. The "non-allergic" group did not respond to corticosteroid therapy. As a result of his enquiry he concluded that it is possible to identify patients who have an "allergic" component in their airways obstruction by comparing the response in their F.E.V.$_1$ to inhalation of atropine methonitrate with that induced by isoprenaline. In this test the magnitude of increase in F.E.V.$_1$ one hour after the inhalation of atropine is compared with the magnitude of increase five minutes after inhalation of isoprenaline; these time intervals are appropriate for an optimum improvement in the F.E.V.$_1$ to each drug. Patients who should respond to corticosteroid therapy ("allergic" factors in operation) have a bigger rise in F.E.V.$_1$ after isoprenaline than after atropine. Patients with "non-allergic" airways obstruction tend to have a greater increase in F.E.V.$_1$ with atropine methonitrate than they do with isoprenaline. Effective corticosteroid treatment of the patient with "allergic" airways obstruction will, however, diminish his isoprenaline responsiveness and in this case the result of the test should be viewed with caution.

It is now generally recognized that asthma cannot be regarded as more of a nuisance than a serious illness. The older view that asthma rarely kills is quite untenable. This attitude probably arose because within the experience of any physician death from asthma was indeed a rare event. However, as Speizer and Doll (1968) have shown, in the age-group 5–34 years (when certification of death from asthma is presumably at its most accurate) deaths in England and Wales due to asthma have been between approximately 0·5 and 1·0 per 100,000 persons since the late nineteenth century, until a striking increase began a decade ago. This rise in mortality, which has been greatest in children aged 10 to 14, has been fairly conclusively related to the introduction and increased usage of aerosol bronchodilators rather than to alterations in the incidence or intrinsic severity of the disease, to any change in its diagnostic classification, or to corticosteroid therapy (Speizer et al., 1968a and b; Inman and Adelstein, 1969). This type of bronchodilator preparation was introduced into British clinical practice in 1960; sales increased rapidly up to 1966 and then declined. Inman and Adelstein (1969) have clearly correlated the rise and fall in sales of aerosol bronchodilators (particularly those containing isoprenaline) with asthma mortality. By 1967 they were able to demonstrate a reduction in mortality from asthma in every age-group over nine years; since 1967 the fall in death rate in patients aged 5 to 34 has been particularly striking and has continued to the first quarter of 1969.

Management of patients with airways obstruction. The first essential is a complete diagnosis wherever possible and, guided by the various criteria discussed above, this is usually feasible. The application of a blanket-term such as "obstructive airways disease" to patients with chronic airways obstruction is to be deprecated if it reduces the physician's efforts to find reversible processes.

The second essential is the adequate recording of patients' data in their notes. A regular record should be kept of weight and, in children, height; in children it is necessary to plot both of these on charts depicting normal growth curves so that deviations from normal are readily detected. A regular reading of the F.E.V.$_1$ or P.F.R. should be made. This is far more informative than the descriptions of auscultatory minutiae which so often adorn the hospital notes of these cases.

It should, however, be realized that there is day-to-day variability in measurements of the F.E.V.$_1$ which will not be seen in the relatively infrequent measurements made at hospital visits. Apparent failure to demonstrate an objective improvement in such measurements must therefore not immediately be interpreted as proof that no benefit has accrued from treatment; more frequent observations might show a definite response. A patient's own observations may therefore still be valid and should always be noted. Daily measurements of P.F.R. by patients themselves are feasible and have been shown by Epstein *et al.* (1969) to be valuable in assessing the response to treatment.

Another possible reason for failure of the F.E.V.$_1$ to reflect genuine improvement should also be noted. Woolcock and Read (1965) showed how the grossly overdistended lungs of the asthmatic may relax to a lower (more normal) volume during recovery, with significant symptomatic improvement yet without necessarily being accompanied by an increase in F.E.V.$_1$. Nevertheless, a rise in F.E.V.$_1$ is usual in these circumstances, and despite fallacies such as the ones just described the F.E.V.$_1$ remains a most valuable and convenient measure of ventilatory function.

Occasional measurements of the blood gases should be made, especially when F.E.V.$_1$ levels below 1·5 litres are recorded.

Finally, certain aspects of treatment and some of its hazards will be considered, under the following headings:

1. *Prophylaxis.* Cigarette smoking and atmospheric pollution are serious public health problems the successful solution of which should lead to a striking reduction in the incidence of chronic bronchitis and emphysema. Unfortunately, cigarette smoking is a habit usually formed early in life and it appears that anti-smoking propaganda has little effect on smoking habits, even among schoolchildren (Holland and Elliott, 1968).

The prophylaxis of asthma requires avoidance of allergens or effective hyposensitization. In rare instances, as with aspirin-induced asthma (Samter and Beers, 1968), the patient may be able to avoid offending allergens though this is usually impossible since these tend to be widespread in the environment. Efforts can be made to minimize contact with allergens, however; regular vacuum-cleaning of mattresses plus the covering of pillows or mattresses with polythene will reduce the intensity of contact with dust. Hyposensitization to house dust is of dubious value (British Tuberculosis

Association, 1968) though the development of extracts from house-dust mites may conceivably increase the effectiveness of such treatment. Clinical experience suggests that treatment by hyposensitization is of greatest benefit when directed at specific seasonal hypersensitivity to pollens.

2. *Antibiotic and chemotherapy.* Numerous clinical trials of chemotherapy have been conducted, given either long-term for the prophylaxis of "infective" exacerbations of chronic bronchitis or short-term for their treatment. These have been reviewed by Stuart-Harris (1968). Results have often been conflicting and statistically validated proof of benefit from antibiotic therapy has not always been forthcoming (Elmes *et al.*, 1965). However, most physicians agree with Pines *et al.* (1968) that it would be unethical not to give antibiotics to seriously ill patients. In their investigation Pines *et al.* (1968) concluded that penicillin and streptomycin combined were superior to ampicillin in the treatment of severe, acute purulent exacerbations of bronchitis.

A working party report to the M.R.C. (1966) on chemoprophylaxis in early chronic obstructive bronchitis indicated that continuous treatment from mid-September to mid-April each year made no material difference to the frequency of exacerbations although their duration might be diminished. One important finding from this investigation was the apparent failure of treatment to influence the rate of decline in F.E.V.$_1$.

Despite such observations a reasonable compromise at the present time appears to be the prompt administration of a broad spectrum antibiotic to patients with chronic airways obstruction, whatever the cause, on suspicion of an upper or lower "respiratory infection". Although such episodes may be of viral aetiology or even non-infective, an antibiotic may limit secondary bacterial growth in the lower respiratory tract.

3. *Bronchodilator drugs.* Aerosol bronchodilators have been incriminated in the increased mortality from asthma over the past decade. Probable reasons for sudden death in asthma are hypoxia and ventricular fibrillation. Paradoxically, despite symptomatic relief from the use of a bronchodilator (associated with a rise in F.E.V.$_1$), there may be no improvement in the arterial P_{O_2} and this may actually fall. This has been shown to occur at times with subcutaneous adrenaline (Rees *et al.*, 1967a) and intravenous amino-phylline (Rees *et al.*, 1967b) as well as with inhaled isoprenaline (Palmer and Diament, 1967).

This paradox may be explained on a basis of alteration in ventilation-perfusion ratios within the lungs. It is known that in very severe asthma the response to isoprenaline is very poor so that the greatest bronchodilator effect (rise in F.E.V.$_1$) is seen in moderately severe obstruction. It also appears that within the lungs less severely obstructed bronchioles respond to broncho-dilator better than those which are more severely obstructed. Yet the time-constants of the least obstructed lung units are such that they already have a high ratio of ventilation to perfusion. Dilatation of the air passages to these units leads to an even higher ventilation-perfusion ratio, which is achieved at the expense of the most severely obstructed lung units where there has been little or no bronchodilatation. A fall in ventilation-perfusion ratio in the latter units will lead to a greater degree of arterial hypoxaemia. This may occur despite an overall increase in F.E.V.$_1$ so that although the breathing feels easier the patient may be more hypoxic than before.

Despite these drawbacks, bronchodilator drugs remain a valuable form of treatment. Providing the patient realizes the potential hazards associated with aerosols and can be trusted not to take the drug repeatedly when a response is not forthcoming, then he should be allowed to use them. There is at present no quicker way to abort an asthmatic attack than the early use of an isoprenaline aerosol.

It remains to be seen, however, whether the latest bronchodilator, salbutamol, which appears to be devoid of the cardiac stimulant effect of isoprenaline and has a longer duration of action, lives up to its early promise and becomes the bronchodilator of first choice (Choo-Kang et al., 1969).

4. *Corticosteroid therapy.* There is no doubt about the potential benefit which corticosteroids offer the asthmatic individual, both in terms of improvement in the quality of life and in recovery from attacks of status asthmaticus. Yet there is no proof of a substantial decrease in mortality since these drugs were introduced. Indeed, they were for some years suspected of contributing to the increase in mortality now attributed to over-use of bronchodilator aerosols.

The main indications for the use of corticosteroids are status asthmaticus and when there is serious disruption of the wellbeing and social life of the patient through loss of sleep, schooling, work or weight. Treatment should be short-term if possible, though long-term treatment may be safely employed if it is required (Walsh and Grant, 1966; Maunsell et al., 1968).

Should long-term therapy with corticosteroids be necessary, then the minimum effective dosage must be found and in an adult this is frequently about 7 or 8 mg of prednisone daily. The availability of 1 mg strength prednisone tablets as well as the 5-mg tablets permits very precise adjustment of the dose; and whenever the total daily dosage is being reduced below 15 mg it is desirable to do so in steps of 1 mg.

In a child, however, long-term maintenance treatment with steroids may suppress growth (Friedman and Strang, 1966) and ACTH is to be preferred. It appears that growth retardation in the asthmatic child, whether or not he is receiving corticosteroids, is due not to suppression of pituitary growth hormone output but probably to "end-organ" resistance to the action of growth hormone (Morris et al., 1968a and b; Sanders and Norman, 1969).

Corticosteroid therapy is usually necessary at some stage in two asthma-syndromes. One is intrinsic asthma of late onset, which is most often seen in women around the menopause. The other is the syndrome of broncho-pulmonary aspergillosis in which an atopic subject also develops a Type III allergic response, usually to *Aspergillus fumigatus* (Henderson, 1968). In the latter condition asthmatic attacks become increasingly intractable and may be associated with systemic symptoms such as anorexia, weight loss and fever; the E.S.R. may be raised, blood eosinophilia is common and the radiological appearances are often characteristic (Fig. 17.8). The plain film usually shows evidence of pulmonary infiltration, and a bronchogram may reveal a characteristic type of bronchiectasis (Scadding, 1967) with a normal bronchial tree beyond the ectatic segment. These lesions have been attributed to an intense Type III precipitin-mediated reaction in the bronchial wall. Plugs of mucus coughed up by the patient may contain some *Aspergillus* mycelium though this is often difficult to demonstrate. The use of corticosteroids is usually essential to prevent progressive lung damage when the clinical picture is fully developed.

5. *Disodium cromoglycate.* This drug has established a place in the treatment of asthma and appears to be of greatest benefit to young people with extrinsic asthma. A number of clinical trials have confirmed its effectiveness (Howell and Altounyan, 1967; Smith and Devey, 1968; Robertson *et al.*, 1969a) though symptomatic benefit has not always been accompanied by an increase in F.E.V.$_1$, a feature which has led some to doubt the drug's value (Grant *et al.*, 1967). Disodium cromoglycate is neither a bronchodilator nor an antihistamine and does not have corticosteroid-like effects. It appears to interfere with the release of pharmacologically active substances which result from antigen-antibody reactions, and it has been shown to inhibit the allergic reactions provoked by inhalation of antigens in subjects with Type III responses as well as in those with Type I allergy (Pepys *et al.*, 1968). Protection from exercise-induced asthma has also been reported (Davies, 1968).

The drug is poorly absorbed and is administered by inhalation in powder form. It appears to be remarkably non-toxic, the only cause for complaint being irritation of the throat after inhalation of the powder.

Personal experience suggests that about 40 per cent of asthmatic patients derive appreciable benefit from cromoglycate and another 15 per cent report some improvement. If long-term corticosteroids are being given con-currently the dosage may be reduced, but steroids should be discontinued with the utmost caution.

REFERENCES

ALTOUNYAN, R. E. C. (1964). Variation of drug action on airway obstruction in man. *Thorax*, **19**, 406.

BRITISH TUBERCULOSIS ASSOCIATION (1968). Treatment of house dust allergy. *Brit. med. J.*, **3**, 774.

CIBA GUEST SYMPOSIUM (1959). Terminology, definitions, and classification of chronic pulmonary emphysema and related conditions. *Thorax*, **14**, 286.

CHOO-KANG, Y. F. J., SIMPSON, W. T. & GRANT, I. W. B. (1969). Controlled comparison of the bronchodilator effects of three beta-adrenergic stimulant drugs administered by inhalation to patients with asthma. *Brit. med. J.*, **2**, 287.

COTES, J. E. (1968). *Lung Function. Assessment and Application in Medicine*. Oxford: Blackwell.

COTES, J. E., ROSSITER, C. E., HIGGINS, I. T. T. & GILSON, J. C. (1966). Average normal values for the forced expiratory volume in white Caucasian males. *Brit. med. J.*, **1**, 1016.

COURT, S. D. M. (1968). Epidemiology and natural history of respiratory infections in children. *J. clin. Path.*, **21**, suppl no. 2, 30.

DAVIES, S. E. (1968). Effect of disodium cromoglycate on exercise-induced asthma. *Brit. med. J.*, **3**, 593.

DORNHORST, A. C. (1955). Respiratory insufficiency. *Lancet*, **1**, 1185.

ELMES, P. C., KING, T. K. C., LANGLANDS, J. H. M., MACKAY, J. A., WALLACE, W. F. M., WADE, O. L. & WILSON, T. S. (1965). Value of ampicillin in the hospital treatment of exacerbations of chronic bronchitis. *Brit. med. J.*, **2**, 904.

EPSTEIN, S. W., FLETCHER, C. M. & OPPENHEIMER, E. A. (1969). Daily peak flow measurements in the assessment of steroid therapy for airway obstruction. *Brit. med. J.*, **1**, 223.

ERIKSSON, S. (1964). Pulmonary emphysema and alpha l-antitrypsin deficiency. *Acta med. Scand.*, **175**, 197.

FLETCHER, C. M. (1968). Bronchial infection and reactivity in chronic bronchitis. *J. Roy. coll. Phycns Lond.*, **2**, 183.

FLETCHER, C. M., ELMES, P. C., FAIRBAIRN, A. S. & WOOD, C. H. (1959). The significance of respiratory symptoms and the diagnosis of chronic bronchitis in a working population. *Brit. med. J.*, **2**, 257.

FLETCHER, C. M., HUGH-JONES, P., McNICOL, M. W. & PRIDE, N. B. (1963). The diagnosis of pulmonary emphysema in the presence of chronic bronchitis. *Quart. J. Med.*, **32**, 33.

FLINDT, M. L. H. (1969). Pulmonary disease due to inhalation of derivatives of *Bacillus subtilis* containing proteolytic enzyme. *Lancet*, **1**, 1177.

FRIEDMAN, M. & STRANG, L. B. (1966). Effect of long-term corticosteroids and corticotrophin on the growth of children. *Lancet*, **2**, 568.

GARDNER, P. S., TURK, D. C., AHERNE, W. A., BIRD, T., HOLDAWAY, M. D. & COURT, S. D. M. (1967). Deaths associated with respiratory tract infection in childhood. *Brit. med. J.*, **4**, 316.

GRANT, I. W. B., CHANNELL, S. & DREVER, J. C. (1967). Disodium cromoglycate in asthma. *Lancet*, **2**, 673.

GRIST, N. R. (1968). Group discussion: Virus infections in chronic bronchitis. 1. In acute exacerbations. *J. clin. Path.*, **21**, suppl. no. 2, 98.

HENDERSON, A. H. (1968). Allergic aspergillosis: review of 32 cases. *Thorax*, **23**, 501.

HOGG, J. C., MACKLEM, P. T. & THURLBECK, W. M. (1968). Site and nature of airway obstruction in chronic obstructive lung disease. *N. Eng. J. Med.*, **278**, 1355.

HOLLAND, W. W. & ELLIOTT, A. (1968). Cigarette smoking, respiratory symptoms and anti-smoking propaganda: an experiment. *Lancet*, **1**, 41.

HOLLAND, W. W., HALIL, T., BENNETT, A. E. & ELLIOTT, A. (1969). Factors influencing the onset of chronic respiratory disease. *Brit. med. J.*, **2**, 205.

HOWARD, P. (1967). Evolution of the ventilatory capacity in chronic bronchitis. *Brit. med. J.*, **3**, 392.

HOWARD, P. & ASTIN, T. W. (1969). Precipitous fall of the forced expiratory volume. *Thorax*, **24**, 492.

HOWELL, J. B. L. & ALTOUNYAN, R. E. C. (1967). A double-blind trial of disodium cromoglycate in the treatment of allergic bronchial asthma. *Lancet*, **2**, 539.

INMAN, W. H. W. & ADELSTEIN, A. M. (1969). Rise and fall of asthma mortality in England and Wales in relation to use of pressurised aerosols. *Lancet*, **2**, 279.

JONES, N. L. (1966). Pulmonary gas exchange during exercise in patients with chronic airway obstruction. *Clin. Sci.*, **31**, 39.

JONES, N. L., BURROWS, B. & FLETCHER, C. M. (1967). Serial studies of 100 patients with chronic airway obstruction in London and Chicago. *Thorax*, **22**, 327.

LAMB, D. & REID, L. (1969). Goblet cell increase in rat bronchial epithelium after exposure to cigarette and cigar tobacco smoke. *Brit. med. J.*, **1**, 33.

Lancet (1966). Hazards of di-isocyanates, **1**, 32.

LANE, D. J., HOWELL, J. B. L. & GIBLIN, B. (1968). Relation between airways obstruction and CO_2 tension in chronic obstructive airways disease. *Brit. med. J.*, **3**, 707.

LEOPOLD, J. G. & GOUGH, J. (1957). The centrilobular form of hypertrophic emphysema and its relation to chronic bronchitis. *Thorax*, **12**, 219.

LOWE, C. R. (1969). Industrial bronchitis. *Brit. med. J.*, **1**, 463.

MCDERMOTT, M. & COLLINS, M. M. (1965). Acute effects of smoking on lung airway resistance in normal and bronchitic subjects. *Thorax*, **20**, 562.

MCDONALD, J. C., WILSON, J. S., THORBURN, W. B., HOLLAND, W. W. & ANDREWS, B. E. (1958). Acute respiratory disease in the R.A.F., 1955-7. *Brit. med. J.*, **2**, 721.

MCNEILL, R. S., NAIRN, J. R., MILLAR, J. S. & INGRAM, C. G. (1966). Exercise-induced asthma. *Quart. J. Med.*, **35**, 55.

MACKLEM, P. T., FRASER, R. G. & BROWN, W. G. (1965). Bronchial pressure measurements in emphysema and bronchitis. *J. clin. Invest.*, **44**, 897.

MAUNSELL, K., PEARSON, R. S. B. & LIVINGSTONE, J. L. (1968). Long-term corticosteroid treatment of asthma. *Brit. med. J.*, **1**, 661.

MEDICAL RESEARCH COUNCIL committee on the aetiology of chronic bronchitis (1965). Definition and classification of chronic bronchitis. *Lancet*, **1**, 775.

MEDICAL RESEARCH COUNCIL working party report (1966). Value of chemoprophylaxis and chemotherapy in early chronic bronchitis. *Brit. med. J.*, **1**, 1317.

MILLER, F. J. W., COURT, S. D. M., WALTON, W. S. & KNOX, E. G. (1960). *Growing up in Newcastle upon Tyne*. London: Oxford University Press.

MORRIS, H. G., JORGENSEN, J. R. & JENKINS, S. A. (1968a). Plasma growth hormone concentration in corticosteroid-treated children. *J. clin. Invest.*, **47**, 427.

MORRIS, H. G., JORGENSEN, J. R., ELRICK, H. & GOLDSMITH, R. E. (1968b). Metabolic effects of human growth hormone in corticosteroid-treated children. *J. clin. Invest.*, **47**, 436.

PALMER, K. N. V. & DIAMENT, M. L. (1967). Effect of aerosol isoprenaline on blood-gas tensions in severe bronchial asthma. *Lancet*, **2**, 1232.

PEPYS, J., HARGREAVE, F. E., CHAN, M. & MCCARTHY, D. S. (1968). Inhibitory effect of disodium cromoglycate on allergen-inhalation tests. *Lancet*, **2**, 134.

PHIBBS, B., HOLMES, R. W. & LOWE, C. R. (1968). Transient myocardial ischaemia: the significance of dyspnoea. *Amer. J. med. Sci.*, **256**, 210.

PINES, A., RAAFAT, H., PULCINSKI, K., GREENFIELD, J. S. B. & SOLARI, M. (1968). Antibiotic regimens in severe and acute purulent exacerbations of chronic bronchitis. *Brit. med. J.*, **2**, 735.

REES, H. A., MILLAR, J. S. & DONALD, K. W. (1967a). Adrenaline in bronchial asthma. *Lancet*, **2**, 1164.

REES, H. A., BORTHWICK, R. C., MILLAR, J. S. & DONALD, K. W. (1967b). Aminophylline in bronchial asthma, *Lancet*, **2**, 1167.

REID, L. (1954). Pathology of chronic bronchitis. *Lancet*, **1**, 275.

REID, L. (1960). Measurement of the bronchial mucous gland layer. A diagnostic yardstick in chronic bronchitis. *Thorax*, **15**, 132.

ROBERTSON, D. G., EPSTEIN, S. W. & WARRELL, D. A. (1969a). Trial of disodium cromoglycate in bronchial asthma. *Brit. med. J.*, **1**, 552.

ROBERTSON, D. G., WARRELL, D. A., NEWTON-HOWES, J. S. & FLETCHER, C. M. (1969b). Bronchial reactivity to cigarette and cigar smoke. *Brit. med. J.*, **3**, 269.

SAMTER, M. & BEERS, R. F. (1968). Intolerance to aspirin. Clinical studies and consideration of its pathogenesis. *Ann. intern. Med.*, **68**, 975.

SANDERS, S. S. & NORMAN, A. P. (1969). Growth hormone secretion in growth-retarded asthmatic children. *Brit. med. J.*, **3**, 25.

SCADDING, J. G. (1967). The bronchi in allergic aspergillosis. *Scand. J. resp. Dis.* **48**, 372.

SEATON, A., DAVIES, G., GAZIANO, D. & HUGHES, R. O. (1969). Exercise-induced asthma. *Brit. med. J.*, **3**, 556.

SMITH, J. M. & DEVEY, G. F. (1968). Clinical trial of disodium cromoglycate in treatment of asthma in children. *Brit. med. J.*, **2**, 340.

SPEIZER, F. E. & DOLL, R. (1968). A century of asthma deaths in young people. *Brit. med. J.*, **3**, 245.

SPEIZER, F. E., DOLL, R. & HEAF, P. (1968a). Observations on recent increase in mortality from asthma. *Brit. med. J.*, **1**, 335.

SPEIZER, F. E., DOLL, R., HEAF, P. & STRANG, L. B. (1968b). Investigation into use of drugs preceding death from asthma. *Brit. med. J.* **1**, 339.

STUART-HARRIS, C. H. (1968). Chronic bronchitis. *Abstr. World. Med.* **42**, 649.

TARKOFF, M. P., KUEPPERS, F. & MILLER, W. F. (1968). Pulmonary emphysema and alpha l-antitrypsin deficiency. *Amer. J. Med.*, **45**, 220.

UNITED STATES DEPARTMENT OF HEALTH, EDUCATION AND WELFARE (1967). The health consequences of smoking. P.H.S. Publication, no. 1696, Washington.

VOORHORST, R., SPIEKSMA, F. TH. M., VAREKAMP, H., LEOUPEN, M. J. & LYKLEMA, A. W. (1967). The house dust mite (*Dermatophagoides pteronyssinus*) and the allergens it produces. Identity with the house-dust antigen. *J. Allergy*, **39**, 325.

WALSH, S. D. & GRANT, I. W. B. (1966). Corticosteroids in treatment of chronic asthma. *Brit. med. J.*, **2**, 796.

WILHELMSEN, L., ORHA, I. & TIBBLIN, G. (1969). Decrease in ventilatory capacity between ages of 50 and 54 in representative sample of Swedish men. *Brit. med. J.*, **3**, 553.

WOOLCOCK, A. J. & READ, J. (1965). Improvement in bronchial asthma not reflected in forced expiratory volume. *Lancet*, **2**, 1323.

WORLD HEALTH ORGANIZATION (1961). Chronic corpulmonale. Report of an expert committee. W.H.O. Techn. Rep. Series No. 213, Geneva.

Index